THE PHYSICS OF RADIATION THERAPY

THIRD EDITION

THE PHYSICS OF
RADIATION THERAPY

THIRD EDITION

FAIZ M. KHAN, Ph.D.

Professor Emeritus
Department of Therapeutic Radiology
University of Minnesota Medical School
Minneapolis, Minnesota

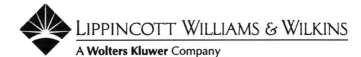

LIPPINCOTT WILLIAMS & WILKINS
A **Wolters Kluwer** Company

Philadelphia · Baltimore · New York · London
Buenos Aires · Hong Kong · Sydney · Tokyo

Acquisitions Editor: Jonathan Pine
Developmental Editors: Michael Standen, Lisa R. Kairis
Production Editor: Thomas Boyce
Manufacturing Manager: Benjamin Rivera
Cover Designer: QT Design
Compositor: TechBooks
Printer: Maple Press

© **2003 by LIPPINCOTT WILLIAMS & WILKINS**
530 Walnut Street
Philadelphia, PA 19106 USA
LWW.com

Printed in the USA

First edition: 1984
Second edition: 1993

Library of Congress Cataloging-in-Publication Data
Khan, Faiz M.
    The physics of radiation therapy / Faiz M. Khan.—3rd ed.
        p.   cm.
    Includes bibliographical references and index.
    ISBN 0-7817-3065-1
    1. Medical physics.   2. Radiotherapy.   I. Title.
R895.K44   2003
615.8′42′0153—dc21
                                        2002040690

Care has been taken to confirm the accuracy of the information presented and to describe generally accepted practices. However, the author and publisher are not responsible for errors or omissions or for any consequences from application of the information in this book and make no warranty, expressed or implied, with respect to the currency, completeness, or accuracy of the contents of the publication. Application of this information in a particular situation remains the professional responsibility of the practitioner.

The author and publisher have exerted every effort to ensure that drug selection and dosage set forth in this text are in accordance with current recommendations and practice at the time of publication. However, in view of ongoing research, changes in government regulations, and the constant flow of information relating to drug therapy and drug reactions, the reader is urged to check the package insert for each drug for any change in indications and dosage and for added warnings and precautions. This is particularly important when the recommended agent is a new or infrequently employed drug.

Some drugs and medical devices presented in this publication have Food and Drug Administration (FDA) clearance for limited use in restricted research settings. It is the responsibility of the health care provider to ascertain the FDA status of each drug or device planned for use in their clinical practice.

10 9 8 7 6 5 4 3 2 1

To very special people in my life:
my wife, Kathy, and my daughters, Sarah, Yasmine, and Rachel

CONTENTS

PREFACE TO THE FIRST EDITION

Most textbooks on radiological physics present a broad field which includes physics of radiation therapy, diagnosis, and nuclear medicine. The emphasis is on the basic physical principles which form a common foundation for these areas. Consequently, the topics of practical interest are discussed only sparingly or completely left out. The need is felt for a book solely dedicated to radiation therapy physics with emphasis on the practical details.

This book is written primarily with the needs of residents and clinical physicists in mind. Therefore, greater emphasis is given to the practice of physics in the clinic. For the residents, the book provides both basic radiation physics and physical aspects of treatment planning, using photon beams, electron beams, and brachytherapy sources. For the clinical physicist, additionally, current information is provided on dosimetry.

Except for some sections in the book dealing with the theory of absorbed dose measurements, the book should also appeal to the radiotherapy technologists. Of particular interest to them are the sections on treatment techniques, patient setups, and dosimetric calculations.

Since the book is designed for a mixed audience, a careful balance had to be maintained between theory and practical details. A conscious effort was made to make the subject palatable to those not formally trained in physics (e.g., residents and technicians) without diminishing the value of the book to the physicist. This object was hopefully achieved by a careful selection of the topics, simplification of the mathematical formalisms, and ample references to the relevant literature.

In developing this text, I have been greatly helped by my physics colleagues, Drs. Jeff Williamson, Chris Deibel, Barry Werner, Ed Cytacki, Bruce Gerbi, and Subhash Sharma. I wish to thank them for reviewing the text in its various stages of development. My great appreciation goes to Sandi Kuitunen who typed the manuscript and provided the needed organization for this lengthy project. I am also thankful to Kathy Mitchell and Lynne Olson who prepared most of the illustrations for the book.

Finally, I greatly value my association with Dr. Seymour Levitt, the chairman of this department, from whom I got much of the clinical philosophy I needed as a physicist.

Faiz M. Khan

PREFACE TO THE SECOND EDITION

The second edition is written with the same objective as the first, namely to present radiation oncology physics as it is practiced in the clinic. Basic physics is discussed to provide physical rationale for the clinical procedures.

As the practice of physics in the clinic involves teamwork among physicists, radiation oncologists, dosimetrists, and technologists, the book is intended for this mixed audience. A delicate balance is created between the theoretical and the practical to retain the interest of all these groups.

All the chapters in the previous edition were reviewed in the light of modern developments and revised as needed. In the basic physics part of the book, greater details are provided on radiation generators, detectors, and particle beams. Chapter 8 on radiation dosimetry has been completely revised and includes derivation of the AAPM TG-2 1 protocol from basic principles. I am thankful to David Rogers for taking the time to review the chapter.

Topics of dose calculation, imaging, and treatment planning have been augmented with current information on interface dosimetry, inhomogeneity corrections, field junctions, asymmetric collimators, multileaf collimators, and portal-imaging systems. The subject of three-dimensional treatment planning is discussed only briefly, but it will be presented more comprehensively in a future book on treatment planning.

The electron chapter was updated in the light of the AAPM TG-25 report. The brachytherapy chapter was revised to include the work by the Interstitial Collaborative Working Group, a description of remote afterloaders, and a commentary on brachytherapy dose specification.

Chapter 16 on radiation protection was revised to include more recent NCRP guidelines and the concept of effective dose equivalent. An important addition to the chapter is the summary outline of the NRC regulations, which I hope will provide a quick review of the subject while using the federal register as a reference for greater details.

Chapter 17 on quality assurance is a new addition to the book. Traditionally, this subject is interspersed with other topics. However, with the current emphasis on quality assurance by the hospital accrediting bodies and the regulatory agencies, this topic has assumed greater importance and an identity of its own. Physical aspects of quality assurance are presented, including structure and process, with the objective of improving outcome.

I acknowledge the sacrifice that my family had to make in letting me work on this book without spending quality time with them. I am thankful for their love and understanding.

I am also appreciative of the support that I have received over the years from the chairman of my department, Dr. Seymour Levitt, in all my professional pursuits.

Last but not least I am thankful to my assistant, Sally Humphreys, for her superb typing and skillful management of this lengthy project.

Faiz M. Khan

PREFACE

New technologies have greatly changed radiation therapy in the last decade or so. As a result, clinical practice in the new millennium is a mixture of standard radiation therapy and special procedures based on current developments in imaging technology, treatment planning, and treatment delivery. The third edition represents a revision of the second edition with a significant expansion of the material to include current topics such as 3-D conformal radiation therapy, IMRT, stereotactic radiation therapy, high dose rate brachytherapy, seed implants, and intravascular brachytherapy. A chapter on TBI is also added to augment the list of these special procedures.

It is realized that not all institutions have the resources to practice state-of-the-art radiation therapy. So, both the conventional and the modern radiation therapy procedures are given due attention instead of keeping only the new and discarding the old. Based on content, the book is organized into three parts: Basic Physics, Classical Radiation Therapy, and Modern Radiation Therapy.

A new AAPM protocol, TG-51, for the calibration of megavoltage photon and electron beams was published in September, 1999, followed by the IAEA protocol, TRS-398, in 2000. Chapter 8 has been extensively revised to update the dosimetry formalism in the light of these developments.

I have enjoyed writing the Third Edition, partly because of my retirement as of January 2001. I simply had more time to research, think, and meditate.

I greatly value my association with Dr. Seymour Levitt who was Chairman of my department from 1970 to 2000. I owe a lot to him for my professional career as a medical physicist.

I greatly appreciate the departmental support I have received from the faculty and the current Chairwoman, Dr. Kathryn Dusenbery. My continued involvement with teaching of residents and graduate students has helped me keep abreast of current developments in the field. I enjoyed my interactions with the physics staff: Dr. Bruce Gerbi, Dr. Pat Higgins, Dr. Parham Alaei, Randi Weaver, Jane Johnson, and Sue Nordberg. I acknowledge their assistance in the preparations of book material such as illustrations and examples of clinical data.

My special thanks go to Gretchen Tuchel who typed the manuscript and managed this project with great professional expertise.

Faiz M. Khan

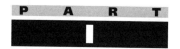

BASIC PHYSICS

1

STRUCTURE OF MATTER

1.1. THE ATOM

All matter is composed of individual entities called elements. Each element is distinguishable from the others by the physical and chemical properties of its basic component—the atom. Originally thought to be the "smallest" and "indivisible" particle of matter, the atom is now known to have a substructure and can be "divided" into smaller components. Each atom consists of a small central core, the nucleus, where most of the atomic mass is located and a surrounding "cloud" of electrons moving in orbits around the nucleus. Whereas the radius of the atom (radius of the electronic orbits) is approximately 10^{-10} m, the nucleus has a much smaller radius, namely, about 10^{-14} m. Thus, for a particle of size comparable to nuclear dimensions, it will be quite possible to penetrate several atoms of matter before a collision happens. As will be pointed out in the chapters ahead, it is important to keep track of those particles that have not interacted with the atoms (the primary beam) and those that have suffered collisions (the scattered beam).

1.2. THE NUCLEUS

The properties of atoms are derived from the constitution of their nuclei and the number and the organization of the orbital electrons.

The nucleus contains two kinds of fundamental particles: protons and neutrons. Whereas protons are positively charged, neutrons have no charge. Because the electron has a negative *unit charge* (1.60×10^{-19} coulombs) and the proton has a positive unit charge, the number of protons in the nucleus is equal to the number of electrons outside the nucleus, thus making the atom electrically neutral.

An atom is completely specified by the formula $_Z^A X$, where X is the chemical symbol for the element; A is the *mass number*, defined as the number of nucleons (neutrons and protons in the nucleus); and Z is the *atomic number*, denoting the number of protons in the nucleus (or the number of electrons outside the nucleus). An atom represented in such a manner is also called a *nuclide*. For example, $_1^1 H$ and $_2^4 He$ represent atoms or nuclei or nuclides of hydrogen and helium, respectively.

On the basis of different proportions of neutrons and protons in the nuclei, atoms have been classified into the following categories: *isotopes*, atoms having nuclei with the same number of protons but different number of neutrons; *isotones*, having the same number of neutrons but different number of protons; *isobars*, with the same number of nucleons but different number of protons; and *isomers*, containing the same number of protons as well as neutrons. The last category, namely isomers, represents identical atoms except that they differ in their nuclear energy states. For example, $_{54}^{131m} Xe$ (*m* stands for metastable state) is an isomer of $_{54}^{131} Xe$.

Certain combinations of neutrons and protons result in stable (nonradioactive) nuclides than others. For instance, stable elements in the low atomic number range have an almost equal number of neutrons, N, and protons, Z. However, as Z increases beyond about 20, the neutron-to-proton ratio for stable nuclei becomes greater than 1 and increases with Z. This is evident in Fig. 1.1, which shows a plot of the ratios of neutrons to protons in stable nuclei.

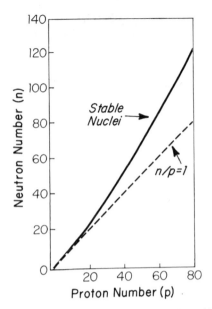

FIG. 1.1. A plot of neutrons versus protons in stable nuclei.

Nuclear stability has also been analyzed in terms of even and odd numbers of neutrons and protons. Of about 300 different stable isotopes, more than half have even numbers of protons and neutrons and are known as even-even nuclei. This suggests that nuclei gain stability when neutrons and protons are mutually paired. On the other hand, only four stable nuclei exist that have both odd Z and odd N, namely $_1^2H$, $_3^6Li$, $_5^{10}B$, and $_7^{14}N$. About 20% of the stable nuclei have even Z and odd N and about the same proportion have odd Z and even N.

1.3. ATOMIC MASS AND ENERGY UNITS

Masses of atoms and atomic particles are conveniently given in terms of atomic mass unit (amu). An amu is defined as 1/12 of the mass of a $_6^{12}C$ nucleus, a carbon isotope. Thus the nucleus of $_6^{12}C$ is arbitrarily assigned the mass equal to 12 amu. In basic units of mass,

$$1 \, amu = 1.66 \times 10^{-27} \, kg$$

The mass of an atom expressed in terms of amu is known as *atomic mass* or *atomic weight*. Another useful term is *gram atomic weight,* which is defined as the mass in grams numerically equal to the atomic weight. According to Avogadro's law, every gram atomic weight of a substance contains the same number of atoms. The number, referred to as *Avogadro's number* (N_A) has been measured by many investigators, and its currently accepted value is 6.0228×10^{23} atoms per gram atomic weight.

From the previous definitions, one can calculate other quantities of interest such as the number of atoms per gram, grams per atom, and electrons per gram. Considering helium as an example, its atomic weight (A_W) is equal to 4.0026.

Therefore,

$$\text{Number atoms/g} = \frac{N_A}{A_W} = 1.505 \times 10^{23}$$

$$\text{Grams/atom} = \frac{A_W}{N_A} = 6.646 \times 10^{-24}$$

$$\text{Number electrons/g} = \frac{N_A \cdot Z}{A_W} = 3.009 \times 10^{23}$$

The masses of atomic particles, according to the atomic mass unit, are electron = 0.000548 amu, proton = 1.00727 amu, and neutron = 1.00866 amu.

Because the mass of an electron is much smaller than that of a proton or neutron and protons and neutrons have nearly the same mass, equal to approximately 1 amu, all the atomic masses in units of amu are very nearly equal to the mass number. However, it is important to point out that the mass of an atom is not exactly equal to the sum of the masses of constituent particles. The reason for this is that, when the nucleus is formed, a certain mass is destroyed and converted into energy that acts as a "glue" to keep the nucleons together. This mass difference is called the *mass defect*. Looking at it from a different perspective, an amount of energy equal to the mass defect must be supplied to separate the nucleus into individual nucleons. Therefore, this energy is also called the *binding energy of the nucleus*.

The basic unit of energy is the joule (J) and is equal to the work done when a force of 1 newton acts through a distance of 1 m. The newton, in turn, is a unit of force given by the product of mass (1 kg) and acceleration (1 m/sec^2). However, a more convenient energy unit in atomic and nuclear physics is the electron volt (eV), defined as the kinetic energy acquired by an electron in passing through a potential difference of 1 V. It can be shown that the work done in this case is given by the product of potential difference and the charge on the electron. Therefore, we have:

$$1\,eV = 1\,V \times 1.602 \times 10^{-19}\,C = 1.602 \times 10^{-19}\,J$$

Multiples of this unit are:

$$1\,keV = 1,000\,eV$$

$$1\,\text{million eV (MeV)} = 10^6\,eV$$

According to the Einstein's *principle of equivalence of mass and energy*, a mass m is equivalent to energy E and the relationship is given by:

$$E = mc^2 \tag{1.1}$$

where c is the velocity of light (3×10^8 m/sec). For example, a mass of 1 kg, if converted to energy, is equivalent to:

$$E = 1\,kg \times (3 \times 10^8\,\text{m/sec})^2$$

$$= 9 \times 10^{16}\,J = 5.62 \times 10^{29}\,MeV$$

The mass of an electron at rest is sometimes expressed in terms of its energy equivalent (E_0). Because its mass is 9.1×10^{-31} kg, we have from Equation 1.1:

$$E_0 = 0.511\,MeV$$

Another useful conversion is that of amu to energy. It can be shown that:

$$1\,amu = 931\,MeV$$

1.4. DISTRIBUTION OF ORBITAL ELECTRONS

According to the model proposed by Niels Bohr in 1913, the electrons revolve around the nucleus in specific orbits and are prevented from leaving the atom by the centripetal force of attraction between the positively charged nucleus and the negatively charged electron.

On the basis of classical physics, an accelerating or revolving electron must radiate energy. This would result in a continuous decrease of the radius of the orbit with the electron eventually spiraling into the nucleus. However, the data on the emission or absorption of radiation by elements reveal that the change of energy is not continuous but discrete. To explain the observed line spectrum of hydrogen, Bohr theorized that the sharp lines of the spectrum represented electron jumps from one orbit down to another with the emission of light of a particular frequency or a quantum of energy. He proposed two

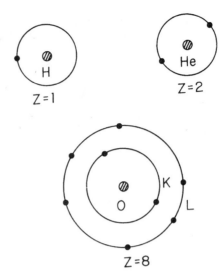

FIG. 1.2. Electron orbits for hydrogen, helium, and oxygen.

fundamental postulates: (a) electrons can exist only in those orbits for which the angular momentum of the electron is an integral multiple of $h/2\pi$, where h is the Planck's constant (6.62×10^{-34} J-sec); and (b) no energy is gained or lost while the electron remains in any one of the permissible orbits.

The arrangement of electrons outside the nucleus is governed by the rules of quantum mechanics and the Pauli exclusion principle (not discussed here). Although the actual configuration of electrons is rather complex and dynamic, one may simplify the concept by assigning electrons to specific orbits. The innermost orbit or shell is called the K shell. The next shells are L, M, N, and O. The maximum number of electrons in an orbit is given by $2n^2$, where n is the orbit number. For example, a maximum of 2 electrons can exist in the first orbit, 8 in the second, and 18 in the third. Figure 1.2 shows the electron orbits of hydrogen, helium, and oxygen atoms.

Electron orbits can also be considered as energy levels. The energy in this case is the potential energy of the electrons. With the opposite sign it may also be called the *binding energy* of the electron.

1.5. ATOMIC ENERGY LEVELS

It is customary to represent the energy levels of the orbital electrons by what is known as the *energy level diagram* (Fig. 1.3). The binding energies of the electrons in various shells depend on the magnitude of Coulomb force of attraction between the nucleus and the orbital electrons. Thus the binding energies for the higher Z atoms are greater because of the greater nuclear charge. In the case of tungsten ($Z = 74$), the electrons in the K, L, and M shells have binding energies of about 69,500, 11,000, and 2,500 eV, respectively. The so-called valence electrons, which are responsible for chemical reactions and bonds between atoms as well as the emission of optical radiation spectra, normally occupy the outer shells. If energy is imparted to one of these valence electrons to raise it to a higher energy (higher potential energy but lower binding energy) orbit, this will create a state of atomic instability. The electron will fall back to its normal position with the emission of energy in the form of optical radiation. The energy of the emitted radiation will be equal to the energy difference of the orbits between which the transition took place.

If the transition involved inner orbits, such as K, L, and M shells where the electrons are more tightly bound (because of larger Coulomb forces), the absorption or emission of energy will involve higher energy radiation. Also, if sufficient energy is imparted to an

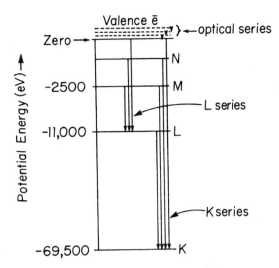

FIG. 1.3. A simplified energy level diagram of the tungsten atom (not to scale). Only few possible transitions are shown for illustration. Zero of the energy scale is arbitrarily set at the position of the valence electrons when the atom is in the unexcited state.

inner orbit electron so that it is completely ejected from the atom, the vacancy or the hole created in that shell will be almost instantaneously filled by an electron from a higher level orbit, resulting in the emission of radiation. This is the mechanism for the production of *characteristic x-rays*.

1.6. NUCLEAR FORCES

As discussed earlier, the nucleus contains neutrons that have no charge and protons with positive charge. But how are these particles held together, in spite of the fact that electrostatic repulsive forces exist between particles of similar charge? Earlier, in section 1.3, the terms *mass defect* and *binding energy of the nucleus* were mentioned. It was then suggested that the energy required to keep the nucleons together is provided by the mass defect. However, the nature of the forces involved in keeping the integrity of the nucleus is quite complex and will be discussed here only briefly.

There are four different forces in nature. These are, in the order of their strengths: (a) strong nuclear force, (b) electromagnetic force, (c) weak nuclear force, and (d) gravitational force. Of these, the gravitational force involved in the nucleus is very weak and can be ignored. The electromagnetic force between charged nucleons is quite strong, but it is repulsive and tends to disrupt the nucleus. A force much larger than the electromagnetic force is the strong nuclear force that is responsible for holding the nucleons together in the nucleus. The weak nuclear force is much weaker and appears in certain types of radioactive decay (e.g., β decay).

The strong nuclear force is a *short-range force* that comes into play when the distance between the nucleons becomes smaller than the nuclear diameter ($\sim 10^{-14}$ m). If we assume that a nucleon has zero potential energy when it is an infinite distance apart from the nucleus, then as it approaches close enough to the nucleus to be within the range of nuclear forces, it will experience strong attraction and will "fall" into the *potential well* (Fig. 1.4A). This potential well is formed as a result of the mass defect and provides the nuclear binding energy. It acts as a *potential barrier* against any nucleon escaping the nucleus.

In the case of a positively charged particle approaching the nucleus, there will be a potential barrier due to the Coulomb forces of repulsion, preventing the particle from approaching the nucleus. If, however, the particle is able to get close enough to the nucleus so as to be within the range of the strong nuclear forces, the repulsive forces will be overcome

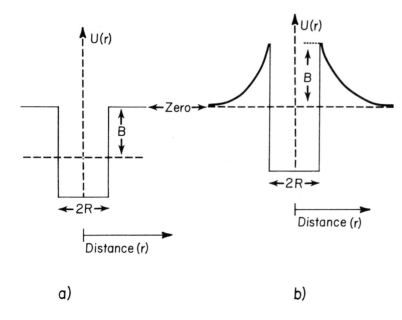

a)

b)

FIG. 1.4. Energy level diagram of a particle in a nucleus: **a,** particle with no charge; **b,** particle with positive charge; *U(r)* is the potential energy as a function of distance *r* from the center of the nucleus. *B* is the barrier height; *R* is the nuclear radius.

and the particle will be able to enter the nucleus. Figure 1.4B illustrates the potential barrier against a charged particle such as an α particle (traveling $^4_2$He nucleus) approaching a $^{238}_{92}$U nucleus. Conversely, the barrier serves to prevent an α particle escaping from the nucleus. Although it appears, according to the classical ideas, that an α particle would require a minimum energy equal to the *height of the potential barrier* (30 MeV) in order to penetrate the $^{238}_{92}$U nucleus or escape from it, the data show that the barrier can be crossed with much lower energies. This has been explained by a complex mathematical theory known as wave mechanics, in which particles are considered associated with de Broglie waves.

1.7. NUCLEAR ENERGY LEVELS

The shell model of the nucleus assumes that the nucleons are arranged in shells, representing discrete energy states of the nucleus similar to the atomic energy levels. If energy is imparted to the nucleus, it may be raised to an excited state, and when it returns to a lower energy state, it will give off energy equal to the energy difference of the two states. Sometimes the energy is radiated in steps, corresponding to the intermediate energy states, before the nucleus settles down to the stable or ground state.

Figure 1.5 shows an energy level diagram with a decay scheme for a cobalt-60 ($^{60}_{27}$Co) nucleus which has been made radioactive in a reactor by bombarding stable $^{59}_{27}$Co atoms with neutrons. The excited $^{60}_{27}$Co nucleus first emits a particle, known as β^- particle and

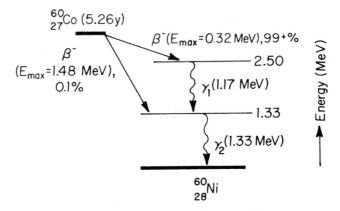

FIG. 1.5. Energy level diagram for the decay of $^{60}_{27}$Co nucleus.

then, in two successive jumps, emits packets of energy, known as photons. The emission of a β^- particle is the result of a nuclear transformation in which one of the neutrons in the nucleus disintegrates into a proton, an electron, and a neutrino. The electron and neutrino are emitted instantaneously and share the released energy with the recoiling nucleus. The process of β decay will be discussed in the next chapter.

1.8. PARTICLE RADIATION

The term *radiation* applies to the emission and propagation of energy through space or a material medium. By particle radiation, we mean energy propagated by traveling corpuscles that have a definite rest mass and within limits have a definite momentum and defined position at any instant. However, the distinction between particle radiation and electromagnetic waves, both of which represent modes of energy travel, became less sharp when, in 1925, de Broglie introduced a hypothesis concerning the dual nature of matter. He theorized that not only do photons (electromagnetic waves) sometimes appear to behave like particles (exhibit momentum) but material particles such as electrons, protons, and atoms have some type of wave motion associated with them (show refraction and other wave-like properties).

Besides protons, neutrons, and electrons discussed earlier, many other atomic and subatomic particles have been discovered. These particles can travel with high speeds, depending on their kinetic energy, but never attain exactly the speed of light in a vacuum. Also, they interact with matter and produce varying degrees of energy transfer to the medium.

The so-called elementary particles have either zero or unit charge (equal to that of an electron). All other particles have charges that are whole multiples of the electronic charge. Some elementary particles of interest in radiological physics are listed in Table 1.1. Their properties and clinical applications will be discussed later in this book.

1.9. ELECTROMAGNETIC RADIATION

A. Wave Model

Electromagnetic radiation constitutes the mode of energy propagation for such phenomena as light waves, heat waves, radio waves, microwaves, ultraviolet rays, x-rays, and γ rays. These radiations are called "electromagnetic" because they were first described, by Maxwell, in terms of oscillating electric and magnetic fields. As illustrated in Fig. 1.6, an electromagnetic wave can be represented by the spatial variations in the intensities of an electric field (E) and a magnetic field (H), the fields being at right angles to each other at any given instant. Energy is propagated with the speed of light (3×10^8 m/sec in vacuum)

TABLE 1.1. ELEMENTARY PARTICLES[a]

Particle	Symbol	Charge	Mass
Electron	e^-, β^-	−1	0.000548 amu
Positron	e^+, β^+	+1	0.000548 amu
Proton	$p, {}_1^1H^+$	+1	1.00727 amu
Neutron	$n, {}_0^1n$	0	1.00866 amu
Neutrino	ν	0	$<1/2{,}000\ m_0$[b]
Mesons	Π^+, Π^-	+1, −1	273 m_0
	Π°	0	264 m_0
	μ^+, μ^-	+1, −1	207 m_0
	K^+, K^-	1, −1	967 m_0
	K°	0	973 m_0

[a] This is only a partial list. Many other elementary particles besides the common ones listed above have been discovered.
[b] m_0 = rest mass of an electron.

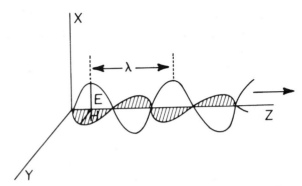

FIG. 1.6. Graph showing electromagnetic wave at a given instant of time. *E* and *H* are, respectively, the peak amplitudes of electric and magnetic fields. The two fields are perpendicular to each other.

in the *Z* direction. The relationship between wavelength (λ), frequency (ν), and velocity of propagation (c) is given by:

$$c = \nu\lambda \tag{1.2}$$

In the above equation, c should be expressed in meters/second; λ, in meters; and ν, in cycles/second or hertz.

Figure 1.7 shows a spectrum of electromagnetic radiations with wavelengths ranging anywhere from 10^7 (radio waves) to 10^{-13} m (ultrahigh energy x-rays). Since wavelength and frequency are inversely related, the frequency spectrum corresponding to the above range will be $3 \times 10^1 - 3 \times 10^{21}$ cycles/sec. Only a very small portion of the electromagnetic spectrum constitutes visible light bands. The wavelengths of the wave to which the human eye responds range from 4×10^{-7} (blue light) to 7×10^{-7} m (red).

The wave nature of the electromagnetic radiation can be demonstrated by experiments involving phenomena such as interference and diffraction of light. Similar effects have been observed with x-rays using crystals which possess interatomic spacing comparable to the x-ray wavelengths. However, as the wavelength becomes very small or the frequency becomes very large, the dominant behavior of electromagnetic radiations can only be explained by considering their particle or quantum nature.

B. Quantum Model

To explain the results of certain experiments involving interaction of radiation with matter, such as the photoelectric effect and the Compton scattering, one has to consider

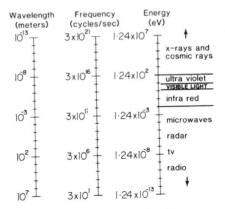

FIG. 1.7. The electromagnetic spectrum. Ranges are approximate.

electromagnetic radiations as particles rather than waves. The amount of energy carried by such a packet of energy, or photon, is given by:

$$E = h\nu \tag{1.3}$$

where E is the energy (joules) carried by the photon, h is the Planck's constant (6.62×10^{-34} J-sec), and ν is the frequency (cycles/second). By combining equations 1.2 and 1.3, we have:

$$E = \frac{hc}{\lambda} \tag{1.4}$$

If E is to be expressed in electron volts (eV) and λ in meters (m), then, since 1 eV = 1.602×10^{-19} J,

$$E = \frac{1.24 \times 10^{-6}}{\lambda} \tag{1.5}$$

The above equations indicate that as the wavelength becomes shorter or the frequency becomes larger, the energy of the photon becomes greater. This is also seen in Fig. 1.7.

2

NUCLEAR TRANSFORMATIONS

2.1. RADIOACTIVITY

Radioactivity, first discovered by Henri Becquerel in 1896, is a phenomenon in which radiation is given off by the nuclei of the elements. This radiation can be in the form of particles, electromagnetic radiation, or both.

Figure 2.1 illustrates a method in which radiation emitted by radium can be separated by a magnetic field. Since α particles (helium nuclei) are positively charged and β^- particles (electrons) are negatively charged, they are deflected in opposite directions. The difference in the radii of curvature indicates that the α particles are much heavier than β particles. On the other hand, γ rays, which are similar to x-rays except for their nuclear origin, have no charge and, therefore, are unaffected by the magnetic field.

It was mentioned in the first chapter (section 1.6) that there is a potential barrier preventing particles from entering or escaping the nucleus. Although the particles inside the nucleus possess kinetic energy, this energy, in a stable nucleus, is not sufficient for any of the particles to penetrate the nuclear barrier. However, a radioactive nucleus has excess energy that is constantly redistributed among the nucleons by mutual collisions. As a matter of probability, one of the particles may gain enough energy to escape from the nucleus, thus enabling the nucleus to achieve a state of lower energy. Also, the emission of a particle may still leave the nucleus in an excited state. In that case, the nucleus will continue stepping down to the lower energy states by emitting particles or γ rays until the stable or the ground state has been achieved.

2.2. DECAY CONSTANT

The process of radioactive *decay* or *disintegration* is a statistical phenomenon. Whereas it is not possible to know when a particular atom will disintegrate, one can accurately predict, in a large collection of atoms, the proportion that will disintegrate in a given time. The mathematics of radioactive decay is based on the simple fact that the number of atoms disintegrating per unit time, $(\Delta N/\Delta t)$ is proportional to the number of radioactive atoms, (N) present. Symbolically,

$$\frac{\Delta N}{\Delta t} \infty N \quad \text{or} \quad \frac{\Delta N}{\Delta t} = -\lambda N \tag{2.1}$$

where λ is a constant of proportionality called the *decay constant*. The minus sign indicates that the number of the radioactive atoms decreases with time.

If ΔN and Δt are so small that they can be replaced by their corresponding differentials, dN and dt, then Equation 2.1 becomes a differential equation. The solution of this equation yields the following equation:

$$N = N_0 e^{-\lambda t} \tag{2.2}$$

where N_0 is the initial number of radioactive atoms and e is the number denoting the base of the natural logarithm ($e = 2.718$). Equation 2.2 is the well-known exponential equation for radioactive decay.

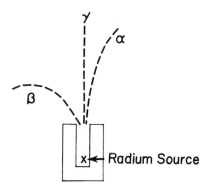

FIG. 2.1. Diagrammatic representation of the separation of three types of radiation emitted by radium under the influence of magnetic field (applied perpendicular to the plane of the paper).

2.3. ACTIVITY

The rate of decay is referred to as the *activity* of a radioactive material. If $\Delta N/\Delta t$ in Equation 2.1 is replaced by A, the symbol for activity, then:

$$A = -\lambda N \tag{2.3}$$

Similarly, Equation 2.2 can be expressed in terms of activity:

$$A = A_0 e^{-\lambda t} \tag{2.4}$$

where A is the activity remaining at time t, and A_0 is the original activity equal to λN_0.

The unit of activity is the curie (Ci), defined as:

$$1 \text{ Ci} = 3.7 \times 10^{10} \text{ disintegrations/sec (dps)}[1]$$

Fractions of this unit are:

$$1 \text{ mCi} = 10^{-3} \text{ Ci} = 3.7 \times 10^7 \text{ dps}$$
$$1 \text{ } \mu\text{Ci} = 10^{-6} \text{ Ci} = 3.7 \times 10^4 \text{ dps}$$
$$1 \text{ nCi} = 10^{-9} \text{ Ci} = 3.7 \times 10^1 \text{ dps}$$
$$1 \text{ pCi} = 10^{-12} \text{ Ci} = 3.7 \times 10^{-2} \text{ dps}$$

The SI unit for activity is becquerel (Bq). The becquerel is a smaller but more basic unit than the curie and is defined as:

$$1 \text{ Bq} = 1 \text{ dps} = 2.70 \times 10^{-11} \text{ Ci}$$

2.4. THE HALF-LIFE AND THE MEAN LIFE

The term *half-life* ($T_{1/2}$) of a radioactive substance is defined as the time required for either the activity or the number of radioactive atoms to decay to half the initial value. By substituting $N/N_0 = 1/2$ in Equation 2.2 or $A/A_0 = 1/2$ in Equation 2.4, at $t = T_{1/2}$, we have:

$$\frac{1}{2} = e^{-\lambda \cdot T_{1/2}} \quad \text{or} \quad T_{1/2} = \frac{\ln 2}{\lambda}$$

---

[1] This definition is based on the rate of decay of 1 g of radium which was originally measured to be 3.7×10^{10} dps. Although the recent measurements have established the decay rate as 3.61×10^{10} dps/g of radium, the original definition of curie remains unchanged.

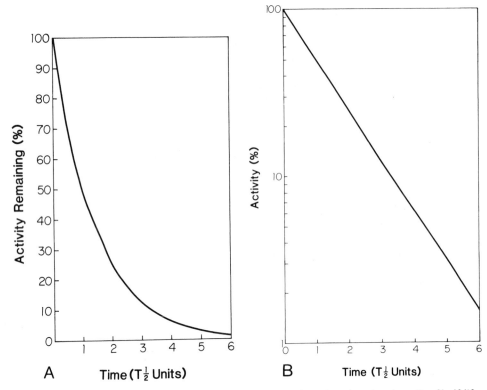

FIG. 2.2. General decay curve. Activity as a percentage of initial activity plotted against time in units of half-life. **A,** plot on linear graph; **B,** plot on semilogarithmic graph.

where ln 2 is the natural logarithm of 2 having a value of 0.693. Therefore,

$$T_{1/2} = \frac{0.693}{\lambda} \tag{2.5}$$

Figure 2.2A illustrates the exponential decay of a radioactive sample as a function of time, expressed in units of half-life. It can be seen that after one half-life, the activity is $1/2$ the initial value, after two half-lives, it is $1/4$, and so on. Thus, after n half-lives, the activity will be reduced to $1/2^n$ of the initial value.

Although an exponential function can be plotted on a linear graph (Fig. 2.2A), it is better plotted on a semilog paper because it yields a straight line, as demonstrated in Fig. 2.2B. This general curve applies to any radioactive material and can be used to determine the fractional activity remaining if the elapsed time is expressed as a fraction of half-life.

The *mean* or *average life* is the average lifetime for the decay of radioactive atoms. Although, in theory, it will take an infinite amount of time for all the atoms to decay, the concept of average life (T_a) can be understood in terms of an imaginary source that decays at a constant rate equal to the initial activity and produces the same total number of disintegrations as the given source decaying exponentially from time $t = 0$ to $t = \infty$. Because the initial activity $= \lambda N_0$ (from Equation 2.3) and the total number of disintegrations must be equal to N_0, we have:

$$T_a \, \lambda N_0 \; = \; N_0 \quad \text{or} \quad T_a \; = \; \frac{1}{\lambda} \tag{2.6}$$

Comparing Equations 2.5 and 2.6, we obtain the following relationship between half-life and average life:

$$T_a \; = \; 1.44 \; T_{1/2} \tag{2.7}$$

Example 1

1. Calculate the number of atoms in 1 g of ^{226}Ra.
2. What is the activity of 1 g of ^{226}Ra (half-life = 1,622 years)?

   1. In section 1.3, we showed that:

$$\text{Number of atoms/g} = \frac{N_A}{A_W}$$

where N_A = Avogadro's number = 6.02×10^{23} atoms per gram atomic weight and A_W is the atomic weight. Also, we stated in the same section that A_W is very nearly equal to the mass number. Therefore, for ^{226}Ra

$$\text{Number of atoms/g} = \frac{6.02 \times 10^{23}}{226} = 2.66 \times 10^{21}$$

   2. Activity = λN (Equation 2.3, ignoring the minus sign). Since $N = 2.66 \times 10^{21}$ atoms/g (example above) and:

$$\lambda = \frac{0.693}{T_{1/2}}$$

$$= \frac{0.693}{(1,622 \text{ years}) \times (3.15 \times 10^7 \text{ sec/year})}$$

$$= 1.356 \times 10^{-11}/\text{sec}$$

Therefore,

$$\text{Activity} = 2.66 \times 10^{21} \times 1.356 \times 10^{-11} \text{ dps/g}$$

$$= 3.61 \times 10^{10} \text{ dps/g}$$

$$= 0.975 \text{ Ci/g}$$

   The activity per unit mass of a radionuclide is termed the *specific activity*. As shown in the previous example, the specific activity of radium is slightly less than 1 Ci/g, although the curie was originally defined as the decay rate of 1 g of radium. The reason for this discrepancy, as mentioned previously, is the current revision of the actual decay rate of radium without modification of the original definition of the curie.

   High specific activity of certain radionuclides can be advantageous for a number of applications. For example, the use of elements as tracers in studying biochemical processes requires that the mass of the incorporated element should be so small that it does not interfere with the normal metabolism and yet it should exhibit measurable activity. Another example is the use of radioisotopes as teletherapy sources. One reason why cobalt-60 is preferable to cesium-137, in spite of its lower half-life (5.26 years for ^{60}Co versus 30.0 years for ^{137}Cs) is its much higher specific activity. The interested reader may verify this fact by actual calculations. (It should be assumed in these calculations that the specific activities are for pure forms of the nuclides.)

Example 2

1. Calculate the decay constant for cobalt-60 ($T_{1/2}$ = 5.26 years) in units of month^{-1}.
2. What will be the activity of a 5,000-Ci ^{60}Co source after 4 years?

   1. From Equation 2.5, we have:

$$\lambda = \frac{0.693}{T_{1/2}}$$

since $T_{1/2} = 5.26$ years $= 63.12$ months. Therefore,

$$\lambda = \frac{0.693}{63.12} = 1.0979 \times 10^{-2} \, month^{-1}$$

2. $t = 4$ years $= 48$ months. From Equations 2.4, we have:

$$A = A_0 e^{-\lambda t}$$
$$= 5,000 \times e^{-1.0979 \times 10^{-2} \times 48}$$
$$= 2,952 \, Ci$$

Alternatively:

$$t = 4 \, years = \frac{4}{5.26} T_{1/2} = 0.760 \, T_{1/2}$$

Therefore,

$$A = 5,000 \times \frac{1}{2^{0.760}} = 29.52 \, Ci$$

Alternatively: reading the fractional activity from the universal decay curve given in Fig. 2.2 at time $= 0.76 \, T_{1/2}$ and then multiplying it with the initial activity, we get the desired answer.

Example 3

When will 5 mCi of ^{131}I ($T_{1/2} = 8.05$ days) and 2 mCi of ^{32}P ($T_{1/2} = 14.3$ days) have equal activities? for ^{131}I:

$$A_0 = 5 \, mCi$$

and

$$\lambda = \frac{0.693}{8.05} = 8.609 \times 10^{-2} \, day^{-1}$$

For ^{32}P:

$$A_0 = 2 \, mCi$$

and

$$\lambda = \frac{0.693}{14.3} = 4.846 \times 10^{-2} \, day^{-1}$$

Suppose the activities of the two nuclides are equal after t days. Then, from Equation 2.4,

$$5 \times e^{-8.609 \times 10^{-2} \times t} = 2 \times e^{-4.846 \times 10^{-2} \times t}$$

Taking the natural log of both sides,

$$\ln 5 - 8.609 \times 10^{-2} \times t = \ln 2 - 4.846 \times 10^{-2} \times t$$
$$or \; 1.609 - 8.609 \times 10^{-2} \times t = 0.693 - 4.846 \times 10^{-2} \times t$$
$$or \; t = 24.34 \, days$$

Alternatively, one may plot the activity of each sample as a function of time. The activities of the two samples will be equal at the time when the two curves intersect each other.

2.5. RADIOACTIVE SERIES

There are a total of 103 elements known today. Of these, the first 92 (from $Z = 1$ to $Z = 92$) occur naturally. The others have been produced artificially. In general, the elements with lower Z tend to be stable whereas the ones with higher Z are radioactive. It

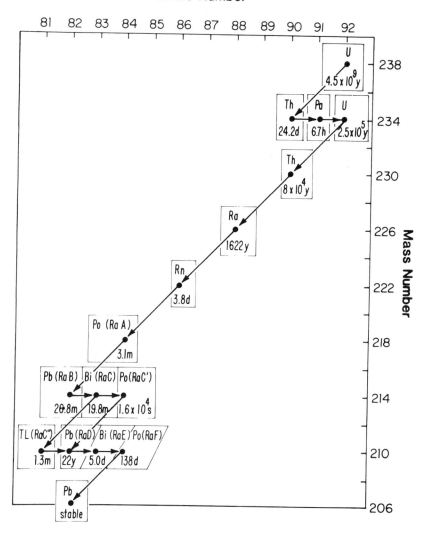

Atomic Number

FIG. 2.3. The uranium series. (Data from U.S. Department of Health, Education, and Welfare. *Radiological health handbook,* rev. ed. Washington, DC: U.S. Government Printing Office, 1970.)

appears that as the number of particles inside the nucleus increases, the forces that keep the particles together become less effective and, therefore, the chances of particle emission are increased. This is suggested by the observation that all elements with Z greater than 82 (lead) are radioactive.

All naturally occurring radioactive elements have been grouped into three series: the uranium series, the actinium series, and the thorium series. The uranium series originates with ^{238}U having a half-life of 4.51×10^9 years and goes through a series of transformations involving the emission of α and β particles. γ rays are also produced as a result of some of these transformations. The actinium series starts from ^{235}U with a half-life of 7.13×10^8 years and the thorium series begins with ^{232}Th with half-life of 1.39×10^{10} years. All the series terminate at the stable isotopes of lead with mass numbers 206, 207, and 208, respectively. As an example and because it includes radium as one of its decay products, the uranium series is represented in Fig. 2.3.

2.6. RADIOACTIVE EQUILIBRIUM

Many radioactive nuclides undergo successive transformations in which the original nuclide, called the *parent,* gives rise to a radioactive product nuclide, called the *daughter.* The naturally occurring radioactive series provides examples of such transitions. If the half-life of the parent is longer than that of the daughter, then after a certain time, a condition of *equilibrium* will be achieved, that is, the ratio of daughter activity to parent activity

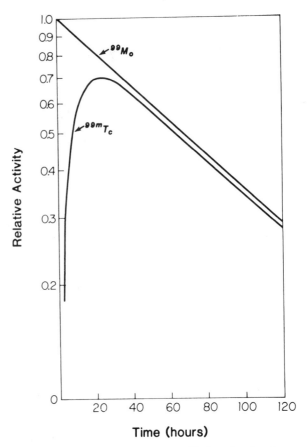

FIG. 2.4. Illustration of transient equilibrium by the decay of ^{99}Mo to ^{99m}Tc. It has been assumed that only 88% of the ^{99}Mo atoms decay to ^{99m}Tc.

will become constant. In addition, the apparent decay rate of the daughter nuclide is then governed by the half-life or disintegration rate of the parent.

Two kinds of radioactive equilibria have been defined, depending on the half-lives of the parent and the daughter nuclides. If the half-life of the parent is not much longer than that of the daughter, then the type of equilibrium established is called the *transient equilibrium.* On the other hand, if the half-life of the parent is much longer than that of the daughter, then it can give rise to what is known as the *secular equilibrium.*

Figure 2.4 illustrates the transient equilibrium between the parent ^{99}Mo ($T_{1/2} = 67$ h) and the daughter ^{99m}Tc ($T_{1/2} = 6$ h). The secular equilibrium is illustrated in Fig. 2.5 showing the case of ^{222}Rn ($T_{1/2} = 3.8$ days) achieving equilibrium with its parent, ^{226}Ra ($T_{1/2} = 1,622$ years).

A general equation can be derived relating the activities of the parent and daughter:

$$A_2 = A_1 \frac{\lambda_2}{\lambda_2 - \lambda_1} \left(1 - e^{-(\lambda_2 - \lambda_1)t}\right) \tag{2.8}$$

where A_1 and A_2 are the activities of the parent and the daughter, respectively. λ_1 and λ_2 are the corresponding decay constants. In terms of the half-lives, T_1 and T_2, of the parent and daughter, respectively, the above equation can be rewritten as:

$$A_2 = A_1 \frac{T_1}{T_1 - T_2} \left(1 - e^{-0.693 \frac{T_1 - T_2}{T_1 T_2} t}\right) \tag{2.9}$$

Equation 2.9, when plotted, will initially exhibit a growth curve for the daughter before approaching the decay curve of the parent (Figs. 2.4 and 2.5). In the case of a transient equilibrium, the time t to reach the equilibrium value is very large compared with the half-life of the daughter. This makes the exponential term in Equation 2.9 negligibly small.

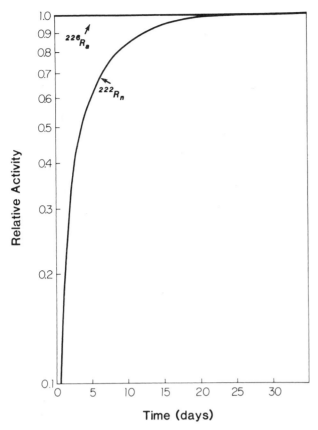

FIG. 2.5. Illustration of secular equilibrium by the decay of ^{226}Ra to ^{222}Rn.

Thus, after the transient equilibrium has been achieved, the relative activities of the two nuclides is given by:

$$\frac{A_2}{A_1} = \frac{\lambda_2}{\lambda_2 - \lambda_1} \tag{2.10}$$

or in terms of half-lives:

$$\frac{A_2}{A_1} = \frac{T_1}{T_1 - T_2} \tag{2.11}$$

A practical example of the transient equilibrium is the ^{99}Mo generator producing ^{99m}Tc for diagnostic procedures. Such a generator is sometimes called "cow" because the daughter product, in this case ^{99m}Tc, is removed or "milked" at regular intervals. Each time the generator is completely milked, the growth of the daughter and the decay of the parent are governed by Equation 2.9. It may be mentioned that not all the ^{99}Mo atoms decay to ^{99m}Tc. Approximately 12% promptly decay to ^{99}Tc without passing through the metastable state of ^{99m}Tc (1). Thus the activity of ^{99}Mo should be effectively reduced by 12% for the purpose of calculating ^{99m}Tc activity, using any of Equations 2.8–2.11.

Since in the case of a secular equilibrium, the half-life of the parent substance is very long compared with the half-life of the daughter, λ_2 is much greater than λ_1. Therefore, λ_1 can be ignored in Equation 2.8:

$$A_2 = A_1(1 - e^{-\lambda_2 t}) \tag{2.12}$$

Equation 2.12 gives the initial buildup of the daughter nuclide, approaching the activity of the parent asymptotically (Fig. 2.5). At the secular equilibrium, after a long time, the product $\lambda_2 t$ becomes large and the exponential term in Equation 2.12 approaches zero.

Thus at secular equilibrium and thereafter:

$$A_2 = A_1 \qquad (2.13)$$

or

$$\lambda_2 N_2 = \lambda_1 N_1 \qquad (2.14)$$

Radium source in a sealed tube or needle (to keep in the radon gas) is an excellent example of secular equilibrium. After an initial time (approximately 1 month), all the daughter products are in equilibrium with the parent and we have the relationship:

$$\lambda_1 N_1 = \lambda_2 N_2 = \lambda_3 N_3 = \ldots \qquad (2.15)$$

2.7. MODES OF RADIOACTIVE DECAY

A. α Particle Decay

Radioactive nuclides with very high atomic numbers (greater than 82) decay most frequently with the emission of an α particle. It appears that as the number of protons in the nucleus increases beyond 82, the Coulomb forces of repulsion between the protons become large enough to overcome the nuclear forces that bind the nucleons together. Thus the unstable nucleus emits a particle composed of two protons and two neutrons. This particle, which is in fact a helium nucleus, is called the α particle.

As a result of α decay, the atomic number of the nucleus is reduced by two and the mass number is reduced by four. Thus a general reaction for α decay can be written as:

$$^A_Z X \rightarrow \, ^{A-4}_{Z-2} Y + \, ^4_2 \text{He} + Q$$

where Q represents the total energy released in the process and is called the *disintegration energy*. This energy, which is equivalent to the difference in mass between the parent nucleus and product nuclei, appears as kinetic energy of the α particle and the kinetic energy of the product nucleus. The equation also shows that the charge is conserved, because the charge on the parent nucleus is Ze (where e is the electronic charge); on the product nucleus it is $(Z - 2)e$ and on the α particle it is $2e$.

A typical example of α decay is the transformation of radium to radon:

$$^{226}_{88}\text{Ra} \xrightarrow[\text{1,622 years}]{T_{1/2}} \, ^{222}_{86}\text{Rn} + \, ^4_2\text{He} + 4.87 \text{ MeV}$$

Since the momentum of the α particle must be equal to the recoil momentum of the radon nucleus and since the radon nucleus is much heavier than the α particle, it can be shown that the kinetic energy possessed by the radon nucleus is negligibly small (0.09 MeV) and that the disintegration energy appears almost entirely as the kinetic energy of the α particle (4.78 MeV).

It has been found that the α particles emitted by radioactive substances have kinetic energies of about 5 to 10 MeV. From a specific nuclide, they are emitted with discrete energies.

B. β Particle Decay

The process of radioactive decay, which is accompanied by the ejection of a positive or a negative electron from the nucleus, is called the β decay. The negative electron, or negatron, is denoted by β^-, and the positive electron, or positron, is represented by β^+. Neither of these particles exists as such inside the nucleus but is created at the instant of the decay process. The basic transformations may be written as:

$$^1_0\text{n} \rightarrow \, ^1_1\text{p} + \, ^{\;\;0}_{-1}\beta + \bar{v} (\beta^- \text{ decay})$$

$$^1_1\text{p} \rightarrow \, ^1_0\text{n} + \, ^{\;\;0}_{+1}\beta + v (\beta^+ \text{ decay})$$

where ^1_0n, ^1_1p, $\bar{v}$, and v stand for neutron, proton, antineutrino, and neutrino, respectively. The last two particles, namely antineutrino and neutrino, are identical particles but with opposite spins. They carry no charge and practically no mass.

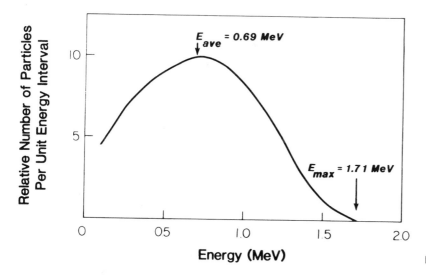

FIG. 2.6. β ray energy spectrum from ^{32}P.

B.1. Negatron Emission

The radionuclides with an excessive number of neutrons or a high neutron-to-proton (n/p) ratio lie above the region of stability (Fig. 1.1). These nuclei tend to reduce the n/p ratio to achieve stability. This is accomplished by emitting a negative electron. The direct emission of a neutron to reduce the n/p ratio is rather uncommon and occurs with some nuclei produced as a result of fission reactions.

The general equation for the negatron or β^- decay is written as:

$$^A_Z X \rightarrow \; ^A_{Z+1}Y + \; ^0_{-1}\beta + \bar{v} + Q$$

where Q is the disintegration energy for the process. This energy is provided by the difference in mass between the initial nucleus $^A_Z X$ and the sum of the masses of the product nucleus $^A_{Z+1}Y$ and the particles emitted.

The energy Q is shared between the emitted particles (including γ rays if emitted by the daughter nucleus) and the recoil nucleus. The kinetic energy possessed by the recoil nucleus is negligible because of its much greater mass compared with the emitted particles. Thus practically the entire disintegration energy is carried by the emitted particles. If there were only one kind of particle involved, all the particles emitted in such a disintegration would have the same energy equal to Q, thus yielding a sharp line spectrum. However, the observed spectrum in the β decay is continuous, which suggests that there is more than one particle emitted in this process. For these reasons, Wolfgang Pauli (1931) introduced the hypothesis that a second particle, later known as the neutrino,[2] accompanied each β particle emitted and shared the available energy.

The experimental data show that the β particles are emitted with all energies ranging from zero to the maximum energy characteristic of the β transition. Figure 2.6 shows the distribution of energy among the β particles of ^{32}P. The overall transition is:

$$^{32}_{15}P \xrightarrow[\text{14.3 days}]{T_{1/2}} \; ^{32}_{16}S + \; ^0_{-1}\beta + \bar{v} + 1.7 \text{ MeV}$$

As seen in Fig. 2.6, the endpoint energy of the β-ray spectrum is equal to the disintegration energy and is designated by E_{max}, the maximum electron energy. Although the shape of the energy spectrum and the values for E_{max} are characteristic of the particular nuclide, the average energy of the β particles from a β emitter is approximately $E_{max}/3$.

The neutrino has no charge and practically no mass. For that reason the probability of its interaction with matter is very small and its detection is extremely difficult. However, Fermi successfully presented the theoretical evidence of the existence of the neutrino and

---

[2] Neutrino is the generic name for the two specific particles, neutrino and antineurino.

predicted the shape of the β-ray spectra. Recently, the existence of neutrinos has been verified by direct experiments.

B.2. Positron Emission

Positron-emitting nuclides have a deficit of neutrons, and their n/p ratios are lower than those of the stable nuclei of the same atomic number or neutron number (Fig. 1.1). For these nuclides to achieve stability, the decay mode must result in an increase of the n/p ratio. One possible mode is the β decay involving the emission of a positive electron or positron. The overall decay reaction is as follows:

$$_Z^A X \rightarrow \ _{Z-1}^A Y + \ _{+1}^0\beta + v + Q$$

As in the case of the negatron emission, discussed previously, the disintegration energy Q is shared by the positron, the neutrino, and any γ rays emitted by the daughter nucleus. Also, like the negatrons, the positrons are emitted with a spectrum of energies.

A specific example of positron emission is the decay of $_{11}^{22}$Na:

$$_{11}^{22}\text{Na} \xrightarrow[\text{2.60 years}]{T_{1/2}} \ _{10}^{22}\text{Ne} + \ _{+1}^0\beta + v + 1.82 \text{ MeV}$$

The released energy, 1.82 MeV, is the sum of the maximum kinetic energy of the positron, 0.545 MeV, and the energy of the γ ray, 1.275 MeV.

An energy level diagram for the positron decay of $_{11}^{22}$Na is shown in Fig. 2.7. The arrow representing β^+ decay starts from a point $2m_0c^2$ ($= 1.02$ MeV) below the energy state of the parent nucleus. This excess energy, which is the equivalent of two electron masses, must be available as part of the transition energy for the positron emission to take place. In other words, the energy levels of the parent and the daughter nucleus must be separated by more than 1.20 MeV for the β^+ decay to occur. Also, it can be shown that the energy released is given by the atomic mass difference between the parent and the daughter nuclides minus the $2m_0c^2$. The positron is unstable and eventually combines with another electron, producing annihilation of the particles. This event results in two γ ray photons, each of 0.51 MeV, thus converting two electron masses into energy.

C. Electron Capture

The electron capture is a phenomenon in which one of the orbital electrons is captured by the nucleus, thus transforming a proton into a neutron:

$$_1^1\text{p} + \ _{-1}^0\text{e} \rightarrow \ _0^1\text{n} + v$$

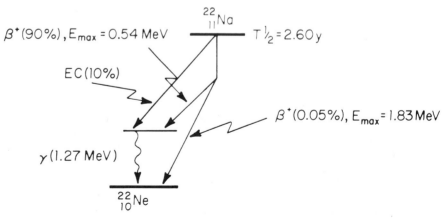

FIG. 2.7. Energy level diagram for the positron decay of $_{11}^{22}$Na to $_{10}^{22}$Ne.

The general equation of the nuclear decay is:

$$_{Z}^{A}X + _{-1}^{0}e \rightarrow _{Z-1}^{A}Y + v + Q$$

The electron capture is an alternative process to the positron decay. The unstable nuclei with neutron deficiency may increase their n/p ratio to gain stability by electron capture. As illustrated in Fig. 2.7, $_{11}^{22}$Na decays 10% of the time by K electron capture. The resulting nucleus is still in the excited state and releases its excess energy by the emission of a γ ray photon. In general, the γ decay follows the particle emission almost instantaneously (less than 10^{-9} sec).

The electron capture process involves mostly the K shell electron because of its closeness to the nucleus. The process is then referred to as *K capture*. However, other L or M capture processes are also possible in some cases.

The decay by electron capture creates an empty hole in the involved shell that is then filled with another outer orbit electron, thus giving rise to the characteristic x-rays. There is also the emission of *Auger electrons,* which are monoenergetic electrons produced by the absorption of characteristic x-rays by the atom and reemission of the energy in the form of orbital electrons ejected from the atom. The process can be crudely described as internal photoelectric effect (to be discussed in later chapters) produced by the interaction of the electron capture characteristic x-rays with the same atom.

D. Internal Conversion

The emission of γ rays from the nucleus is one mode by which a nucleus left in an excited state after a nuclear transformation gets rid of excess energy. There is another competing mechanism, called internal conversion, by which the nucleus can lose energy. In this process, the excess nuclear energy is passed on to one of the orbital electrons, which is then ejected from the atom. The process can be crudely likened to an internal photoelectric effect in which the γ ray escaping from the nucleus interacts with an orbital electron of the same atom. The kinetic energy of the internal conversion electron is equal to energy released by the nucleus minus the binding energy of the orbital electron involved.

As discussed in the case of the electron capture, the ejection of an orbital electron by internal conversion will create a vacancy in the involved shell, resulting in the production of characteristic photons or Auger electrons.

D.1. Isomeric Transition

In most radioactive transformations, the daughter nucleus loses the excess energy immediately in the form of γ rays or by internal conversion. However, in the case of some nuclides, the excited state of the nucleus persists for an appreciable time. In that case, the excited nucleus is said to exist in the *metastable* state. The metastable nucleus is an *isomer* of the final product nucleus which has the same atomic and mass number but different energy state. An example of such a nuclide commonly used in nuclear medicine is ^{99m}Tc, which is an isomer of ^{99}Tc. As discussed earlier (section 2.6), ^{99m}Tc is produced by the decay of ^{99}Mo ($T_{1/2} = 67$ hours) and itself decays to ^{99}Tc with a half-life of 6 hours.

2.8. NUCLEAR REACTIONS

A. The α,p Reaction

The first nuclear reaction was observed by Rutherford in 1919 in an experiment in which he bombarded nitrogen gas with α particles from a radioactive source. Rutherford's original transmutation reaction can be written as:

$$_{7}^{14}N + _{2}^{4}He \rightarrow _{8}^{17}O + _{1}^{1}H + Q$$

where Q generally represents the energy released or absorbed during a nuclear reaction. If Q is positive, energy has been released and the reaction is called *exoergic,* and if Q is negative, energy has been absorbed and the reaction is *endoergic*. Q is also called *nuclear reaction energy* or disintegration energy (as defined earlier in decay reactions) and is equal to the difference in the masses of the initial and final particles. As an example, Q may be calculated for the previous reaction as follows:

Mass of Initial Particles (amu)	Mass of Final Particles (amu)
$^{14}_{7}N = 14.003074$	$^{17}_{8}O = 16.999133$
$^{4}_{2}He = \dfrac{4.002603}{18.005677}$	$^{1}_{1}H = \dfrac{1.007825}{18.006958}$

The total mass of final particles is greater than that of the initial particles.

Difference in masses, $\Delta m = 0.001281$ amu

Since 1 amu $= 931$ MeV, we get:

$$Q = -0.001281 \times 931 = -1.19\,\text{MeV}$$

Thus the above reaction is endoergic, that is, at least 1.19 MeV of energy must be supplied for the reaction to take place. This minimum required energy is called the *threshold energy* for the reaction and must be available from the kinetic energy of the bombarding particle.

A reaction in which an α particle interacts with a nucleus to form a *compound nucleus* which, in turn, disintegrates immediately into a new nucleus by the ejection of a proton is called an α,p reaction. The first letter, α, stands for the bombarding particle and the second letter, p, stands for the ejected particle, in this case a proton. The general reaction of this type is written as:

$$^{A}_{Z}X + {}^{4}_{2}He \rightarrow {}^{A+3}_{Z+1}Y + {}^{1}_{1}H + Q$$

A simpler notation to represent the previous reaction is $^{A}X(\alpha,\text{p})^{A+3}Y$. (It is not necessary to write the atomic number Z with the chemical symbol, since one can be determined by the other.)

B. The α,n Reaction

The bombardment of a nucleus by α particles with the subsequent emission of neutrons is designated as an α,n reaction. An example of this type of reaction is $^{9}Be(\alpha,\text{n})^{12}C$. This was the first reaction used for producing small neutron sources. A material containing a mixture of radium and beryllium has been commonly used as a neutron source in research laboratories. In this case, the α particles emitted by radium bombard the beryllium nuclei and eject neutrons.

C. Proton Bombardment

The most common reaction consists of a proton being captured by the nucleus with the emission of a γ ray. The reaction is known as p,γ. Examples are:

$$^{7}Li(\text{p},\gamma)^{8}Be \quad \text{and} \quad {}^{12}C(\text{p},\gamma)^{13}N$$

Other possible reactions produced by proton bombardment are of the type p,n; p,d; and p,α. The symbol d stands for the deuteron ($^{2}_{1}H$).

D. Deuteron Bombardment

The deuteron particle is a combination of a proton and a neutron. This combination appears to break down in most deuteron bombardments with the result that the compound nucleus emits either a neutron or a proton. The two types of reactions can be written as

$$_Z^A X(d,n)_{Z+1}^{A+1} Y \quad \text{and} \quad _Z^A X(d,p)_Z^{A+1} X.$$

An important reaction that has been used as a source of high energy neutrons is produced by the bombardment of beryllium by deuterons. The equation for the reaction is:

$$_1^2 H + _4^9 Be \rightarrow _5^{10} B + _0^1 n$$

The process is known as *stripping*. In this process the deuteron is not captured by the nucleus but passes close to it. The proton is stripped off from the deuteron and the neutron continues to travel with high speed.

E. Neutron Bombardment

Neutrons, because they possess no electric charge, are very effective in penetrating the nuclei and producing nuclear reactions. For the same reason, the neutrons do not have to possess high kinetic energies in order to penetrate the nucleus. As a matter of fact, *slow* neutrons or *thermal* neutrons (neutrons with average energy equal to the energy of thermal agitation in a material, which is about 0.025 eV at room temperature) have been found to be extremely effective in producing nuclear transformations. An example of a slow neutron capture is the n,α reaction with boron:

$$_5^{10} B + _0^1 n \rightarrow _3^7 Li + _2^4 He$$

The previous reaction forms the basis of neutron detection. In practice, an ionization chamber (to be discussed later) is filled with boron gas such as BF_3. The α particle released by the n,α reaction with boron produces the ionization detected by the chamber.

The most common process of neutron capture is the n,γ reaction. In this case the compound nucleus is raised to one of its excited states and then immediately returns to its normal state with the emission of a γ ray photon. These γ rays, called *capture γ rays,* can be observed coming from a hydrogenous material such as paraffin used to slow down (by multiple collisions with the nuclei) the neutrons and ultimately capture some of the slow neutrons. The reaction can be written as follows:

$$_1^1 H + _0^1 n \rightarrow _1^2 H + \gamma$$

Because the thermal neutron has negligible kinetic energy, the energy of the capture γ ray can be calculated by the mass difference between the initial particles and the product particles, assuming negligible recoil energy of $_1^2 H$.

Products of the n,γ reaction, in most cases, have been found to be radioactive, emitting β particles. Typical examples are:

$$_{27}^{59} Co + _0^1 n \rightarrow _{27}^{60} Co + \gamma$$

followed by:

$$_{27}^{60} Co \xrightarrow[\text{5.3 years}]{T_{1/2}} _{28}^{60} Ni + _{-1}^0 \beta + \gamma_1 + \gamma_2;$$

$$_{79}^{197} Au + _0^1 n \rightarrow _{79}^{198} Au + \gamma$$

followed by:

$$_{79}^{198} Au \xrightarrow[\text{2.7 days}]{T_{1/2}} _{80}^{198} Hg + _{-1}^0 \beta$$

Another type of reaction produced by neutrons, namely the n,p reaction, also yields β emitters in most cases. This process with slow neutrons has been observed in the case of nitrogen:

$$_7^{14} N + _0^1 n \rightarrow _6^{14} C + _1^1 H$$

followed by:

$$\ce{^{14}_{6}C} \xrightarrow[\text{5,700 years}]{T_{1/2}} \ce{^{14}_{7}N} + \ce{^{0}_{-1}\beta}$$

The example of a fast neutron n,p reaction is the production of ^{32}P:

$$\ce{^{32}_{16}S} + \ce{^{1}_{0}n} \rightarrow \ce{^{32}_{15}P} + \ce{^{1}_{1}H}$$

followed by:

$$\ce{^{32}_{15}P} \xrightarrow[\text{14.3 days}]{T_{1/2}} \ce{^{32}_{16}S} + \ce{^{0}_{-1}\beta}$$

It should be pointed out that whether a reaction will occur with fast or slow neutrons depends on the magnitude of the mass difference between the expected product nucleus and the bombarded nucleus. For example, in the case of an n,p reaction, if this mass difference exceeds 0.000840 amu (mass difference between a neutron and a proton), then only fast neutrons will be effective in producing the reaction.

F. Photo Disintegration

An interaction of a high energy photon with an atomic nucleus can lead to a nuclear reaction and to the emission of one or more nucleons. In most cases, this process of photo disintegration results in the emission of neutrons by the nuclei. An example of such a reaction is provided by the nucleus of ^{63}Cu bombarded with a photon beam:

$$\ce{^{63}_{29}Cu} + \gamma \rightarrow \ce{^{62}_{29}Cu} + \ce{^{1}_{0}n}$$

The above reaction has a definite threshold, 10.86 MeV. This can be calculated by the definition of *threshold energy,* namely, the difference between the rest energy of the target nucleus and that of the residual nucleus plus the emitted nucleon(s). Because the rest energies of many nuclei are known to a very high accuracy, the photodisintegration process can be used as a basis for energy calibration of machines producing high energy photons.

In addition to the γ,n reaction, other types of photodisintegration processes have been observed. Among these are γ,p, γ,d, γ,t, and γ,α, where d stands for deuteron ($\ce{^{2}_{1}H}$) and t stands for triton ($\ce{^{3}_{1}H}$).

G. Fission

This type of reaction is produced by bombarding certain high atomic number nuclei by neutrons. The nucleus, after absorbing the neutron, splits into nuclei of lower atomic number as well as additional neutrons. A typical example is the fission of ^{235}U with slow neutrons:

$$\ce{^{235}_{92}U} + \ce{^{1}_{0}n} \rightarrow \ce{^{236}_{92}U} \rightarrow \ce{^{141}_{56}Ba} + \ce{^{92}_{36}Kr} + 3\ce{^{1}_{0}n} + Q$$

The energy released Q can be calculated, as usual, by the mass difference between the original and the final particles and, in the above reaction, averages more than 200 MeV. This energy appears as the kinetic energy of the product particles as well as γ rays. The additional neutrons released in the process may also interact with other ^{235}U nuclei, thereby creating the possibility of a *chain reaction*. However, a sufficient mass or, more technically, the *critical mass* of the fissionable material is required to produce the chain reaction.

As seen in the above instance, the energy released per fission is enormous. The process, therefore, has become a major energy source as in the case of nuclear reactors.

H. Fusion

Nuclear fusion may be considered the reverse of nuclear fission; that is, low mass nuclei are combined to produce one nucleus. A typical reaction is:

$$\ce{^{2}_{1}H} + \ce{^{3}_{1}H} \rightarrow \ce{^{4}_{2}He} + \ce{^{1}_{0}n} + Q$$

Because the total mass of the product particles is less than the total mass of the reactants, energy Q is released in the process. In the above example, the loss in mass is about 0.0189 amu, which gives $Q = 17.6$ MeV.

For the fusion reaction to occur, the nuclei must be brought sufficiently close together so that the repulsive coulomb forces are overcome and the short-range nuclear forces can initiate the fusion reaction. This is accomplished by heating low Z nuclei to very high temperatures (greater than 10^7 K) which are comparable with the inner core temperature of the sun. In practice, fission reactions have been used as starters for the fusion reactions.

2.9. ACTIVATION OF NUCLIDES

Elements can be made radioactive by various nuclear reactions, some of which have been described in the preceding section. The *yield* of a nuclear reaction depends on parameters such as the number of bombarding particles, the number of target nuclei, and the probability of the occurrence of the nuclear reaction. This probability is called the *cross-section* and is usually given in units of *barns,* where a barn is 10^{-24} cm^2. The cross-section of nuclear reaction depends on the nature of the target material as well as the type of the bombarding particles and their energy.

Another important aspect of activation is the *growth of activity.* It can be shown that in the activation of isotopes the activity of the transformed sample grows exponentially. If both the activation and decay of the material are considered, the actual growth of activity follows a net growth curve that reaches a maximum value, called *saturation activity,* after several half-lives. When that happens, the rate of activation equals the rate of decay.

As mentioned earlier, the slow (thermal) neutrons are very effective in activating nuclides. High fluxes of slow neutrons (10^{10} to 10^{14} neutrons/cm^2/sec) are available in a nuclear reactor where neutrons are produced by fission reactions.

2.10. NUCLEAR REACTORS

In nuclear reactors, the fission process is made self-sustaining by chain reaction in which some of the fission neutrons are used to induce still more fissions. The nuclear "fuel" is usually ^{235}U, although thorium and plutonium are other possible fuels. The fuel, in the form of cylindrical rods, is arranged in a lattice within the reactor core. Because the neutrons released during fission are fast neutrons, they have to be slowed down to thermal energy (about 0.025 eV) by collisions with nuclei of low Z material. Such materials are called *moderators.* Typical moderators include graphite, beryllium, water, and heavy water (water with heavy hydrogen $^2_1$H as part of the molecular structure). The fuel rods are immersed in the moderators. The reaction is "controlled" by inserting rods of material that efficiently absorbs neutrons, such as cadmium or boron. The position of these control rods in the reactor core determines the number of neutrons available to induce fission and thus control the fission rate or power output.

One of the major uses of nuclear reactors is to produce power. In this case, the heat generated by the absorption of γ rays and neutrons is used for the generation of electrical power. In addition, because reactors can provide a large and continuous supply of neutrons, they are extremely valuable for producing radioisotopes used in nuclear medicine, industry, and research.

REFERENCE

1. U.S. Department of Health, Education, and Welfare. *Radiological health handbook,* rev. ed. Washington, DC: U.S. Government Printing Office, 1970.

PRODUCTION OF X-RAYS

X-rays were discovered by Roentgen in 1895 while studying cathode rays (stream of electrons) in a gas discharge tube. He observed that another type of radiation was produced (presumably by the interaction of electrons with the glass walls of the tube) that could be detected outside the tube. This radiation could penetrate opaque substances, produce fluorescence, blacken a photographic plate, and ionize a gas. He named the new radiation *x-rays*.

Following this historic discovery, the nature of x-rays was extensively studied and many other properties were unraveled. Our understanding of their nature was greatly enhanced when they were classified as one form of electromagnetic radiation (section 1.9).

3.1. THE X-RAY TUBE

Figure 3.1 is a schematic representation of a conventional x-ray tube. The tube consists of a glass envelope which has been evacuated to high vacuum. At one end is a cathode (negative electrode) and at the other an anode (positive electrode), both hermetically sealed in the tube. The cathode is a tungsten filament which when heated emits electrons, a phenomenon known as *thermionic emission*. The anode consists of a thick copper rod at the end of which is placed a small piece of tungsten target. When a high voltage is applied between the anode and the cathode, the electrons emitted from the filament are accelerated toward the anode and achieve high velocities before striking the target. The x-rays are produced by the sudden deflection or acceleration of the electron caused by the attractive force of the tungsten nucleus. The physics of x-ray production will be discussed later, in section 3.4. The x-ray beam emerges through a thin glass window in the tube envelope. In some tubes, thin beryllium windows are used to reduce inherent filtration of the x-ray beam.

A. The Anode

The choice of tungsten as the target material in conventional x-ray tubes is based on the criteria that the target must have high atomic number and high melting point. As will be discussed in section 3.4, the efficiency of x-ray production depends on the atomic number, and for that reason, tungsten with $Z = 74$ is a good target material. In addition, tungsten, which has a melting point of 3,370°C, is the element of choice for withstanding intense heat produced in the target by the electronic bombardment.

Efficient removal of heat from the target is an important requirement for the anode design. This has been achieved in some tubes by conduction of heat through a thick copper anode to the outside of the tube where it is cooled by oil, water, or air. Rotating anodes have also been used in diagnostic x-rays to reduce the temperature of the target at any one spot. The heat generated in the rotating anode is radiated to the oil reservoir surrounding the tube. It should be mentioned that the function of the oil bath surrounding an x-ray tube is to insulate the tube housing from high voltage applied to the tube as well as absorb heat from the anode.

Some stationary anodes are *hooded* by a copper and tungsten shield to prevent stray electrons from striking the walls or other nontarget components of the tube. These are secondary electrons produced from the target when it is being bombarded by the primary

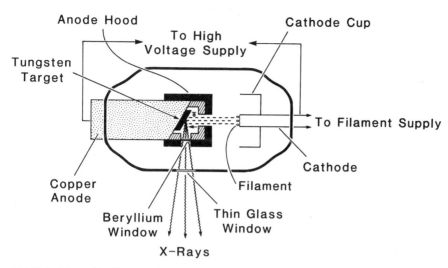

FIG. 3.1. Schematic diagram of a therapy x-ray tube with hooded anode.

electron beam. Whereas copper in the hood absorbs the secondary electrons, the tungsten shield surrounding the copper shield absorbs the unwanted x-rays produced in the copper.

An important requirement of the anode design is the optimum size of the target area from which the x-rays are emitted. This area, which is called the *focal spot*, should be as small as possible for producing sharp radiographic images. However, smaller focal spots generate more heat per unit area of target and, therefore, limit currents and exposure. In therapy tubes, relatively larger focal spots are acceptable since the radiographic image quality is not the overriding concern.

The apparent size of the focal spot can be reduced by the principle of *line focus*, illustrated in Fig. 3.2. The target is mounted on a steeply inclined surface of the anode. The apparent side *a* is equal to $A \sin \theta$, where *A* is the side of the actual focal spot at an angle θ with respect to the electron beam. Since the other side of the actual focal spot is perpendicular to the electron, its apparent length remains the same as the original. The dimensions of the actual focal spot are chosen so that the apparent focal spot results in an approximate square. Therefore, by making the target angle θ small, side *a* can be reduced to a desired size. In diagnostic radiology, the target angles are quite small (6–17 degrees) to produce apparent focal spot sizes ranging from 0.1×0.1 to 2×2 mm. In most therapy

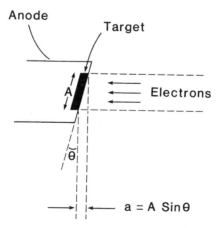

FIG. 3.2. Diagram illustrating the principle of line focus. The side *A* of the actual focal spot is reduced to side *a* of the apparent focal spot. The other dimension (perpendicular to the plane of the paper) of the focal spot remains unchanged.

tubes, however, the target angle is larger (about 30 degrees) and the apparent focal spot ranges between 5 × 5 to 7 × 7 mm.

Since the x-rays are produced at various depths in the target, they suffer varying amounts of attenuation in the target. There is greater attenuation for x-rays coming from greater depths than those from near the surface of the target. Consequently, the intensity of the x-ray beam decreases from the cathode to the anode direction of the beam. This variation across the x-ray beam is called the *heel effect*. The effect is particularly pronounced in diagnostic tubes because of the low x-ray energy and steep target angles. The problem can be minimized by using a compensating filter to provide differential attenuation across the beam in order to compensate for the heel effect and improve the uniformity of the beam.

B. The Cathode

The cathode assembly in a modern x-ray tube (Coolidge tube) consists of a wire filament, a circuit to provide filament current, and a negatively charged focusing cup. The function of the cathode cup is to direct the electrons toward the anode so that they strike the target in a well-defined area, the focal spot. Since size of focal spot depends on filament size, the diagnostic tubes usually have two separate filaments to provide "dual-focus," namely one small and one large focal spot. The material of the filament is tungsten, which is chosen because of its high melting point.

3.2. BASIC X-RAY CIRCUIT

The actual circuit of a modern x-ray machine is very complex. In this section, however, we will consider only the basic aspects of the x-ray circuit. For more detailed information the reader is referred to the literature.

A simplified diagram of a self-rectified therapy unit is shown in Fig. 3.3. The circuit can be divided into two parts: the high-voltage circuit to provide the accelerating potential for the electrons and the low-voltage circuit to supply heating current to the filament. Since the voltage applied between the cathode and the anode is high enough to accelerate all the electrons across to the target, the filament temperature or filament current controls the tube current (the current in the circuit due to the flow of electrons across the tube) and hence the x-ray intensity.

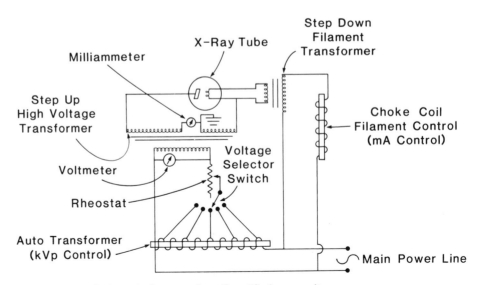

FIG. 3.3. Simplified circuit diagram of a self-rectified x-ray unit.

The filament supply for electron emission usually consists of 10 V at about 6 A. As shown in Fig. 3.3, this can be accomplished by using a step-down transformer in the AC line voltage. The filament current can be adjusted by varying the voltage applied to the filament. Since a small change in this voltage or filament current produces a large change in electron emission or the current (Fig. 3.10), a special kind of transformer is used which eliminates normal variations in line voltage.

The high voltage to the x-ray tube is supplied by the step-up transformer (Fig. 3.3). The primary of this transformer is connected to an *autotransformer* and a *rheostat*. The function of the autotransformer is to provide a stepwise adjustment in voltage. The device consists of a coil of wire wound on an iron core and operates on the principle of inductance. When an alternating line voltage is applied to the coil, potential is divided between the turns of the coil. By using a selector switch, a contact can be made to any turn, thus varying the output voltage which is measured between the first turn of the coil and the selector contact.

The rheostat is a variable resister, i.e., a coil of wire wound on some cylindrical object with a sliding contact to introduce as much resistance in the circuit as desired and thus vary the voltage in a continuous manner. It may be mentioned that, whereas there is appreciable power loss in the rheostat because of the resistance of the wires, the power loss is small in the case of the inductance coil since the wires have low resistance.

The voltage input to the high-tension transformer or the x-ray transformer can be read on a voltmeter in the primary part of its circuit. The voltmeter, however, is calibrated so that its reading corresponds to the kilovoltage which will be generated by the x-ray transformer secondary coil in the output part of the circuit and applied to the x-ray tube. The tube voltage can be measured by the *sphere gap* method in which the voltage is applied to two metallic spheres separated by an air gap. The spheres are slowly brought together until a spark appears. There is a mathematical relationship between the voltage, the diameter of the spheres, and the distance between them at the instant that the spark first appears.

The tube current can be read on a milliammeter in the high-voltage part of the tube circuit. The meter is actually placed at the midpoint of the x-ray transformer secondary coil, which is grounded. The meter, therefore, can be safely placed at the operator's console.

The alternating voltage applied to the x-ray tube is characterized by the peak voltage and the frequency. For example, if the line voltage is 220 V at 60 cycles/sec, the peak voltage will be $220\sqrt{2} = 311$ V, since the line voltage is normally expressed as the root mean square value. Thus, if this voltage is stepped up by an x-ray transformer of turn ratio 500:1, the resultant peak voltage applied to the x-ray tube will be $220\sqrt{2} \times 500 = 155,564$ V $= 155.6$ kV.

Since the anode is positive with respect to the cathode only through half the voltage cycle, the tube current flows through that half of the cycle. During the next half-cycle, the voltage is reversed and the current cannot flow in the reverse direction. Thus the tube current as well as the x-rays will be generated only during the half-cycle when the anode is positive. A machine operating in this manner is called the *self-rectified* unit. The variation with time of the voltage, tube current, and x-ray intensity[1] is illustrated in Fig. 3.4.

3.3. VOLTAGE RECTIFICATION

The disadvantage of the self-rectified circuit is that no x-rays are generated during the *inverse* voltage cycle (when the anode is negative relative to the cathode), and therefore, the output of the machine is relatively low. Another problem arises when the target gets

---

[1] Intensity is defined as the time variation of energy fluence or total energy carried by particles (in this case, photons) per unit area per unit time. The term is also called energy flux density.

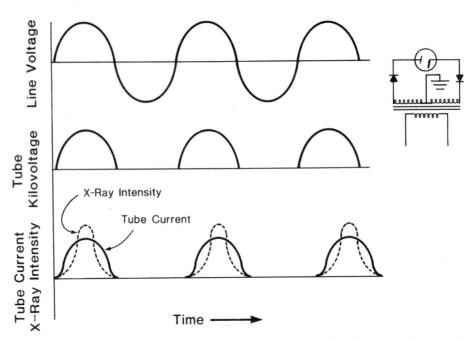

FIG. 3.4. Graphs illustrating the variation with time of the line voltage, the tube kilovoltage, the tube current, and the x-ray intensity for self- or half-wave rectification. The half-wave rectifier circuit is shown on the right. Rectifier indicates the direction of conventional current (opposite to the flow of electrons).

hot and emits electrons by the process of thermionic emission. During the inverse voltage cycle, these electrons will flow from the anode to the cathode and bombard the cathode filament. This can destroy the filament.

The problem of tube conduction during inverse voltage can be solved by using voltage rectifiers. Rectifiers placed in series in the high-voltage part of the circuit prevent the tube from conducting during the inverse voltage cycle. The current will flow as usual during the cycle when the anode is positive relative to the cathode. This type of rectification is called *half-wave rectification* and is illustrated in Fig. 3.4.

The high-voltage rectifiers are either valve or solid state type. The valve rectifier is similar in principle to the x-ray tube. The cathode is a tungsten filament and the anode is a metallic plate or cylinder surrounding the filament. The current[2] flows only from anode to the cathode but the valve will not conduct during the inverse cycle even if the x-ray target gets hot and emits electrons.

A valve rectifier can be replaced by solid state rectifiers. These rectifiers consist of conductors which have been coated with certain semiconducting elements such as selenium, silicon, and germanium. These semiconductors conduct electrons in one direction only and can withstand reverse voltage up to a certain magnitude. Because of their very small size, thousands of these rectifiers can be stacked in series in order to withstand the given inverse voltage.

Rectifiers can also be used to provide *full-wave* rectification. For example, four rectifiers can be arranged in the high-voltage part of the circuit so that the x-ray tube cathode is negative and the anode is positive during both half-cycles of voltage. This is schematically shown in Fig. 3.5. The electronic current flows through the tube via ABCDEFGH when the transformer end A is negative and via HGCDEFBA when A is positive. Thus the electrons flow from the filament to the target during both half-cycles of the transformer voltage. As a result of full-wave rectification, the effective tube current is higher since the current flows during both half-cycles.

---

[2] Here the current means conventional current. The electronic current will flow from the cathode to the anode.

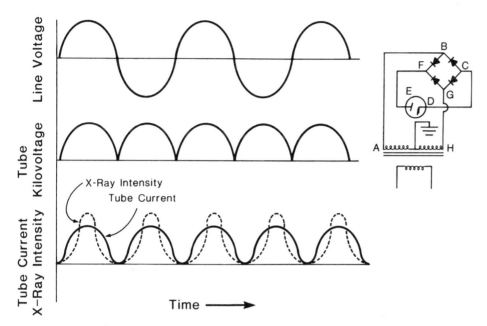

FIG. 3.5. Graphs illustrating the variation with time of the line voltage, the tube kilovoltage, the tube current, and the x-ray intensity for full-wave rectification. The rectifier circuit is shown on the right. The *arrow* symbol on the rectifier diagram indicates the direction of conventional current flow (opposite to the flow of electronic current).

In addition to rectification, the voltage across the tube may be kept nearly constant by a smoothing condenser (high capacitance) placed across the x-ray tube. Such constant potential circuits are commonly used in x-ray machines for therapy.

3.4. PHYSICS OF X-RAY PRODUCTION

There are two different mechanisms by which x-rays are produced. One gives rise to *bremsstrahlung x-rays* and the other *characteristic x-rays*. These processes were briefly mentioned earlier (sections 1.5 and 3.1) but now will be presented in greater detail.

A. Bremsstrahlung

The process of bremsstrahlung (braking radiation) is the result of radiative "collision" (interaction) between a high-speed electron and a nucleus. The electron while passing near a nucleus may be deflected from its path by the action of Coulomb forces of attraction and lose energy as bremsstrahlung, a phenomenon predicted by Maxwell's general theory of electromagnetic radiation. According to this theory, energy is propagated through space by electromagnetic fields. As the electron, with its associated electromagnetic field, passes in the vicinity of a nucleus, it suffers a sudden deflection and acceleration. As a result, a part or all of its energy is dissociated from it and propagates in space as electromagnetic radiation. The mechanism of bremsstrahlung production is illustrated in Fig. 3.6.

Since an electron may have one or more bremsstrahlung interactions in the material and an interaction may result in partial or complete loss of electron energy, the resulting bremsstrahlung photon may have any energy up to the initial energy of the electron. Also, the direction of emission of bremsstrahlung photons depends on the energy of the incident electrons (Fig. 3.7). At electron energies below about 100 keV, x-rays are emitted more or less equally in all directions. As the kinetic energy of the electrons increases, the direction of x-ray emission becomes increasingly forward. Therefore, *transmission-type targets* are used in megavoltage x-ray tubes (accelerators) in which the electrons bombard the target from one side and the x-ray beam is obtained on the other side. In the low voltage x-ray tubes,

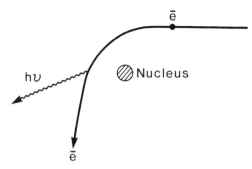

FIG. 3.6. Illustration of bremsstrahlung process.

it is technically advantageous to obtain the x-ray beam on the same side of the target, i.e., at 90 degrees with respect to the electron beam direction.

The energy loss per atom by electrons depends on the square of the atomic number (Z^2). Thus the probability of bremsstrahlung production varies with Z^2 of the target material. However the efficiency of x-ray production depends on the first power of atomic number and the voltage applied to the tube. The term *efficiency* is defined as the ratio of output energy emitted as x-rays to the input energy deposited by electrons. It can be shown (1,2) that:

$$\text{Efficiency} = 9 \times 10^{-10} ZV$$

where V is tube voltage in volts. From the above equation it can be shown that the efficiency of x-ray production with tungsten target ($Z = 74$) for electrons accelerated through 100 kV is less than 1%. The rest of the input energy ($\sim$99%) appears as heat. The accuracy of above equation is limited to a few MV.

B. Characteristic X-rays

Electrons incident on the target also produce characteristic x-rays. The mechanism of their production is illustrated in Fig. 3.8. An electron, with kinetic energy E_0, may interact with the atoms of the target by ejecting an orbital electron, such as a K, L, or M electron, leaving the atom *ionized*. The original electron will recede from the collision with energy

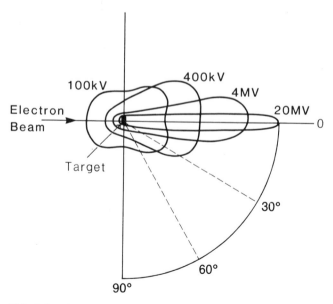

FIG. 3.7. Schematic illustration of spatial distribution of x-rays around a thin target.

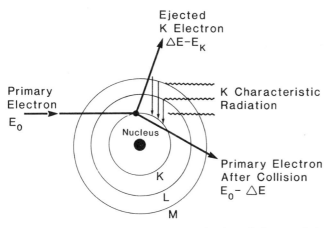

FIG. 3.8. Diagram to explain the production of characteristic radiation.

$E_0 - \Delta E$, where ΔE is the energy given to the orbital electron. A part of ΔE is spent in overcoming the binding energy of the electron and the rest is carried by the ejected electron. When a vacancy is created in an orbit, an outer orbital electron will fall down to fill that vacancy. In so doing, the energy is radiated in the form of electromagnetic radiation. This is called characteristic radiation, i.e., characteristic of the atoms in the target and of the shells between which the transitions took place. With higher atomic number targets and the transitions involving inner shells such as K, L, M, and N, the characteristic radiations emitted are of high enough energies to be considered in the x-ray part of the electromagnetic spectrum. Table 3.1 gives the major characteristic radiation produced in a tungsten target.

It should be noted that, unlike bremsstrahlung, characteristic radiation or x-rays are emitted at discrete energies. If the transition involved an electron descending from the L shell to the K shell, then the photon emitted will have energy $h\nu = E_K - E_L$, where E_K and E_L are the electron-binding energies of the K shell and the L shell, respectively.

The threshold energy that an incident electron must possess in order to first strip an electron from the atom is called *critical absorption energy*. These energies for some elements are given in Table 3.2.

3.5. X-RAY ENERGY SPECTRA

X-ray photons produced by an x-ray machine are heterogenous in energy. The energy spectrum shows a continuous distribution of energies for the bremsstrahlung photons superimposed by characteristic radiation of discrete energies. A typical spectral distribution is shown in Fig. 3.9.

If no filtration, inherent or added, of the beam is assumed, the calculated energy spectrum will be a straight line (shown as dotted lines in Fig. 3.9) and mathematically given by Kramer's equation (3):

$$I_E = KZ(E_m - E) \tag{3.1}$$

where I_E is the intensity of photons with energy, E, Z is the atomic number of the target, E_m is the maximum photon energy, and K is a constant. As pointed out earlier, the maximum possible energy that a bremsstrahlung photon can have is equal to the energy of the incident electron. The maximum energy in kiloelectron volts is numerically equal to the applied kilovolts peak (kVp). However, the intensity of such photons is zero as predicted by the previous equation, that is, $I_E = 0$ when $E = E_m$.

The unfiltered energy spectrum discussed previously is considerably modified as the photons experience inherent filtration (absorption in the target, glass walls of the tube, or thin beryllium window). The inherent filtration in conventional x-ray tubes is usually equivalent to about 0.5- to 1.0-mm aluminum. Added filtration, placed externally to the

TABLE 3.1. PRINCIPAL CHARACTERISTIC X-RAY ENERGIES FOR TUNGSTEN

Series	Lines	Transition	Energy (keV)
K Series	$K\beta_2$	$N_{III} - K$	69.09
	$K\beta_1$	$M_{III} - K$	67.23
	$K\alpha_1$	$L_{III} - K$	59.31
	$K\alpha_2$	$L_{II} - K$	57.97
L Series	$L\gamma_1$	$N_{IV} - L_{II}$	11.28
	$L\beta_2$	$N_V - L_{III}$	9.96
	$L\beta_1$	$M_{IV} - L_{II}$	9.67
	$L\alpha_1$	$M_V - L_{III}$	8.40
	$L\alpha_2$	$M_{IV} - L_{III}$	8.33

Data from U.S. Department of Health, Education, and Welfare. Radiological health handbook. Rev. ed. Washington, DC: U.S. Government Printing Office, 1970.

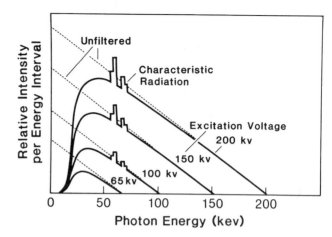

FIG. 3.9. Spectral distribution of x-rays calculated for a thick tungsten target using Equation 3.1. *Dotted curves* are for no filtration and the *solid curves* are for a filtration of 1-mm aluminum. (Redrawn from Johns HE, Cunningham JR. *The physics of radiology,* 3rd ed. Springfield, IL: Charles C Thomas, 1969, with permission.)

tube, further modifies the spectrum. It should be noted that the filtration affects primarily the initial low-energy part of the spectrum and does not affect significantly the high-energy photon distribution.

The purpose of the *added filtration* is to enrich the beam with higher-energy photons by absorbing the lower-energy components of the spectrum. As the filtration is increased, the transmitted beam *hardens,* i.e., it achieves higher average energy and therefore greater penetrating power. Thus the addition of filtration is one way of improving the penetrating power of the beam. The other method, of course, is by increasing the voltage across the tube. Since the total intensity of the beam (area under the curves in Fig. 3.9) decreases with increasing filtration and increases with voltage, a proper combination of voltage and filtration is required to achieve desired hardening of the beam as well as acceptable intensity.

The shape of the x-ray energy spectrum is the result of the alternating voltage applied to the tube, multiple bremsstrahlung interactions within the target and filtration in the beam. However, even if the x-ray tube were to be energized with a constant potential, the x-ray beam would still be heterogeneous in energy because of the multiple bremsstrahlung processes that result in different energy photons.

Because of the x-ray beam having a spectral distribution of energies, which depends on voltage as well as filtration, it is difficult to characterize the beam quality in terms of energy, penetrating power, or degree of beam hardening. A rule of thumb is often used which states that the average x-ray energy is approximately one-third of the maximum energy or kVp. Of course, the one-third rule is a rough approximation since filtration significantly alters the average energy. Another quantity, known as *half-value layer,* has been defined to describe the quality of an x-ray beam. This topic is discussed in detail in Chapter 7.

TABLE 3.2. CRITICAL ABSORPTION ENERGIES (keV)

Level	Element											
	H	C	O	Al	Ca	Cu	Sn	I	Ba	W	Pb	U
Z	1	6	8	13	20	29	50	53	56	74	82	92
K	0.0136	0.283	0.531	1.559	4.038	8.980	29.190	33.164	37.41	69.508	88.001	115.59
L				0.087	0.399	1.100	4.464	5.190	5.995	12.090	15.870	21.753

Data from U.S. Department of Health, Education, and Welfare. Radiological health handbook. Rev. ed. Washington, DC: U.S. Government Printing Office, 1970.

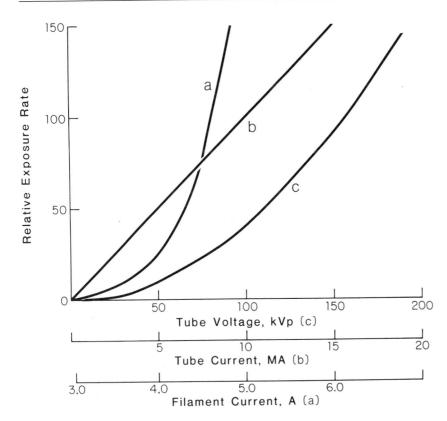

FIG. 3.10. Illustration of typical operating characteristics. Plots of relative exposure rate versus **a,** filament current at a given kVp; **b,** tube current at a given kVp; and **c,** tube voltage at a given tube current.

3.6. OPERATING CHARACTERISTICS

In this section, the relationships between x-ray output, filament current, tube current, and tube voltage are briefly discussed.

The filament current affects the emission of electrons from the filament and, therefore, the tube current. Figure 3.10A shows the typical relationship between the relative exposure rate and the filament current measured in amperes (A). The figure shows that under typical operating conditions (filament current of 5 to 6 A), a small change in filament current produces a large change in relative exposure rate. This means that the constancy of filament current is critical to the constancy of the x-ray output.

The *output* of an x-ray machine can also be expressed in terms of the ionization it produces in air. This quantity, which is a measure of ionization per unit mass of air, is called *exposure*. In Figure 3.10B, the exposure rate is plotted as a function of the tube current. There is a linear relationship between exposure rate and tube current. As the current or milliamperage is doubled, the output is also doubled.

The increase in the x-ray output with increase in voltage, however, is much greater than that given by a linear relationship. Although the actual shape of the curve (Fig. 3.10C) depends on the filtration, the output of an x-ray machine varies approximately as a square of kilovoltage.

REFERENCES

1. Botden P. Modern trends in diagnostic radiologic instrumentation. In: Moseley R, Rust J, eds. *The reduction of patient dose by diagnostic instrumentation.* Springfield, IL: Charles C Thomas, 1964:15.
2. Hendee WR. *Medical radiation physics,* 2nd ed. Chicago: Year Book Medical Publishers, 1979.
3. Kramers HA. On the theory of x-ray absorption and the continuous x-ray spectrum. *Phil Mag* 1923;46:836.

CLINICAL RADIATION GENERATORS

4.1. KILOVOLTAGE UNITS

Up to about 1950, most of the external beam radiotherapy was carried out with x-rays generated at voltages up to 300 kVp. Subsequent development of higher-energy machines and the increasing popularity of the cobalt-60 units in the 1950s and the 1960s resulted in a gradual demise of the conventional kilovoltage machines. However, these machines have not completely disappeared. Even in the present era of the megavoltage beams, there is still some use for the lower-energy beams, especially in the treatment of superficial skin lesions.

In Chapter 3, we discussed in general the principle and operation of an x-ray generator. In this chapter, we will consider in particular the salient features of the therapy machines.

On the basis of beam quality and their use, the x-ray therapy in the kilovoltage range has been divided into subcategories (1,2). The following ranges are more in accordance with the National Council on Radiation Protection (2).

A. Grenz-ray Therapy

The term *grenz-ray therapy* is used to describe treatment with beams of very soft (low-energy) x-rays produced at potentials below 20 kV. Because of the very low depth of penetration (Fig. 4.1, line a), such radiations are no longer used in radiation therapy.

B. Contact Therapy

A *contact therapy* or *endocavitary* machine operates at potentials of 40 to 50 kV and facilitates irradiation of accessible lesions at very short source (focal spot) to surface distances (SSD). The machine operates typically at a tube current of 2 mA. Applicators available with such machines can provide an SSD of 2.0 cm or less. A filter of 0.5- to 1.0-mm thick aluminum is usually interposed in the beam to absorb the very soft component of the energy spectrum.

Because of very short SSD and low voltage, the contact therapy beam produces a very rapidly decreasing depth dose[1] in tissue. For that reason, if the beam is incident on a patient, the skin surface is maximally irradiated but the underlying tissues are spared to an increasing degree with depth. The dose versus depth curve or simply the depth-dose curve of a typical contact therapy beam is shown in Fig. 4.1, line b. It is readily seen that this quality of radiation is useful for tumors not deeper than 1 to 2 mm. The beam is almost completely absorbed with 2 cm of soft tissue.

C. Superficial Therapy

The term *superficial therapy* applies to treatment with x-rays produced at potentials ranging from 50 to 150 kV. Varying thicknesses of filtration (usually 1- to 6-mm aluminum) are added to harden the beam to a desired degree. As mentioned in section 3.5, the degree of hardening or beam quality can be expressed as the half-value layer (HVL). The HVL is

---

[1] The term *dose*, or *absorbed dose*, is defined as the energy absorbed per unit mass of the irradiated material.

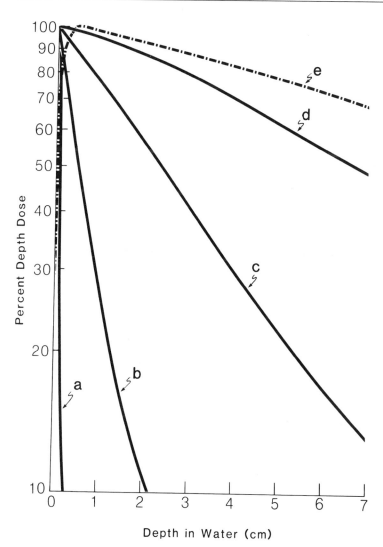

FIG. 4.1. Depth dose curves in water or soft tissues for various quality beams. **Line a:** Grenz rays, HVL = 0.04 mm Al, field diameter ≃ 33 cm, SSD = 10 cm. **Line b:** Contact therapy, HVL = 1.5 mm Al, field diameter = 2.0 cm, SSD = 2 cm. **Line c:** Superficial therapy, HVL = 3.0 mm Al, field diameter = 3.6 cm, SSD = 20 cm. **Line d:** Orthovoltage, HVL = 2.0 mm Cu, field size = 10 × 10 cm, SSD = 50 cm. **Line e:** Cobalt-60 γ rays, field size = 10 × 10 cm, SSD = 80 cm. (Plotted from data in Cohen M, Jones DEA, Green D, eds. Central axis depth dose data for use in radiotherapy. *Br J Radiol* 1978[suppl 11]. The British Institute of Radiology, London, with permission.)

defined as the thickness of a specified material that, when introduced into the path of the beam, reduces the exposure rate by one-half. Typical HVLs used in the superficial range are 1.0- to 8.0-mm Al.

The superficial treatments are usually given with the help of applicators or cones attachable to the diaphragm of the machine. The SSD typically ranges between 15 and 20 cm. The machine is usually operated at a tube current of 5 to 8 mA.

As seen in Fig. 4.1, line c, a superficial beam of the quality shown is useful for irradiating tumors confined to about 5-mm depth (∼90% depth dose). Beyond this depth, the dose dropoff is too severe to deliver adequate depth dose without considerable overdosing of the skin surface.

D. Orthovoltage Therapy or Deep Therapy

The term *orthovoltage therapy*, or *deep therapy*, is used to describe treatment with x-rays produced at potentials ranging from 150 to 500 kV. Most orthovoltage equipment is operated at 200 to 300 kV and 10 to 20 mA. Various filters have been designed to achieve half-value layers between 1 and 4 mm Cu. An orthovoltage machine is shown in Fig. 4.2.

Although cones can be used to collimate the beam into a desired size, a movable diaphragm, consisting of lead plates, permits a continuously adjustable field size. The SSD is usually set at 50 cm.

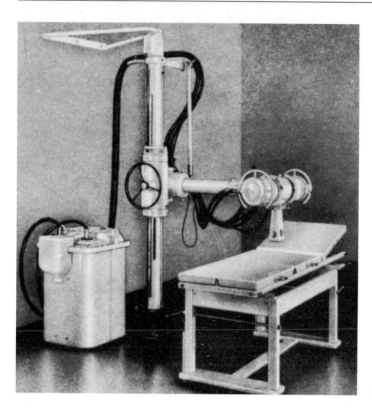

FIG. 4.2. Photograph of Sieman's Stabilapan.

Figure 4.1, line d shows a depth dose curve for a moderately filtered orthovoltage beam. Although the actual depth dose distribution would depend on many conditions such as kilovoltage, HVL, SSD, and field size, some generalizations can be made from this curve about the orthovoltage beam characteristics. The maximum dose occurs close to the skin surface, with 90% of that value occurring at a depth of about 2 cm. Thus, in a single field treatment, adequate dose cannot be delivered to a tumor beyond this depth. However, by increasing beam filtration or HVL and combining two or more beams directed at the tumor from different directions, a higher dose to deeper tumors is delivered. As will be discussed in further detail in Chapter 11, there are severe limitations to the use of orthovoltage beam in treating lesions deeper than 2 to 3 cm. The greatest limitation is the skin dose, which becomes prohibitively large when adequate doses are to be delivered to deep-seated tumors. In the early days of radiation therapy, when orthovoltage was the highest energy available, treatments were given until radiation tolerance of the skin was reached. Although methods were developed to use *multiple beams* and other techniques to keep the skin dose under tolerance limits, the problem of high skin dose remained an overriding concern in the orthovoltage era. With the availability of cobalt teletherapy, the *skin-sparing* properties of higher energy radiation (Fig. 4.1, line e) became the major reason for the modern trend to megavoltage beams.

Although skin dose and depth dose distribution have been presented here as two examples of the limitations posed by low-energy beams, there are other properties such as increased absorbed dose in bone and increased scattering that make orthovoltage beams unsuitable for the treatment of tumors behind bone.

E. Supervoltage Therapy

X-ray therapy in the range of 500 to 1,000 kV has been designated as *high-voltage therapy* or *supervoltage therapy*. In a quest for higher-energy x-ray beams, considerable progress was made during the postwar years toward developing higher-voltage machines. The major problem at that time was insulating the high-voltage transformer. It soon became apparent that conventional transformer systems were not suitable for producing potential much

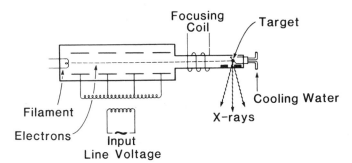

FIG. 4.3. Diagram of a resonant transformer unit.

above 300 kVp. However, with the rapidly advancing technology of the times, new approaches to the design of high-energy machines were found. One of these machines is the resonant transformer, in which the voltage is stepped up in a very efficient manner.

E.1. Resonant Transformer Units

Resonant transformer units have been used to generate x-rays from 300 to 2,000 kV. The schematic diagram of the apparatus is shown in Fig. 4.3. In this apparatus, the secondary of the high-voltage transformer (without the iron core) is connected in parallel with capacitors distributed lengthwise inside the x-ray tube. The combination of the transformer secondary and the capacitance in parallel exhibits the phenomenon of resonance. At the resonant frequency, the oscillating potential attains very high amplitude. Thus the peak voltage across the x-ray tube becomes very large when the transformer is tuned to resonate at the input frequency. Since the electrons attain high energies before striking the target, a transmission-type target (section 3.4) may be used to obtain the x-ray beam on the other side of the target. The electrical insulation is provided by pressurized Freon gas.

F. Megavoltage Therapy

X-ray beams of energy 1 MV or greater can be classified as megavoltage beams. Although the term strictly applies to the x-ray beams, the γ ray beams produced by radionuclides are also commonly included in this category if their energy is 1 MeV or greater. Examples of clinical megavoltage machines are accelerators such as Van de Graaff generator, linear accelerator, betatron and microtron, and teletherapy γ ray units such as cobalt-60.

4.2. VAN DE GRAAFF GENERATOR

The Van de Graaff machine is an electrostatic accelerator designed to accelerate charged particles. In radiotherapy, the unit accelerates electrons to produce high-energy x-rays, typically at 2 MV.

Figure 4.4 shows a schematic diagram illustrating the basic principle of a Van de Graaff generator. In this machine, a charge voltage of 20 to 40 kV is applied across a moving belt of insulating material. A corona discharge takes place and electrons are sprayed onto the belt. These electrons are carried to the top where they are removed by a collector connected to a spherical dome. As the negative charges collect on the sphere, a high potential is developed between the sphere and the ground. This potential is applied across the x-ray tube consisting of a filament, a series of metal rings, and a target. The rings are connected to resistors to provide a uniform drop of potential from the bottom to the top. X-rays are produced when the electrons strike the target.

Van de Graaff machines are capable of reaching energies up to 10 MV, limited only by size and required high-voltage insulation. Normally the insulation is provided by a mixture

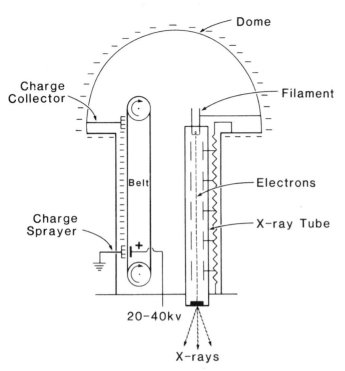

FIG. 4.4. A Van de Graaff generator.

of nitrogen and CO_2. The generator is enclosed in a steel tank and is filled with the gas mixture at a pressure of about 20 atm.

Van de Graaff and resonant transformer (section 4.1.E) units for clinical use are no longer produced commercially. The reason for their demise is the emergence of technically better machines such as cobalt-60 units and linear accelerators.

4.3. LINEAR ACCELERATOR

The linear accelerator (linac) is a device that uses high-frequency electromagnetic waves to accelerate charged particles such as electrons to high energies through a linear tube. The high-energy electron beam itself can be used for treating superficial tumors, or it can be made to strike a target to produce x-rays for treating deep-seated tumors.

There are several types of linear accelerator designs, but the ones used in radiation therapy accelerate electrons either by traveling or stationary electromagnetic waves of frequency in the microwave region (~3,000 megacycles/sec). The difference between traveling wave and stationary wave accelerators is the design of the accelerator structure. Functionally, the traveling wave structures require a terminating, or "dummy," load to absorb the residual power at the end of the structure, thus preventing a backward reflected wave. On the other hand, the standing wave structures provide maximum reflection of the waves at both ends of the structure so that the combination of forward and reverse traveling waves will give rise to stationary waves. In the standing wave design, the microwave power is coupled into the structure via side coupling cavities rather than through the beam aperture. Such a design tends to be more efficient than the traveling wave designs since axial, beam transport cavities, and the side cavities can be independently optimized (3). However, it is more expensive and requires installation of a *circulator* (or isolator) between the power source and the structure to prevent reflections from reaching the power source. For further details on this subject and linear accelerator operation the reader is referred to Karzmark, Nunan, and Tanabe (3).

Figure 4.5 is a block diagram of a medical linear accelerator showing major components and auxiliary systems. A *power supply* provides direct current (DC) power to the *modulator,* which includes the *pulse-forming network* and a switch tube known as *hydrogen*

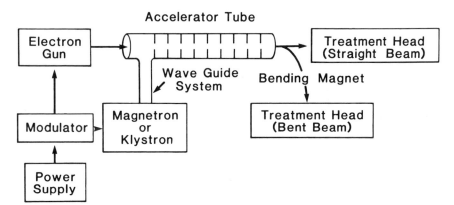

FIG. 4.5. A block diagram of typical medical linear accelerator.

thyratron. High-voltage pulses from the modulator section are flat-topped DC pulses of a few microseconds in duration. These pulses are delivered to the *magnetron* or *klystron*[2] and simultaneously to the electron gun. Pulsed microwaves produced in the magnetron or klystron are injected into the accelerator tube or structure via a *waveguide* system. At the proper instant electrons, produced by an *electron gun,* are also pulse injected into the *accelerator structure.*

The accelerator structure (or accelerator waveguide) consists of a copper tube with its interior divided by copper discs or diaphragms of varying aperture and spacing. This section is evacuated to a high vacuum. As the electrons are injected into the accelerator structure with an initial energy of about 50 keV, the electrons interact with the electromagnetic field of the microwaves. The electrons gain energy from the sinusoidal electric field by an acceleration process analogous to that of a surf rider.

As the high-energy electrons emerge from the exit window of the accelerator structure, they are in the form of a pencil beam of about 3 mm in diameter. In the low-energy linacs (up to 6 MV) with relatively short accelerator tube, the electrons are allowed to proceed straight on and strike a target for x-ray production. In the higher-energy linacs, however, the accelerator structure is too long and, therefore, is placed horizontally or at an angle with respect to the horizontal. The electrons are then bent through a suitable angle (usually about 90 or 270 degrees) between the accelerator structure and the target. The precision bending of the electron beam is accomplished by the *beam transport system* consisting of bending magnets, focusing coils, and other components.

A. The Magnetron

The magnetron is a device that produces microwaves. It functions as a high-power oscillator, generating microwave pulses of several microseconds' duration and with a repetition rate of several hundred pulses per second. The frequency of the microwaves within each pulse is about 3,000 MHz.

The magnetron has a cylindrical construction, having a central cathode and an outer anode with resonant cavities machined out of a solid piece of copper (Fig. 4.6). The space between the cathode and the anode is evacuated. The cathode is heated by an inner filament and the electrons are generated by thermionic emission. A static magnetic field is applied perpendicular to the plane of the cross-section of the cavities and a pulsed DC electric field is applied between the cathode and the anode. The electrons emitted from the cathode are accelerated toward the anode by the action of the pulsed DC electric field. Under the simultaneous influence of the magnetic field, the electrons move in complex spirals

---

[2] Magnetron and klystron are both devices for producing microwaves. Whereas magnetrons are generally less expensive than klystrons, the latter have a long life span. In addition, klystrons are capable of delivering higher-power levels required for high-energy accelerators and are preferred as the beam energy approaches 20 MeV or higher.

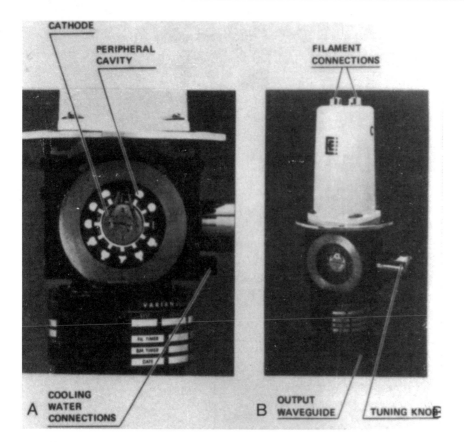

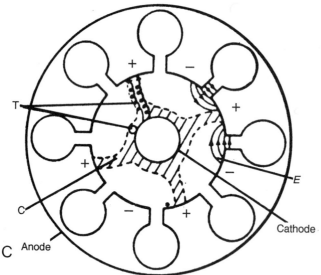

FIG. 4.6. A, B: Cutaway magnetron pictures. **C:** Cross-sectional diagram showing principle of magnetron operation. (From Karzmark CJ, Morton RJ. *A primer on theory and operation of linear accelerators in radiation therapy.* Rockville, MD: U.S. Department of Health and Human Services, Bureau of Radiological Health, 1981, with permission.)

toward the resonant cavities, radiating energy in the form of microwaves. The generated microwave pulses are led to the accelerator structure via the waveguide.

Typically, magnetrons operate at 2 MW peak power output to power low-energy linacs (6 MV or less). Although most higher-energy linacs use klystrons, accelerators of energy as high as 25 MeV have been designed to use magnetrons of about 5 MW power.

B. The Klystron

The klystron is not a generator of microwaves but rather a microwave amplifier. It needs to be driven by a low-power microwave oscillator.

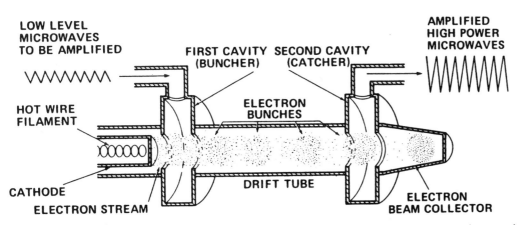

FIG. 4.7. Cross-sectional drawing of a two-cavity klystron. (From Karzmark CJ, Morton RJ. *A primer on theory and operation of linear accelerators in radiation therapy.* Rockville, MD: U.S. Department of Health and Human Services, Bureau of Radiological Health, 1981, with permission.)

Figure 4.7 shows a cross-sectional drawing of an elementary two-cavity klystron. The electrons produced by the cathode are accelerated by a negative pulse of voltage into the first cavity, called the buncher cavity, which is energized by low-power microwaves. The microwaves set up an alternating electric field across the cavity. The velocity of the electrons is altered by the action of this electric field to a varying degree by a process known as *velocity modulation*. Some electrons are speeded up while others are slowed down and some are unaffected. This results in bunching of electrons as the velocity-modulated beam passes through a field-free space in the drift tube.

As the electron bunches arrive at the catcher cavity (Fig. 4.7), they induce charges on the ends of the cavity and thereby generate a retarding electric field. The electrons suffer deceleration, and by the principle of conservation of energy, the kinetic energy of electrons is converted into high-power microwaves.

C. The Linac X-ray Beam

Bremsstrahlung x-rays are produced when the electrons are incident on a target of a high-Z material such as tungsten. The target is water cooled and is thick enough to absorb most of the incident electrons. As a result of bremsstrahlung-type interactions (section 3.4.A), the electron energy is converted into a spectrum of x-ray energies with maximum energy equal to the incident electron energy. The average photon energy of the beam is approximately one third of the maximum energy.

It is customary for some of the manufacturers to designate their linear accelerators that have both electron and x-ray treatment capabilities by the maximum energy of the electron beam available. For example, the Varian Clinac 18 unit produces electron beams of energy 6, 9, 12, 15, and 18 MeV and x-rays of energy 10 MV. The electron beam is designated by million electron volts because it is almost monoenergetic before incidence on the patient surface. The x-ray beam, on the other hand, is heterogeneous in energy and is designated by megavolts, as if the beam were produced by applying that voltage across an x-ray tube.

D. The Electron Beam

As mentioned previously, the electron beam, as it exits the window of the accelerator tube is a narrow pencil about 3 mm in diameter. In the electron mode of linac operation, this beam, instead of striking the target, is made to strike an electron *scattering foil* to spread the beam as well as get a uniform electron fluence across the treatment field. The scattering foil consists of a thin metallic foil, usually of lead. The thickness of the foil is such that most of the electrons are scattered instead of suffering bremsstrahlung. However, a small fraction of the total energy is still converted into bremsstrahlung and appears as x-ray contamination of the electron beam.

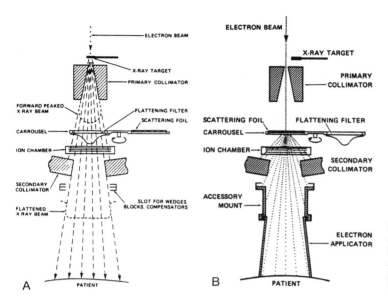

FIG. 4.8. Components of treatment head. **A:** X-ray therapy mode. **B:** Electron therapy mode. (From Karzmark CJ, Morton RJ. A primer on theory and operation of linear accelerators in radiation therapy. Rockville, MD: U.S. Department of Health and Human Services, Bureau of Radiological Health, 1981, with permission.)

In some linacs, the broadening of the electron beam is accomplished by electromagnetic scanning of the electron pencil beam over a large area. Although this minimizes the x-ray contamination, some x-rays are still produced by electrons striking the collimator walls or other high atomic number materials in the electron collimation system.

E. Treatment Head

The treatment head (Fig. 4.8) consists of a thick shell of high-density shielding material such as lead, tungsten, or lead-tungsten alloy. It contains an x-ray target, scattering foil, flattening filter, ion chamber, fixed and movable collimator, and light localizer system. The head provides sufficient shielding against leakage radiation in accordance with radiation protection guidelines (see Chapter 16).

F. Target and Flattening Filter

In section 3.4.A, we discussed the angular distribution of x-rays produced by electrons of various energies incident on a target. Since linear accelerators produce electrons in the megavoltage range, the x-ray intensity is peaked in the forward direction. To make the beam intensity uniform across the field, a *flattening filter* is inserted in the beam (Fig. 4.8A). This filter is usually made of lead, although tungsten, uranium, steel, aluminum, or a combination has also been used or suggested. The choice of target and flattening filter materials has been discussed by Podgorsak et al. (4).

G. Beam Collimation and Monitoring

The treatment beam is first collimated by a *fixed primary collimator* located immediately beyond the x-ray target. In the case of x-rays, the collimated beam then passes through the flattening filter. In the electron mode, the filter is moved out of the way (Fig. 4.8B).

The flattened x-ray beam or the electron beam is incident on the *dose monitoring chambers*. The monitoring system consists of several ion chambers or a single chamber with multiple plates. Although the chambers are usually transmission type, i.e., flat parallel plate chambers to cover the entire beam, cylindrical thimble chambers have also been used in some linacs.

The function of the ion chamber is to monitor dose rate, integrated dose, and field symmetry. Since the chambers are in a high-intensity radiation field and the beam is pulsed, it is important to make sure that the ion collection efficiency of the chambers remains unchanged with changes in the dose rate. Bias voltages in the range of 300 to 1,000 V are applied across the chamber electrodes, depending on the chamber design. Contrary to the beam calibration chambers, the monitor chambers in the treatment head are usually sealed so that their response is not influenced by temperature and pressure of the outside air. However, these chambers have to be periodically checked for leaks.

After passing through the ion chambers, the beam is further collimated by a continuously *movable x-ray collimator*. This collimator consists of two pairs of lead or tungsten blocks (jaws) which provide a rectangular opening from 0 × 0 to the maximum field size (40 × 40 cm or a little less) projected at a standard distance such as 100 cm from the x-ray source (focal spot on the target). The collimator blocks are constrained to move so that the block edge is always along a radial line passing through the target.

The field size definition is provided by a *light localizing system* in the treatment head. A combination of mirror and a light source located in the space between the chambers and the jaws projects a light beam as if emitting from the x-ray focal spot. Thus the light field is congruent with the radiation field. Frequent checks are required to ensure this important requirement of field alignment.

Whereas the x-ray collimation systems of most medical linacs are similar, the *electron collimation systems* vary widely. Since electrons scatter readily in air, the beam collimation must be achieved close to the skin surface of the patient. There is a considerable scattering of electrons from the collimator surfaces including the movable jaws. Dose rate can change by a factor of two or three as the collimator jaws are opened to maximum field size limits. If the electrons are collimated by the same jaws, as for x-rays, there will be an extremely stringent requirement on the accuracy of the jaw opening, since output so critically depends on the surface area of the collimator. This problem has been solved by keeping the x-ray collimator wide open and attaching an auxiliary collimator for electrons in the form of trimmers extended down to the skin surface. In other systems, the auxiliary electron collimator consists of a set of attachable cones of various sizes.

The dose distribution in an electron field is significantly influenced by the collimation system provided with the machine because of electron scattering.

H. Gantry

Most of the linear accelerators currently produced are constructed so that the source of radiation can rotate about a horizontal axis (Fig. 4.9). As the gantry rotates, the collimator axis (supposedly coincident with the central axis of the beam) moves in a vertical plane. The point of intersection of the collimator axis and the axis of rotation of the gantry is known as the *isocenter*.

The isocentric mounting of the radiation machines has advantages over the units that move only up and down. The latter units are not suitable for *isocentric treatment* techniques in which beams are directed from different directions but intersect at the same point, the isocenter, placed inside the patient. However, the nonisocentric units are usually swivel mounted, that is, the treatment head can be swiveled or rotated in any direction while the gantry can move only upward or downward. Although these units are not as flexible, they are mechanically simpler, more reliable, and less expensive than the isocentric models.

4.4. BETATRON

The operation of the betatron is based on the principle that an electron in a changing magnetic field experiences acceleration in a circular orbit. Figure 4.10 shows a schematic drawing of the machine. The accelerating tube is shaped like a hollow doughnut and is placed between the poles of an alternating current magnet. A pulse of electrons is introduced into this evacuated doughnut by an injector at the instant that the alternating current cycle begins. As the magnetic field rises, the electrons experience acceleration continuously and spin with increasing velocity around the tube. By the end of the first quarter cycle of

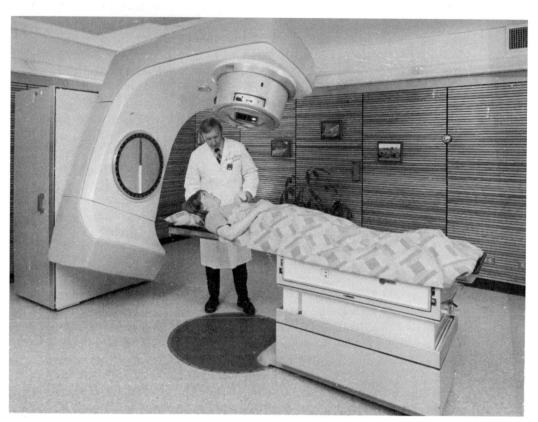

FIG. 4.9. Photograph of a linear accelerator, isocentrically mounted. (Courtesy of Varian Associates, Palo Alto, California.)

the alternating magnetic field, the electrons have made several thousand revolutions and achieved maximum energy. At this instant or earlier, depending on the energy desired, the electrons are made to spiral out of the orbit by an additional attractive force. The high-energy electrons then strike a target to produce x-rays or a scattering foil to produce a broad beam of electrons.

Betatrons were first used for radiotherapy in the early 1950s. They preceded the introduction of linear accelerators by a few years. Although the betatrons can provide x-ray and electron therapy beams over a wide range of energies, from less than 6 to more than 40 MeV, they are inherently low-electron-beam current devices. The x-ray dose rates and field size capabilities of medical betatrons are low compared with medical linacs and even modern cobalt units. However, in the electron therapy mode, the beam current is adequate to provide a high dose rate. The reason for this difference between x-ray and electron dose

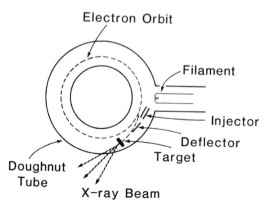

FIG. 4.10. Diagram illustrating the operation of a betatron.

rates is that the x-ray production via bremsstrahlung as well as beam flattening requires a much larger primary electron beam current (about 1,000 times) than that required for the electron therapy beam.

The availability of medium energy linacs with high x-ray does rates, large field sizes, and electron therapy energies up to 20 MeV has given the linacs a considerable edge in popularity over the betatrons. Moreover, many radiation therapists regard the small field size and dose rate capabilities of the betatron as serious disadvantages to the general use of the device. Thus a significant increase in betatron installations in this country, paralleling medical linacs, seems unlikely.

4.5. MICROTRON

The microtron is an electron accelerator that combines the principles of both the linear accelerator and the cyclotron (section 4.6). In the microtron, the electrons are accelerated by the oscillating electric field of one or more microwave cavities (Fig. 4.11A,B). A magnetic field forces the electrons to move in a circular orbit and return to the cavity. As the electrons receive higher and higher energy by repeated passes through the cavity, they describe orbits of increasing radius in the magnetic field. The cavity voltage, frequency, and magnetic field are so adjusted that the electrons arrive each time in the correct phase at the cavity. Because the electrons travel with an approximately constant velocity (almost the speed of light), the above condition can be maintained if the path length of the orbits increases with one

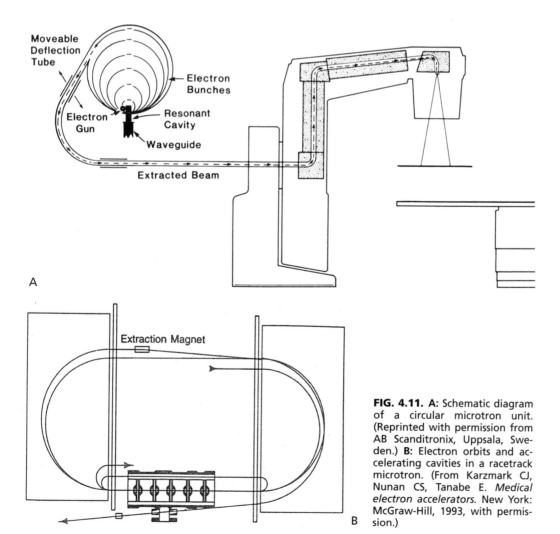

FIG. 4.11. A: Schematic diagram of a circular microtron unit. (Reprinted with permission from AB Scanditronix, Uppsala, Sweden.) **B:** Electron orbits and accelerating cavities in a racetrack microtron. (From Karzmark CJ, Nunan CS, Tanabe E. *Medical electron accelerators.* New York: McGraw-Hill, 1993, with permission.)

microwave wavelength per revolution. The microwave power source is either a klystron or a magnetron.

The extraction of the electrons from an orbit is accomplished by a narrow deflection tube of steel that screens the effect of the magnetic field. When the beam energy is selected, the deflection tube is automatically moved to the appropriate orbit to extract the beam.

The principal advantages of the microtron over a linear accelerator of comparable energy are its simplicity, easy energy selection, and small beam energy spread as well as the smaller size of the machine. Because of the low energy spread of the accelerated electrons and small beam emittance (product of beam diameter and divergence), the beam transport system is greatly simplified. These characteristics have encouraged the use of a single microtron to supply a beam to several treatment rooms.

Although the method of accelerating electrons used in the microtron was proposed as early as in 1944 by Veksler (5), the first microtron for radiotherapy (a 10-MeV unit) was described by Reistad and Brahme (6) in 1972. Later, a 22-MeV microtron (7) was developed by AB Scanditronix and installed at the University of Umeå, Sweden. This particular model (MM 22) produced two x-rays beams of energy 6 or 10 and 21 MV and 10 electron beams of 2, 5, 7, 9, 11, 13, 16, 18, 20, and 22 MeV.

The circular microtron, as described above and shown schematically in Fig. 4.11A, is a bulky structure because it requires a large magnetic gap to accommodate accelerating cavity and large diameter magnetic field to accommodate the large number of spaced orbits with limited energy gain per orbit. These constraints are removed by a racetrack microtron, which uses a standing wave linac structure (instead of a single cavity) to accelerate the electrons (Fig. 4.11B). The parameters of a 50-MeV racetrack microtron developed at the Royal Institute of Technology, Stockholm, are given by Rosander et al. (8). A review is also provided by Karzmark et al. (3).

4.6. CYCLOTRON

The cyclotron is a charged particle accelerator, mainly used for nuclear physics research. In radiation therapy, these machines have been used as a source of high-energy protons for proton beam therapy. More recently, the cyclotrons have been adopted for generating neutron beams. In the latter case, the deuterons ($^2_1H^+$) are accelerated to high energies and then made to strike a suitable target to produce neutrons by nuclear reactions. One such reaction occurs when a beam of deuterons, accelerated to a high energy (~15 to 50 MeV), strikes a target of low atomic number, such as beryllium. Neutrons are produced by a process called stripping (section 2.8.D). Another important use of the cyclotron in medicine is as a particle accelerator for the production of certain radionuclides.

A schematic diagram illustrating the principle of cyclotron operation is shown in Fig. 4.12. The machine consists essentially of a short metallic cylinder divided into two

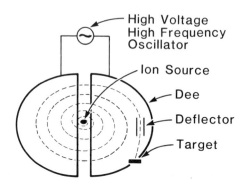

FIG. 4.12. Diagram illustrating the principle of operation of a cyclotron.

sections, usually referred to as *D*s. These Ds are highly evacuated and placed between the poles of a direct current magnet (not shown), producing a constant magnetic field. An alternating potential is applied between the two Ds. Positively charged particles such as protons or deuterons are injected into the chamber at the center of the two Ds. Under the action of the magnetic field, the particles travel in a circular orbit. The frequency of the alternating potential is adjusted so that as the particle passes from one D to the other, it is accelerated by the electric field of the right polarity. With each pass between the Ds, the particle receives an increment of energy and the radius of its orbit increases. Thus, by making many revolutions, the particle such as a deuteron achieves kinetic energy as high as 30 MeV.

There is a limit to the energy that a particle can attain by the above process. According to the theory of relativity, as the particle reaches high velocity (in the relativistic range), further acceleration causes the particle to gain in mass. This tends to slow down the particle, which can then get out of step with the frequency of the alternating potential applied to the Ds. This problem has been solved in the synchrotrons where the frequency of the potential is adjusted to compensate for the decrease in particle velocity.

4.7. MACHINES USING RADIONUCLIDES

Radionuclides such as radium-226, cesium-137, and cobalt-60 have been used as sources of γ rays for teletherapy.[3] These γ rays are emitted from the radionuclides as they undergo radioactive disintegration.

Of all the radionuclides, ^{60}Co has proved to be the most suitable for external beam radiotherapy. The reasons for its choice over radium and cesium are higher possible specific activity (curies per gram), greater radiation output per curie and higher average photon energy. These characteristics for the three radionuclides are compared in Table 4.1. In addition, radium is much more expensive and has greater self-absorption of its radiation than either cesium or cobalt.

A. Cobalt-60 Unit

A.1. Source

The ^{60}Co source is produced by irradiating ordinary stable ^{59}Co with neutrons in a reactor. The nuclear reaction can be represented by ^{59}Co(n,γ) ^{60}Co.

The ^{60}Co source, usually in the form of a solid cylinder, discs, or pallets, is contained inside a stainless-steel capsule and sealed by welding. This capsule is placed into another steel capsule which is again sealed by welding. The double-welded seal is necessary to prevent any leakage of the radioactive material.

The ^{60}Co source decays to ^{60}Ni with the emission of β particles ($E_{max} = 0.32$ MeV) and two photons per disintegration of energies 1.17 and 1.33 MeV (decay scheme given in Fig. 1.5). These γ rays constitute the useful treatment beam. The β particles are absorbed in the cobalt metal and the stainless-steel capsules resulting in the emission of bremsstrahlung x-rays and a small amount of characteristic x-rays. However, these x-rays of average energy around 0.1 MeV do not contribute appreciably to the dose in the patient because they are strongly attenuated in the material of the source and the capsule. The other "contaminants" to the treatment beam are the lower-energy γ rays produced by the interaction of the primary γ radiation with the source itself, the surrounding capsule, the source housing, and the collimator system. The scattered components of the beam contribute significantly (~10%) to the total intensity of the beam (9). All these secondary interactions thus, to

---

[3] *Teletherapy* is a general term applied to external beam treatments in which the source of radiation is at a large distance from the patient.

TABLE 4.1. TELETHERAPY SOURCE CHARACTERISTICS

Radionuclide	Half-Life (yr)	γ-Ray Energy MeV	Γ Value[a] $\left(\dfrac{Rm^2}{Ci-h}\right)$	Specific Activity Achieved in Practice (Ci/g)
Radium-226 (filtered by 0.5 mm Pt)	1,622	0.83 (avg.)	0.825	~0.98
Cesium-137	30.0	0.66	0.326	~50
Cobalt-60	5.26	1.17, 1.33	1.30	~200

[a]Exposure rate constant (Γ) is discussed in Chapter 8. The higher the Γ value, the greater will be the exposure rate or output per curie of the teletherapy source.

some extent, result in heterogeneity of the beam. In addition, electrons are also produced by these interactions and constitute what is usually referred to as the *electron contamination* of the photon beam.

A typical teletherapy ^{60}Co source is a cylinder of diameter ranging from 1.0 to 2.0 cm and is positioned in the cobalt unit with its circular end facing the patient. The fact that the radiation source is not a point source complicates the beam geometry and gives rise to what is known as the geometric penumbra.

A.2. Source Housing

The housing for the source is called the *sourcehead* (Fig. 4.13). It consists of a steel shell filled with lead for shielding purposes and a device for bringing the source in front of an opening in the head from which the useful beam emerges.

Also, a heavy metal alloy sleeve is provided to form an additional primary shield when the source is in the *off* position.

A number of methods have been developed for moving the source from the off position to the *on* position. These methods have been discussed in detail by Johns and Cunningham (10). It will suffice here to mention briefly four different mechanisms: (a) the source mounted on a rotating wheel inside the sourcehead to carry the source from the off position to the on position; (b) the source mounted on a heavy metal drawer plus its ability to slide horizontally through a hole running through the sourcehead—in the on position the source faces the aperture for the treatment beam and in the off position the source moves to its shielded location and a light source mounted on the same drawer occupies the on position of the source; (c) mercury is allowed to flow into the space immediately below the source to shut off the beam; and (d) the source is fixed in front of the aperture and the beam can be turned on and off by a shutter consisting of heavy metal jaws. All of the above mechanisms incorporate a safety feature in which the source is returned automatically to the off position in case of a power failure.

A.3. Beam Collimation and Penumbra

A collimator system is designed to vary the size and shape of the beam to meet the individual treatment requirements. The simplest form of a continuously adjustable diaphragm consists of two pairs of heavy metal blocks. Each pair can be moved independently to obtain a square or a rectangle-shaped field. Some collimators are multivane type, i.e., multiple blocks to control the size of the beam. In either case, if the inner surface of the blocks is made parallel to the central axis of the beam, the radiation will pass through the edges of the collimating blocks resulting in what is known as the *transmission penumbra*. The extent of this penumbra will be more pronounced for larger collimator openings because of greater obliquity of the rays at the edges of the blocks. This effect has been minimized in some designs by shaping the collimator blocks so that the inner surface of the blocks remains always parallel to the edge of the beam. In these collimators, the blocks are hinged to the top of the collimator housing so that the slope of the blocks is

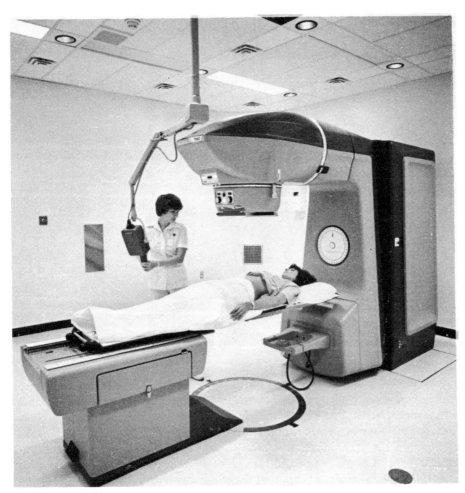

FIG. 4.13. Photograph of cobalt unit, Theratron 780. (Courtesy of Atomic Energy of Canada, Ltd., Ottawa, Canada.)

coincident with the included angle of the beam. Although the transmission penumbra can be minimized with such an arrangement, it cannot be completely removed for all field sizes.

The term *penumbra,* in a general sense, means the region, at the edge of a radiation beam, over which the dose rate changes rapidly as a function of distance from the beam axis (10). The transmission penumbra, mentioned above, is the region irradiated by photons which are transmitted through the edge of the collimator block.

Another type of penumbra, known as the *geometric penumbra,* is illustrated in Fig. 4.14. The geometric width of the penumbra (P_d) at any depth (d) from the surface of a patient can be determined by considering similar triangles ABC and DEC. From geometry, we have:

$$\frac{DE}{AB} = \frac{CE}{CA} = \frac{CD}{CB} = \frac{MN}{OM} = \frac{OF + FN - OM}{OM} \tag{4.1}$$

If $AB = s$, the source diameter, $OM = \text{SDD}$, the source to diaphragm distance, $OF = \text{SSD}$, the source to surface distance, then from the previous equation, the penumbra (DE) at depth d is given by:

$$P_d = \frac{s(\text{SSD} + d - \text{SDD})}{\text{SDD}} \tag{4.2}$$

The penumbra at the surface can be calculated by substituting $d = 0$ in Equation 4.2.

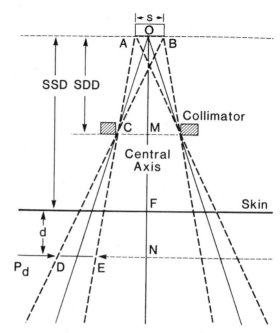

FIG. 4.14. Diagram for calculating geometric penumbra.

As Equation 4.2 indicates, the penumbra width increases with increase in source diameter, SSD, and depth but decreases with an increase in SDD. The geometric penumbra, however, is independent of field size as long as the movement of the diaphragm is in one plane, that is, SDD stays constant with increase in field size.

Because SDD is an important parameter in determining the penumbra width, this distance can be increased by extendable *penumbra trimmers*. These trimmers consist of heavy metal bars to attenuate the beam in the penumbra region, thus "sharpening" the field edges. The penumbra, however, is not eliminated completely but reduced since SDD with the trimmers extended is increased. The new SDD is equal to the source to trimmer distance. An alternative way of reducing the penumbra is to use secondary blocks, placed close to the patient, for redefining or shaping the field. As will be discussed in Chapter 13, the blocks should not be placed closer than 15 to 20 cm from the patient because of excessive electron contaminants produced by the block carrying tray.

The combined effect of the transmission and geometric penumbras is to create a region of dose variation at the field edges. A dose profile of the beam measured across the beam in air at a given distance from the source would show dosimetrically the extent of the penumbra. However, at a depth in the patient the dose variation at the field border is a function of not only geometric and transmission penumbras but also the scattered radiation produced in the patient. Thus, dosimetrically, the term *physical penumbra* width has been defined as the lateral distance between two specified isodose curves[4] at a specified depth (11).

4.8. HEAVY PARTICLE BEAMS

Whereas x-rays and electrons are the main radiations used in radiotherapy, heavy particle beams offer special advantages with regard to dose localization and therapeutic gain (greater effect on tumor than on normal tissue). These particles include neutrons, protons, deuterons, α particles, negative pions, and heavy ions accelerated to high energies. Their

---

[4] An isodose curve is a line passing through points of equal dose.

use in radiation therapy is still experimental, and because of the enormous cost involved, only a few institutions have been able to acquire these modalities for clinical trials. From the literature, which is full of encouraging as well as discouraging reports about their efficacy, it appears that the role of heavy particles in radiation therapy is not yet established. However, the radiobiological interest in the field remains as strong as ever.

A. Neutrons

High-energy neutron beams for radiotherapy are produced by deuterium tritium (D-T) generators, cyclotrons, or linear accelerators. The bombarding particles are either deuterons or protons and the target material is usually beryllium, except in the D-T generator in which tritium is used as the target.

A.1. D-T Generator

A low-energy deuteron beam (100–300 keV) incident on a tritium target yields neutrons by the following reaction:

$$^{2}_{1}\text{H} + {}^{3}_{1}\text{H} \rightarrow {}^{4}_{2}\text{He} + {}^{1}_{0}n + 17.6\,\text{MeV} \tag{4.3}$$

The disintegration energy of 17.6 MeV is shared between the helium nucleus (α particle) and the neutron, with about 14 MeV given to the neutron. The neutrons thus produced are essentially monoenergetic and isotropic (same yield in all directions). The major problem is the lack of sufficient dose rate at the treatment distance. The highest dose rate that has been achieved so far is about 15 cGy/min at 1 m. The advantage of D-T generators over other sources is that its size is small enough to allow isocentric mounting on a gantry.

A.2. Cyclotron

Deuterons accelerated to high energies ($\sim$15–50 MeV) by a cyclotron bombard a low atomic number target such as beryllium to produce neutrons according to a *stripping* reaction (see section 2.8.D):

$$^{2}_{1}\text{H} + {}^{9}_{4}\text{Be} \rightarrow {}^{10}_{5}\text{B} + {}^{1}_{0}n$$

Neutrons are produced mostly in the forward direction with a spectrum of energies, as shown in Fig. 4.15. The average neutron energy is about 40% to 50% of the deuteron energy.

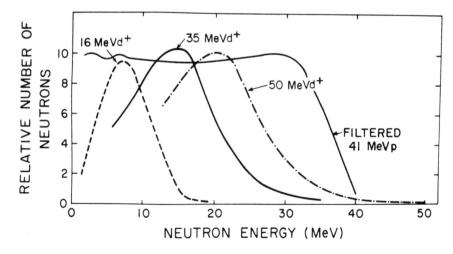

FIG. 4.15. Neutron spectra produced by deuterons on beryllium target. (From Raju MR. *Heavy particle radiotherapy.* New York: Academic Press, 1980. Data from Hall EJ, Roizin-Towle L, Attix FH. Radiobiological studies with cyclotron-produced neutrons currently used for radiotherapy. *Int J Radiol-Oncol Biol Phys* 1975;1:33, and Graves RG, Smathers JB, Almond PR, et al. Neutron energy spectra of d(49)-Be and P(41)-Be neutron radiotherapy sources. *Med Phys* 1979;6:123; with permission.)

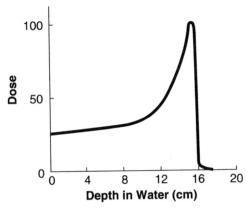

FIG. 4.16. Depth dose distribution characteristic of heavy charged particles, showing Bragg peak.

The bombarding particles can also be protons accelerated to high energies by a cyclotron or a linear accelerator. The neutron spectrum produced by 41 MeV protons is shown in Fig. 4.15. A hydrogenous material filter (e.g., polyethylene) is used to reduce the number of low-energy neutrons in the spectrum.

B. Protons and Heavy Ions

Proton beams for therapeutic application range in energy from 150 to 250 MeV. These beams can be produced by a cyclotron or a linear accelerator. The major advantage of high-energy protons and other heavy charged particles is their characteristic distribution of dose with depth (Fig. 4.16). As the beam traverses the tissues, the dose deposited is approximately constant with depth until near the end of the range where the dose peaks out to a high value followed by a rapid falloff to zero. The region of high dose at the end of the particle range is called the Bragg peak.

Figure 14.17 shows the range energy relationship for protons. The approximate range for other particles with the same initial velocity can be calculated by the following relationship:

$$R_1 / R_2 = (M_1 / M_2) \cdot (Z_2 / Z_1)^2 \tag{4.4}$$

where R_1 and R_2 are particle ranges, M_1 and M_2 are the masses, and Z_1 and Z_2 are the charges of the two particles being compared. Thus from the range energy data for protons one can calculate the range of other particles.

The energy of heavy charged particles or stripped nuclei is often expressed in terms of kinetic energy per nucleon (specific kinetic energy) or MeV/u where u is the mass number of the nucleus. Particles with the same MeV/u have approximately the same velocity and range. For example, 150 MeV protons, 300 MeV deuterons, and 600 MeV helium ions all have approximately the same range of about 16 cm in water. However, for ions heavier than helium, the range for the same MeV/u is somewhat less than that for protons. As predicted by Equation 4.4, the range is dependent on A/Z^2, where A is the atomic number and Z is the nuclear charge. Since A/Z^2 decreases as the ions get heavier, the range of heavier ions is less than the range of lighter ions for the same MeV/u.

C. Negative Pions

The existence of pi mesons was theoretically predicted by Yukawa in 1935 when he postulated that protons and neutrons in the nucleus are held together by a mutual exchange of pi mesons. A pi meson (or pion) has a mass 273 times that of electron and may have a positive charge, a negative charge, or may be neutral. The charged pions decay into mu

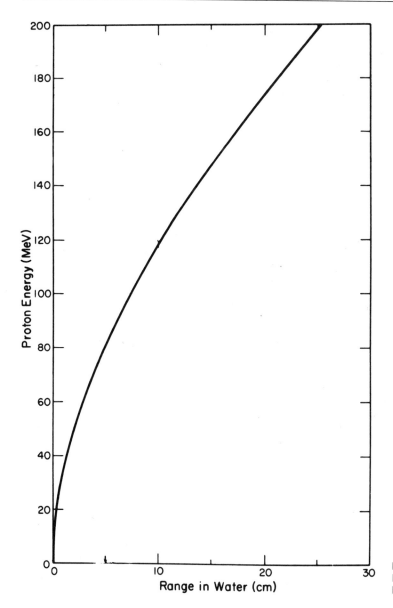

FIG. 4.17. Range energy relationship for protons. (From Raju MR. *Heavy particle radiotherapy.* New York: Academic Press, 1980, with permission.)

mesons and neutrinos with a mean life of 2.54×10^{-8} seconds and the neutral pions decay into pairs of photons with a mean life of about 10^{-16} seconds.

$$\pi^+ \rightarrow \mu^+ + \nu$$
$$\pi^- \rightarrow \mu^- + \bar{\nu}$$
$$\pi^0 \rightarrow h\nu_1 + h\nu_2$$

Only negative pions have been used for radiation therapy.

Beams of negative pions can be produced in a nuclear reaction. Protons of energy in the range of 400 to 800 MeV, produced in a cyclotron or a linear accelerator are usually used for pion beam production for radiotherapy. Beryllium is a suitable target material. Pions of positive, negative, and zero charge with a spectrum of energies are produced and negative pions of suitable energy are extracted from the target using bending and focusing magnets. Pions of energy close to 100 MeV are of interest in radiation therapy, providing a range in water of about 24 cm.

The Bragg peak exhibited by pions is more pronounced than other heavy particles because of the additional effect of nuclear disintegration by π^- capture. This phenomenon, commonly known as *star formation,* occurs when a pion is captured by a nucleus in the medium near the end of its range. A pion capture results in the release of several other particles such as protons, neutrons, and α particles.

Although pion beams have attractive radiobiologic properties, they suffer from the problems of low dose rates, beam contamination, and high cost.

REFERENCES

1. Paterson R. *The treatment of malignant disease by radium and x-rays.* Baltimore: Williams & Wilkins, 1963.
2. National Council on Radiation Protection. *Medical x-ray and gamma ray protection for energies up to 10 MeV.* NCRP report 34. Washington, DC: National Council on Radiation Protection and Measurements, 1970.
3. Karzmark CJ, Nunan CS, Tanabe E. *Medical electron accelerators.* New York: McGraw-Hill, 1993.
4. Podgorsak EB, Rawlinson JA, Johns HE. X-ray depth doses from linear accelerators in the energy range from 10 to 32 MeV. *AJR* 1975;123:182.
5. Veksler VJ. A new method for acceleration of relativistic particles. *Dokl Akad Nauk SSSR* 1944;43:329.
6. Reistad D, Brahme A.The microtron, a new accelerator for radiation therapy. In: *The Third ICMP Executive Committee, ed. Digest of the 3rd international conference on medical physics.* Götenborg, Sweden: Chalmers University of Technology, 1972:23.5.
7. Svensson H, Johnsson L, Larsson LG, et al. A 22 MeV microtron for radiation therapy. *Acta Radiol Ther Phys Biol* 1977;16:145.
8. Rosander S, Sedlacek M, Werholm O. The 50 MeV racetrack microtron at the Royal Institute of Technology, Stockholm. *Nucl Inst Meth* 1982;204:1–20.
9. Cormack DV, Johns HE. Spectral distribution of scattered radiation from a kilocurie cobalt 60 unit. *Br J Radiol* 1958;31:497.
10. Johns HE, Cunningham JR. *The physics of radiology,* 3rd ed. Springfield, IL: Charles C Thomas, 1969:120.
11. International Commission on Radiation Units. Determination of absorbed dose in a patient irradiated by beams of x- or gamma rays in radiotherapy procedures. ICRU report 24. Washington, DC: International Commission on Radiation Units and Measurements, 1976:54.

INTERACTIONS OF IONIZING RADIATION

When an x- or γ ray beam passes through a medium, interaction between photons and matter can take place with the result that energy is transferred to the medium. The initial step in the energy transfer involves the ejection of electrons from the atoms of the absorbing medium. These high-speed electrons transfer their energy by producing ionization and excitation of the atoms along their paths. If the absorbing medium consists of body tissues, sufficient energy may be deposited within the cells, destroying their reproductive capacity. However, most of the absorbed energy is converted into heat, producing no biologic effect.

5.1. IONIZATION

The process by which a neutral atom acquires a positive or a negative charge is known as *ionization*. Removal of an orbital electron leaves the atom positively charged, resulting in an ion pair. The stripped electron, in this case, is the negative ion and the residual atom is the positive ion. In some cases, an electron may be acquired by a neutral atom and the negatively charged atom then becomes the negative ion.

Charged particles such as electrons, protons, and α particles are known as *directly ionizing radiation* provided they have sufficient kinetic energy to produce ionization by collision[1] as they penetrate matter. The energy of the incident particle is lost in a large number of small increments along the ionization track in the medium, with an occasional interaction in which the ejected electron receives sufficient energy to produce a secondary track of its own, known as a δ *ray*. If, on the other hand, the energy lost by the incident particle is not sufficient to eject an electron from the atom but is used to raise the electrons to higher energy levels, the process is termed *excitation*.

The uncharged particles such as neutrons and photons are *indirectly ionizing radiation* because they liberate directly ionizing particles from matter when they interact with matter.

Ionizing photons interact with the atoms of a material or *absorber* to produce high-speed electrons by three major processes: photoelectric effect, Compton effect, and pair production. Before considering each process in detail, we shall discuss the mathematical aspects of radiation absorption.

5.2. PHOTON BEAM DESCRIPTION

An x-ray beam emitted from a target or a γ ray beam emitted from a radioactive source consists of a large number of photons, usually with a variety of energies. A beam of photons can be described by many terms, some of which are defined as follows:

---

[1] The process of collision is an interaction between the electromagnetic fields associated with the colliding particle and orbital electron. Actual physical contact between the particles is not required.

1. The fluence (Φ) of photons is the quotient dN by da, where dN is the number of photons that enter an imaginary sphere of cross-sectional area da.

$$\Phi = \frac{dN}{da} \tag{5.1}$$

2. *Fluence rate or flux density* (ϕ) is the fluence per unit time.

$$\phi = \frac{d\Phi}{dt} \tag{5.2}$$

where dt is the time interval.

3. *Energy fluence* (Ψ) is the quotient of dE_{fl} by da, where dE_{fl} is the sum of the energies of all the photons that enter a sphere of cross-sectional area da.

$$\Psi = \frac{dE_{fl}}{da} \tag{5.3}$$

For a monoenergetic beam, dE_{fl} is just the number of photons dN times energy $h\nu$ carried by each photon:

$$dE_{fl} = dN \cdot h\nu \tag{5.4}$$

4. *Energy fluence rate, energy flux density, or intensity* (ψ) is the energy fluence per unit time:

$$\psi = \frac{d\Psi}{dt} \tag{5.5}$$

5.3. PHOTON BEAM ATTENUATION

An experimental arrangement designed to measure the attenuation characteristics of a photon beam is shown in Fig. 5.1. A narrow beam of monoenergetic photons is incident on an absorber of variable thickness. A detector is placed at a fixed distance from the source and sufficiently farther away from the absorber so that only the *primary* photons (those photons that passed through the absorber without interacting) are measured by the detector. Any photon scattered by the absorber is not supposed to be measured in this arrangement. Thus, if a photon interacts with an atom, it is either completely absorbed or scattered away from the detector.

Under these conditions, the reduction in the number of photons (dN) is proportional to the number of incident photons (N) and to the thickness of the absorber (dx). Mathematically,

$$dN \propto N dx$$

or

$$dN = -\mu N dx \tag{5.6}$$

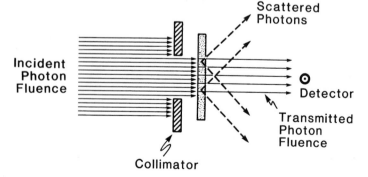

FIG. 5.1. Diagram to illustrate an experimental arrangement for studying narrow beam attenuation through an absorber. Measurements are under "good geometry," i.e., scattered photons are not measured.

where μ is the constant of proportionality, called the *attenuation coefficient*. The minus sign indicates that the number of photons decreases as the absorber thickness increases. The above equation can also be written in terms of intensity (I):

$$dI = -\mu I dx$$

or

$$\frac{dI}{I} = -\mu dx \tag{5.7}$$

If thickness x is expressed as a length, then μ is called the *linear attenuation coefficient*. For example, if the thickness is measured in centimeters, the units of μ are 1/cm, or cm^{-1}.

Equation 5.7 is identical to Equation 2.1, which describes radioactive decay, and μ is analogous to decay constant λ. As before, the differential equation for attenuation can be solved to yield the following equation:

$$I(x) = I_0 e^{-\mu x} \tag{5.8}$$

where $I(x)$ is the intensity transmitted by a thickness x and I_0 is the intensity incident on the absorber. If $I(x)$ is plotted as a function of x for a narrow monoenergetic beam, a straight line will be obtained on semilogarithmic paper (Fig. 5.2A), showing that the attenuation of a monoenergetic beam is described by an exponential function.

The term analogous to half-life (section 2.4) is the *half-value layer* (HVL) defined as the thickness of an absorber required to attenuate the intensity of the beam to half its original value. That means that when $x =$ HVL, $I/I_0 = 1/2$, by definition. Thus from

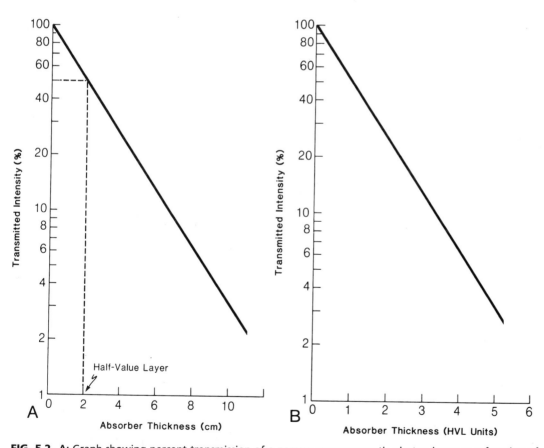

FIG. 5.2. A: Graph showing percent transmission of a narrow monoenergetic photon beam as a function of absorber thickness. For this quality beam and absorber material, HVL = 2 cm and $\mu = 0.347$ cm^{-1}. **B:** Universal attenuation curve showing percent transmission of a narrow monoenergetic beam as a function of absorber thickness in units of half-value layer (HVL).

Equation 5.8 it can be shown that:

$$\text{HVL} = \frac{0.693}{\mu} \qquad (5.9)$$

As mentioned previously, exponential attenuation strictly applies to a monoenergetic beam. Figure 5.2B is a general attenuation curve for a monoenergetic beam or a beam whose half-value layer does not change with absorber thickness. Such a curve may be used to calculate the number of HVLs required to reduce the transmitted intensity to a given percentage of the incident intensity.

A practical beam produced by an x-ray generator, however, consists of a spectrum of photon energies. Attenuation of such a beam is no longer quite exponential. This effect is seen in Fig. 5.3, in which the plot of transmitted intensity on semilogarithmic paper is not a straight line. The slope of the attenuation curve decreases with increasing absorber thickness because the absorber or *filter* preferentially removes the lower-energy photons. As shown in Fig. 5.3, the first HVL is defined as that thickness of material which reduces the

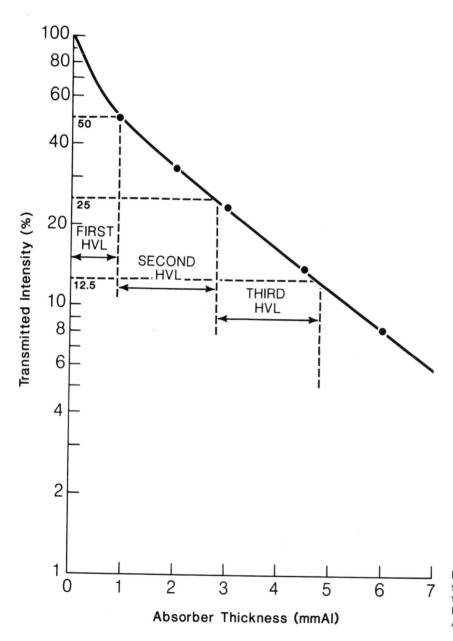

FIG. 5.3. Schematic graph showing transmission of an x-ray beam with a spectrum of photon energies through an aluminum absorber. First HVL = 0.99 mm Al, second HVL = 1.9 mm Al, third HVL = 2.0 mm Al.

incident beam intensity by 50%. The second HVL reduces the beam to 50% of its intensity after it has been transmitted through the first HVL. Similarly, the third HVL represents the quality of the beam after it has been transmitted through the absorber of thickness equal to two HVLs. In general, for a heterogeneous beam, the first HVL is less than the subsequent HVLs. As the filter thickness increases, the average energy of the transmitted beam increases or the beam becomes increasingly *harder*. Thus, by increasing the filtration in such an x-ray beam, one increases the penetrating power or the half-value layer of the beam.

5.4. COEFFICIENTS

A. Attenuation Coefficient

In the previous section, we discussed the linear attenuation coefficient μ, which has units of cm^{-1}. In general, this coefficient depends on the energy of the photons and the nature of the material. Since the attenuation produced by a thickness x depends on the number of electrons presented in that thickness, μ depends on the density of the material. Thus, by dividing μ by density ρ, the resulting coefficient (μ/ρ) will be independent of density; μ/ρ is known as the *mass attenuation coefficient*. This is a more fundamental coefficient than the linear coefficient, since the density has been factored out and its dependence on the nature of the material does not involve density but rather the atomic composition.

The mass attenuation coefficient has units of cm^2/g because $\mu/\rho = cm^{-1}/(g/cm^3)$. When using μ/ρ in the attenuation Equation 5.8, the thickness should be expressed as ρx, which has units of g/cm^2, because $\mu x = (\mu/\rho)(\rho x)$ and $\rho x = (g/cm^3)(cm)$.

In addition to the cm and g/cm^2 units, the absorber thickness can also be expressed in units of $electrons/cm^2$ and $atoms/cm^2$. The corresponding coefficients for the last two units are *electronic attenuation coefficient* $(_e\mu)$ and *atomic attenuation coefficient* $(_a\mu)$, respectively.

$$_e\mu = \frac{\mu}{\rho} \cdot \frac{1}{N_0} \; cm^2/electron \tag{5.10}$$

$$_a\mu = \frac{\mu}{\rho} \cdot \frac{Z}{N_0} \; cm^2/atom \tag{5.11}$$

where Z is the atomic number and N_0 is the number of electrons per gram and N_0 is given by:

$$N_0 = \frac{N_A \cdot Z}{A_W} \tag{5.12}$$

where N_A is Avogadro's number and A_W is the atomic weight (see section 1.3).

The attenuation process or the attenuation coefficient represents the fraction of photons removed per unit thickness. The transmitted intensity $I(x)$ in Equation 5.8 is caused by photons that did not interact with the material. Those photons which produced interactions will transfer part of their energy to the material and result in part or all of that energy being absorbed.

B. Energy Transfer Coefficient

When a photon interacts with the electrons in the material, a part or all of its energy is converted into kinetic energy of electrons. If only a part of the photon energy is given to the electron, the photon itself is scattered with reduced energy. The scattered photon may interact again with a partial or complete transfer of energy to the electrons. Thus a photon may experience one or multiple interactions in which the energy lost by the photon is converted into kinetic energy of electrons.

If we consider a photon beam traversing a material, the fraction of photon energy transferred into kinetic energy of charged particles per unit thickness of absorber is given by the *energy transfer coefficient* (μ_{tr}). This coefficient is related to μ as follows:

$$\mu_{tr} = \frac{\overline{E}_{tr}}{h\nu}\mu \tag{5.13}$$

where $\overline{E}_{tr}$ is the average energy transferred into kinetic energy of charged particles per interaction. The *mass energy transfer coefficient* is given by μ_{tr}/ρ.

C. Energy Absorption Coefficient

Most of the electrons set in motion by the photons will lose their energy by inelastic collisions (ionization and excitation) with atomic electrons of the material. A few, depending on the atomic number of the material, will lose energy by bremsstrahlung interactions with the nuclei. The bremsstrahlung energy is radiated out of the local volume as x-rays and is not included in the calculation of locally absorbed energy.

The *energy absorption coefficient* (μ_{en}) is defined as the product of energy transfer coefficient and $(1 - g)$ where g is the fraction of the energy of secondary charged particles that is lost to bremsstrahlung in the material.

$$\mu_{en} = \mu_{tr}(1 - g) \tag{5.14}$$

As before, the mass energy absorption coefficient is given by μ_{en}/ρ.

For most interactions involving soft tissues or other low Z material in which electrons lose energy almost entirely by ionization collisions, the bremsstrahlung component is negligible. Thus $\mu_{en} = \mu_{tr}$ under those conditions. These coefficients can differ appreciably when the kinetic energies of the secondary particles are high and material traversed has a high atomic number.

The energy absorption coefficient is an important quantity in radiotherapy since it allows the evaluation of energy absorbed in the tissues, a quantity of interest in predicting the biologic effects of radiation.

5.5. INTERACTIONS OF PHOTONS WITH MATTER

Attenuation of a photon beam by an absorbing material is caused by five major types of interactions. One of these, photo disintegration, was considered in section 2.8F. This reaction between photon and nucleus is only important at very high photon energies (>10 MeV). The other four processes are coherent scattering, the photoelectric effect, the Compton effect, and the pair production. Each of these processes can be represented by its own attenuation coefficient, which varies in its particular way with the energy of the photon and with the atomic number of the absorbing material. The total attenuation coefficient is the sum of individual coefficients for these processes:

$$\mu/\rho = \sigma_{coh}/\rho + \tau/\rho + \sigma_c/\rho + \pi/\rho \tag{5.15}$$

where σ_{coh}, τ, σ_c, and π are attenuation coefficients for coherent scattering, photoelectric effect, Compton effect, and pair production, respectively.

5.6. COHERENT SCATTERING

The coherent scattering, also known as classical scattering or Rayleigh scattering, is illustrated in Fig. 5.4. The process can be visualized by considering the wave nature of electromagnetic radiation. This interaction consists of an electromagnetic wave passing near the electron and setting it into oscillation. The oscillating electron reradiates the energy at the same frequency as the incident electromagnetic wave. These scattered x-rays

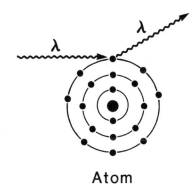

Atom

FIG. 5.4. Diagram illustrating the process of coherent scattering. The scattered photon has the same wavelength as the incident photon. No energy is transferred.

have the same wavelength as the incident beam. Thus no energy is changed into electronic motion and no energy is absorbed in the medium. The only effect is the scattering of the photon at small angles. The coherent scattering is probable in high atomic number materials and with photons of low energy. The process is only of academic interest in radiation therapy.

5.7. PHOTOELECTRIC EFFECT

The photoelectric effect is a phenomenon in which a photon interacts with an atom and ejects one of the orbital electrons from the atom (Fig. 5.5). In this process, the entire energy hv of the photon is first absorbed by the atom and then transferred to the atomic electron. The kinetic energy of the ejected electron (called the photoelectron) is equal to $hv - E_B$, where E_B is the binding energy of the electron. Interactions of this type can take place with electrons in the K, L, M, or N shells.

After the electron has been ejected from the atom, a vacancy is created in the shell, thus leaving the atom in an excited state. The vacancy can be filled by an outer orbital electron with the emission of characteristic x-rays (section 3.4B). There is also the possibility of emission of Auger electrons (section 2.7C), which are monoenergetic electrons produced by the absorption of characteristic x-rays internally by the atom. Because the K shell binding energy of soft tissues is only about 0.5 keV, the energy of the characteristic photons produced in biologic absorbers is very low and can be considered to be locally absorbed. For higher-energy photons and higher atomic number materials, the characteristic photons are of higher energy and may deposit energy at large distances compared with the range

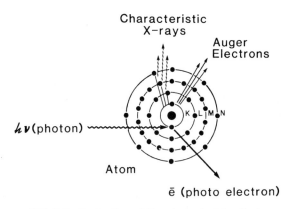

FIG. 5.5. Illustration of the photoelectric effect.

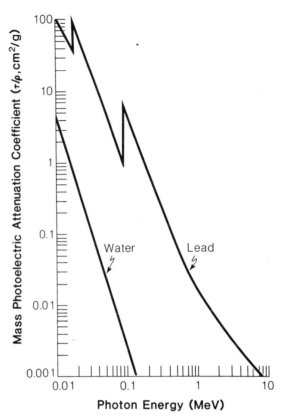

FIG. 5.6. Mass photoelectric attenuation coefficient (τ/ρ) plotted against photon energy. Curves for water ($Z_{\text{eff}} = 7.42$) and lead ($Z = 82$). (Data from Grodstein GW. X-ray attenuation coefficients from 10 keV to 100 MeV. Pub. No. 583. Washington, DC: U.S. Bureau of Standards, 1957.)

of the photoelectron. In such cases, the local energy absorption is reduced by the energy emitted as characteristic radiation (also called fluorescent radiation) which is considered to be remotely absorbed.

The probability of photoelectric absorption depends on the photon energy as illustrated in Fig. 5.6, where the mass photoelectric attenuation coefficient (τ/ρ) is plotted as a function of photon energy. Data are shown for water, representing a low atomic number material similar to tissue, and for lead, representing a high atomic number material. On logarithmic paper, the graph is almost a straight line with a slope of approximately -3; therefore, we get the following relationship between τ/ρ and photon energy:

$$\tau/\rho \propto 1/E^3 \qquad (5.16)$$

The graph for lead has discontinuities at about 15 and 88 keV. These are called *absorption edges* and correspond to the binding energies of L and K shells. A photon with energy less than 15 keV does not have enough energy to eject an L electron. Thus, below 15 keV, the interaction is limited to the M or higher-shell electrons. When the photon has an energy that just equals the binding energy of the L shell, resonance occurs and the probability of photoelectric absorption involving the L shell becomes very high. Beyond this point, if the photon energy is increased, the probability of photoelectric attenuation decreases approximately as $1/E^3$ until the next discontinuity, the K absorption edge. At this point on the graph, the photon has 88 keV energy, which is just enough to eject the K electron. As seen in Fig. 5.6, the absorption probability in lead at this critical energy increases dramatically, by a factor of about 10.

The discontinuities or absorption edges for water are not shown in the graph because the K absorption edge for water occurs at very low photon energies ($\sim$0.5 keV).

The data for various materials indicate that photoelectric attenuation depends strongly on the atomic number of the absorbing material. The following approximate relationship holds:

$$\tau/\rho \propto Z^3 \tag{5.17}$$

This relationship forms the basis of many applications in diagnostic radiology. The difference in Z of various tissues such as bone, muscle, and fat amplifies differences in x-ray absorption, provided the primary mode of interaction is photoelectric. This Z^3 dependence is also exploited when using contrast materials such as $BaSO_4$ mix and Hypaque. In therapeutic radiology, the low-energy beams produced by superficial and orthovoltage machines cause unnecessary high absorption of x-ray energy in bone as a result of this Z^3 dependence; this problem will be discussed later in section 5.10. By combining Equations 5.16 and 5.17, we have:

$$\tau/\rho \propto Z^3/E^3 \tag{5.18}$$

The angular distribution of electrons emitted in a photoelectric process depends on the photon energy. For a low-energy photon, the photoelectron is emitted most likely at 90 degrees relative to the direction of the incident photon. As the photon energy increases, the photoelectrons are emitted in a more forward direction.

5.8. COMPTON EFFECT

In the Compton process, the photon interacts with an atomic electron as though it were a "free" electron. The term *free* here means that the binding energy of the electron is much less than the energy of the bombarding photon. In this interaction, the electron receives some energy from the photon and is emitted at an angle θ (Fig. 5.7). The photon, with reduced energy, is scattered at an angle ϕ.

The Compton process can be analyzed in terms of a collision between two particles, a photon and an electron. By applying the laws of conservation of energy and momentum, one can derive the following relationships:

$$E = h\nu_0 \frac{\alpha(1 - \cos\phi)}{1 + \alpha(1 - \cos\phi)} \tag{5.19}$$

$$h\nu' = h\nu_0 \frac{1}{1 + \alpha(1 - \cos\phi)} \tag{5.20}$$

$$\cos\theta = (1 + \alpha)\tan\phi/2 \tag{5.21}$$

where $h\nu_0$, $h\nu'$, and E are the energies of the incident photon, scattered photon, and electron, respectively and, $\alpha = h\nu_0/m_0c^2$, where m_0c^2 is the rest energy of the electron (0.511 MeV). If $h\nu_0$ is expressed in MeV, then $\alpha = h\nu_0/0.511$.

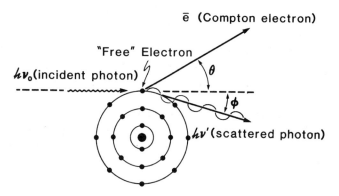

FIG. 5.7. Diagram illustrating the Compton effect.

A. Special Cases of Compton Effect

A.1. Direct Hit

If a photon makes a direct hit with the electron, the electron will travel forward ($\theta = 0$ degrees) and the scattered photon will travel backward ($\phi = 180$ degrees) after the collision. In such a collision, the electron will receive maximum energy E_{max} and the scattered photon will be left with minimum energy $h\nu'_{min}$. One can calculate E_{max} and $h\nu'_{min}$ by substituting $\cos\phi = \cos 180$ degrees $= -1$ in Equations 5.19 and 5.20.

$$E_{max} = h\nu_0 \frac{2\alpha}{1 + 2\alpha} \tag{5.22}$$

$$h\nu'_{min} = h\nu_0 \frac{1}{1 + 2\alpha} \tag{5.23}$$

A.2. Grazing Hit

If a photon makes a grazing hit with the electron, the electron will be emitted at right angles ($\theta = 90$ degrees) and the scattered photon will go in the forward direction ($\phi = 0$ degrees). By substituting $\cos\phi = \cos 0$ degrees $= 1$ in Equations 5.19 and 5.20, one can show that for this collision $E = 0$ and $h\nu' = h\nu_0$.

A.3. 90-Degree Photon Scatter

If a photon is scattered at right angles to its original direction ($\phi = 90$ degrees), one can calculate E and $h\nu'$ from Equations 5.19 and 5.20 by substituting $\cos\phi = \cos 90$ degrees $= 0$. The angle of the electron emission in this case will depend on α, according to Equation 5.21.

Examples

Some useful examples will now be given to illustrate application of the Compton effect to practical problems.

a. *Interaction of a low-energy photon.* If the incident photon energy is much less than the rest energy of the electron, only a small part of its energy is imparted to the electron, resulting in a scattered photon of almost the same energy as the incident photon. For example, suppose $h\nu_0 = 51.1$ keV; then $\alpha = h\nu_0/m_0 c^2 = 0.0511$ MeV/0.511 MeV $= 0.1$. From Equations 5.22 and 5.23,

$$E_{max} = 51.1 \, (\text{keV}) \frac{2(0.1)}{1 + 2(0.1)} = 8.52 \, \text{keV} \tag{5.24}$$

$$h\nu'_{min} = 51.1 \, (\text{keV}) \frac{1}{1 + 2(0.1)} = 42.58 \, \text{keV} \tag{5.25}$$

Thus, for a low-energy photon beam, the Compton scattered photons have approximately the same energy as the original photons. Indeed, as the incident photon energy approaches zero, the Compton effect becomes the classical scattering process described in section 5.6.

b. *Interaction of a high energy photon.* If the incident photon has a very high energy (much greater than the rest energy of the electron), the photon loses most of its energy to the Compton electron and the scattered photon has much less energy. Suppose $h\nu_0 = 5.11$ MeV; then $\alpha = 10.0$. From Equations 5.22 and 5.23,

$$E_{max} = 5.11 \, (\text{MeV}) \frac{2(10)}{1 + 2(10)} = 4.87 \, \text{MeV} \tag{5.26}$$

$$hv'_{min} = 5.11 \, (\text{MeV}) \frac{1}{1 + 2(10)} = 0.24 \, \text{MeV} \qquad (5.27)$$

In contrast to example (a) above, the scattered photons produced by high-energy photons carry away only a small fraction of the initial energy. Thus, at high photon energy, the Compton effect causes a large amount of energy absorption compared with the Compton interactions involving low-energy photons.

c. *Compton scatter at $\phi = 90$ degrees and 180 degrees.* In designing radiation protection barriers (walls) to attenuate scattered radiation, one needs to know the energy of the photons scattered at different angles. The energy of the photons scattered by a patient under treatment at 90 degrees with respect to the incident beam is of particular interest in calculating barrier or wall thicknesses against scattered radiation.

By substituting $\phi = 90$ degrees in Equation 5.20, we obtain:

$$hv' = \frac{hv_0}{1 + \alpha} \qquad (5.28)$$

For high-energy photons with $\alpha \gg 1$, the previous equation reduces to:

$$hv' \approx \frac{hv_0}{\alpha} \qquad (5.29)$$

or

$$hv' = m_0 c^2 = 0.511 \, \text{MeV}$$

Similar calculations for scatter at $\phi = 180$ degrees will indicate $hv' = 0.255$ MeV. Thus, if the energy of the incident photon is high ($\alpha \gg 1$), we have the following important generalizations: (a) the radiation scattered at right angles is independent of incident energy and has a maximum value of 0.511 MeV; (b) the radiation scattered backwards is independent of incident energy and has a maximum value of 0.255 MeV.

The maximum energy of radiation scattered at angles between 90 and 180 degrees will lie between the above energy limits. However, the energy of the photons scattered at angles less than 90 degrees will be greater than 0.511 MeV and will approach the incident photon energy for the condition of forward scatter. Because the energy of the scattered photon plus that of the electron must equal the incident energy, the electron may acquire any energy between zero and E_{max} (given by Equation 5.22).

B. Dependence of Compton Effect on Energy and Atomic Number

It was mentioned previously that the Compton effect is an interaction between a photon and a free electron. Practically, this means that the energy of the incident photon must be large compared with the electron binding energy. This is in contrast to the photoelectric effect which becomes most probable when the energy of the incident photon is equal to or slightly greater than the binding energy of the electron. Thus, as the photon energy increases beyond the binding energy of the K electron, the photoelectric effect decreases rapidly with energy (Equation 5.16) (Fig. 5.6) and the Compton effect becomes more and more important. However, as shown in Fig. 5.8, the Compton effect also *decreases with increasing photon energy.*

Because the Compton interaction involves essentially free electrons in the absorbing material, *it is independent of atomic number Z.* It follows that the Compton mass attenuation coefficient (σ/ρ) is independent of Z and depends only on the number of electrons per gram. Although the number of electrons per gram of elements decreases slowly but systemically with atomic number, most materials except hydrogen can be considered as having approximately the same number of electrons per gram (Table 5.1). Thus, σ/ρ is *nearly the same for all materials.*

From the previous discussion, it follows that if the energy of the beam is in the region where the Compton effect is the only possible mode of interaction, approximately the same

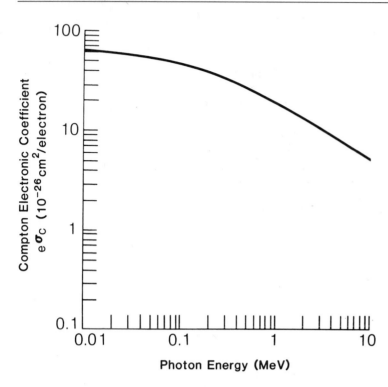

FIG. 5.8. A plot of Compton electronic coefficient $_e\sigma$ against photon energy. The mass coefficient (σ/ρ) is obtained by multiplying the electronic coefficient with the number of electrons per gram for a given material. (Data from Hubbell JH. Proton cross sections attenuation coefficients and energy absorption coefficients from 10 keV to 100 GeV. Pub. No. 29. Washington, DC: U.S. National Bureau of Standards, 1969.)

attenuation of the beam will occur in any material of equal density thickness,[2] expressed as g/cm^2. For example, in the case of a ^{60}Co γ ray beam that interacts by Compton effect, the attenuation per g/cm^2 for bone is nearly the same as that for soft tissue. However, 1 cm of bone will attenuate more than 1 cm of soft tissue, because bone has a higher electron density,[3] ρ_e (number of electrons per cubic centimeter), which is given by density times the number of electrons per gram. If the density of bone is assumed to be 1.85 g/cm^3 and that of soft tissue 1 g/cm^3, then the attenuation produced by 1 cm of bone will be equivalent to that produced by 1.65 cm of soft tissue:

$$(1 \text{ cm}) \frac{(\rho_e)_{\text{bone}}}{(\rho_e)_{\text{muscle}}} = (1 \text{ cm}) \times \frac{1.85(\text{g/cm}^3) \times 3.00 \times 10^{23}(\text{electrons/g})}{1.00(\text{g/cm}^3) \times 3.36 \times 10^{23}(\text{electrons/g})}$$

$$= 1.65 \text{ cm}$$

5.9. PAIR PRODUCTION

If the energy of the photon is greater than 1.02 MeV, the photon may interact with matter through the mechanism of pair production. In this process (Fig. 5.9), the photon interacts strongly with the electromagnetic field of an atomic nucleus and gives up all its energy in the process of creating a pair consisting of a negative electron (e$^-$) and a positive electron (e$^+$). Because the rest mass energy of the electron is equivalent to 0.51 MeV, a minimum energy of 1.02 MeV is required to create the pair of electrons. Thus the *threshold energy* for the pair production process is 1.02 MeV. The photon energy in excess of this threshold is shared between the particles as kinetic energy. The total kinetic energy available for the

---

[2] Density thickness is equal to the linear thickness multiplied by density, i.e., cm $\times$ g/cm^3 = g/cm^2.
[3] In the literature, the term *electron density* has been defined both as the number of electrons per gram and as the number of electrons per cubic centimeter. The reader should be aware of this possible source of confusion.

TABLE 5.1. NUMBER OF ELECTRONS PER GRAM OF VARIOUS MATERIALS

Material	Density (g/cm³)	Atomic Number	Number of Electrons per Gram
Hydrogen	0.0000899	1	6.00×10^{23}
Carbon	2.25	6	3.01×10^{23}
Oxygen	0.001429	8	3.01×10^{23}
Aluminum	2.7	13	2.90×10^{23}
Copper	8.9	29	2.75×10^{23}
Lead	11.3	82	2.38×10^{23}
		Effective Atomic Number	
Fat	0.916	5.92	3.48×10^{23}
Muscle	1.00	7.42	3.36×10^{23}
Water	1.00	7.42	3.34×10^{23}
Air	0.001293	7.64	3.01×10^{23}
Bone	1.85	13.8	3.00×10^{23}

Data from Johns HE, Cunningham JR. The physics of radiology. 3rd ed. Springfield, IL: Charles C Thomas, 1969.

electron-positron pair is given by $(h\nu - 1.02)$ MeV. The particles tend to be emitted in the forward direction relative to the incident photon.

The most probable distribution of energy is for each particle to acquire half the available kinetic energy, although any energy distribution is possible. For example, in an extreme case, it is possible that one particle may receive all the energy while the other receives no energy.

The pair production process is an example of an event in which energy is converted into mass, as predicted by Einstein's equation $E = mc^2$. The reverse process, namely the conversion of mass into energy, takes place when a positron combines with an electron to produce two photons, called the annihilation radiation.

A. Annihilation Radiation

The positron created as a result of pair production process loses its energy as it traverses the matter by the same type of interactions as an electron does, namely by ionization, excitation, and bremsstrahlung. Near the end of its range, the slowly moving positron combines with one of the free electrons in its vicinity to give rise to two annihilation photons, each having 0.51 MeV energy. Because momentum is conserved in the process, the two photons are ejected in opposite directions (Fig. 5.10).

B. Variation of Pair Production with Energy and Atomic Number

Because the pair production results from an interaction with the electromagnetic field of the nucleus, the probability of this process increases rapidly with atomic number. The

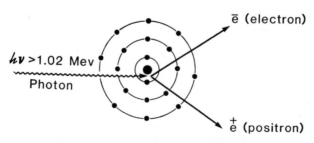

FIG. 5.9. Diagram illustrating the pair production process.

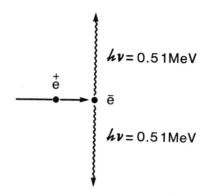

FIG. 5.10. Diagram illustrating the production of annihilation radiation.

attenuation coefficient for pair production (Π) varies with Z^2 per atom, Z per electron, and approximately Z per gram. In addition, for a given material, the likelihood of this interaction increases as the logarithm of the incident photon energy above the threshold energy; these relationships are shown in Fig. 5.11. To remove the major dependence of the pair production process on atomic number, the coefficients per atom have been divided by Z^2 before plotting. For energies up to about 20 MeV, the curves are almost coincident for all materials, indicating that $_a\Pi \propto Z^2$. At higher energies, the curves for higher Z materials fall below the low Z materials because of the screening of the nuclear charge by the orbital electrons.

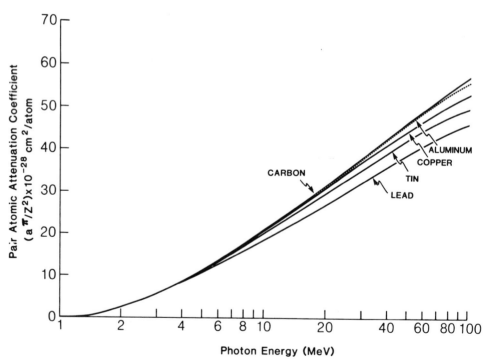

FIG. 5.11. Plot of pair atomic attenuation coefficient divided by the square of the atomic number as a function of photon energy for carbon ($Z = 6$) and lead ($Z = 82$). The mass attenuation coefficient can be obtained by multiplying a^π/Z^2 obtained from the graph, first by Z^2 and then by the number of atoms per gram of the absorber. (Data from Hubbell JH. Proton cross sections attenuation coefficients and energy absorption coefficients from 10 keV to 100 GeV. Pub. No. 29. Washington, DC: U.S. National Bureau of Standards, 1969.)

5.10. RELATIVE IMPORTANCE OF VARIOUS TYPES OF INTERACTIONS

The total mass attenuation coefficient (μ/ρ) is the sum of the four individual coefficients:

$$(\mu/\rho) = \underset{\text{photoelectric}}{(\tau/\rho)} + \underset{\text{coherent}}{(\sigma_{\text{coh}}/\rho)} + \underset{\text{compton}}{(\sigma/\rho)} + \underset{\text{pair}}{(\Pi/\rho)} \qquad (5.30)$$

$$\underset{\text{total}}{}$$

As noted previously, coherent scattering is only important for very low photon energies (<10 keV) and high Z materials. At therapeutic energies, it is often omitted from the sum.

Figure 5.12 is the plot of total coefficient $(\mu/\rho)_{\text{total}}$ vs. energy for two different materials, water and lead, representative of low and high atomic number materials. The mass attenuation coefficient is large for low energies and high atomic number media because of the predominance of photoelectric interactions under these conditions.

The attenuation coefficient decreases rapidly with energy until the photon energy far exceeds the electron binding energies and the Compton effect becomes the predominant mode of interaction. In the Compton range of energies, the μ/ρ of lead and water do not differ greatly, since this type of interaction is independent of atomic number. The coefficient, however, decreases with energy until pair production begins to become important. The dominance of pair production occurs at energies much greater than the threshold energy of 1.02 MeV.

The relative importance of various types of interactions is presented in Table 5.2. These data for water will also be true for soft tissue. The photon energies listed in column 1 of Table 5.2 represent monoenergetic beams. As discussed in Chapter 3, an x-ray tube operating at a given peak voltage produces radiation of all energies less than the peak energy. As a rough approximation and for the purposes of Table 5.2, one may consider the average energy of an x-ray beam to be equivalent to one-third of the peak energy. Thus a 30-keV monoenergetic beam in column 1 should be considered as equivalent to an x-ray beam produced by an x-ray tube operated at about 90 kVp. Of course, the

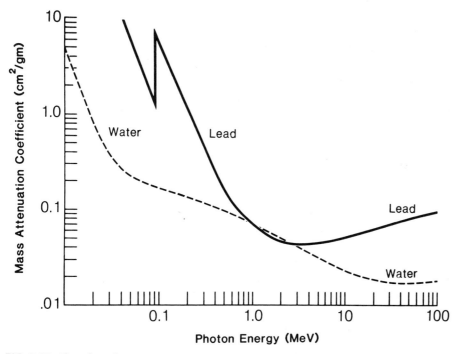

FIG. 5.12. Plot of total mass attenuation coefficient (μ/ρ) as a function of photon energy for lead and water. (Reprinted with permission from Johns HE, Cunningham JR. *The physics of radiology,* 3rd ed. Springfield, IL: Charles C Thomas, 1969.)

**TABLE 5.2. RELATIVE IMPORTANCE OF PHOTOELEC-
TRIC (τ), COMPTON (σ), AND PAIR PRODUCTION (Π)
PROCESSES IN WATER**

Photon Energy (MeV)	Relative Number of Interactions (%)		
	τ	σ	Π
0.01	95	5	0
0.026	50	50	0
0.060	7	93	0
0.150	0	100	0
4.00	0	94	6
10.00	0	77	23
24.00	0	50	50
100.00	0	16	84

Data from Johns HE, Cunningham JR. The physics of radiology.
3rd ed. Springfield, IL: Charles C Thomas, 1969.

accuracy of this approximation is limited by the effects of filtration on the energy spectrum of the beam.

5.11. INTERACTIONS OF CHARGED PARTICLES

Whereas photons interact with matter by photoelectric, Compton, or pair production process, charged particles (electrons, protons, α particles, and nuclei) interact principally by ionization and excitation. Radiative collisions in which the charged particle interacts by the bremsstrahlung process are possible but are much more likely for electrons than for heavier charged particles.

The charged particle interactions or collisions are mediated by Coulomb force between the electric field of the traveling particle and electric fields of orbital electrons and nuclei of atoms of the material. Collisions between the particle and the atomic electrons result in ionization and excitation of the atoms. Collisions between the particle and the nucleus result in radiative loss of energy or bremsstrahlung. Particles also suffer scattering without significant loss of energy. Because of much smaller mass, electrons suffer greater multiple scattering than do heavier particles.

In addition to the Coulomb force interactions, heavy charged particles give rise to nuclear reactions, thereby producing radioactive nuclides. For example, a proton beam passing through tissue produces short-lived radioisotopes ^{11}C, ^{13}N, and ^{15}O, which are positron emitters.

The rate of kinetic energy loss per unit path length of the particle (dE/dx) is known as the stopping power (S). The quantity S/ρ is called the mass stopping power, where ρ is the density of the medium and is usually expressed in MeV cm^2/g.

A. Heavy Charged Particles

The rate of energy loss or stopping power caused by ionization interactions for charged particles is proportional to the square of the particle charge and inversely proportional to the square of its velocity. Thus, as the particle slows down, its rate of energy loss increases and so does the ionization or absorbed dose to the medium. As was seen in Fig. 4.16, the dose deposited in water increases at first very slowly with depth and then very sharply near the end of the range, before dropping to an almost zero value. This peaking of dose near the end of the particle range is called the *Bragg peak*.

Because of the Bragg peak effect and minimal scattering, protons and heavier charged particle beams provide a much sought-after advantage in radiotherapy—the ability to concentrate dose inside the target volume and minimize dose to surrounding normal tissues.

B. Electrons

Interactions of electrons when passing through matter are quite similar to those of heavy particles. However, because of their relatively small mass, the electrons suffer greater multiple scattering and changes in direction of motion. As a consequence, the Bragg peak is not observed for electrons. Multiple changes in direction during the slowing down process smears out the Bragg peak.

In water or soft tissue, electrons, like other charged particles, lose energy predominantly by ionization and excitation. This results in deposition of energy or absorbed dose in the medium. As stated earlier, the ionization process consists of stripping electrons from the atoms. If the energy transferred to the orbital electron is not sufficient to overcome the binding energy, it is displaced from its stable position and then returns to it; this effect is called *excitation*. Furthermore, in the process of ionization, occasionally the stripped electron receives sufficient energy to produce an ionization track of its own. This ejected electron is called a secondary electron, or a δ ray.

Again, because of its small mass, an electron may interact with the electromagnetic field of a nucleus and be decelerated so rapidly that a part of its energy is lost as bremsstrahlung. The rate of energy loss as a result of bremsstrahlung increases with the increase in the energy of the electron and the atomic number of the medium. The topic of electron interactions will be discussed further in Chapter 14.

5.12. INTERACTIONS OF NEUTRONS

Like x-rays and γ rays, neutrons are indirectly ionizing. However, their mode of interaction with matter is different. Neutrons interact basically by two processes: (a) recoiling protons from hydrogen and recoiling heavy nuclei from other elements, and (b) nuclear disintegrations. The first process may be likened to a billiard-ball collision in which the energy is redistributed after the collision between the colliding particles. The energy transfer is very efficient if the colliding particles have the same mass, e.g., a neutron colliding with a hydrogen nucleus. On the other hand, the neutron loses very little energy when colliding with a heavier nucleus. Thus the most efficient absorbers of a neutron beam are the hydrogenous materials such as paraffin wax or polyethylene. Lead, which is a very good absorber for x-rays, is a poor shielding material against neutrons.

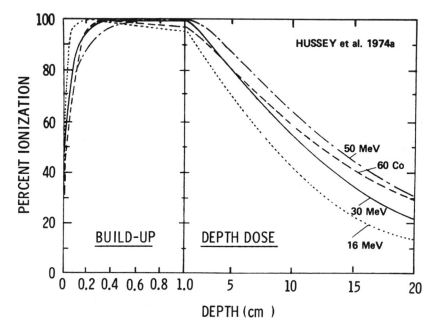

FIG. 5.13. Depth-dose distribution of neutrons produced by deutrons on beryllium, compared with a cobalt-60 γ beam. (From Raju MR. *Heavy particle radiotherapy.* New York: Academic Press, 1980. Data from Hussey DH, Fletcher GH, Caderao JB. Experience with fast neutron therapy using the Texas A&M variable energy cyclotron. *Cancer* 1974;34:65.)

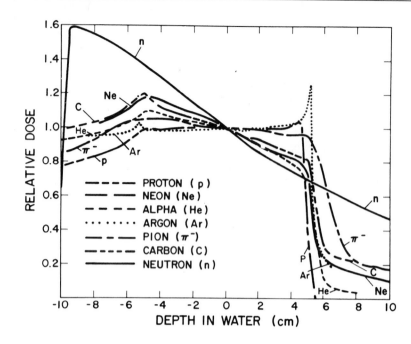

FIG. 5.14. Depth-dose distribution for various heavy particle beams with modulated Bragg peak at a depth of 10 cm and normalized at the peak center. (From Raju MR. *Heavy particle radiotherapy.* New York: Academic Press, 1980.)

Dose deposited in tissue from a high-energy neutron beam is predominantly contributed by recoil protons. Because of the higher hydrogen content, the dose absorbed in fat exposed to a neutron beam is about 20% higher than in muscle. Nuclear disintegrations produced by neutrons result in the emission of heavy charged particles, neutrons, and γ rays and give rise to about 30% of the tissue dose. Because of such diverse secondary radiation produced by neutron interactions, the neutron dosimetry is relatively more complicated than the other types of clinical beams.

5.13. COMPARATIVE BEAM CHARACTERISTICS

No one kind of radiation beam is ideal for radiation therapy. Whereas x-rays and electrons are the most useful beams, particle beams have some unique physical and radiobiologic

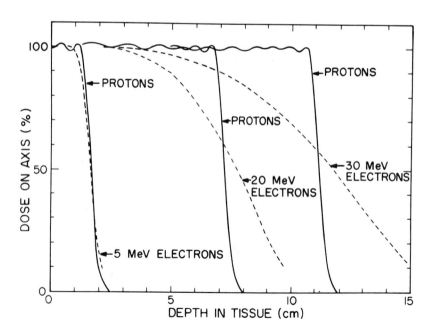

FIG. 5.15. Comparison of depth-dose distribution for protons and electrons. (From Koehler AM, Preston WM. Protons in radiation therapy. *Radiology* 1972;104:191, with permission.)

characteristics that have attracted the attention of many investigators. For details the reader is referred to reference 1.

Physical advantages of a radiation therapy beam are derived from the depth-dose distributions and scatter characteristics. Figures 5.13, 5.14, and 5.15 compare the depth-dose characteristics of various beams. It is seen that the depth dose distribution of neutron beams is qualitatively similar to the ^{60}Co γ rays. The heavy charged particle beams, the Bragg peaks of which were modulated using filters (as is typically done in clinical situations), show a flat dose distribution at the peak region and a sharp dose dropoff beyond the range. Electron beams also show a constant dose region up to about half the particle range and a sharp dose dropoff beyond that point. However, for higher electron energies, the characteristic falloff in dose becomes more gradual. Protons, on the other hand, maintain a sharp cutoff in dose beyond the range, irrespective of energy.

REFERENCE

1. Raju MR. *Heavy particle radiotherapy.* New York: Academic Press, 1980.

6

MEASUREMENT OF IONIZING RADIATION

6.1. INTRODUCTION

In the early days of x-ray usage for diagnosis and therapy, attempts were made to measure ionizing radiation on the basis of chemical and biologic effects. For instance, radiation effects on photographic emulsions, changes in the color of some chemical compounds, and reddening of the human skin could be related to the amount of radiation absorbed. However, these effects were poorly understood at the time and could only provide crude estimation of radiation dose. For example, in radiotherapy, a unit called skin erythema dose (SED) was defined as that amount of x or γ radiation that just produced reddening of the human skin. However, the unit has many drawbacks. Skin erythema depends on many conditions, such as the type of skin, the quality of radiation, the extent of skin exposed, dose fractionation (dose per fraction and interval between fractions), and differences between early and delayed skin reactions.

Although the SED was later discarded in favor of a more precisely measurable unit such as the roentgen, the skin erythema was used by physicians as an approximate index of response to the radiation treatments. This happened in the orthovoltage era when the skin was the limiting organ to the delivery of tumoricidal doses. The reliance on skin reaction for the assessment of radiation response had to be abandoned when megavoltage beams with the skin-sparing properties became the main tools of radiation therapy.

In 1928, the International Commission on Radiation Units and Measurements (ICRU) adopted the roentgen as the unit of measuring x and γ radiation exposure. The unit is denoted by R.

6.2. THE ROENTGEN

The roentgen is a unit of exposure. The quantity *exposure* is a measure of ionization produced in air by photons. The ICRU (1) defines exposure *(X)* as the quotient of dQ by dm where dQ is the absolute value of the total charge of the ions of one sign produced in air when all the electrons (negatrons and positrons) liberated by photons in air of mass dm are completely stopped in air.

$$X = \frac{dQ}{dm} \tag{6.1}$$

The Systems Internationale d'Unites (SI) unit for exposure is coulomb per kilogram (C/kg) but the special unit is roentgen (R).[1]

$$1R = 2.58 \times 10^{-4} \text{ C/kg air}$$

---

[1] Roentgen was originally defined as $1R = 1$ electrostatic unit (esu)/cm^3 air at standard temperature and pressure (STP) ($0°C$, 760 mm Hg). The current definition of $1R = 2.58 \times 10^{-4}$ C/kg air is equivalent to the original if the charge is expressed in coulombs (1 esu $= 3.333 \times 10^{-10}$ C) and the volume of air is changed to mass (1 cm^3 of air at STP weighs 1.293×10^{-6} kg).

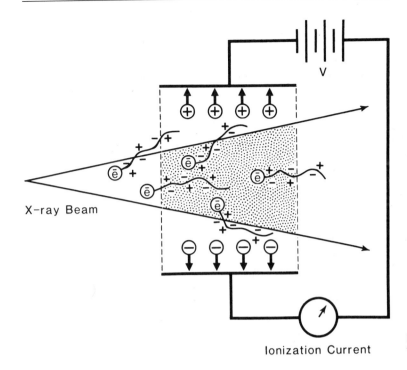

FIG. 6.1. Diagram illustrating electronic equilibrium in a free-air chamber.

The definition of roentgen is illustrated in Fig. 6.1. An x-ray beam in passing through air sets in motion electrons by photoelectric effect, Compton effect, or pair production. These high-speed electrons produce ionization along their tracks. Because of the electric field produced by the voltage applied across the ion-collection plates, the positive charges move toward the negative plate and the negative charges move toward the positive plate. This constitutes a current. The collected charge of either sign can be measured by an electrometer.

According to the definition of roentgen, the electrons produced by photons in a specified volume (shaded in Fig. 6.1) must spend all their energies by ionization in air enclosed by the plates (region of ion collection) and the total ionic charge of either sign should be measured. However, some electrons produced in the specified volume deposit their energy outside the region of ion collection and thus are not measured. On the other hand, electrons produced outside the specified volume may enter the ion-collecting region and produce ionization there. If the ionization loss is compensated by the ionization gained, a condition of *electronic equilibrium* exists. Under this condition, the definition of roentgen is effectively satisfied. This is the principle of free-air ionization chamber, described below.

6.3. FREE-AIR IONIZATION CHAMBER

The free-air, or standard, ionization chamber is an instrument used in the measurement of the roentgen according to its definition. Generally, such a primary standard is used only for the calibration of secondary instruments designed for field use. The free-air chamber installations are thus confined principally to some of the national standards laboratories.

A free-air chamber is represented schematically in Fig. 6.2. An x-ray beam, originating from a focal spot S, is defined by the diaphragm D, and passes centrally between a pair of parallel plates. A high-voltage (field strength of the order of 100 V/cm) is applied between the plates to collect ions produced in the air between the plates. The ionization is measured for a length L defined by the limiting lines of force to the edges of the collection plate C. The lines of force are made straight and perpendicular to the collector by a guard ring G.

As discussed previously, electrons produced by the photon beam in the specified volume (shaded in Fig. 6.2) must spend all their energy by ionization of air between the

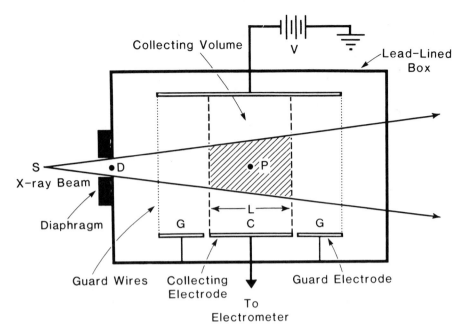

FIG. 6.2. A schematic diagram of a free-air chamber.

plates. Such a condition can exist only if the range of the electrons liberated by the incident photons is less than the distance between each plate and the specified volume. In addition, for electronic equilibrium to exist, the beam intensity (photon fluence per unit time) must remain constant across the length of the specified volume, and the separation between the diaphragm and the ion-collecting region must exceed the electron range in air.

If ΔQ is the charge collected in Coulombs and ρ is the density (kg/m^3) of air, then the exposure X_p at the center of the specified volume (point P) is:

$$X_p = \frac{\Delta Q}{\rho \cdot A_p \cdot L} \cdot \frac{1}{2.58 \times 10^{-4}} \text{ roentgens} \qquad (6.2)$$

where A_p is the cross-sectional area (in meters squared) of the beam at point P and L (in meters) is the length of the collecting volume. In practice, it is more convenient to state the exposure (X) at the position of the diaphragm. Suppose f_1 and f_2 are the distances of the x-ray source to the diaphragm and point P, respectively. Because the intensity at point P and at the diaphragm are related by an inverse square law factor $(f_1/f_2)^2$, which also relates the area of the beams at the diaphragm and at point P, exposure X_D at the diaphragm is given by:

$$X_D = \frac{\Delta Q}{\rho \cdot A_D \cdot L} \cdot \frac{1}{2.58 \times 10^{-4}} \text{ roentgens} \qquad (6.3)$$

where A_D is the diaphragm aperture area.

Accurate measurements with a free-air ionization chamber require considerable care. A few corrections that are usually applied include (a) correction for air attenuation; (b) correction for recombination of ions; (c) correction for the effects of temperature, pressure, and humidity on the density of air; and (d) correction for ionization produced by scattered photons. For details of various corrections the reader is referred to National Bureau of Standards handbook (2).

There are limitations on the design of a free-air chamber for the measurement of roentgens for high-energy x-ray beams. As the photon energy increases, the range of the electrons liberated in air increases rapidly. This necessitates an increase in the separation of the plates to maintain electronic equilibrium. Too large a separation, however, creates problems of nonuniform electric field and greater ion recombination. Although the plate separation can be reduced by using air at high pressures, the problems still remain in regard to air attenuation, photon scatter, and reduction in the efficiency of ion collection. Because of these problems, there is an upper limit on the photon energy above which the roentgen cannot be accurately measured. This limit occurs at about 3 MeV.

6.4. THIMBLE CHAMBERS

Free-air ionization chambers are too delicate and bulky for routine use. Their main function is in the standardizing laboratories where they can be used to calibrate field instruments such as a thimble chamber.

The principle of the thimble chamber is illustrated in Fig. 6.3. In Fig. 6.3A, a spherical volume of air is shown with an air cavity at the center. Suppose this sphere of air is irradiated uniformly with a photon beam. Also, suppose that the distance between the outer sphere and the inner cavity is equal to the maximum range of electrons generated in air. If the number of electrons entering the cavity is the same as that leaving the cavity, electronic equilibrium exists. Suppose also that we are able to measure the ionization charge produced in the cavity by the electrons liberated in the air surrounding the cavity. Then by knowing the volume or mass of air inside the cavity, we can calculate the charge per unit mass or the beam exposure at the center of the cavity. Now if the air wall in Fig. 6.3A is compressed into a solid shell as in Fig. 6.3B, we get a thimble chamber. Although the thimble wall is solid, it is air equivalent, i.e., its effective atomic number is the same as that of air. In addition, the thickness of the thimble wall is such that the electronic equilibrium occurs inside the cavity, just as it did in Fig. 6.3A. As before, it follows that the wall thickness must be equal to or greater than the maximum range of the electrons liberated in the thimble wall.

Since the density of the solid air-equivalent wall is much greater than that of free air, the thicknesses required for electronic equilibrium in the thimble chamber are considerably reduced. For example, in the 100 to 250 kVp x-ray range, the wall thickness of the thimble (assuming unit density) is about 1 mm, and in the case of ^{60}Co γ rays (average $h\nu \approx$ 1.25 MeV), it is approximately 5 mm. In practice, however, a thimble chamber is constructed with wall thicknesses of 1 mm or less and this is supplemented with close-fitting caps of Plexiglas or other plastic to bring the total wall thickness up to that needed for electronic equilibrium for the radiation in question.

A. Chamber Wall

Figure 6.3C shows a typical thimble ionization chamber. The wall is shaped like a sewing thimble—hence the name. The inner surface of the thimble wall is coated by a special

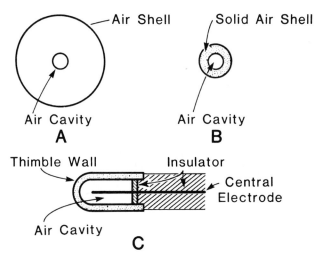

FIG. 6.3. Schematic diagram illustrating the nature of the thimble ionization chamber. **A:** Air shell with air cavity. **B:** Solid air shell with air cavity. **C:** The thimble chamber.

material to make it electrically conducting. This forms one electrode. The other electrode is a rod of low atomic number material such as graphite or aluminum held in the center of the thimble but electrically insulated from it. A suitable voltage is applied between the two electrodes to collect the ions produced in the air cavity.

As mentioned previously, most of the ionization produced in the cavity air arises from electrons liberated in the surrounding wall (for at least up to 2 MeV photons). For the thimble chamber to be equivalent to a free-air chamber, the thimble wall should be air equivalent. This condition would ensure that the energy spectrum of electrons liberated in the thimble wall is similar to that in air.

For the thimble chamber to be air equivalent, the effective atomic number of the wall material and the central electrode must be such that the system as a whole behaves like a free-air chamber. Most commonly used wall materials are made either of graphite (carbon), Bakelite, or a plastic coated on the inside by a conducting layer of graphite or of a conducting mixture of Bakelite and graphite. The effective atomic number of the wall is generally a little less than that of air. It is closer to that of carbon ($Z = 6$). As a consequence, such a wall should give rise to less ionization in the air cavity than a free-air wall. However, the usually greater atomic number of the central electrode, its dimensions, and the placement geometry within the thimble can provide compensation for the lower atomic number of the wall.

B. Effective Atomic Number

It is instructive to discuss the term *effective atomic number* ($\overline{Z}$) in a greater detail. $\overline{Z}$ is the atomic number of an element with which photons interact the same way as with the given composite material. Since photoelectric effect is highly Z dependent (section 5.7), $\overline{Z}$ is considered for photoelectric interactions. Mayneord (3) has defined the effective atomic number of a compound as follows:

$$\overline{Z} = (a_1 Z_1^{2.94} + a_2 Z_2^{2.94} + a_3 Z_3^{2.94} + \ldots + a_n Z_n^{2.94})^{1/2.94} \tag{6.4}$$

where $a_1, a_2, a_3, \ldots a_n$ are the fractional contributions of each element to the total number of electrons in the mixture.

Example 1. Calculation of $\overline{Z}$ for Air

Composition by weight: nitrogen 75.5%, oxygen 23.2%, and argon 1.3%

Number of electrons/g of air: $\frac{N_A Z}{A_w} \times$ (fraction by weight)

$$\text{Nitrogen} = \frac{6.02 \times 10^{23} \times 7}{14.007} \times 0.755 = 2.27 \times 10^{23}$$

$$\text{Oxygen} = \frac{6.02 \times 10^{23} \times 8}{15.999} \times 0.232 = 0.7 \times 10^{23}$$

$$\text{Argon} = \frac{6.02 \times 10^{23} \times 18}{39.94} \times 0.013 = 0.04 \times 10^{23}$$

Total number of electrons/g of air = 3.01×10^{23} (Table 5.1)

$$a_1 \text{ for nitrogen} = \frac{2.27}{3.01} = 0.754$$

$$a_2 \text{ for oxygen} = \frac{0.70}{3.01} = 0.233$$

$$a_3 \text{ for argon} = \frac{0.04}{3.01} = 0.013$$

$$\overline{Z}_{\text{air}} = ((0.754) \times 7^{2.94} + (0.233) \times 8^{2.94} + (0.013) \times 18^{2.94})^{1/2.94} = 7.67$$

C. Chamber Calibration

A thimble chamber could be used directly to measure exposure if (a) it were air equivalent, (b) its cavity volume were accurately known, and (c) its wall thickness was sufficient to provide electronic equilibrium. Under the above conditions, the exposure X is given by:

$$X = \frac{Q}{\rho \cdot v} \cdot \frac{1}{A} \qquad (6.5)$$

where Q is the ionization charge liberated in the cavity air of density ρ and volume v; A is the fraction of the energy fluence transmitted through the air-equivalent wall of equilibrium thickness. The factor A is slightly less than 1.00 and is used here to calculate the exposure for the energy fluence that would exist at the point of measurement in the absence of the chamber.

There are practical difficulties in designing a chamber that would rigorously satisfy the conditions of Equation 6.5. It is almost impossible to construct a thimble chamber that is exactly air equivalent, although with a proper combination of wall material and the central electrode one can achieve acceptable air equivalence in a limited photon energy range. In addition, it is difficult to determine accurately the chamber volume directly. Therefore, in actual practice, the thimble chambers are always calibrated against a free-air chamber for x-rays up to a few hundred kilovolts (2). At higher energies (up to ^{60}Co γ rays), the thimble chambers are calibrated against a standard cavity chamber with nearly air-equivalent walls (e.g., graphite) and accurately known volume (4). In any case, the exposure calibration of a thimble chamber removes the need for knowing its cavity volume (see Chapter 8).

Although adequate wall thickness is necessary to achieve electronic equilibrium, the wall produces some attenuation of the photon flux. Figure 6.4 shows the effect of wall thickness on the chamber response. When the wall thickness is much less than that required for equilibrium or maximum ionization, too few electrons are generated in the wall, and thus the chamber response is low. Beyond the equilibrium thickness, the chamber response is again reduced because of increased attenuation of the beam in the wall. The true exposure (without attenuation) can be obtained by extrapolating linearly the attenuation curve beyond the maximum back to zero thickness, as shown in Fig. 6.4. If the chamber response is normalized to the maximum reading, then the extrapolated value for zero wall thickness gives the correction factor $1/A$ used in Equation 6.5. The correction for zero wall thickness, however, is usually allowed for in the exposure calibration of the chamber and is inherent in the calibration factor. Thus, when the calibration factor is applied to the chamber reading (corrected for changes in temperature and pressure of cavity air), it converts the value into true exposure in free air (without chamber). The exposure value thus obtained is free from the wall attenuation or the perturbing influence of the chamber.

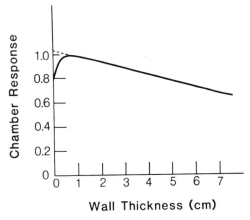

FIG. 6.4. The effect of wall thickness on chamber response (schematic).

D. Desirable Chamber Characteristics

A practical ion chamber for exposure measurement should have the following characteristics.

1. There should be minimal variation in sensitivity or exposure calibration factor over a wide range of photon energies.
2. There should be suitable volume to allow measurements for the expected range of exposures. The sensitivity (charge measured per roentgen) is directly proportional to the chamber sensitive volume. For example, the reading obtained for a given exposure with a 30-cm^3 chamber will be approximately 50 times higher than that obtained with a 0.6-cm^3 chamber. However, the ratio may not be exactly 50, because a chamber response also depends on the chamber design, as discussed previously.
3. There should be minimal variation in sensitivity with the direction of incident radiation. Although this kind of variation can be minimized in the design of the chamber, care is taken to use the chamber in the same configuration with respect to the beam as specified under chamber calibration conditions.
4. There should be minimal stem "leakage." A chamber is known to have stem leakage if it records ionization produced anywhere other than its sensitive volume. The problem of stem leakage is discussed later in this chapter.
5. The chamber should have been calibrated for exposure against a standard instrument for all radiation qualities of interest.
6. There should be minimal ion recombination losses. If the chamber voltage is not high enough or regions of low electric field strength occur inside the chamber, such as in the vicinity of sharply concave surfaces or corners, ions may recombine before contributing to the measured charge. The problem becomes severe with high-intensity or pulsed beams.

6.5. PRACTICAL THIMBLE CHAMBERS

A. Condenser Chambers

A condenser chamber is a thimble ionization chamber connected to a condenser. Figure 6.5 shows a Victoreen condenser chamber, manufactured by Victoreen Instrument Company. The thimble at the right-hand end consists of an approximately air equivalent wall (Bakelite, nylon, or other composition) with a layer of carbon coated on the inside to make it electrically conducting. The conducting layer makes contact with the metal stem. The central electrode (aluminum rod) is connected to a conducting layer of carbon coated on the inside of a hollow polystyrene insulator. This arrangement of an outer metal shield and an inner conducting layer with an insulator in between constitutes an electrical condenser capable of storing charge. The central wire and the thimble's inner conducting surface together also act as a condenser. Thus the chamber has a total capacitance (C) between the central electrode and the outer metal sheath which is given by:

$$C = C_c + C_t \tag{6.6}$$

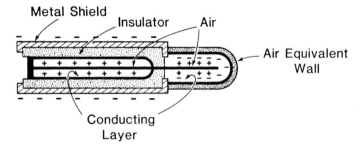

FIG. 6.5. Schematic diagram of a typical condenser chamber.

where C_c and C_t are the capacitance of the condenser and thimble, respectively. Usually C_c is much greater than C_t.

The device for charging the condenser chamber and measuring its charge is an electrometer (described later in this section). When fully charged, the potential difference between the carbon layer of the thimble wall and the central electrode is of the order of 400 V. When the chamber is exposed to radiation, electrons are generated in the thimble wall and produce ionization of the air in the thimble cavity. The negative ions are attracted to the positive central electrode and the positive ions are attracted to the negative inner wall. As ions are collected, the charge on the electrodes is reduced. The reduction in charge is proportional to the exposure.

In general, all the ionization measured is produced in the air volume within the thimble. Although the ionization is also produced in the air within the hollow portion of the stem, these ions recombine since they are in a field-free region.

Figure 6.6 shows several Victoreen condenser chambers designed with different sensitivities. The chambers are designated by the maximum exposure that can be measured. For example, a 100-R chamber is capable of measuring exposures up to 100 R. This chamber has a sensitive volume of about 0.45 cm³. A 25-R chamber has a volume of about 1.8 cm³, which is four times that of 100-R chamber and, therefore, about four times as sensitive, since chamber sensitivity is directly proportional to sensitive volume (see Equation 6.11).

A.1. Chamber Sensitivity

Suppose a chamber with volume v is given an exposure X. The charge Q collected is given by:

$$Q = X \cdot \rho_{\text{air}} \cdot v \qquad (6.7)$$

where ρ_{air} is the density of air and $\rho_{\text{air}} \cdot v$ is the mass of the air volume. The Equation 6.7 is in accordance with the definition of exposure, given by Equation 6.1 as well as Equation

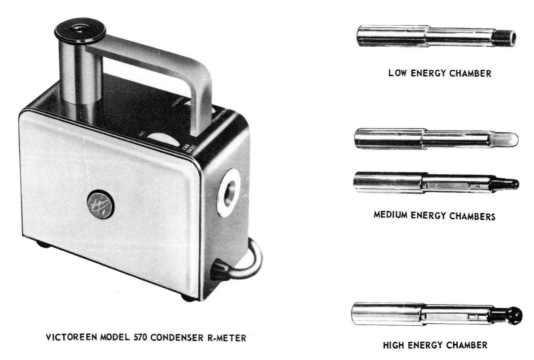

LOW ENERGY CHAMBER

MEDIUM ENERGY CHAMBERS

HIGH ENERGY CHAMBER

VICTOREEN MODEL 570 CONDENSER R-METER

FIG. 6.6. A set of Victoreen condenser chambers with a string electrometer. (Courtesy of Victoreen, Inc., Melbourne, Florida.)

6.5 if A is assumed equal to 1. Using appropriate units,

$$Q\,(\text{coulombs}) = X(R) \cdot (2.58 \times 10^{-4}\,\text{C/kg}_{\text{air}}) \cdot \rho_{\text{air}}(\text{kg/m}^3) \cdot v(\text{m}^3)$$

If air is assumed to be at standard temperature and pressure (0°C and 760 mm Hg), $\rho_{\text{air}} = 1.29\,\text{kg/m}^3$. Then,

$$Q = 3.33 \times 10^{-4}\,X \cdot v \qquad (6.8)$$

If C is the total capacitance of the chamber (Equation 6.6) in farads, then the voltage drop V across the chamber is:

$$V = \frac{Q}{C} = \frac{3.33 \times 10^{-4}\,X \cdot v}{C} \qquad (6.9)$$

The voltage drop per roentgen is:

$$\frac{V}{X} = 3.33 \times 10^{-4}\frac{v}{C} \qquad (6.10)$$

The voltage drop per roentgen is known as the *sensitivity* of the chamber. Thus the chamber sensitivity is directly proportional to the chamber volume and inversely to the chamber capacitance.

If the chamber is connected to an electrometer of capacitance C_e used to measure the charge, then the sensitivity of the chamber is modified:

$$\frac{V}{X} = \frac{3.33 \times 10^{-4}v}{C + C_e} \qquad (6.11)$$

A.2. Stem Effect

Figure 6.7 shows an arrangement used for measuring exposure with a condenser chamber. A chamber is oriented with the axis of the chamber at a right angle to the direction of the beam. Different lengths of the chamber stem are included in the field, depending on the field size. However, the calibration of the thimble chamber against a standard chamber is performed with a fixed field that may cover the entire stem or only a small portion of the stem. If the irradiation of the stem gives rise to ionization that can be measured by the chamber, the chamber reading depends on the amount of the stem in the beam. Thus a correction will be necessary whenever the length of the stem irradiated differs from that irradiated at the time of the chamber calibration.

Stem effect can be caused by two problems: (a) measurable ionization in the body of the stem and (b) ionization of the air between the end of the chamber and the metal cap. As discussed earlier, the ionization produced in air in the central hollow portion of the stem is normally not measured since this is a field-free region and the ions produced there

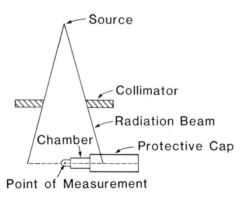

FIG. 6.7. Geometry of exposure measurements with a condenser chamber.

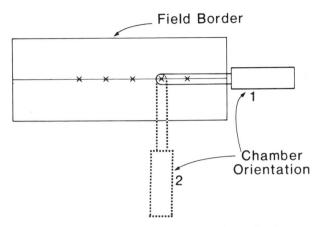

FIG. 6.8. Geometry of stem correction determination.

recombine. However, electrons ejected from the metal stem and the insulator could reach the central electrode and reduce its charge. This kind of stem leakage is usually small and occurs only with high-energy radiation (~2 MeV or higher). The stem leakage caused by ionization of the air surrounding the stem end is eliminated or minimized by a metal cap which fits over the end of the chamber and covers up the central electrode. In addition, the end cap attenuates the radiation and reduces the stem ionization. This cap must be in place during irradiation (Fig. 6.6). If the cap does not fit properly over the chamber end, some charge can be collected in the air adjacent to the end of the electrode, thus causing stem leakage. Correction for the stem effect may be as large as 10%. For further details concerning condenser chamber stem leakage, see Adams (5).

The stem correction may be determined as illustrated in Fig. 6.8. Measurements are made with the chamber oriented in each of the two positions shown. A number of points in the field are selected for such measurements and correction factors are obtained as a function of the stem length exposed relative to the amount of the stem exposed during calibration. Figure 6.9 presents data for a particular chamber which had been calibrated for ^{60}Co exposure with the center of the chamber sensitive volume at the center of a 10 × 10-cm field. It appears that in this case the major stem effect is occurring at the stem end where the protective cap seals the chamber.

B. Farmer Chamber

Condenser chambers are suitable for measuring exposure rate in air for relatively lower-energy beams (≤2 MeV). Although there are no basic limitations to their use for

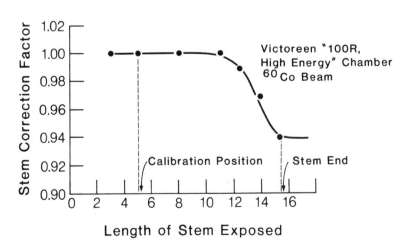

FIG. 6.9. Plot of stem correction factor (multiplicative) as a function of stem length, measured from center of sensitive volume.

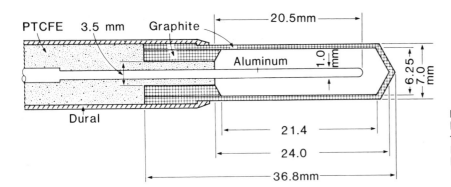

PTCFE   3.5 mm   Graphite

20.5mm

Aluminum

1.0 mm

6.25 — 7.0 mm

Dural

21.4

24.0

36.8mm

FIG. 6.10. Farmer graphite/aluminum chamber. Nominal air volume, 0.6 ml. PTCFE, polytrichlorofluorethylene. (Redrawn from Aird EGA, Farmer FT. The design of a thimble chamber for the Farmer dosimeter. *Phys Med Biol* 1972;17:169.)

higher-energy radiation, the design of the stem and excessive stem leakage create dosimetric problems, especially when making measurements in phantoms. In 1955, Farmer (6) designed a chamber which provided a stable and reliable secondary standard for x-rays and γ rays for all energies in the therapeutic range. This chamber connected to a specific electrometer (to measure ionization charge) is known as the Baldwin-Farmer substandard dosimeter.

The original design of the Farmer chamber was later modified by Aird and Farmer (7) to provide better (flatter) energy response characteristics and more constancy of design from one chamber to another. This chamber is shown schematically in Fig. 6.10. Actual dimensions of the thimble and the central electrode are indicated on the diagram. The thimble wall is made of pure graphite and the central electrode is of pure aluminum. The insulator consists of polytrichlorofluorethylene. The collecting volume of the chamber is nominally 0.6 cm^3.

There are three electrodes in a well-guarded ion chamber: the central electrode or the collector, the thimble wall and the guard electrode. The collector delivers the current to a charge measuring device, an electrometer. The electrometer is provided with a dual polarity HV source to hold the collector at a high bias voltage (e.g., 300 V). The thimble is at ground potential and the guard is kept at the same potential as the collector. Most often the collector is operated with a positive voltage to collect negative charge although either polarity should collect the same magnitude of ionization charge, if the chamber is designed with minimal polarity effects (to be discussed later).

The guard electrode serves two different purposes. One is to prevent leakage current from the high voltage electrode (the collector) and the other is to define the ion collecting volume. In a plane-parallel ion chamber (to be discussed later) the plane-collecting electrode is surrounded by a wide margin of guard ring to prevent undue curvature of the electric field over the collector. In such a chamber, when graphite coatings are used as collecting surfaces on an insulator, the collector can be separated from the guard ring by a scratch through the graphite coating.

The energy response of the chamber designed by Aird and Farmer is shown in the form of a plot of calibration factor as a function of beam half-value layer (Fig. 6.11). The response is almost constant from 0.3 mm Cu HVL upward and within 4% from 0.05 mm

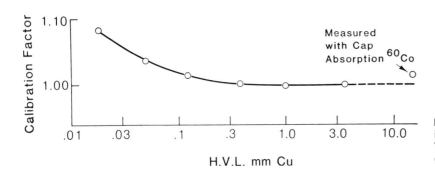

FIG. 6.11. Energy response of the chamber shown in Fig. 6.10. (Redrawn from Aird EGA, Farmer FT. The design of a thimble chamber for the Farmer dosimeter. *Phys Med Biol* 1972;17:169.)

Cu upward. Aird and Farmer found the total stem leakage of this chamber to be about 0.4% when irradiated with 4-MV x-rays with the whole stem in the beam.

Farmer chambers, like the one described above and other Farmer-type chambers are commercially available. The latter chambers are constructed similar to the original Farmer chamber but vary with respect to the composition of the wall material or the central electrode. The user of any such chamber is cautioned against using a chamber the characteristics of which have not been evaluated and found acceptable. For further details of chamber design and characteristics the reader is referred to Boag (8).

6.6. ELECTROMETERS

A. String Electrometer

The electrometer is basically a charge measuring device. The string electrometer is a type of electrometer that operates on the principle of a gold-leaf electroscope. Such electrometers are commonly used for the measurement of charge on a condenser chamber. Figure 6.12 shows the mechanism of a string electrometer used in a Victoreen R meter. The device consists of a string (platinum wire) stretching along a support rod and maintained under tension by a quartz loop attached at one end of the rod. A deflection electrode is mounted near the middle of the string. When the support rod and the platinum wire are positively charged, a negative charge is induced on the deflection electrode. The deflection electrode attracts the wire that moves a distance that depends on the amount of charge on the wire. The deflection of the wire is viewed through a small microscope that shows a shadow of the wire projected on an illuminated scale.

To operate the instrument, the condenser chamber is inserted into the electrometer. This connects the central electrode of the chamber with the support rod and the wire. The chamber and the electrometer are then charged until the shadow of the wire coincides with the zero end of the scale (fully charged position). The voltage across the chamber electrodes at this instant is about 400 V. The chamber is then removed from the electrometer and exposed to radiation. The ionization produced in the thimble air of the chamber reduces

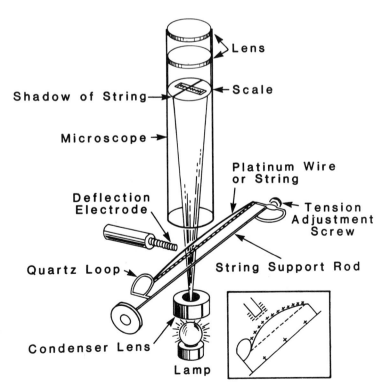

FIG. 6.12. Schematic diagram of Victoreen electrometer. (Adapted from a diagram by Victoreen, Inc.)

the charge on the central electrode. As the chamber is reconnected to the electrometer, the reduction in charge is shared by the chamber and the electrometer. The attraction between the wire and the deflection electrode is decreased and the string shadow moves upscale. The reading on the scale reflects the amount of radiation received by the chamber. The exposure in roentgens can be calculated by multiplying the reading with several correction factors such as temperature and pressure correction, chamber calibration factor for the given quality of radiation, and stem correction.

B. Other Electrometers

The condenser chambers described earlier are detached from the electrometer during exposure and then reattached to measure the charge. Other exposure-measuring devices are available in which the chamber remains connected to the electrometer during exposure. The cable is long enough so that the electrometer is placed outside the room at the control console of the radiation generator. This arrangement is more convenient than that of the detachable condenser chamber in which the operator must carry the chamber to the room, return to the control console, operate the machine, and then go back in the room to retrieve the chamber for charge measurement. In calibrating a radiation unit, this amounts to a large number of trips, going in and out of the room.

B.1. Operational Amplifiers

Since the ionization current or charge to be measured is very small, special electrometer circuits have been designed to measure it accurately. The most commonly used electrometers use *negative-feedback operational amplifiers*. Figure 6.13 schematically shows three simplified circuits that are used to measure ionization in the integrate mode, rate mode, and direct-reading dosimeter mode. The operational amplifier is designated as a triangle with two input points. The negative terminal is called the inverting terminal and the positive

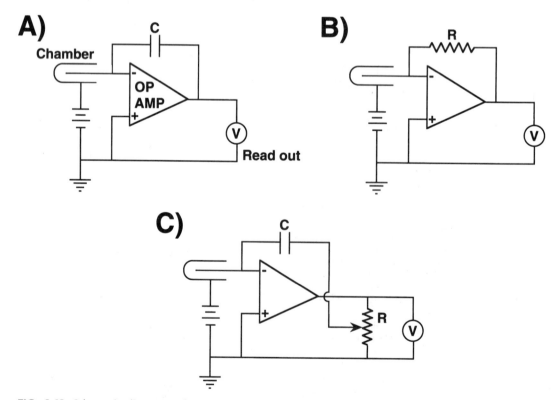

FIG. 6.13. Schematic diagrams of ion chambers connected to negative-feedback operational amplifiers. **A:** Integrate mode. **B:** Rate mode. **C:** Direct-exposure reading mode.

one as the noninverting position. This terminology implies that a negative voltage applied to the inverting terminal will give a positive amplified voltage and a positive voltage applied to the noninverting terminal will give a positive amplified voltage. A negative-feedback connection is provided, which contains either a capacitor or a resistor.

The operational amplifier has a high open-loop gain ($> 10^4$) and a high input impedence ($> 10^{12}$ ohm). Because of this, the output voltage is dictated by the feedback element, independent of the open-loop gain, and the potential between the positive and negative inputs of the amplifier (called the error voltage) is maintained very low (< 100 mV). For example, if the ionization current is 10^{-8} A and the resistor in the feedback circuit of Fig. 6.13B is 10^9 ohm, the output voltage will be current times the resistance or 10 V. Assuming open-loop gain of 10^4, the error voltage between the input terminals of the amplifier will be 10^{-3} V or 1 mV. This leads to a very stable operation, and the voltage across the feedback element can be accurately measured with the closed-loop gain of almost unity.

In the integrate mode (Fig. 6.13A), the charge Q collected by the ion chamber is deposited on the feedback capacitor C. The voltage V across C is read by a voltmeter and is given by Q/C, where C is the capacity. Measurement of this voltage is essentially the measurement of ionization charge.

In the rate mode (Fig. 6.13B), the capacitor is replaced by a resistance R. Irradiation of the chamber causes an ionization current I to flow through the resistor, generating a voltage $V = IR$ across the resistance. The measurement of this voltage reflects the magnitude of the ionization current.

For total capacitative or resistive feedback circuits, the closed-loop gain of the operational amplifier is unity, i.e., the output voltage is given by the voltage across the feedback element. If a variable fraction of the output voltage is fed back to the input as by a voltage divider (Fig. 6.13C), the electrometer can be converted into a direct exposure-reading (R or R/min) instrument for a given chamber and a given quality of radiation.

Special electrometer circuits have been designed to measure accurately ionization currents, even as low as 10^{-15} A. The reader is referred to Johns (9) for further details.

Several combinations of chambers and electrometers using *operational amplifiers* are commercially available. Figure 6.14 shows one of such systems. A Farmer 0.6-cm^3 ion chamber is connected through a long shielded cable to a Keithley 616 electrometer. The system can be used to measure integrated charge or ionization current. Both the chamber and the electrometer are calibrated so that the reading can be converted into exposure.

6.7. SPECIAL CHAMBERS

A cylindrical thimble chamber is most often used for exposure calibration of radiation beams when the dose gradient across the chamber volume is minimal. It is not suitable for surface dose measurements. As will be discussed in Chapter 13, high-energy photon beams exhibit a *dose buildup* effect, that is, a rapid increase of dose with depth in the first few millimeters. To measure the dose at a point in this buildup region or at the surface, the detector must be very thin so that there is no dose gradient across its sensitive volume. In addition, the chamber must not significantly perturb the radiation field. Special chambers have been designed to achieve the above requirements.

A. Extrapolation Chamber

Failla (10) designed an ionization chamber for measuring surface dose in an irradiated phantom in 1937. He called this chamber an extrapolation chamber (Fig. 6.15). The beam enters through a thin foil which is carbon coated to form the upper electrode. The lower or the collecting electrode is a small coin-shaped region surrounded by a guard ring and is connected to an electrometer. The electrode spacing can be varied accurately by micrometer screws. By measuring the ionization per unit volume as a function of electrode spacing, one can estimate the superficial dose by extrapolating the ionization curves to zero electrode spacing.

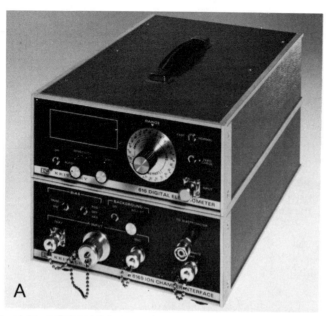

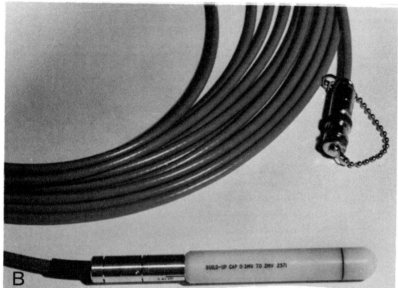

FIG. 6.14. A photograph of a Farmer 0.6-cm^3 ion chamber with a Keithley 616 electrometer. (Courtesy of Keithley Instruments, Inc., Cleveland, Ohio.)

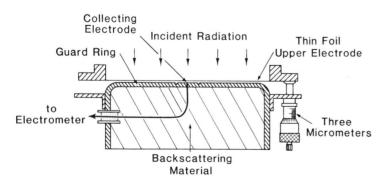

FIG. 6.15. Extrapolation ion chamber by Failla. (Redrawn from Boag JW. Ionization chambers. In: Attix FH, Roesch WC, eds. *Radiation dosimetry,* Vol 2. New York: Academic Press, 1969:1.)

The extrapolation chambers of the type described above have been used for special dosimetry, e.g., the measurement of dose in the superficial layers of a medium and the dosimetry of electrons and β particles.

B. Parallel-plate Chambers

Parallel-plate chambers are similar to the extrapolation chambers except for the variable electrode spacing. The electrode spacing of the parallel-plate chambers is small ($\sim$2 mm) but fixed. A thin wall or window (e.g., foils of 0.01- to 0.03-mm-thick Mylar, polystyrene, or mica) allows measurements practically at the surface of a phantom without significant wall attenuation. By adding layers of phantom material on top of the chamber window, one can study the variation in dose as a function of depth, at shallow depths where cylindrical chambers are unsuitable because of their larger volume.

The small electrode spacing in a parallel-plate chamber minimizes cavity perturbations in the radiation field. This feature is especially important in the dosimetry of electron beams where cylindrical chambers may produce significant perturbations in the electron field.

6.8. ION COLLECTION

A. Saturation

As the voltage difference between the electrodes of an ion chamber exposed to radiation is increased, the ionization current increases at first almost linearly and later more slowly. The curve finally approaches a saturation value for the given exposure rate (Fig. 6.16). The initial increase of ionization current with voltage is caused by incomplete ion collection at low voltages. The negative and the positive ions tend to recombine unless they are quickly separated by the electric field. This recombination can be minimized by increasing the field strength (V/cm).

If the voltage is increased much beyond saturation, the ions, accelerated by the electric field, can gain enough energy to produce ionization by collision with gas molecules. This results in a rapid multiplication of ions, and the current, once again, becomes strongly dependent on the applied voltage. The chamber should be used in the saturation region so that small changes in the voltage do not result in changes in the ionic current.

B. Collection Efficiency

As previously discussed, the maximum field that can be applied to the chamber is limited by the onset of ionization by collision. Depending on the chamber design and the ionization

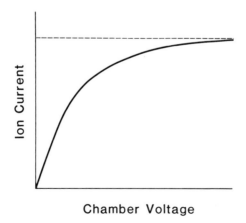

FIG. 6.16. Saturation curve for an ion chamber.

intensity, a certain amount of ionization loss by recombination can be expected. Especially at very high ionization intensity, such as is possible in the case of pulsed beams, significant loss of charge by recombination may occur even at maximum possible chamber voltages. Under these conditions, the *recombination losses* may have to be accepted and the correction applied for these losses.

The *collection efficiency,* defined as the ratio of the number of ions collected to the number produced, may be determined either by calculation (8,11) or by measurements (11). Experimentally, the measured current is plotted against the inverse of the polarizing voltage in the region of losses below 5%. The "ideal" saturation current is then determined by linear interpolation of the curve to infinite polarizing voltage. Another, simpler, method, called the two-voltage testing technique, has been described by Boag and Currant (12) for determining the efficiency of ion collection. In this method, measurements are made at two different voltages, one given working voltage and the other much lower voltage. By combining the two readings in accordance with the theoretical formula by Boag and Currant (12), one can obtain the collection efficiency at the given voltage.

A more practical method of determining ion recombination correction (P_{ion}) is to measure ionization at two bias voltages, V_1 and V_2, so that $V_1 = 2V_2$. The ratio of the two readings is related to P_{ion}. Figure 6.17 is based on the work by Boag (13) and Almond (14) and may be used to determine P_{ion} for a chamber for continuous radiation (e.g., ^{60}Co), pulsed radiation, or pulsed scanning beams produced by accelerators.

Whenever possible, the voltage on the chamber should be arranged to give less than 1% loss of charge by recombination, that is, collection efficiency of better than 99%. In a 0.6-cm³ Farmer-type chamber, this is generally achieved if the collection voltage is about 300 V or higher and a dose per pulse in the chamber cavity is 0.1 cGy or less.

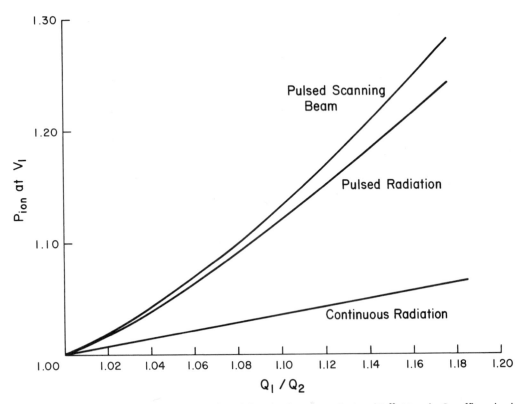

FIG. 6.17. Ion recombination correction factors (P_{ion}) for continuous radiation (Co⁶⁰, Van de Graaff), pulsed radiation (accelerator-produced x-rays and electron beams), and pulsed scanning beams. These data are applicable when $V_1 = 2V_2$. (From AAPM. A protocol for the determination of absorbed dose from high-energy photon and electron beams. *Med Phys* 1983;10:741, with permission.)

6.9. CHAMBER POLARITY EFFECTS

It is sometimes found that for a given exposure the ionic charge collected by an ion chamber changes in magnitude as the polarity of the collecting voltage is reversed. There are many possible causes of such polarity effects, some of which have been reviewed by Boag (8). With the chamber operating under saturation conditions, major causes of the polarity effects include the following:

a. High energy electrons such as Compton electrons ejected by high-energy photons constitute a current (also called the *Compton current*) independent of gas ionization. This may add to or reduce the collector current, depending on the polarity of the collecting electrode. In addition, some of these electrons may stop in the collector but may not be entirely balanced by ejection of recoil electrons from the collector. The previous effects are minimized by making the central electrode very thin. Errors due to these causes are likely to be appreciable for parallel-plate chambers with small electrode spacing. However, the true ionization current in this case can be determined by taking the mean of two currents obtained by reversing the chamber polarity.

b. *Extracameral* current, for example, current collected outside the sensitive volume of the chamber, may cause the polarity effect. Such current may be collected at inadequately screened collector circuit points. Also, irradiation of the cable connecting the chamber with the electrometer can cause extracameral current as well as the Compton current discussed above. The errors caused by these effects can be minimized but not eliminated by reversing the chamber polarity and taking the mean value of the collector current.

In general, the chamber polarity effects are relatively more severe for measurements in electron beams than photon beams, and in addition, the effect increases with decreasing electron energy. Therefore, it is important to determine polarity effects of a chamber at various depths in a phantom. The polarity effect is very much dependent on chamber design and irradiation conditions. Several commercially available chambers have been studied for this effect (15,16) and the reader is referred to these reports for further details.

Many of the polarity effects and stem leakage can be minimized in the design of the chamber and the associated circuitry. Also, the adequacy of chamber voltage is an important factor in minimizing some of the other polarity effects (not mentioned here but discussed by Boag [8]). Finally, it is recommended that the difference between the ionization currents measured at positive and negative polarizing potential should be less than 0.5% for any radiation beam quality.

6.10. ENVIRONMENTAL CONDITIONS

If the ion chamber is not sealed, its response is affected by air temperature and pressure. In fact, most chambers are unsealed and communicate to the outside atmosphere. Because the density of air depends on the temperature and pressure, in accordance with the gas laws, the density of air in the chamber volume will likewise depend on these atmospheric conditions. The density or the mass of air in the chamber volume will increase as the temperature decreases or pressure increases. Since exposure is given by the ionization charge collected per unit mass of air (section 6.2), the chamber reading for a given exposure will increase as the temperature decreases or as the pressure increases.

Standard laboratories calibrate chambers under the conditions present at the time of calibration. This factor is then converted to specific atmospheric conditions, namely, 760 mm Hg pressure and 22°C temperature. The correction $C_{T,P}$ for conditions other than the above reference conditions can be calculated.

$$C_{T,P} = \left(\frac{760}{P}\right) \times \left(\frac{273.2 + t}{295.2}\right) \tag{6.12}$$

where P is the pressure in millimeters of mercury and t is temperature in degrees Celsius.

The second bracketed term gives the ratio of temperature *t* to the reference temperature (22°C), both converted to the absolute scale of temperature (in degrees Kelvin) by adding 273.2 to the Celsius temperatures.

6.11. MEASUREMENT OF EXPOSURE

Exposure in units of roentgen can be measured with a thimble chamber having an exposure calibration factor N_C traceable to the National Institute of Standards and Technology (NIST) for a given quality of radiation. The chamber is held at the desired point of measurement in the same configuration as used in the chamber calibration (Fig. 6.7). Precautions are taken to avoid media, other than air, in the vicinity of the chamber which might scatter radiation. Suppose a reading *M* is obtained for a given exposure. This can be converted to roentgens as follows:

$$X = M \cdot N_C \cdot C_{T,P} \cdot C_s \cdot C_{st} \qquad (6.13)$$

where $C_{T,P}$ is the correction for temperature and pressure (Equation 6.12), C_s is the correction for loss of ionization as a result of recombination (section 6.8), and C_{st} is the stem leakage correction (section 6.5). The quantity *X* given by Equation 6.13 is the exposure that would be expected in free air at the point of measurement in the absence of the chamber. In other words, the correction for any perturbation produced in the beam by the chamber is inherent in the chamber calibration factor N_C.

For lower-energy radiation such as in the superficial and orthovoltage range, the thimble chambers are usually calibrated and used without a buildup cap. For higher energies such as cobalt-60, a Lucite buildup cap is used unless the chamber wall is already thick enough to provide electronic equilibrium (e.g., Victoreen high-energy chambers). In either case, the correction to zero wall thickness (section 6.4) is inherent in the chamber calibration factor N_C.

REFERENCES

1. International Commission on Radiation Units and Measurements. Radiation quantities and units. Report No. 33. Washington, DC: ICRU, 1980.
2. Wyckoff HO, Attix FH. Design of free-air ionization chambers. National Bureau of Standards Handbook No. 64. Washington, DC: U.S. Government Printing Office, 1957.
3. Mayneord WV. The significance of the röntgen. *Acta Int Union Against Cancer* 1937;2:271.
4. Loftus TP, Weaver JT. Standardization of ^{60}Co and ^{137}Cs gamma-ray beams in terms of exposure. *J Res Natl Bur Stand (US)* 1974;78A(Phys Chem):465.
5. Adams GD. On the use of thimble chambers in phantoms. *Radiology* 1962;78:77.
6. Farmer FT. A substandard x-ray dose-meter. *Br J Radiol* 1955;28:304.
7. Aird EGA, Farmer FT. The design of a thimble chamber for the Farmer dosimeter. *Phys Med Biol* 1972;17:169.
8. Boag JW. Ionization chambers. In: Attix FH, Roesch WC, eds. *Radiation dosimetry*, Vol 2. New York: Academic Press, 1969:1.
9. Johns HE, Cunningham JR. *The physics of radiology*, 4th ed. Springfield, IL: Charles C Thomas, 1983.
10. Failla G. The measurement of tissue dose in terms of the same unit for all ionizing radiations. *Radiology* 1937;29:202.
11. International Commission on Radiation Units and Measurements. Physical aspects of irradiation. Report No. 10b. Handbook 85. Washington, DC: NBS, 1964.
12. Boag JW, Currant J. Current collection and ionic recombination in small cylindrical ionization chambers exposed to pulsed radiation. *Br J Radiol* 1980;53:471.
13. Boag JW. The recombination correction for an ionization chamber exposed to pulsed radiation in a 'swept beam' technique. *Phys Med Biol* 1982;27:201.
14. Almond PR. Use of a Victoreen 500 electrometer to determine ionization chamber collection efficiencies. *Med Phys* 1981;8:901.
15. Mattsson LO, Johansson KA, Svensson H. Calibration and use of plane-parallel ionization chambers for the determination of absorbed dose in electron beams. *Acta Radiol Oncol* 1981;20:385.
16. Gerbi BJ, Khan FM. The polarity effect for commercially available plane-parallel ionization chambers. *Med Phys* 1987;14:210.

QUALITY OF X-RAY BEAMS

In Chapter 5, we described x-ray beam in terms of photon fluence and energy fluence. Such a description requires the knowledge of the number and energy of the photons in the beam. In this chapter, we will characterize an x-ray beam in terms of its ability to penetrate materials of known composition. The penetrating ability of the radiation is often described as the *quality* of the radiation.

An ideal way to describe the quality of an x-ray beam is to specify its spectral distribution, that is, energy fluence in each energy interval as shown in Fig. 3.9. However, spectral distributions are difficult to measure and, furthermore, such a complete specification of the beam quality is not necessary in most clinical situations. Since the biologic effects of x-rays are not very sensitive to the quality of the beam, in radiotherapy one is interested primarily in the penetration of the beam into the patient rather than its detailed energy spectrum. Thus a crude but simpler specification of the beam quality is often used, namely the *half-value layer*.

7.1. HALF-VALUE LAYER

As defined earlier (Chapter 5), the term half-value layer (HVL) is the thickness of an absorber of specified composition required to attenuate the intensity of the beam to half its original value. Although all beams can be described in terms of their HVL, the quality of a γ ray beam is usually stated in terms of the energy of the γ rays or its nuclide of origin which has a known emission spectrum. For example, the quality of a γ ray beam emitted from a ^{60}Co source can be stated in terms of 1.17 and 1.33 MeV (average 1.25 MeV) or simply cobalt-60 beam. Because all x-ray beams produced by radiation generators are heterogeneous in energy, that is, possess continuous energy spectra that depend on the peak voltage, target material, and beam filtration, they are usually described by the HVL, a single parameter specifying the overall penetrating ability of the beam.

In the case of low-energy x-ray beams (below megavoltage range), it is customary to describe quality in terms of HVL together with kVp, although HVL alone is adequate for most clinical applications. On the other hand, in the megavoltage x-ray range, the quality is specified by the peak energy and rarely by the HVL. The reason for this convention is that in the megavoltage range the beam is so heavily filtered through the transmission type target and the flattening filter that any additional filtration does not significantly alter the beam quality or its HVL. Thus for a "hard" beam with a fixed filtration, the x-ray energy spectrum is a function primarily of the peak energy and so is the beam quality. The average energy of such a beam is approximately one third of the peak energy.

7.2. FILTERS

In section 3.5, we briefly discussed the energy spectrum of an x-ray beam. The x-rays produced by an x-ray generator show a continuous distribution of energies of bremsstrahlung photons on which is superimposed discrete lines of characteristic radiation (Fig. 7.1). Curve A in Fig. 7.1 schematically represents the energy spectrum of a 200-kVp x-ray beam filtered by a 1-mm-thick aluminum filter. This distribution includes the effects of attenuation in

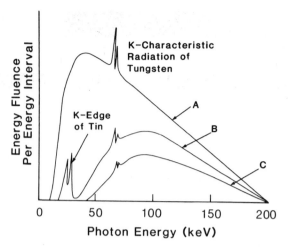

FIG. 7.1. Schematic graph showing changes in spectral distribution of 200 kVp x-ray beam with various filters. *Curve A* is for Al, *curve B* is for Sn + Al, and *curve C* is for Sn + Cu + Al.

the glass envelope of the x-ray tube, the surrounding oil, and the exit window of the tube housing as well. This so-called *inherent filtration* is equivalent to approximately 1-mm Al in most x-ray tubes.

The K characteristic x-rays produced in the tungsten target possess discrete energies between 58 and 69 keV (Table 3.1). Other emission lines of tungsten, however, have much lower energies and are not shown in Fig. 7.1 because they are effectively removed by the inherent filtration as well as the added filtration.

The energy fluence of the K lines of tungsten can be preferentially reduced using a tin filter. Because the K absorption edge of tin is at about 29.2 keV (Table 3.2), it strongly absorbs photons above 29.2 keV by the photoelectric process. However, lower-energy photons cannot eject the K electrons. As seen in curve B of Fig. 7.1, the energy fluence in the region from 30 to 70 keV is considerably reduced relative to either the higher-energy part of the spectrum or the spectrum below 29 keV. Because the L absorption edge of tin is only 4.5 keV, there is little reduction in the spectrum below 29 keV. In addition to the above effects, tin produces its own characteristic radiation by the photoelectric process involving the K shell, and these lines are superimposed on the spectrum below the tin absorption edge.

To absorb preferentially the energy fluence below the K edge of tin, including the characteristic x-rays of tin, a copper filter is quite efficient. The K edge of copper is at 9 keV, and therefore, the photons below 29 keV are strongly absorbed by the copper filter as seen in curve C of Fig. 7.1 The very low energy characteristic x-rays produced by copper can be effectively absorbed by adding an aluminum filter next to the copper filter.

Combination filters containing plates of tin, copper, and aluminum have been designed to increase the resulting half-value layer of the orthovoltage beams without reducing the beam intensity to unacceptably low values. Such filters are called *Thoraeus filters* (1) and are described in Table 7.1. It is important that the combination filters

TABLE 7.1. THORAEUS FILTERS USED WITH ORTHO-VOLTAGE X-RAYS

Filter	Composition
Thoraeus I	0.2 mm Sn + 0.25 mm Cu + 1 mm Al
Thoraeus II	0.4 mm Sn + 0.25 mm Cu + 1 mm Al
Thoraeus III	0.6 mm Sn + 0.25 mm Cu + 1 mm Al

be arranged in the proper order, with the highest atomic number material nearest the x-ray target. Thus a Thoraeus filter is inserted with tin facing the x-ray tube and the aluminum facing the patient, with the copper sandwiched between the tin and the aluminum plates.

In the diagnostic and superficial x-ray energy range (section 4.1), primarily aluminum filters are used to harden the beam. The half-value layers of these beams are also expressed in terms of millimeters of aluminum. In the orthovoltage range, however, combination filters are often used to obtain half-value layers in the range of about 1 to 4 mm Cu. For cesium and cobalt teletherapy machines, on the other hand, filters are not needed because the beams are almost monoenergetic.

Although a megavoltage x-ray beam has a spectrum of energies, the beam is hardened by the inherent filtration of the transmission target as well as by transmission through the flattening filter. Thus no additional filtration is required to improve the beam quality. It may be mentioned that the primary purpose of the flattening filter is to make the beam intensity uniform in cross-section rather than to improve the beam quality.

7.3. MEASUREMENT OF BEAM QUALITY PARAMETERS

A. Half-Value Layer

As discussed in section 5.3, the half-value layer of a beam is related to the linear attenuation coefficient (μ) by the following equation:

$$\text{HVL} = \frac{0.693}{\mu} \tag{7.1}$$

Like the attenuation coefficient, the half-value layer must be measured under narrow-beam or "good" geometry conditions. Such a geometry can be achieved by using a narrow beam and a large distance between the absorber and the detector such as an ion chamber (Fig. 5.1). Under these conditions, the exposure reading is mainly a result of the photons that are transmitted through the absorber without interaction and practically no scattered photons are detected by the chamber. The attenuation data are obtained by measuring transmitted exposure through absorbers of varying thickness but constant composition. These data are then plotted on a semilogarithmic graph paper to determine HVL. If the beam has a low filtration or contains an appreciable amount of low-energy component in the spectrum, the slope of the attenuation curve decreases with increasing absorber thickness (Fig. 5.3). Thus different half-value layer beams can be obtained from such a beam by using different filters. In general, the HVL increases with increasing filter thickness as the beam becomes increasingly "harder," that is, contains a greater proportion of higher-energy photons. Beyond a certain thickness, however, additional filtration may result in "softening" of the beam by Compton scattering.

Because an increase in filtration is accompanied by a reduction in the available exposure rate, the filtration is carefully chosen to obtain a suitable HVL as well as acceptable beam output. In addition, as discussed in the previous section, certain filters are more efficient than others in selectively removing low-energy photons from the beam, including characteristic x-rays which are undesirable for therapy because of their low energy.

B. Peak Voltage

Neither the HVL nor the tube potential nor both provide sufficient information regarding the spectral distribution of the radiation. However, for most clinical purposes, these two parameters give an appropriate specification of radiation quality. It has been recommended (2) that the quality of the clinical beams in the superficial and orthovoltage range be specified by the HVL and the kVp in preference to the HVL alone.

The determination of x-ray tube potential is difficult because the high-tension circuits of most x-ray equipment are sealed and hence are not easily accessible for direct voltage measurement. Indirect methods, therefore, are often used to measure the kVp without approach to the high-tension circuits. However, if access to the high-voltage terminals can be achieved, direct measurements can be made by precision voltage dividers or a sphere-gap apparatus.

B.1. Direct Measurement

Voltage Divider. If the high-tension leads of the x-ray tube are accessible, then the effective voltage across the tube can be measured directly by a voltage divider. The voltage divider is a circuit in which several high resistances are connected in series to form a resistance tower which is placed across the high-tension leads. The total potential is thus divided among the separate resisters. The effective voltage between any two points is given by the effective current through the tower times the resistance between the two points. The ratio of total resistance to the output resistance between two selected points gives the calibration factor, which when multiplied by the observed output voltage across those points gives the total voltage across the voltage divider. For further details of the method, the reader is referred to Gilbertson and Fingerhut (3) and Giarratano et al. (4).

Sphere-Gap Method. The sphere-gap method is one of the oldest methods of determining the kVp. Each high-voltage lead of the x-ray tube is connected to a polished metallic sphere by a cable adapter. The distance between the two spheres is reduced until an electric spark passes between them. By knowing the critical distance, corrected for air density and humidity, one can calculate the peak voltage across the x-ray tube.

B.2. Indirect Measurement

Fluorescence Method. The fluorescence method is based on two principles (5). First, the peak photon energy is given by the peak potential, i.e., hv_{max} in keV is numerically equal to the kVp. Second, K edge absorption is a threshold phenomenon in which K orbit fluorescence (characteristic x-ray production) occurs when the photon energy is just equal to or greater than the binding energy of the K shell electron. Hence, by using materials of several different K absorption edges, one can calibrate the kVp dial on the machine.

Figure 7.2 illustrates an experimental arrangement for the procedure. A secondary radiator (attenuator), the K absorption edge of which is accurately known, is placed at an angle of 45 degrees to the central axis of the beam. While one ionization chamber, placed behind the radiator, measures the transmitted x-rays, a second chamber, placed at an angle of 90 degrees to the beam axis, measures scattered and fluorescent radiation. This chamber is shielded to prevent the reception of radiation other than that from the radiator. Furthermore, a differential filter (low *Z* absorber) is used in front of this chamber to minimize the effect of low-energy scattered x-rays.

When the tube voltage is below the K edge, both the transmitted and the scattered radiation increase at a faster rate. Because of a sudden increase in absorption at and beyond the K edge, the transmitted radiation decreases and the secondary radiation increases as a result of the production of characteristic fluorescent radiation. Thus, if the ratio of the transmitted to the secondary radiation is plotted against the tube potential, a break in the curve is observed at the K edge threshold (Fig. 7.3). The applied kVp at that point is numerically equal to the K edge absorption energy expressed in keV.

Attenuation Method. The attenuation method, described by Morgan (6) and Newell and Henny (7), is based on the observation that the slope of the transmission curve of an x-ray beam at high filtration depends on the peak kilovoltage. The apparatus consists of a detector such as an ion chamber with two caps of copper or aluminum of different thicknesses. The instrument is first calibrated by determining the ratio of the detector response with the two caps in place as a function of kVp of x-ray beams produced by a

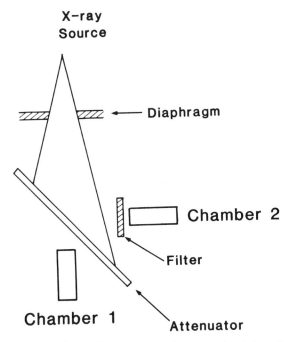

FIG. 7.2. Experimental arrangement for measuring tube voltage by K fluorescence method. Chamber 1 measures radiation transmitted through the attenuator and chamber 2 measures characteristic as well as scattered x-rays. The filter in front of chamber 2 absorbs most of the scattered radiation from the attenuator.

generator of accurately known peak potentials. Accordingly, an unknown kVp of an x-ray beam can be estimated from the calibration curve by determining the ratio of the detector response for the same two caps. This method, however, has a limited accuracy and depends strongly on the wave form of the x-ray tube potential.

Penetrameter. The operation of the penetrameter consists of comparing transmission through two materials with x-ray absorptions that change differently with photon energy. The original penetrameter was designed by Benoist (8) in 1901. The design was optimized in 1966 by Stanton et al. (9). Their device consists of a rectangular central reference block of polyethylene, on both sides of which are identical metal step wedges. Aluminum wedges

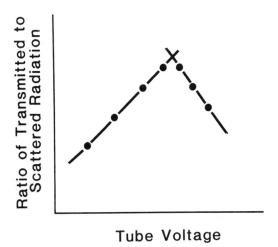

FIG. 7.3. Plot of the transmitted (chamber 1 reading) to scattered radiation (chamber 2 reading) as a function of tube kilovoltage. The discontinuity occurs in the curve at the tube voltage numerically equal to the K edge threshold of the attenuator.

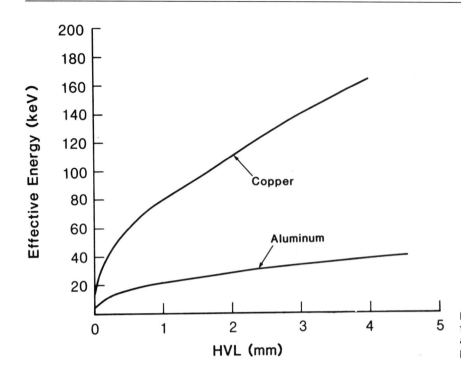

FIG. 7.4. Plot of effective energy as a function of half-value layer. Data calculated from attenuation coefficients of monoenergetic photon beams.

are recommended for the low kilovolt range and brass wedges for the higher kilovolt. The central polyethylene block is surrounded on its sides by lead scatter shields.

For kilovoltage measurement, the penetrameter is radiographed in the beam with heavy filtration and scatter shielding. The optical density ratios of adjacent wedge and reference areas are used to obtain the "matching step position." If the instrument has been calibrated against known potentials, the desired peak voltage can be read from the calibration curve.

Another penetrameter is known as the Ardran-Crooks cassette (10). This device consists of a film which is covered partly with a slow intensifying screen and partly with a fast screen. A copper step system is superimposed on the fast screen, while the slow screen is kept uncovered to serve as a reference. A sheet of lead allows only small (0.5-cm diameter) beam to pass through each copper step and the uncovered slow screen. When a radiograph is taken, the match of a step density with the reference depends on the kilovoltage. By using an appropriate calibration curve, one can determine the desired kilovolts. A commercial version of the Ardran-Crooks penetrameter is known as the Wisconsin Test Cassette.[1]

C. Effective Energy

Because x-ray beams used in radiology are always heterogeneous in energy, it is convenient sometimes to express the quality of an x-ray beam in terms of the effective energy. The *effective (or equivalent) energy* of an x-ray beam is the energy of photons in a monoenergetic beam which is attenuated at the same rate as the radiation in question. Since the attenuation curve for a given material is characterized by the slope or the linear attenuation coefficient (μ), the effective energy is determined by finding the energy of monoenergetic photons which have the same μ as the given beam. In general, however, the μ or the effective energy of a heterogeneous beam varies with the absorber thickness (Fig. 5.3).

Because μ and HVL are interrelated (Equation 7.1), the effective energy may also be defined as the energy of a monoenergetic photon beam having the same HVL as the given beam. Figure 7.4 shows the relationship between effective energy and half-value layer for x-ray beams in the superficial and orthovoltage range. These data were calculated by using

---

[1] Available Radiation Measurements, Inc., Middleton, Wisconsin.

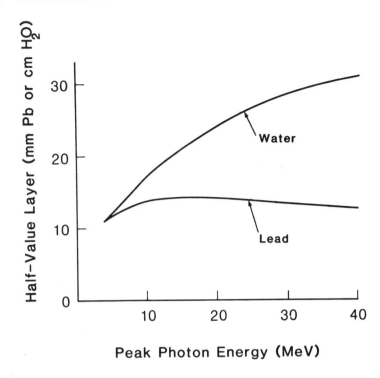

FIG. 7.5. Half-value layer as a function of peak photon energy for water and lead. *Note:* Since these data were calculated from thin-target Schiff (12) spectra, HVL values plotted here are slightly lower than those measured in practical radiotherapy machines. (Data from Nath R, Schulz RJ. On the choice of material for half-value-layer measurements for megavoltage x-rays. *Med Phys* 1977;4:132, with permission.)

Equation 7.1 to obtain μ and finding the energy of a monoenergetic photon beam with the same μ given in the Appendix.

Although lead is commonly used to express half-value layers for the megavoltage beams, it is not necessarily the best choice for characterizing the beam quality in this energy range. It has been shown that the low atomic number materials such as water are more sensitive to changes in spectral quality of megavoltage x-rays than the high atomic number materials such as lead (11). This can be seen in Fig. 7.5 in which HVL is plotted as a function of peak photon energy. The HVL in terms of lead begins to decrease with increase in energy beyond about 20 MV. This is because the mass attenuation coefficient of lead first decreases and then increases with increase in energy, whereas for water it monotonically decreases (see section 5.10).

D. Mean Energy

The spectral distribution of a radiation field (particles or photons) is characterized by the distribution of fluence or energy fluence with respect to energy. Suppose $\Phi(E)$ denotes fluence Φ of photons with energy between 0 and E. The differential distribution (Φ_E) of the fluence with respect to energy is given by:

$$\Phi_E = \frac{d\Phi(E)}{dE}$$

The product $\Phi_E dE$ is the fluence of photons with energies lying between E and $E + dE$. The total fluence (Φ) is given by:

$$\int_0^{E_{\max}} \Phi_E dE$$

The mean energy ($\overline{E}$) of a photon beam can be calculated as:

$$\overline{E} = \frac{\int_0^{E_{\max}} \Phi_E E \cdot dE}{\int_0^{E_{\max}} \Phi_E \cdot dE} \tag{7.2}$$

The mean energy can also be calculated from the energy fluence (Ψ_E) distribution.

$$\overline{E} = \frac{\int_0^{E_{max}} \Psi_E E \cdot dE}{\int_0^{E_{max}} \Psi_E dE} \tag{7.3}$$

The above two expressions, however, lead to different values of $\overline{E}$ because $\Phi_E \neq \Psi_E$. Thus it is important to specify the type of distribution used in calculating the mean energy.

7.4. MEASUREMENT OF MEGAVOLTAGE BEAM ENERGY

The complete energy spectrum of a megavoltage x-ray beam can be obtained by calculation using thin target bremsstrahlung spectra (12), scintillation spectrometry (13,14), and photoactivation (15). However, for the characterization of a megavoltage x-ray beam by a single energy parameter, namely, by its maximum energy, one needs to determine the energy of the electron beam before incidence on the target. Several methods for determining this energy are discussed in Chapter 14.

The most practical method of determining the megavoltage beam energy is by measuring percent depth dose distribution, tissue-air ratios, or tissue-maximum ratios (Chapter 10) and comparing them with the published data such as those from the Hospital Physicist's Association (16). Although clinically relevant, the method is only approximate since depth dose distributions are relatively insensitive to small changes in the peak energy.

A sensitive method of monitoring x-ray beam spectral quality has been proposed by Nath and Schulz (17) and is referred to as the *photoactivation ratio* (PAR) method. The basic procedure involves irradiating a pair of foils that can be activated by the photodisintegration process (section 2.8F). The choice of foils must be such that one of them is sensitive to higher energies than the other in the energy spectrum of the x-ray beam. After irradiation, the induced radioactivity in the foils is measured using a scintillation counter. The ratio of induced activities gives the PAR which can be related to the peak photon energy. The PAR method provides a more sensitive method of measuring x-ray spectral quality than the conventional method of measuring HVL in water.

7.5. MEASUREMENT OF ENERGY SPECTRUM

Although the HVL is a practical parameter characterizing therapeutic beams, it is only approximate and cannot be used in systems that are sensitive to spectral distribution of photons. For example, some radiation detectors show a large variation in response with different photon energies (e.g., film, diodes), and even ion chambers are more or less energy dependent, depending on their design. In such instances, spectral distribution is the relevant parameter of beam quality. In this and other investigative work, it is important to determine experimentally spectral distributions of photon beams. There are many references dealing with spectrometry (12–15), and the interested reader is referred to those papers. Only one method, namely scintillation spectrometry, will be briefly described here.

The scintillation spectrometer consists of a crystal or phosphor, usually sodium iodide, attached to a photomultiplier tube (Fig. 7.6). When a photon beam is incident on the crystal, electrons are ejected which travel in the crystal and produce ionization and excitation of the crystal atoms. As a result, photons of energy in the optical or ultraviolet region are produced along the electron tracks. These light photons, on striking the photosensitive surface (photocathode) of a photomultiplier tube, eject low-energy photoelectrons which are collected and multiplied about a million times by the photomultiplier dynodes. This results in an output pulse which is proportional to the energy of the original x-ray photon entering the crystal. A multichannel pulse height analyzer is used to sort out electronically different-size pulses. Each channel corresponds to a particular input photon energy and accumulates counts or number of photons with a particular energy. The spectrum is then displayed in terms of photons per unit energy interval as a function of photon energy (Fig. 7.6).

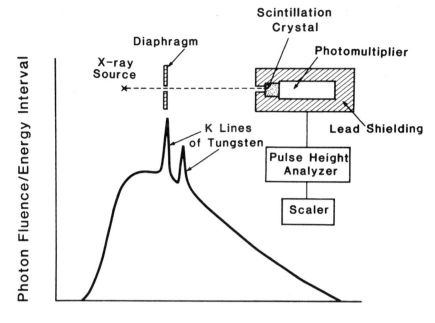

FIG. 7.6. Energy spectrum of an x-ray beam determined by scintillation spectrometer (shown in the inset).

REFERENCES

1. Thoraeus R. A study of the ionization method for measuring the intensity and absorption of x-rays and of different filters used in therapy. *Acta Radiol* 1932;15[suppl].
2. International Commission on Radiation Units and Measurements. Physical aspects of irradiation. Report 10b. Washington, DC: U.S. National Bureau of Standards, 1964.
3. Gilbertson JD, Fingerhut AG. Standardization of diagnostic x-ray generators. *Radiology* 1969; 93:1033.
4. Giarratano JC, Waggener RG, Hevezi JM, et al. Comparison of voltage-divider, modified Ardran-Crooks cassette and Ge (Li) spectrometer methods to determine the peak kilovoltage (kVp) of diagnostic x-ray units. *Med Phys* 1976;3:142.
5. Greening J. The measurement of ionization methods of the peak kilovoltage across x-ray tubes. *Br J Appl Phys* 1955;6:73.
6. Morgan R. A simple method of measuring peak voltage in diagnostic roentgen equipment. *AJR* 1944;52:308.
7. Newell RR, Henny GC. Inferential kilovoltmeter: measuring x-ray kilovoltage by absorption in two filters. *Radiology* 1955;64:88.
8. Glasser O, Quimby EH, Taylor LS, et al. *Physical foundations of radiology*, 3rd ed. New York: Paul B. Hoeber, 1961:241.
9. Stanton L, Lightfoot DA, Mann S. A penetrameter method for field kV calibration of diagnostic x-ray machines. *Radiology* 1966;87:87.
10. Ardran GM, Crooks HE. Checking diagnostic x-ray beam quality. *Br J Radiol* 1968;41:193.
11. Nath R, Schulz RJ. On the choice of material for half-value-layer measurements for megavoltage x-rays. *Med Phys* 1977;4:132.
12. Schiff LI. Energy-angle distribution of thin target bremsstrahlung. *Phys Rev* 1951;83:252.
13. Skarsgard LD, Johns HE. Spectral flux density of scattered and primary radiation generated at 250 kV. *Radiat Res* 1961;14:231.
14. Epp ER, Weiss H. Experimental study of the photon energy spectrum of primary diagnostic x-rays. *Phys Med Biol* 1966;11:225.
15. Nath R, Schulz RJ. Determination of high energy x-ray spectra by photoactivation. *Med Phys* 1976;3:133.
16. Hospital Physicist's Association. Central axis depth dose data for use in radiotherapy. *Br J Radiol* 1983;17[suppl].
17. Nath R, Schulz RJ. Photoactivation ratios for specification of high-energy x-ray quality: part I and II. *Med Phys* 1977;4:36.

MEASUREMENT OF ABSORBED DOSE

8.1. RADIATION ABSORBED DOSE

In Chapter 6, the quantity exposure and its unit, the roentgen (C/kg), were discussed. It was then pointed out that exposure applies only to x and γ radiations, is a measure of ionization in air only, and cannot be used for photon energies above about 3 MeV. The quantity *absorbed dose* has been defined to describe the quantity of radiation for all types of ionizing radiation, including charged and uncharged particles; all materials; and all energies. Absorbed dose is a measure of the biologically significant effects produced by ionizing radiation.

The current definition of *absorbed dose,* or simply *dose,* is the quotient $d\bar{\epsilon}/dm$, where $d\bar{\epsilon}$ is the mean energy imparted by ionizing radiation to material of mass dm (1). The old unit of dose is *rad* (an acronym for radiation absorbed dose) and represents the absorption of 100 ergs of energy per gram of absorbing material.

$$1 \text{ rad} = 100 \text{ ergs/g} = 10^{-2} \text{ J/kg} \tag{8.1}$$

The *SI unit* for absorbed dose is the *gray* (Gy) and is defined as:

$$1 \text{ Gy} = 1 \text{ J/kg} \tag{8.2}$$

Thus the relationship between gray and rad is:

$$1 \text{ Gy} = 100 \text{ rad} \tag{8.3}$$

or

$$1 \text{ rad} = 10^{-2} \text{ Gy} \tag{8.4}$$

Because gray is a larger unit than rad, there is a practical difficulty in switching from rad to grays. For instance, if a patient receives treatments of 175 rad/day, the dose will have to be recorded as 1.75 grays. Because most people prefer numbers without decimals as well as a common resistance to change to the SI units in this country, the adoption of the SI system has been delayed. However, for some, the change is inevitable and the rad is routinely converted into grays. A subunit, centigray (cGy), has often been used as being equivalent to rad.

8.2. RELATIONSHIP BETWEEN KERMA, EXPOSURE, AND ABSORBED DOSE

A. Kerma

The quantity kerma (K) (*k*inetic *e*nergy *r*eleased in the *m*edium) is defined as "the quotient of dE_{tr} by dm, where dE_{tr} is the sum of the initial kinetic energies of all the charged ionizing particles (electrons and positrons) liberated by uncharged particles (photons) in a material of mass dm" (1).

$$K = \frac{dE_{tr}}{dm} \tag{8.5}$$

The unit for kerma is the same as for dose, that is, J/kg. The name of its SI unit is gray (Gy) and its special unit is rad.

For a photon beam traversing a medium, kerma at a point is directly proportional to the photon energy fluence Ψ and is given by:

$$K = \Psi \left(\frac{\overline{\mu}_{tr}}{\rho} \right) \tag{8.6}$$

where $\overline{\mu}_{tr}/\rho$ is the mass energy transfer coefficient for the medium averaged over the energy fluence spectrum of photons. As discussed in section 5.4,

$$\left(\frac{\overline{\mu}_{en}}{\rho} \right) = \left(\frac{\overline{\mu}_{tr}}{\rho} \right) (1 - \overline{g}) \tag{8.7}$$

where $\overline{\mu}_{en}/\rho$ is the averaged mass energy absorption coefficient and $\overline{g}$ is the average fraction of an electron energy lost to radiative processes. Therefore,

$$K = \Psi \left(\frac{\overline{\mu}_{en}}{\rho} \right) \Big/ (1 - \overline{g}) \tag{8.8}$$

A major part of the initial kinetic energy of electrons in low atomic number materials (e.g., air, water, soft tissue) is expended by inelastic collisions (ionization and excitation) with atomic electrons. Only a small part is expended in the radiative collisions with atomic nuclei (bremsstrahlung). Kerma can thus be divided into two parts:

$$K = K^{col} + K^{rad} \tag{8.9}$$

where K^{col} and K^{rad} are the collision and the radiation parts of kerma, respectively. From Equations 8.8 and 8.9,

$$K^{col} = \Psi \left(\frac{\overline{\mu}_{en}}{\rho} \right) \tag{8.10}$$

and

$$K^{rad} = \Psi \left(\frac{\overline{\mu}_{en}}{\rho} \right) \cdot \left(\frac{\overline{g}}{1 - \overline{g}} \right) \tag{8.11}$$

B. Exposure and Kerma

In Chapter 6, the quantity exposure was defined as dQ/dm where dQ is the total charge of the ions of one sign produced in air when all the electrons (negatrons and positrons) liberated by photons in (dry) air of mass dm are completely stopped in air.

Exposure is the ionization equivalent of the collision kerma in air. It can be calculated from K^{col} by knowing the ionization charge produced per unit of energy deposited by photons. The mean energy required to produce an ion pair in dry air is almost constant for all electron energies and has a value of $\overline{W} = 33.97$ eV/ion pair (2). If e is the electronic charge ($= 1.602 \times 10^{-19}$ C), then $\frac{\overline{W}}{e}$ is the average energy required per unit charge of ionization produced. Since 1 eV $= 1.602 \times 10^{-19}$ J, $\frac{\overline{W}}{e} = 33.97$ J/C. Exposure (X) is given by:

$$X = (K^{col})_{air} \cdot \left(\frac{e}{\overline{W}} \right) \tag{8.12}$$

From Equations 8.10 and 8.12,

$$X = \Psi_{air} \left(\frac{\overline{\mu}_{en}}{\rho} \right)_{air} \cdot \left(\frac{e}{\overline{W}} \right)_{air} \tag{8.13}$$

The SI unit for exposure is C/kg and the special unit is roentgen (1 R $= 2.58 \times 10^{-4}$ C/kg).

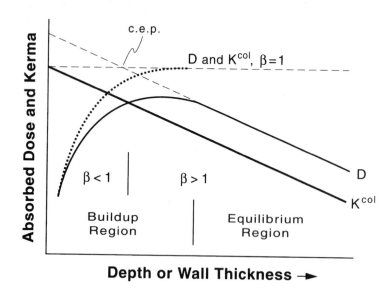

FIG. 8.1. Relationship between absorbed dose (*D*) and collision kerma (K^col) for a megavoltage photon beam. β is the ratio of absorbed dose to collision kerma. The point designated as c.e.p. is the center of electron production (see text). (From Loevinger R. A formalism for calculation of absorbed dose to a medium from photon and electron beams. *Med Phys* 1981;8:1, with permission.)

C. Absorbed Dose and Kerma

Relationship between absorbed dose (*D*) and the collision part of kerma K^{col} is illustrated in Fig. 8.1 when a broad beam of photons enters a medium. Whereas kerma is maximum at the surface and decreases with depth, the dose initially builds up to a maximum value and then decreases at the same rate as kerma. Before the two curves meet, the electron buildup is less than complete, and:

$$\beta = D/K^{col} < 1 \tag{8.14}$$

where β is the quotient of absorbed dose at a given point and the collision part of kerma at the same point.

Because of the increasing range of the electrons, complete electronic equilibrium does not exist within megavoltage photon beams. However, conceptually electronic equilibrium would exist if it were assumed that photon attenuation is negligible throughout the region of interest. Then:

$$\beta = D/K^{col} = 1 \tag{8.15}$$

At depths greater than the maximum range of electrons, there is a region of quasiequilibrium called the transient electron equilibrium in which:

$$\beta = D/K^{col} > 1 \tag{8.16}$$

In the transient equilibrium region, β is greater than unity because of the combined effect of attenuation of the photon beam and the predominantly forward motion of the electrons. Because the dose is being deposited by electrons originating upstream, one can think of a point somewhere upstream at a distance less than the maximum electron range from where the energy is effectively transported by secondary electrons. This point has been called the "center of electron production" (3). Since the effective center of electron production is located upstream relative to the point of interest, the dose is greater than kerma in the region of transient electronic equilibrium.

The relationship between absorbed dose and photon energy fluence Ψ at a point where a transient electron equilibrium exists is given by:

$$D = \beta \cdot (\overline{\mu}_{en}/\rho) \cdot \Psi \tag{8.17}$$

Suppose D_1 is the dose at a point in some material in a photon beam and another material is substituted of a thickness of at least one maximum electron range in all directions from the point, then D_2, the dose in the second material, is related to D_1 by:

$$\frac{D_1}{D_2} = \frac{(\beta \cdot \mu_{en}/\rho)_1 \cdot \Psi_1}{(\beta \cdot \mu_{en}/\rho)_2 \cdot \Psi_2} \tag{8.18}$$

The factor β has been calculated for ^{60}Co and other photon energies for air, water, polystyrene, carbon, and aluminum (4,5). The results show that the value of β varies with energy, not medium. A fixed value of $\beta = 1.005$ has been used for ^{60}Co in conjunction with ion chamber dosimetry (6).

For further details of the relationship between absorbed dose and kerma and its significance in dosimetry, the reader is referred to a paper by Loevinger (4).

8.3. CALCULATION OF ABSORBED DOSE FROM EXPOSURE

A. Absorbed Dose to Air

Determination of absorbed dose from exposure is readily accomplished under conditions of electron equilibrium. However, for energies in the megavoltage range, the electron fluence producing absorbed dose at a point is characteristic of photon energy fluence some distance upstream. Consequently, there may be appreciable photon attenuation in this distance. The calculation of absorbed dose from exposure when rigorous electronic equilibrium does not exist is much more difficult, requiring energy-dependent corrections. Therefore, the determination of exposure and its conversion to absorbed dose is practically limited to photon energies up to ^{60}Co.

In the presence of charged particle equilibrium (CPE), dose at a point in any medium is equal to the collision part of kerma, that is, $\beta = 1$. Dose to air (D_{air}) under these conditions is given by (see Equation 8.12):

$$D_{air} = (K^{col})_{air} = X \cdot \frac{\overline{W}}{e} \tag{8.19}$$

Inserting units

$$D_{air}(J/kg) = X(R) \cdot 2.58 \times 10^{-4} \left(\frac{C/kg}{R}\right) \cdot 33.97(J/C) = 0.876 \times 10^{-2} \left(\frac{J/kg}{R}\right) \cdot X(R)$$

Since 1 rad = 10^{-2} J/kg,

$$D_{air}(rad) = 0.876 \left(\frac{rad}{R}\right) \cdot X(R) \tag{8.20}$$

From Equation 8.20 it is seen that the *roentgen-to-rad conversion factor* for air, under the conditions of electronic equilibrium, is 0.876.

B. Absorbed Dose to Any Medium

In the presence of full charged particle equilibrium, the absorbed dose (D) to a medium can be calculated from the energy fluence Ψ and the weighted mean mass energy absorption coefficient, $\overline{\mu}_{en}/\rho$ (i.e., $\beta = 1$ in Equation 8.17).

$$D = \Psi \cdot \overline{\mu}_{en}/\rho \tag{8.21}$$

Suppose Ψ_{air} is the energy fluence at a point in air and Ψ_{med} is the energy fluence at the same point when a material other than air (medium) is interposed in the beam. Then, under conditions of electronic equilibrium in either case, the dose to air is related to the dose to the medium by the following relationship:

$$\frac{D_{med}}{D_{air}} = \frac{(\overline{\mu}_{en}/\rho)_{med}}{(\overline{\mu}_{en}/\rho)_{air}} \cdot A \tag{8.22}$$

where A is a transmission factor which equals the ratio Ψ_{med}/Ψ_{air} at the point of interest.

From Equations 8.19 and 8.22, we obtain the relationship between exposure to air and absorbed dose to a medium.

$$D_{\mathrm{med}} = X \cdot \frac{\overline{W}_{\mathrm{air}}}{e} \cdot \frac{(\overline{\mu}_{en}/\rho)_{\mathrm{med}}}{(\overline{\mu}_{en}/\rho)_{\mathrm{air}}} \cdot A \qquad (8.23)$$

Again, if we express X in roentgens and D_{med} in rad, we have:

$$D_{\mathrm{med}} = \left[0.876 \frac{(\overline{\mu}_{en}/\rho)_{\mathrm{med}}}{(\overline{\mu}_{en}/\rho)_{\mathrm{air}}} \right] \cdot X \cdot A \qquad (8.24)$$

The quantity in brackets has frequently been represented by the symbol f_{med} so that:

$$D_{\mathrm{med}} = f_{\mathrm{med}} \cdot X \cdot A \qquad (8.25)$$

where

$$f_{\mathrm{med}} = 0.876 \frac{(\overline{\mu}_{en}/\rho)_{\mathrm{med}}}{(\overline{\mu}_{en}/\rho)_{\mathrm{air}}} \qquad (8.26)$$

The quantity f_{med} or simply the *f factor* is sometimes called the roentgen-to-rad conversion factor. As the above equation suggests, this factor depends on the mass energy absorption coefficient of the medium relative to the air. Thus the f factor is a function of the medium composition as well as the photon energy.

A list of f factors for water, bone, and muscle as a function of photon energy is given in Table 8.1. Since for materials with an atomic number close to that of air, for example, water and soft tissue, the ratio $(\overline{\mu}_{en}/\rho)_{\mathrm{med}}/(\overline{\mu}_{en}/\rho)_{\mathrm{air}}$ varies slowly with photon energy (~10% variation from 10 keV and 10 MeV), the f factor for these materials does not vary much over practically the whole therapeutic range of energies. However, bone with a high effective atomic number not only has a much larger f factor between 10 and 100 keV but the f factor drops sharply from its maximum value of 4.24 at 30 keV to about 1.0 at 175 keV. This high peak value and rapid drop of the f factor are the result of the photoelectric process for which the mass energy absorption coefficient varies approximately as Z^3 and $1/E^3$ (see Chapter 5). At higher photon energies where the Compton

TABLE 8.1. *f* FACTORS FOR WATER, BONE, AND MUSCLE UNDER CONDITIONS OF CHARGED PARTICLE EQUILIBRIUM

Photon Energy (keV)	*f* Factor					
	Water		Bone		Muscle	
	(Gy kg/C)	(rad/R)	(Gy kg/C)	(rad/R)	(Gy kg/C)	(rad/R)
10	35.3	0.911	134	3.46	35.7	0.921
15	34.9	0.900	149	3.85	35.7	0.921
20	34.6	0.892	158	4.07	35.6	0.919
30	34.3	0.884	164	4.24	35.6	0.918
40	34.4	0.887	156	4.03	35.7	0.922
50	34.9	0.900	136	3.52	36.0	0.929
60	35.5	0.916	112	2.90	36.3	0.937
80	36.5	0.942	75.1	1.94	36.8	0.949
100	37.1	0.956	56.2	1.45	37.1	0.956
150	37.5	0.967	41.2	1.06	37.2	0.960
200	37.6	0.969	37.9	0.978	37.2	0.961
300	37.6	0.970	36.5	0.941	37.3	0.962
400	37.6	0.971	36.2	0.933	37.3	0.962
600	37.6	0.971	36.0	0.928	37.3	0.962
1,000	37.6	0.971	35.9	0.927	37.3	0.962
2,000	37.6	0.971	35.9	0.927	37.3	0.962

Data from Wyckoff HO. (Communication.) Med Phys 1983;10:715. Calculations are based on energy absorption coefficient data from Hubbell JH. Photon mass attenuation and energy-absorption coefficients from 1 keV to 20 MeV. Int J Appl Radiat Isot 1982;33:1269.

process is the only mode of interaction possible, the f factors are approximately the same for all materials.

Strictly speaking, in the Compton range of energies, the f factor varies as a function of the number of electrons per gram. Since the number of electrons per gram for bone is slightly less than for air, water, or fat, the f factor for bone is also slightly lower than for the latter materials in the Compton region of the megavoltage energies. Of course, the f factor is not defined beyond 3 MeV since the roentgen is not defined beyond this energy.

C. Dose Calibration with Ion Chamber in Air

As discussed in Chapter 6, a cavity ion chamber is exposure calibrated against a free-air ion chamber or a standard cavity chamber, under conditions of electronic equilibrium. For lower-energy radiations such as x-ray beams in the superficial or orthovoltage range, the chamber walls are usually thick enough to provide the desired equilibrium, and therefore, the chamber calibration is provided without a build-up cap. However, in the case of higher-energy radiations such as from cobalt-60, a build-up cap is used over the sensitive volume of the chamber so that the combined thickness of the chamber wall and the build-up cap is sufficient to provide the required equilibrium. This build-up cap is usually made up of acrylic (same as Plexiglas, Lucite, or Perspex) and must be in place when measuring exposure.

Suppose the chamber is exposed to the beam (Fig. 8.2A) and the reading M is obtained (corrected for air temperature and pressure, stem leakage, collection efficiency, etc.). The exposure X is then given by:

$$X = M \cdot N_x \tag{8.27}$$

where N_x is the exposure calibration factor for the given chamber and the given beam quality. The exposure thus obtained is the exposure at point P (center of the chamber sensitive volume) in free air in the absence of the chamber (Fig. 8.2B). In other words, the perturbing influence of the chamber is removed once the chamber calibration factor is applied.

Consider a small amount of soft tissue at point P that is just large enough to provide electronic equilibrium at its center (Fig. 8.2C). The dose at the center of this equilibrium mass of tissue is referred to as the *dose in free space*. The term dose in free space was introduced by Johns and Cunningham (7) who related this quantity to the dose in an extended tissue medium by means of tissue air ratios (to be discussed in Chapter 9).

Equation 8.25 can be used to convert exposure into dose in free space, $D_{\text{f.s.}}$.

$$D_{\text{f.s.}} = f_{\text{tissue}} \cdot X \cdot A_{\text{eq}} \tag{8.28}$$

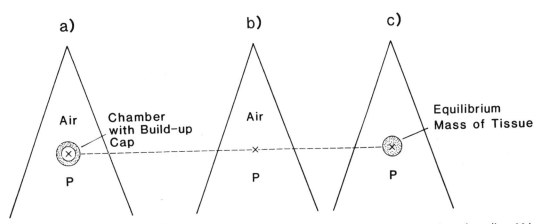

FIG. 8.2. A: Chamber with build-up cap is placed in a radiation beam at point P in air and reading M is obtained. **B:** Exposure in free air at P is calculated using Equation 8.27. **C:** Dose in free space at P is calculated using Equation 8.28.

where A_{eq} is the transmission factor representing the ratio of the energy fluence at the center of the equilibrium mass of tissue to that in free air at the same point. Thus, A_{eq} represents the ratio of the energy fluence at point P in Fig. 8.2C to that at the same point in Fig. 8.2B. For cobalt-60 beam, A_{eq} is close to 0.99 (7) and its value approaches 1.000 as the beam energy decreases to the orthovoltage range.

D. Dose Measurement from Exposure with Ion Chamber in a Medium

Equations 8.27 and 8.28 provide the basis for absorbed dose calculation in any medium from exposure measurement in air. Similar procedure is valid when the exposure measurement is made with the chamber imbedded in a medium. Figure 8.3A shows an arrangement in which the chamber with its build-up cap is surrounded by the medium and exposed to a photon energy fluence Ψ_b at the center of the chamber (point P). If the energy of the beam incident on the chamber is such that a state of electronic equilibrium exists within the air cavity, then the exposure at point P, with the chamber and the build-up cap removed, is given by:

$$X = M \cdot N_x$$

The exposure thus measured is defined in free air at point P due to energy fluence Ψ_c that would exist at P in the air-filled cavity of the size equal to the external dimensions of the buildup cap (Fig. 8.3B). To convert this exposure to absorbed dose at P in the medium, the air in the cavity must be replaced by the medium (Fig. 8.3C) and the following equation is applied:

$$D_{med} = X \cdot f_{med} \cdot A_m$$

or

$$D_{med} = M \cdot N_x \cdot \frac{\overline{W}}{e} \cdot \left(\frac{\overline{\mu_{en}}}{\rho}\right)_{air}^{med} \cdot A_m \tag{8.29}$$

where A_m is the transmission factor for the photon energy fluence at point P when the cavity in Fig. 8.3B is replaced by the medium. If Ψ_m is the energy fluence at P in the medium, the factor A_m is given by Ψ_m/Ψ_c and has been called a displacement factor.

The above equation is similar to Equation 8.28 except that A_m is used instead of A_{eq}. However, the difference between A_m and A_{eq} is small for a tissue equivalent medium since

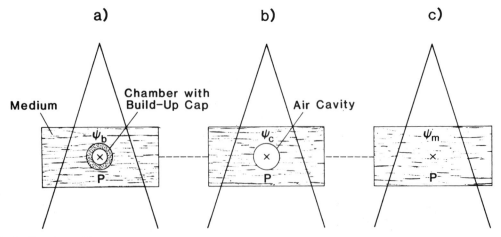

FIG. 8.3. **A:** Chamber with build-up cap with its center at point P in a medium, exposed to a photon beam whose energy fluence is Ψ_b at P. Reading M is obtained. **B:** Exposure at P in air cavity of size equal to the external dimensions of the build-up cap is calculated. Energy fluence at P is Ψ_c. **C:** Absorbed dose at point P in the medium is calculated by Equation 8.29. Ψ_m is the energy fluence at P.

the equilibrium mass of tissue to which A_{eq} applies is only slightly smaller than the mass of the medium displaced by a typical small ion chamber with its build-up cap.

An interesting question arises in regard to the necessity of the build-up cap being left on the chamber when making measurements in a medium. If the chamber has been calibrated for exposure in air with its build-up cap on (to achieve electronic equilibrium) and if a significant part of the cavity ionization is the result of electrons produced in the build-up cap, then replacing the build-up cap with the medium could, in general, alter the chamber reading. This substitution of a layer of medium for the build-up cap could change the electronic and photon fluence incident on the chamber wall by virtue of differences in the composition of the medium and the material of the build-up cap. However, in practical calibration measurements, no significant differences have been observed when exposing the chamber in water with and without the Lucite build-up cap. Day et al. (8) added Perspex sheaths up to 5 mm in thickness to a Baldwin-Farmer ionization chamber irradiated at a depth of 5 cm in a water phantom using radiations from ^{137}Cs to 6 MV. The readings differed by less than 0.5%.

8.4. THE BRAGG-GRAY CAVITY THEORY

As discussed earlier, calculation of absorbed dose from exposure is subject to some major limitations. For instance, it may not be used for photons above 3 MeV and may not be used in cases where electronic equilibrium does not exist. In addition, the term *exposure* applies only to x and γ radiations and for that reason methods of section 8.3 are not valid for particle dosimetry. The Bragg-Gray cavity theory, on the other hand, may be used without such restrictions to calculate dose directly from ion chamber measurements in a medium.

According to the Bragg-Gray theory (9,10), the ionization produced in a gas-filled cavity placed in a medium is related to the energy absorbed in the surrounding medium. When the cavity is sufficiently small so that its introduction into the medium does not alter the number or distribution of the electrons that would exist in the medium without the cavity, then the following Bragg-Gray relationship is satisfied:

$$D_{\mathrm{med}} = J_g \cdot \frac{\overline{W}}{e} \cdot (\overline{S}/\rho)_g^{\mathrm{med}} \qquad (8.30)$$

where D_{med} is the absorbed dose in the medium (in the absence of the cavity), J_g is the ionization charge of one sign produced per unit mass of the cavity gas, and $(\overline{S}/\rho)_g^{\mathrm{med}}$ is a weighted mean ratio of the mass stopping power of the medium to that of the gas for the electrons crossing the cavity. The product of $J_g\left(\frac{\overline{W}}{e}\right)$ is the energy absorbed per unit mass of the cavity gas.

The basic Bragg-Gray relationship has been carefully examined by many investigators and several modifications of the theory have been proposed (11–14). These refinements resulted in more detailed considerations of what is appropriate to use for the mass stopping power ratio in Equation 8.30.

A. Stopping Power

The term *stopping power* refers to the energy loss by electrons per unit path length of a material (for greater details, see section 14.1). An extensive set of calculated values of mass stopping powers has been published (15,16). As mentioned earlier, to use stopping power ratios in the Bragg-Gray formula, it is necessary to determine a weighted mean of the stopping power ratios for the electron spectrum set in motion by the photon spectrum in the materials concerned. Methods for calculating average stopping powers (S) for photon beams have been published (17).

Several authors have worked out the theory of the stopping power ratio for an air-filled cavity in a medium such as water under electron irradiation. A good approximation is provided by the Spencer-Attix formulation (11,18):

$$\overline{L}/\rho = \frac{\displaystyle\int_{\Delta}^{E_0} \Phi(E) \cdot L/\rho(E)\, dE}{\displaystyle\int_{\Delta}^{E_0} \Phi(E)\, dE} \tag{8.31}$$

where $\Phi(E)$ is the distribution of electron fluence in energy and L/ρ is the *restricted mass collision stopping power* with Δ as the cutoff energy.

The "primary electrons" (original electrons or electrons generated by photons) give rise to ionization as well as "secondary electrons" or δ rays. The effects of the latter are accounted for in the Spencer-Attix formulation by using an arbitrary energy limit, Δ, below which energy transfers are considered dissipative, that is, the secondary electron of energy less than Δ is assumed to dissipate its energy near the site of its release. Thus, when the integration is performed (Equation 8.31) to obtain the energy deposited in the cavity by the electron fluence, the lower energy limit should be Δ, greater than zero. For ion chambers it must have a value of the order of the energy of an electron that will just cross the cavity. The value of Δ for most cavity applications in ion chambers will lie between 10 and 20 keV.

The Spencer-Attix formulation of the Bragg-Gray cavity theory uses the following relationship:

$$D_{\text{med}} = J_g \cdot \frac{\overline{W}}{e} \cdot \left(\frac{\overline{L}}{\rho}\right)_g^{\text{med}} \tag{8.32}$$

where $\frac{\overline{L}}{\rho}$ is the average restricted mass collisional stopping power of electrons. Tables A.1 to A.5 in the Appendix give $\frac{\overline{L}}{\rho}$ for various media and various photon and electron energies.

B. Chamber Volume

The quantity J_g in Equation 8.32 can be determined for a chamber of known volume or known mass of air in the cavity if the chamber is connected to a charge-measuring device. However, the chamber volume is usually not known to an acceptable accuracy. An indirect method of measuring J_{air} is to make use of the exposure calibration of the chamber for [60]Co γ ray beam. This in effect determines the chamber volume.

Consider an ion chamber that has been calibrated with a build-up cap for ^{60}Co exposure. Suppose the chamber with this build-up cap is exposed in free air to a ^{60}Co beam and that a transient electronic equilibrium exists at the center of the chamber. Also assume initially that the chamber wall and the build-up cap are composed of the same material (wall). Now, if the chamber (plus the build-up cap) is replaced by a homogeneous mass of wall material with outer dimensions equal to that of the cap, the dose D_{wall} at the center of this mass can be calculated as follows:

$$D_{\text{wall}} = J_{\text{air}} \cdot \left(\frac{\overline{W}}{e}\right) \cdot \left(\frac{\overline{L}}{\rho}\right)_{\text{air}}^{\text{wall}} \cdot (\Phi_{\text{cav}})_{\text{air}}^{\text{wall}} \tag{8.33}$$

where $(\Phi_{\text{cav}})_{\text{air}}^{\text{wall}}$ is the ratio of electron fluence at the reference point P (center of the cavity) with chamber cavity filled with wall material to that with the cavity filled with air. This correction is applied to the Bragg-Gray relation (Equation 8.29) to account for change in electron fluence.

As discussed by Loevinger (4)[1], Φ in the above equation can be replaced by Ψ, provided a transient electron equilibrium exists throughout the region of the wall from

---

[1] Electron fluence at P with the cavity filled with wall material is proportional to Ψ_{wall} at P. With the air cavity in place, the electron fluence at P is proportional to the mean photon energy fluence at the surface of the cavity, which can be taken as equal to Ψ_{air} at the center of the cavity.

which secondary electrons can reach the cavity. Therefore,

$$D_{\text{wall}} = J_{\text{air}} \cdot \left(\frac{\overline{W}}{e}\right) \cdot \left(\frac{\overline{L}}{\rho}\right)^{\text{wall}}_{\text{air}} \cdot (\Psi_{\text{cav}})^{\text{wall}}_{\text{air}} \tag{8.34}$$

If D_{air} is the absorbed dose to air that would exist at the reference point with the chamber removed and under conditions of transient electronic equilibrium in air, we get from Equation 8.18:

$$D_{\text{air}} = D_{\text{wall}} \cdot \left(\beta \frac{\overline{\mu}_{en}}{\rho}\right)^{\text{air}}_{\text{wall}} \cdot (\Psi_{\text{chamb}})^{\text{air}}_{\text{wall}} \tag{8.35}$$

where $(\Psi_{\text{chamb}})^{\text{air}}_{\text{wall}}$ is the ratio that corrects for the change in photon energy fluence when air replaces the chamber (wall plus cap).

From Equations 8.34 and 8.35, we get:

$$D_{\text{air}} = J_{\text{air}} \cdot \left(\frac{\overline{W}}{e}\right) \cdot \left(\frac{\overline{L}}{\rho}\right)^{\text{wall}}_{\text{air}} \cdot \left(\beta \frac{\overline{\mu}_{en}}{\rho}\right)^{\text{air}}_{\text{wall}} \cdot (\Psi_{\text{cav}})^{\text{wall}}_{\text{air}} \cdot (\Psi_{\text{chamb}})^{\text{air}}_{\text{wall}} \tag{8.36}$$

Also D_{air} (under conditions of transient electronic equilibrium in air) can be calculated from exposure measurement in a ^{60}Co beam with a chamber plus build-up cap, which bears an exposure calibration factor N_x for ^{60}Co γ rays.

$$D_{\text{air}} = k \cdot M \cdot N_x \cdot \left(\frac{\overline{W}}{e}\right) \cdot \beta_{\text{air}} \cdot A_{\text{ion}} \cdot P_{\text{ion}} \tag{8.37}$$

where k is the charge per unit mass produced in air per unit exposure (2.58×10^{-4} C kg^{-1} R^{-1}); M is the chamber reading (C or scale division) normalized to standard atmospheric conditions, A_{ion} is the correction for ionization recombination under calibration conditions, and P_{ion} is the ionization recombination correction for the present measurement.

Standard conditions for N_x are defined by the standards laboratories. The National Institute of Standards and Technology (NIST) specifies standard conditions as temperature at 22°C and pressure at 760 mm Hg. Since exposure is defined for dry air, humidity correction of 0.997 (for change in $\overline{W}$ with humidity) is used by NIST, which can be assumed constant in the relative humidity range of 10% to 90% for the measurement conditions with minimal error (19). Thus the user does not need to apply additional humidity correction as long as $\frac{\overline{W}}{e}$ is used for dry air.

From Equations 8.36 and 8.37,

$$J_{\text{air}} = k \cdot M \cdot N_x \cdot (\Psi_{\text{cav}})^{\text{air}}_{\text{wall}} \cdot (\Psi_{\text{chamb}})^{\text{wall}}_{\text{air}} \cdot \beta_{\text{wall}} \cdot A_{\text{ion}} \cdot \left(\frac{\overline{L}}{\rho}\right)^{\text{air}}_{\text{wall}} \cdot \left(\frac{\overline{\mu}_{en}}{\rho}\right)^{\text{wall}}_{\text{air}} \cdot P_{\text{ion}} \tag{8.38}$$

The product $(\Psi_{\text{cav}})^{\text{air}}_{\text{wall}} \cdot (\Psi_{\text{chamb}})^{\text{wall}}_{\text{air}}$ equals $(\Psi_{\text{wall}})^{\text{wall}}_{\text{air}}$ which represents a correction for the change in J_{air} due to attenuation and scattering of photons in the chamber wall and build-up cap. This factor has been designated as A_{wall} in the AAPM protocol (6). Thus, Equation 8.38 becomes:

$$J_{\text{air}} = k \cdot M \cdot N_x \cdot A_{\text{wall}} \cdot \beta_{\text{wall}} \cdot A_{\text{ion}} \cdot \left(\frac{\overline{L}}{\rho}\right)^{\text{air}}_{\text{wall}} \cdot \left(\frac{\overline{\mu}_{en}}{\rho}\right)^{\text{wall}}_{\text{air}} \cdot P_{\text{ion}} \tag{8.39}$$

Now consider a more realistic situation in which the chamber wall and build-up cap are of different materials. According to the two-component model of Almond and Svensson (20), let α be the fraction of cavity air ionization owing to electrons generated in the wall and the remaining $(1 - \alpha)$ from the build-up cap. Equation 8.39 can now be written as:

$$J_{\text{air}} = k \cdot M \cdot N_x \cdot A_{\text{wall}} \cdot \beta_{\text{wall}} \cdot A_{\text{ion}} \left[\alpha \left(\frac{\overline{L}}{\rho}\right)^{\text{air}}_{\text{wall}} \cdot \left(\frac{\overline{\mu}_{en}}{\rho}\right)^{\text{wall}}_{\text{air}} \right.$$
$$\left. + (1 - \alpha) \left(\frac{\overline{L}}{\rho}\right)^{\text{air}}_{\text{cap}} \cdot \left(\frac{\overline{\mu}_{en}}{\rho}\right)^{\text{cap}}_{\text{air}} \right] \cdot P_{\text{ion}} \tag{8.40}$$

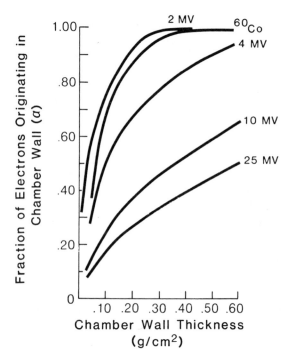

FIG. 8.4. The fraction, α, of cavity ionization due to electrons generated in the chamber wall, plotted as a function of wall thickness. (From Lempert GD, Nath R, Schulz RJ. Fraction of ionization from electrons arising in the wall of an ionization chamber. *Med Phys* 1983;10:1, with permission.)

or

$$J_{air} = k \cdot M \cdot N_x \cdot A_{wall} \cdot \beta_{wall} \cdot A_{ion} \cdot A_\alpha \cdot P_{ion}$$

where A_α is the quantity in the brackets of Equation 8.40.

The fraction *a* has been determined experimentally by dose build-up measurements for various wall thicknesses (Fig. 8.4). In addition, it has been shown (21) that α is independent of wall composition or build-up cap, as long as it is composed of low atomic number material.

Since J_{air} is the charge produced per unit mass of the cavity air, we have:

$$J_{air} = \frac{M \cdot P_{ion}}{\rho_{air} \cdot V_c} \tag{8.41}$$

where V_c is the chamber volume and ρ_{air} is the density of air normalized to standard conditions. Comparing Equations 8.40 and 8.41, we have:

$$V_c = \frac{1}{k \cdot \rho_{air} \cdot N_x \cdot A_{wall} \cdot \beta_{wall} \cdot A_{ion} \cdot A_\alpha} \tag{8.42}$$

C. Effective Point of Measurement

C.1. Plane Parallel Chambers

Since the front plane (toward the source) of the air cavity is flat and is exposed to a uniform fluence of electrons, the point of measurement is at the front surface of the cavity. This would be strictly true if the electrons were monodirectional and forward directed, perpendicular to the cavity face. If a significant part of the cavity ionization is caused by back-scattered electrons, the point of measurement will shift toward the center. If the plane-parallel chamber has a small plate separation and the electron fluence is mostly forward directed, it is reasonable to assume that the point of measurement is the front surface of the cavity.

C. 2. Cylindrical Chambers

Electrons (from an electron beam or generated by photons) transversing a cylindrical chamber of internal radius r will enter the sensitive volume of the chamber (air cavity) at different distances from the center of the chamber. Dutreix and Dutreix (22) showed that theoretically the point of measurement for a cylindrical chamber in a unidirectional beam is displaced by $0.85r$ from the center and toward the source. Derivation of this value is instructive in understanding the concept and is, therefore, presented here.

Figure 8.5 shows a cross-section of a cylindrical chamber exposed to a parallel, uniform, and forwardly directed fluence Φ of electrons. For an electron entering the chamber at point A, the point of measurement is at a distance X above the center. Considering electrons entering the chamber at point A, the effective point of measurement is influenced by the number of electrons entering through a surface area ds at A of the chamber and the track length of these electrons in the cavity. Thus the effective point of measurement, X_{eff}, can be determined by weighting the displacement X by the number of electrons ($\Phi \cdot ds \cos \theta$) entering the chamber and the track length ($2X$).

$$X_{\text{eff}} = \frac{\displaystyle\int_{\theta=0}^{\pi/2} x \cdot (2x) \cdot \Phi \cdot \cos \theta \cdot ds}{\displaystyle\int_{\theta=0}^{\pi/2} 2x \cdot \Phi \cdot \cos \theta \cdot ds} \qquad (8.43)$$

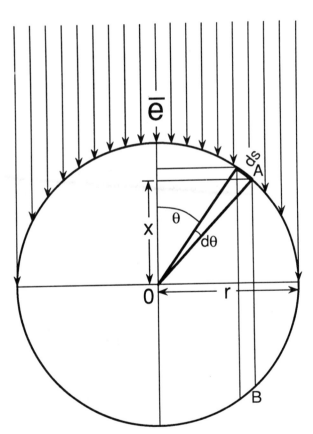

FIG. 8.5. Diagram to illustrate the determination of effective point of measurement for a cylindrical chamber exposed to a unidirectional electron beam.

substituting $X = r \cos\theta$ and $ds = rd\theta$,

$$X_{\text{eff}} = r \left[\frac{\int_0^{\pi/2} \cos^3\theta \, d\theta}{\int_0^{\pi/2} \cos^2\theta \, d\theta} \right] = 8r/3\pi = 0.85r \qquad (8.44)$$

The above theoretical result is modified under actual irradiation conditions as some of the electrons enter the chamber at oblique angles.

The shift in the point of measurement takes place because of the cylindricality of the chamber cavity. If there is a gradient of electron fluence across the cavity (as in the exponential falloff of the depth dose curve), a shift in the point of measurement will result in a "gradient correction" to the dose measured at a point corresponding to the center of the chamber (to be discussed).

8.5. CALIBRATION OF MEGAVOLTAGE BEAMS: TG-21 PROTOCOL

A. Cavity-Gas Calibration Factor (N_{gas})

The AAPM TG-21 protocol (6) for absorbed dose calibration introduced a factor (N_{gas}) to represent calibration of the cavity gas in terms of absorbed dose to the gas in the chamber per unit charge or electrometer reading. For an ionization chamber containing air in the cavity and exposed to a ^{60}Co γ ray beam,[2]

$$N_{\text{gas}} = \frac{D_{\text{air}}}{M \cdot P_{\text{ion}}} = \frac{J_{\text{air}} \cdot \frac{\overline{W}}{e}}{M \cdot P_{\text{ion}}} \qquad (8.45)$$

From Equations 8.40 and 8.45,

$$N_{\text{gas}} = N_x \cdot k \cdot \left(\frac{\overline{W}}{e} \right) \cdot A_{\text{ion}} \cdot A_{\text{wall}} \cdot \beta_{\text{wall}} \left[\alpha \left(\frac{\overline{L}}{\rho} \right)_{\text{wall}}^{\text{air}} \left(\frac{\overline{\mu}_{en}}{\rho} \right)_{\text{air}}^{\text{wall}} \right.$$
$$\left. + (1 - \alpha) \left(\frac{\overline{L}}{\rho} \right)_{\text{cap}}^{\text{air}} \left(\frac{\overline{\mu}_{en}}{\rho} \right)_{\text{air}}^{\text{cap}} \right] \qquad (8.46)$$

As seen in Equation 8.46, N_{gas} is derived from N_x, the exposure calibration for the chamber, and other chamber-related parameters, all determined for the calibration energy, e.g., ^{60}Co. Once N_{gas} is determined, the chamber can be used as a calibrated Bragg-Gray cavity to determine absorbed dose from photon and electron beams of any energy and in phantoms of any composition.

It may be noted that in Equation 8.46 the term in the big brackets is presented differently from the AAPM protocol. This difference remains unexplained, but the two expression give the same value to within 0.05% in the limit of $\alpha = 0$ and $\alpha = 1$ (24).

N_{gas} is unique to each ionization chamber, because it is related to the volume of the chamber. From Equations 8.42 and 8.46, using $\frac{\overline{W}}{e} = 33.97 \, J/C$ and $\rho_{\text{air}} = 1.197 \, \text{kg/m}^3$ at standard conditions (22°C and 1 atm),

$$N_{\text{gas}} = \frac{\frac{\overline{W}}{e}}{\rho_{\text{air}} \cdot V_c} = \frac{28.379}{V_c(\text{m}^3)} \, \text{Gy C}^{-1} \qquad (8.47)$$

As an example, if the volume of the chamber is 0.600 cm^3, its N_{gas} will be 4.73×10^7 Gy/C, as calculated from Equation 8.47. It must be realized, however, that the volume is

---

[2] The TG-21 protocol uses $\frac{\overline{W}}{e}$ value of 33.7 *J/C* which assumes a dry air value of 33.85 *J/C* and corrects it for 50% relative humidity (23). In our derivation we will assume a dry air value of 33.97 *J/C* and no humidity correction, as discussed earlier in relation to Equation 8.37.

not exactly the nominal volume associated with commercial chambers. The latter is usually an approximate value used for designating chamber sensitivity.

B. Chamber as a Bragg-Gray Cavity

In this section, we will discuss the application of the Spencer-Attix formulation of the Bragg-Gray cavity theory to the problem of absorbed dose determination to a medium using a heterogeneous chamber, that is, a chamber with wall material different from the surrounding medium. It will be assumed that the chamber with its build-up cap has been calibrated for cobalt-60 exposure and this provides the basis for the determination of N_{gas}, as discussed in the previous section.

B.1. Photon Beams

Suppose the chamber, with its build-up cap removed (it is recommended not to use build-up cap for in-phantom dosimetry), is placed in a medium and irradiated by a photon beam of given energy. If M is the charge measured, the absorbed dose (D_{air}) to cavity air, at a point at the center of the cavity (P), is given by:

$$D_{air} = M \cdot N_{gas} \cdot P_{ion} \qquad (8.48)$$

where P_{ion} is a correction factor for ion recombination losses.

Dose to medium (D_{med}) is given by the Bragg-Gray relationship using the Spencer-Attix formulation. Using AAPM protocol (6) notation and substituting "air" for "gas" in the chamber,

$$D_{med} = D_{air} \cdot \left(\frac{\overline{L}}{\rho}\right)_{air}^{med} \cdot P_{repl} \cdot P_{wall} \qquad (8.49)$$

where P_{repl} is a replacement factor that corrects for perturbation in the electron and photon fluences at point P as a result of insertion of the cavity in the medium and P_{wall} is a factor which accounts for perturbation caused by the wall being different from the medium.

In general, Equation 8.49 is valid for any energy and any depth in the medium (irrespective of the state of electronic equilibrium) provided P_{repl} and P_{wall} are known for the measurement conditions. Although these correction factors are quite small (usually less than 1%) for typical photon dosimetry conditions, their determination is complex, especially under conditions of nonequilibrium. The AAPM values for P_{repl} and P_{wall} have been derived with the chamber irradiated under the conditions of transient electronic equilibrium (on the descending exponential part of the depth dose curve). The following derivation of these factors will initially assume these conditions but later will consider their applicability to nonequilibrium situations.

Suppose the chamber is positioned at depth in the medium at which transient electronic equilibrium exists. If the chamber wall is thick enough so that the electrons crossing the cavity arise entirely from photons interacting with the wall material, we have:

$$D_{wall} = D_{air} \cdot \left(\frac{\overline{L}}{\rho}\right)_{air}^{wall} \cdot (\Psi_{cav})_{air}^{wall} \qquad (8.50)$$

where D_{wall} is the dose at point P when cavity air is replaced by the wall material and $(\Psi_{cav})_{air}^{wall}$ is the ratio that corrects for the difference in the photon energy fluence at point P when air cavity is replaced by the wall material. The rationale for using $(\Psi_{cav})_{air}^{wall}$ as the perturbation correction factor in this case has been discussed by Loevinger (4).

Dose to point P if the chamber is replaced by the medium is given by:

$$D_{med} = D_{wall} \cdot \left(\beta \frac{\overline{\mu}_{en}}{\rho}\right)_{wall}^{med} \cdot (\Psi_{chamb})_{wall}^{med} \qquad (8.51)$$

or

$$D_{\text{med}} = D_{\text{air}} \cdot \left(\frac{\overline{L}}{\rho} \right)_{\text{air}}^{\text{wall}} \cdot \left(\beta \frac{\overline{\mu}_{en}}{\rho} \right)_{\text{wall}}^{\text{med}} \cdot (\Psi_{\text{cav}})_{\text{air}}^{\text{wall}} \cdot (\Psi_{\text{chamb}})_{\text{wall}}^{\text{med}} \tag{8.52}$$

where $(\Psi_{\text{chamb}})_{\text{wall}}^{\text{med}}$ is the ratio that corrects for the change in photon energy fluence when medium replaces the wall material in a volume that corresponds to the entire chamber (wall plus cavity).

Now if all the electrons crossing the cavity arise from the medium, we effectively have a case of a chamber with medium equivalent wall. Then, under conditions of transient electronic equilibrium,

$$D_{\text{med}} = D_{\text{air}} \cdot \left(\frac{\overline{L}}{\rho} \right)_{\text{air}}^{\text{med}} \cdot (\Psi_{\text{cav}})_{\text{air}}^{\text{med}} \tag{8.53}$$

For a given chamber, suppose a fraction α of the cavity ionization is contributed by electrons from the chamber wall and the remainder $(1 - \alpha)$ by electrons from the medium, then, dose to air in the chamber is given by:

$$D_{\text{air}} = \alpha \cdot D_{\text{air}}(\text{wall}) + (1 - \alpha) \cdot D_{\text{air}}(\text{med}) \tag{8.54}$$

where $D_{\text{air}}(\text{wall})$ and $D_{\text{air}}(\text{med})$ are derived from Equations 8.52 and 8.53. Thus,

$$D_{\text{air}} = D_{\text{med}} \cdot \left[\alpha \left(\frac{\overline{L}}{\rho} \right)_{\text{wall}}^{\text{air}} \cdot \left(\beta \frac{\overline{\mu}_{en}}{\rho} \right)_{\text{med}}^{\text{wall}} \cdot (\Psi_{\text{cav}})_{\text{wall}}^{\text{air}} \cdot (\Psi_{\text{chamb}})_{\text{med}}^{\text{wall}} \right.$$
$$\left. + (1 - \alpha) \left(\frac{\overline{L}}{\rho} \right)_{\text{med}}^{\text{air}} \cdot (\Psi_{\text{cav}})_{\text{med}}^{\text{air}} \right] \tag{8.55}$$

By rearranging Equation 8.55,

$$D_{\text{med}} = D_{\text{air}} \cdot \left(\frac{\overline{L}}{\rho} \right)_{\text{air}}^{\text{med}}$$
$$\cdot (\Psi_{\text{cav}})_{\text{air}}^{\text{med}} \left[\frac{1}{\alpha \left(\frac{\overline{L}}{\rho} \right)_{\text{wall}}^{\text{med}} \cdot \left(\beta \frac{\overline{\mu}_{en}}{\rho} \right)_{\text{med}}^{\text{wall}} \cdot (\Psi_{\text{cav}})_{\text{wall}}^{\text{med}} \cdot (\Psi_{\text{chamb}})_{\text{med}}^{\text{wall}} + 1 - \alpha} \right] \tag{8.56}$$

The product term $(\Psi_{\text{cav}})_{\text{wall}}^{\text{med}} \cdot (\Psi_{\text{chamb}})_{\text{med}}^{\text{wall}}$ may be equated to $(\Psi_{\text{wall}})_{\text{med}}^{\text{wall}}$, a factor that accounts for change in photon energy fluence when wall is replaced by medium.

Then from Equations 8.48, 8.49, and 8.56,

$$D_{\text{med}} = M \cdot N_{\text{gas}} \cdot \left(\frac{\overline{L}}{\rho} \right)_{\text{air}}^{\text{med}} \cdot P_{\text{ion}} \cdot P_{\text{repl}} \cdot P_{\text{wall}} \tag{8.57}$$

where

$$P_{\text{repl}} = (\Psi_{\text{cav}})_{\text{air}}^{\text{med}} \tag{8.58}$$

and

$$P_{\text{wall}} = \frac{1}{\alpha \left(\frac{\overline{L}}{\rho} \right)_{\text{wall}}^{\text{med}} \cdot \left(\beta \frac{\overline{\mu}_{en}}{\rho} \right)_{\text{med}}^{\text{wall}} \cdot (\Psi_{\text{wall}})_{\text{med}}^{\text{wall}} + 1 - \alpha} \tag{8.59}$$

Since β does not change significantly with change in material composition (4), the ratio β_{med}^{wall} can be equated to 1. Equation 8.59 becomes:

$$P_{wall} = \cfrac{1}{\alpha \left(\cfrac{\overline{L}}{\rho}\right)_{wall}^{med} \cdot \left(\cfrac{\overline{\mu}_{en}}{\rho}\right)_{med}^{wall} \cdot (\Psi_{wall})_{med}^{wall} + 1 - \alpha} \qquad (8.60)$$

Equation 8.60 as an expression for P_{wall} differs from the one in the AAPM protocol, since the components α and $(1 - \alpha)$ are applied to D_{air} before calculating D_{med} (see Equation 8.52). Rogers (24) has pointed out that the AAPM expression for P_{wall}, which assigns the two components to D_{med} directly, is not theoretically justified. However, this does not give rise to any significant differences in the results. Also, the previous expression includes $(\Psi_{wall})_{med}^{wall}$, which appears from the theoretical considerations presented here. This factor may approximately be equated to $\left(e^{-\frac{\overline{\mu}_{en}}{\rho} \cdot \rho x}\right)_{wall} \Big/ \left(e^{-\frac{\overline{\mu}_{en}}{\rho} \cdot \rho x}\right)_{med}$ where x is the wall thickness.

An *alternative approach* to deriving P_{repl} is to define $D_{air} = M \cdot N_{gas}$ as the dose to air of an infinitesimally small air cavity located in the medium at a point P', corresponding to the chamber's effective point of measurement (see section 8.4C). Because P_{repl} for this small cavity can be assumed as 1, we have:

$$(D_{med})_{P'} = M \cdot N_{gas} \cdot \left(\frac{\overline{L}}{\rho}\right)_{air}^{med} \cdot P_{ion} \cdot P_{wall} \qquad (8.61)$$

Dose to medium at point P corresponding to the center of the chamber will then be:

$$(D_{med})_P = M \cdot N_{gas} \cdot \left(\frac{\overline{L}}{\rho}\right)_{air}^{med} \cdot \frac{(D_{med})_P}{(D_{med})_{P'}} \cdot P_{ion} \cdot P_{wall} \qquad (8.62)$$

Therefore, P_{repl} for the chamber under consideration is:

$$P_{repl} = \frac{(D_{med})_P}{(D_{med})_{P'}} = \text{gradient correction} \qquad (8.63)$$

This derivation assumes that P_{repl} arises as a result of the displacement of the effective point of measurement of the chamber, and its value depends on the depth dose gradient. This point has been discussed by Khan (25). For a cylindrical chamber, P_{repl} can be calculated from the following equation:

$$P_{repl}(d) = D(d) / D(d - \eta r) \qquad (8.64)$$

where $D(d)$ is the dose at depth d, ηr is the displacement correction, and r is the radius of the cavity. η for photon beams is taken to be equal to 0.6. Equation 8.64 shows that P_{repl} depends not only on energy but also on the depth of measurement.

The AAPM TG-21 protocol recommends P_{repl} factors based on the semiempirical values of Cunningham and Sontag (26). These values are applicable only if a measurement is made at a point on the descending exponential part of the depth dose curve. Moreover, as pointed out by Rogers (24), Cunningham and Sontag's values pertain to the outer diameter of the chamber instead of the inner diameter presented in the protocol data.

The use of chamber displacement correction to determine P_{repl} (Equation 8.64) is useful not only in calibration but also in correcting the entire depth-dose distribution. In the latter case, instead of calculating P_{repl} at individual points, the depth-dose (or depth ionization) curve as a whole is shifted toward the surface by a distance ηr.

B.2. Electron Beams

When a chamber, with its build-up cap removed, is placed in a medium and irradiated by an electron beam, it is usually assumed that the chamber wall does not introduce any perturbation of the electron fluence. This assumption is considered valid for thin-walled

(≤0.5 mm) chambers composed of low atomic number materials (e.g., graphite, acrylic) (15,27). Thus the Bragg-Gray relationship can be applied without the wall perturbation correction, i.e., $P_{wall} = 1$.

For an electron beam of mean energy $\overline{E}_z$ at depth Z of measurement,

$$D_{med} = M \cdot N_{gas} \cdot \left[\left(\frac{\overline{L}}{\rho} \right)_{air}^{med} \cdot (\Phi_{cav})_{air}^{med} \right]_{\overline{E}_z} \cdot P_{ion} \qquad (8.65)$$

or in the notation of the AAPM protocol (6),

$$D_{med} = M \cdot N_{gas} \left[\left(\frac{\overline{L}}{\rho} \right)_{air}^{med} \cdot P_{repl} \right]_{\overline{E}_z} \cdot P_{ion} \qquad (8.66)$$

where P_{repl} is a replacement correction factor to account for three effects: (a) the *in-scatter effect*, which increases the fluence in the cavity since electron scattering out of the cavity is less than that expected in the intact medium; (b) the *obliquity effect*, which decreases the fluence in the cavity because electrons travel relatively straight in the cavity instead of taking oblique paths as they would owing to larger-angle scattering in the medium; and (c) *displacement in the effective point of measurement*, which gives rise to a correction if the point of measurement is on the sloping part of the depth dose curve. The first two effects may be grouped into a *fluence correction* while the third is called the *gradient correction*.

The AAPM TG-21 protocol (6) recommends that the electron beam calibration be made at the point of depth dose maximum. Because there is no dose gradient at that depth, the gradient correction is ignored. P_{repl}, then, constitutes only a fluence correction. Table 8.2 gives P_{repl} for cylindrical chambers as a function of mean electron energy at the depth of measurement and the inner diameter of ion chamber. These values were measured by Johansson et al. (27).

As discussed in an AAPM report (28), a depth ionization curve can be converted into a depth dose curve using Equation 8.66. The parameters $\left(\frac{\overline{L}}{\rho} \right)_{air}^{med}$ and P_{repl} are both energy or depth dependent. The gradient correction, however, is best handled by shifting the point of measurement toward the surface through a distance of $0.5r$ (28,29). For well-designed plane-parallel chambers with adequate guard rings, both fluence and gradient corrections are ignored, i.e., $P_{repl} = 1$; the point of measurement is at the front surface of the cavity.

C. Dose Calibration Parameters

Absorbed dose calibration of a clinical radiation beam requires that a nationally or internationally approved protocol be followed. This is important not only to ensure acceptable

TABLE 8.2. ELECTRON FLUENCE PERTURBATION FACTORS FOR ION CHAMBERS

E_z(MeV)	Inner Diameter (mm)			
	3	5	6	7
2	0.977	0.962	0.956	0.949
3	0.978	0.966	0.959	0.952
5	0.982	0.971	0.965	0.960
7	0.986	0.977	0.972	0.967
10	0.990	0.985	0.981	0.978
15	0.995	0.992	0.991	0.990
20	0.997	0.996	0.995	0.995

From Johansson K, Mattsson L, Lindberg L, Svensson H. Absorbed-dose determination with ionization chambers in electron and photon beams having energies between 1 and 50 MeV. IAEA-SM-222/35. Vienna, 1977;243:270, with permission.

dosimetric accuracy in patient treatments but also to provide consistency of dosimetric data among institutions that provide radiotherapy. In the previous section, derivation of a dose calibration formalism recommended by the AAPM TG-21 protocol was presented. In the process, a few discrepancies or inconsistencies in the protocol were noted. However, their overall impact on the accuracy of the protocol is not serious enough to recommend variance from the protocol. An AAPM task group was formed which was charged with the task of carefully reviewing the protocol and making necessary revisions or updates. In the meantime the user was advised to follow the protocol as it stood. A new protocol, TG-51, was introduced by the AAPM in 1999 (to be discussed later).

As a summary to the previous section, pertinent calibration parameters of the TG-21 protocol are outlined below with a brief description of their function and evaluation.

C.1. Chamber Calibration Factor, N_x

Ion chamber exposure calibration factor (R/C or R/scale division) for ^{60}Co γ rays is provided by the NIST or an Accredited Dosimetry Calibration Laboratory (ADCL). This factor—which is characteristic of the chamber, its volume, and its build-up cap—is determined by exposing it to a ^{60}Co beam of known exposure rate and/or comparing its response with a chamber of known exposure calibration factor for ^{60}Co.

At the NIST, specially constructed spherical, graphite ionization chambers of known volume are used to calibrate the cobalt beam in terms of exposure rate. Details of the procedure are given by Loftus and Weaver (3).

N_X provided by the U.S. calibration laboratories is normalized to 22°C and 760 mm Hg. Calibration of the electrometer (device to measure ionization charge), if detached, is provided separately.

Exposure measured in a cobalt-60 beam is given by:

$$X = M \cdot N_x N_{el} \tag{8.67}$$

where X is the exposure at a point corresponding to the center of the chamber when the chamber is not there; M is the reading corrected for temperature and pressure and N_{el} is the electrometer calibration factor, if separate from the chamber. The above equation functionally defines N_x.

C.2. Cavity-Gas Calibration Factor, N_{gas}

Cavity-gas calibration factor (Gy/C or Gy/scale division) is calculated from N_x and other parameters as discussed earlier. It is defined as dose to the gas in the chamber per unit charge or electrometer reading. D_{gas} is simply given by $J_{gas} \cdot \left(\frac{\overline{W}}{e}\right)$ where J_{gas} is the charge per unit mass of cavity gas and $\frac{\overline{W}}{e}$ is the average energy expended per unit charge of ionization produced in the gas. Since mass of air in the cavity or chamber volume is not accurately known, one has to determine this volume indirectly from N_x (Equation 8.46). However, it may be pointed out that N_{gas} is independent of all properties of the chamber except its cavity volume (Equation 8.47).

If N_{gas} is not provided by the calibration laboratory, the user is required to calculate it. Table 8.3 gives ratios of N_{gas}/N_x for a number of commercially available chambers. It is seen that N_{gas}/N_x does not vary greatly between commonly used chambers. However, the user must follow the protocol to calculate N_{gas} for the given chamber and use Table 8.3 for comparison. Normally, chambers are recalibrated every 2 years and N_{gas} is calculated at each new calibration of the chamber.

C.3. $\frac{\overline{W}}{e}$

For dry air, $\frac{\overline{W}}{e}$ is independent of electron energy above a few kiloelectron volts and its currently accepted value is 33.97 ± 0.06 *J/C*. The TG-21 protocol (6) uses 33.7 *J/C*

TABLE 8.3. RATIOS OF N_{gas}/N_X FOR COMMERCIALLY AVAILABLE CHAMBERS

Chamber: Model No. (Wall-Build-Up Cap)	A_{wall}	α	$(L/\rho)^{wall}_{air}$ $\times (\mu_{en}/\rho)^{air}_{wall}$	$(L/\rho)^{cap}_{air}$ $\times (\mu_{en}/\rho)^{air}_{cap}$	$N_{gas}/(N_X A_{ion})$ (Gy/R)
Capintec: PR-06C, PR-06G (C552–polystyrene)	0.991	0.46	1.000	1.032	8.51×10^{-3}
Capintec: PR-05 (C552–polystyrene)	0.989	0.89	1.000	1.032	8.61×10^{-3}
Capintec: PR-05P (C552–polystyrene)	0.988	0.89	1.000	1.032	8.60×10^{-3}
Exradin: A1, Spokas (C552–C552)					
2-mm build-up cap	0.985	0.86	1.000	1.00	8.61×10^{-3}
4-mm build-up cap	0.976	0.86	1.000	1.00	8.53×10^{-3}
Exradin: T2, Spokas (A150–A150)	0.985	0.73	1.037	1.037	8.30×10^{-3}
Exradin: T1, min Shonka (A150–A150)	0.992	0.74	1.037	1.037	8.36×10^{-3}
Exradin: A3, Shonka–Wycoff (C552)	0.984	1.00	1.000	—	8.60×10^{-3}
NEL Farmer: 2505, '54–'59 (Tufnol–acrylic)	0.992	0.59	1.021	1.020	8.49×10^{-3}
NEL Farmer: 2505, '59–'67 (Tufnol–acrylic)	0.990	0.59	1.021	1.020	8.48×10^{-3}
NEL Farmer: 2505/A, '67–'74 (nylon–acrylic)	0.990	0.53	1.038	1.020	8.40×10^{-3}
NEL Farmer: 2505/3,3A, '71–'79 (graphite–acrylic)	0.990	0.54	1.009	1.020	8.53×10^{-3}
NEL Farmer: 2505/3,3B, '74– (nylon–acrylic)	0.990	0.40	1.038	1.020	8.42×10^{-3}
NEL Farmer: 2571, '79– (graphite–Delrin)	0.990	0.54	1.009	1.019	8.54×10^{-3}
NEL Farmer: 2581, '80– (A150–Lucentine)	0.990	0.39	1.037	1.032	8.37×10^{-3}
NEL NPL Secondary Standard: 2561 (graphite–Delrin)	0.984	0.65	1.009	1.019	8.49×10^{-3}
PTW: N23333, NA 30-351 3-mm build-up cap	0.993	0.51	1.020	1.020	8.50×10^{-3}
PTW: N23333, NA 30-351 NA 30-352, VIC 500-104 (acrylic-acrylic) 4.6-mm build-up cap	0.990	0.48	1.020	1.020	8.48×10^{-3}
PTW: N233331, NA 30-361 (acrylic–acrylic)	0.990	0.79	1.020	1.020	8.48×10^{-3}
PTW: M23332-Normal, NA 30-348 (acrylic–acrylic)	0.993	0.51	1.020	1.020	8.50×10^{-3}
PTW: M23331-Transit, NA 30-349 (acrylic–acrylic)	0.992	0.51	1.020	1.020	8.50×10^{-3}
PTW: N2333641, NA 30-316 (acrylic–acrylic)	0.992	0.65	1.020	1.020	8.50×10^{-3}
Victoreen: 555-100HA (Derlin)	0.990	1.00	1.019	—	8.49×10^{-3}
Victoreen: 550-6, 6A (polystyrene–acrylic)	0.991	0.74	1.032	1.020	8.42×10^{-3}
Far West: IC-17 (A150)	0.983	1.00	1.037	—	8.28×10^{-3}
Far West: IC-17A (A150–A150)	0.984	0.79	1.037	1.037	8.29×10^{-3}
Far West: IC-18 (A150–A150)	0.991	0.86	1.037	1.037	8.35×10^{-3}

From Gastorf R, Humphries L, Rozenfeld M. Cylindrical chamber dimensions and the corresponding values of A_{wall} and $N_{gas}/N_X A_{ion}$). Med Phys 1986;13:751, with permission.

in all its equations because at the time the protocol was written the accepted value of $\frac{\overline{W}}{e}$ for dry air was 33.85 J/C and was corrected for 50% relative humidity to give 33.7 J/C. Whereas users of the TG-21 protocol may stick to the original protocol for consistency reasons, the current understanding is that, since exposure is defined for dry air and N_x is already corrected for humidity effect by the standards laboratory, $\frac{\overline{W}}{e}$ value in the equations discussed earlier should pertain to dry air, i.e., 33.97 J/C.

C.4. Ion Recombination Correction: A_{ion}, P_{ion}

A_{ion} is a factor that corrects for incomplete collection of charge in the chamber at the time of its calibration at the standards laboratory. Because ^{60}Co sources used for chamber calibration usually have low dose rates, A_{ion} can be assumed equal to 1 for most chambers with adequate bias voltage.

P_{ion} corrects for ion recombination loss when the chamber is irradiated in the user's beam. This factor depends on the dose rate (or dose per pulse), chamber geometry and the bias voltage. A method for determining P_{ion} (two-voltage technique) has been discussed in Chapter 6. For a 0.6 cm^3 Farmer type chamber operating at a bias voltage of about 300 V and exposed to dose rates in the clinical range (~500 cGy/min or less), P_{ion} is usually less than 1.005.

C. 5. Wall-Correction Factors: A_{wall}, β_{wall}, P_{wall}

The A_{wall} correction factor occurs in the N_{gas} formula and accounts for attenuation and scatter of photons in the wall and build-up cap of the chamber when exposed in air to ^{60}Co γ ray beam. In Equation 8.36, A_{wall} appears as a ratio of photon energy fluence at the center of the cavity with the chamber and its build-up cap in place in air to that when the chamber is removed, i.e., $(\Psi_{wall})^{wall}_{air}$. This ratio is approximately given by $e^{-(\overline{\mu}_{en}/\rho) \cdot \rho x}$, where $\overline{\mu}_{en}/\rho$ is the average mass energy absorption coefficient for the ^{60}Co beam and ρx is the density thickness, both pertaining to the chamber wall and its build-up cap.

The AAPM protocol (6) provides a table of A_{wall} values for cylindrical chambers as a function of chamber wall (plus build-up cap) thickness and the length of the chamber volume. These values are based on Monte-Carlo calculation by Nath and Schultz (30). Table 8.3 gives A_{wall} for various commercially available chambers, derived from the same data (31).

β_{wall} is the quotient of absorbed dose to collision part of kerma in the wall under the conditions of transient electronic equilibrium. As discussed in section 8.2C, β_{wall} accounts for the difference between the point of interaction ("center of electron production") and the point of energy deposition. Its value is taken to be 1.005 for ^{60}Co.

Although the TG-21 protocol uses β_{wall} in addition to the A_{wall}, it is now understood (23,24,32) that the Monte-Carlo calculated values of A_{wall} include β_{wall}. Thus the use of β_{wall} in the AAPM protocol is an error. However, as pointed out earlier, some of the errors in the TG-21 protocol cancel each other and, therefore, no change was recommended in the protocol until a revised protocol was introduced.

P_{wall} is a correction factor that accounts for the difference between the composition of the chamber wall and the phantom as it pertains to photon beam interactions in the user's beam. This factor depends on beam energy, wall thickness, wall composition, and the fraction α of the cavity ionization contributed by electrons originating in the chamber wall. Calculations indicate that $P_{wall} \simeq 1$ when $\alpha < 0.25$. As can be deduced from Table 8.3, P_{wall} is close to unity for Farmer type chambers (wall thickness <0.1 g/cm^2) and photon energies ≥ 6 MV.

The expression for the calculation of P_{wall}, given by Equation 8.60, is different from the one in the TG-21 protocol. The reasons for the discrepancy have been discussed earlier. Again, because the differences are quite small, no variance is recommended if TG-21 protocol is followed.

C.6. Replacement Correction Factor, P_{repl}

From the previous discussion of this factor, it is evident that P_{repl} corrects for change in J_{air} (ionization charge per unit mass of cavity air) caused by the finite size of the cavity. According to Equation 8.58, if the measurement is made under the conditions of transient electronic equilibrium, P_{repl} is the ratio of photon energy fluence at the center of the cavity when the cavity is filled with medium to that when the cavity is filled with air.

This ratio is also the ratio of electron fluences with and without the cavity. One may call this a fluence correction factor or P_{fl}. However, when the electron fluence is measured with a cylindrical ion chamber, there is a shift in the point of measurement depending on the radius of the cavity (see section 8.4, C.2). Because of this shift upstream, the ionization measured is greater than if there was no shift or cavity radius was zero. The component of P_{repl} caused by the shift in the point of measurement is called the gradient correction or P_{gr}. The magnitude of P_{gr} is dependent on the gradient of the dose and the inner diameter of the ion chamber. Thus P_{repl} may be the thought of having two components, the gradient and fluence correction factor or $P_{repl} = P_{fl}P_{gr}$.

In the case of photon beams, fluence corrections are not needed if the measurements are made at d_{max} or beyond in a broad beam because transient electronic equilibrium exists there (33). Under these conditions, $P_{fl} = 1$ because electron spectrum is not changed by the presence of air cavity. P_{repl} for photon beams can therefore be equated to P_{gr} only if the chamber is positioned on the descending portion of the depth dose curve.

Replacement correction for electron beam calibration is more complex. Presence of the cavity alters the primary electron fluence because air scatters electrons less than the medium. Generally, the fluence correction factor is less 1 and its value depends on the depth in the medium (energy spectrum at the depth of measurement) and the size of the cavity. The gradient correction for electron beam calibration is ignored in TG-21 because the recommended point of measurement is at the depth of dose maximum, where there is no significant dose gradient. However, gradient correction is applied for the measurement of depth dose distribution. In practice, this is accomplished by shifting the entire depth dose curve through a distance of $0.5r$ toward the source, where r is the radius of the cylindrical cavity. In the case of plane-parallel chamber, P_{repl} is equated to unity and no shift correction is used as long as the point of measurement is taken at the proximal surface of the cavity.

C.7. Calibration Phantom

The TG-21 protocol (6) recommends that calibrations be expressed in terms of dose to water. Water, polystyrene, or acrylic phantoms may be used. Since in clinical dosimetry dose to soft tissue or muscle is the quantity of interest, one needs to convert D_{water} to D_{muscle} when dose is specified for patient treatments. This conversion is done by the following relationships:

For photon beams,

$$D_{muscle} = D_{water} \cdot (\overline{\mu}_{en}/\rho)_{water}^{muscle} \tag{8.68}$$

For electron beams,

$$D_{muscle} = D_{water} \cdot (\overline{S}/\rho)_{water}^{muscle} \tag{8.69}$$

The factors $(\overline{\mu}_{en}/\rho)_{water}^{muscle}$ and $(\overline{S}/\rho)_{water}^{muscle}$ vary only slightly with energy and may be equated to 0.99 for all photon and electron beams used clinically.

A calibration phantom must provide at least 5 cm margin laterally beyond field borders and at least 10 cm margin in depth beyond the point of measurement. This is to ensure full scatter conditions. Calibration depths for a megavoltage photon beams are recommended to be between 5- and 10-cm depth, depending on energy. Alternatively, a single depth of 10 cm may be used for all energies between ^{60}Co and 50 MV. Dose rate or dose per monitor unit is then calculated for the reference field size at the reference depth by using depth-dose distribution data.

For electron beams, the calibration depth recommended by TG-21 is the depth of dose maximum for the reference cone (e.g., 10×10 cm) and the given energy. For lower-energy electron beams (<10 MeV), the AAPM protocol recommends the use of plane-parallel chambers. These chambers may be calibrated in comparison with cylindrical chambers, using a calibration set up for a high-energy electron beam. The procedure is somewhat complicated by the fact that plane-parallel chambers are used in plastic phantoms, thereby creating additional uncertainties in the interconversion of dose to water and plastic media.

C.8. Simplified Equations

The TG-21 protocol (6) has worksheets for calculating N_{gas} and dose to water for photon and electron beam calibration. It is important that the user of this protocol complete these worksheets for any new chamber and a new beam to be calibrated. Once all the relevant calibration parameters have been established for the given chamber and the given beam, routine calibration checks can be performed using simplified equations and precalculated tables.

TABLE 8.4. CALIBRATION PARAMETERS FOR PHOTON BEAMS[a]

Energy (MV)	Calibration Depth (cm water)	Percent Depth Dose	$\left(\dfrac{\overline{L}}{\rho}\right)^{water}_{air}$	P_{repl}	F_{muscle}
^{60}Co	5	80.4	1.134	0.992	1.114
6	5	87.0	1.127	0.993	1.108
10	5	91.1	1.117	0.994	1.099
18	10	79.9	1.100	0.994	1.082
24	10	84.5	1.094	0.995	1.078

[a]Water phantom, 10 × 10-cm field at SSD = 100 cm, 0.6-mL PTW Farmer chamber N23333 (see Table 8.3 for characteristics). The mass energy absorption coefficient ratio, $(\overline{\mu}_{en}/\rho)^{muscle}_{water}$, is assumed to be 0.990 for all energies; $P_{wall} = 1$; F_{muscle} is defined by Eq. 8.71.

For photon beams, dose to muscle is given by:

$$D_{muscle} = M \cdot N_{gas} \cdot F_{muscle} \cdot P_{ion} \tag{8.70}$$

where

$$F_{muscle} = (\overline{L}/\rho)^{water}_{air} \cdot (\overline{\mu}_{en}/\rho)^{muscle}_{water} \cdot P_{wall} \cdot P_{repl} \tag{8.71}$$

Table 8.4 gives F_{muscle} values for a specific chamber and a number of photon beam energies. This table is reproduced here as an example and for rough comparisons.

For electron beams, D_{muscle} is given by:

$$D_{muscle} = M \cdot N_{gas} \cdot F_{muscle} \cdot P_{ion} \tag{8.72}$$

where

$$F_{muscle} = (\overline{L}/\rho)^{water}_{air} \cdot \left(\frac{\overline{S}}{\rho}\right)^{muscle}_{water} \cdot P_{repl} \tag{8.73}$$

Table 8.5 gives F_{muscle} values for a given chamber and a number of electron energies. Again these data may be used for rough comparisons if the user's chamber is not very different from Farmer type ion chamber used in these calculations.

In an *SSD type calibration* of a photon beam, a 10 × 10-cm field is placed at an SSD of 100 cm and the chamber is positioned at the recommended depth of calibration (e.g., 10 cm). Dose to muscle[3] per monitor unit is calculated and then converted to D_{muscle} at the reference depth of dose maximum (d_m) by using percent depth dose (P) at the depth of measurement.

$$D_{muscle}(\text{at } d_m) = \frac{D_{muscle}(\text{at the depth of measurement})}{P/100} \tag{8.74}$$

An *isocentric calibration* involves setting up of a 10 × 10-cm field at the recommended depth of calibration (e.g., 10 cm) and a source-to-chamber distance (SCD) of 100 cm. If TMR is the tissue-maximum ratio (discussed in Chapter 10) at the depth of measurement,

$$D_{muscle}(\text{at } d_m) = \frac{D_{muscle}(\text{at the depth of measurement})}{\text{TMR}} \tag{8.75}$$

8.6. AAPM TG-51 PROTOCOL

The TG-51 protocol (34) represents a major upgrade of the TG-21 protocol in several respects: (a) it is based on absorbed-dose-to-water calibration factor, $N^{60Co}_{D,W}$, instead of exposure or air kerma calibration of the ion chamber; (b) the user does not need to

---

[3]Although the AAPM protocol recommends calibration in terms of dose to water, many consider it more convenient to convert D_{water} to D_{muscle} at the time of calibration and set the accelerator in terms of dose to muscle per monitor unit.

TABLE 8.5. CALIBRATION PARAMETERS FOR ELECTRON BEAMS[a]

Energy (MeV)		Depth d_m (cm water)	Mean Energy (MeV) at d_m	$\left(\dfrac{\overline{L}}{\rho}\right)_{air}^{water}$	P_{repl}	F_{muscle}
Nominal	E_0					
6	5.66	1.3	3.2	1.077	0.960	1.020
9	8.62	1.9	5.0	1.052	0.965	1.005
12	11.53	2.1	7.5	1.025	0.974	0.985
15	14.63	2.1	10.5	1.002	0.982	0.971
18	17.59	1.5	14.7	0.979	0.991	0.958
22	20.85	1.5	18.0	0.967	0.993	0.948

[a]Water phantom, field size, 10 × 10 cm cone, SSD = 100 cm, energy derived from broad-beam depth dose distribution (25 × 25 cm field), 0.6-ml PTW Farmer chamber N23333 (see Table 8.3 for characteristics). $(\overline{S}/\rho)_{water}^{muscle}$ is assumed to be 0.987 for all energies, F_{muscle} is defined by Eq. 8.73, E_0 is the mean electron energy at the surface.

calculate any theoretical dosimetry factors; and (c) large tables of stopping-power ratios and mass-energy absorption coefficients are not needed. Although the adoption of TG-51 results in only modest improvement in dosimetric accuracy over the TG-21 protocol (1%–2%), the gain in simplicity is a significant factor from the user's point of view.

The theoretical aspects of TG-51 go back to the TG-21 formalism, especially in the calculation of correction factors such as $\overline{L}/\rho$ ratios, P_{wall}, P_{repl}, P_{ion}, $P_{polarity}$, $P_{gradient}$, $P_{fluence}$, etc. If these factors are normalized to reference conditions of absorbed-dose-to-water in a ^{60}Co beam, the formalism simplifies to the application of a quality conversion factor, which converts the calibration factor for a ^{60}Co beam to that for the user's beam.

The basic TG-51 equation for absorbed calibration is as follows:

$$D_w^Q = M k_Q N_{D,w}^{60_{Co}} \tag{8.76}$$

where D_w^Q is the absorbed dose to water at the reference point of measurement in a beam of quality Q; M is the electrometer reading that has been fully corrected for ion recombination, environmental temperature and pressure, electrometer calibration and chamber polarity effects; k_Q is the quality conversion factor that converts the absorbed-dose-to-water calibration factor for a ^{60}Co beam into the calibration factor for an arbitrary beam of quality Q; and $N_{D,w}^{60_{Co}}$ is the absorbed-dose-to-water calibration factor for the chamber in a ^{60}Co beam under reference conditions.

The reference point of measurement in Equation (8.76) is specified at the reference depth corresponding to the center of cavity for a cylindrical chamber and the front surface of the cavity for a plane parallel chamber. Although the effective point of measurement occurs upstream for a cylindrical chamber, the resulting gradient correction has already been taken into account in the k_Q factor.

A. Beam Quality, Q

1. Photon Beams

The TG-21 protocol specifies photon beam energy in terms of nominal accelerating potential which is shown to be related to "ionization ratio" (6). The ionization ratio is defined as the ratio of ionization charge or dose measured at 20-cm depth to that measured at 10-cm depth for a constant source to detector distance and a 10 × 10 cm^2 field at the plane of the chamber (isocentric geometry). This ionization ratio is the same as what is also known as TPR_{10}^{20} or $TPR_{20,10}$ used by Andreo and Brahme (35) and the International Atomic Energy Agency (IAEA) protocol (36). The AAPM TG-51 (34) protocol has instead recommended %dd(10)$_x$ as the beam quality-specifier. The quantity %dd(10)$_x$ is the photon component of the photon beam percentage depth dose at 10-cm depth in a 10 × 10 cm^2 field on the surface of a water phantom at an SSD of 100 cm. The pros and cons of using TPR_{10}^{20} versus %dd(10)$_x$ have been discussed in the literature (37,38).

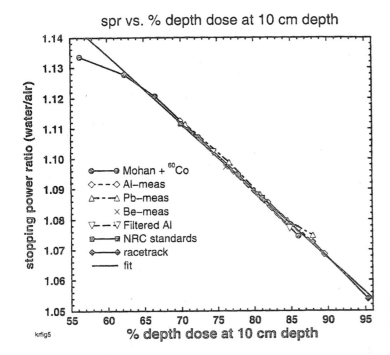

FIG. 8.6. spr vs. % depth dose at 10 cm depth

FIG. 8.6. A plot of water to air stopping power ratios as a function of %dd(10)$_x$. (From Kosunen A, Rogers DWO. Beam quality specification for photon beam dosimetry. *Med Phys* 1993;20:1013–1018, with permission.)

The rationale for %dd(10)$_x$ as a photon beam quality specifier is provided by Kosunen and Rogers (39) who showed that for any x-ray beam above 4 MV, there is a linear relationship between stopping powers ratios and %dd(10)$_x$ for the photon component of the beam (Fig. 8.6). Mathematically,

$$\left(\overline{L}/\rho\right)_{\text{air}}^{w} = 1.2676 - 0.002224(\%dd(10)_x) \qquad (8.77)$$

Determination of %dd(10)$_x$ requires that the photon beam be free of electron contamination. Because it is impossible to remove electron contamination completely from clinical photon beams, the TG-51 protocol recommends that %dd(10)$_x$ be measured by interposing a 1-mm-thick lead (Pb) foil in the beam at a distance of about 50 cm from the phantom surface. This arrangement minimizes the electron contamination incident at the phantom surface as the lead foil acts as an electron filter (40).

For photon beams of energy less than 10 MV, the contribution of dose at $d_{\max}$ from incident electron contamination is minimal for a 10 × 10 cm^2. So the %dd(10) measured in an open beam without lead may be equated to the %dd(10)$_x$. The use of lead foil, however, is recommended for %dd(10)$_x$ measurement for energies of 10 MV or higher.

Calculation of %dd(10)$_x$ for various beam energies involves the following equations, as recommended by TG -51:

$$\%dd(10)_x = \%dd(10) \qquad [\text{for } \%dd(10) \leq 75\%] \qquad (8.78)$$

$$\%dd(10)_x = [0.8905 + 0.00150\%dd(10)_{Pb}]\%dd(10)_{Pb} \ [\text{for } \%dd(10)_{Pb} \geq 73\% \qquad (8.79)$$

It should be noted that the Pb foil is used only when determining the beam quality specifier, %dd(10)$_x$, and must be removed at the conclusion of that determination. In addition, if the measurement of depth doses involves a cylindrical chamber, the depth dose curve must be corrected for gradient effects, that is, shift of the curve upstream by 0.6r$_{\text{cav}}$, where r$_{\text{cav}}$ is the radius of the chamber cavity.

In case the lead foil is not available, an approximate relationship for the determination of %dd(10)$_x$ on an interim basis is recommended by TG-51:

$$\%dd(10)_x = 1.267\%dd(10) - 20.0 \qquad [\text{for } 75\% < \%dd(10) \leq 89\%] \qquad (8.80)$$

The previous equation is based on a global fit to data (33) and in extreme cases may lead to an error in k_Q or absorbed dose of 0.4%.

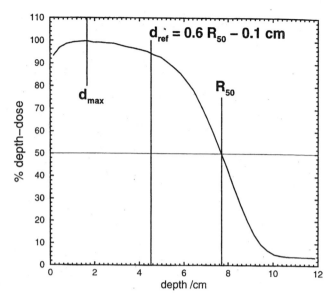

FIG. 8.7. A typical electron beam depth dose curve showing depth of maximum dose (d_{max}), depth of 50% dose (R_{50}) and depth for clinic reference dosimetry (d_{ref}). (From AAPM. AAPM's TG-51 protocol for clinical reference dosimetry of high-energy photon and electron beams. *Med Phys* 1999;26:1847–1870, with permission.)

2. Electron Beams

The beam quality for electron beam dosimetry is specified by R_{50}, the depth in water (in centimeters) at which the percent depth dose is 50% for a "broad beam" (field size at the phantom surface $\geq 10 \times 10$ cm^2 for energies up to 20 MeV or 20×20 cm^2 for all energies in the clinical range) at an SSD of 100 cm. Figure 8.7 shows a typical electron beam depth dose curve with d_{max}, d_{ref} (reference depth of calibration) and R_{50} indicated.

R_{50} for a broad beam (e.g., 20×20 cm^2 field size) may be determined by measurement of dose at two points on central axis: one at d_{max} and the other at depth where the dose falls to 50% of the maximum dose. If a cylindrical ion chamber is used for this measurement, the point of d_{max} should correspond to where the chamber reads maximum ionization on central axis. A point is then located downstream on central axis where the ionization measured is 50% of the maximum value. The depth of 50% ionization (I_{50}) is determined by subtracting $0.5r_{cav}$ from the depth indicated by the center of chamber cavity. The beam quality specifier, R_{50}, is then calculated from I_{50} (41):

$$R_{50} = 1.029\,I_{50} - 0.06\,(\text{cm}) \qquad [\text{for } 2 \leq I_{50} \leq 10 \text{ cm}] \qquad (8.81)$$

or

$$R_{50} = 1.059\,I_{50} - 0.37\,(\text{cm}) \qquad [\text{for } I_{50} > 10 \text{ cm}] \qquad (8.82)$$

Alternatively, R_{50} may be determined from the depth ionization curve (measured with a cylindrical chamber), which has been corrected for gradient effects by shifting the entire curve upstream by $0.5r_{cav}$ (Fig. 8.8) and converting I_{50} to R_{50} by using the above Equations. If a water phantom scanner with ion chamber is used, most systems are equipped with software to convert depth ionization curves into depth-dose curves using appropriate factors (e.g., $(\overline{L}/\rho)^w_{air}$ and P_{repl} or $P_{fl} \cdot P_{gr}$, as a function of depth). This allows a quick determination of important dosimetry parameters such as d_{max}, d_{ref}, R_{50}, and R_p.

If a diode or film is used to determine depth-dose distribution in a water or water equivalent phantom, the detector response as a function of depth gives depth dose curve directly without further corrections (section 14.3B). However, it is important to establish

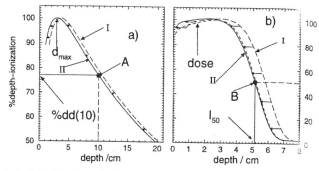

FIG. 8.8. Shifting of depth ionization curves upstream by $0.6r_{cav}$ for photons and $0.5r_{cav}$ for electrons in order to correct for shift in the point of measurement when using a cylindrical ion chamber of cavity radius, r_{cav}. (From AAPM. AAPM's TG-51 protocol for clinical reference dosimetry of high-energy photon and electron beams. *Med Phys* 1999; 26:1847–1870, with permission.)

first by suitable benchmark tests, that these dosimetry systems agree with corrected ion chamber dosimetry.

B. Quality Conversion Factor, k_Q

By definition, k_Q is given by:

$$k_Q = N_{D,w}^Q / {}^{60}Co_{N_{D,w}} \tag{8.83}$$

From TG-21 Equation [8.57]:

$$N_{D,w} = D_w / M P_{ion} = N_{gas} \left(\overline{L}/\rho \right)_{air}^w P_{wall} P_{repl} \tag{8.84}$$

As discussed earlier (section 8.5, C.6), P_{repl} has two components, the gradient and fluence correction factors:

$$P_{repl} = P_{gr} P_{fl} \tag{8.85}$$

Equation 8.84 may be further revised by multiplying the right hand side of the equation by the central electrode correction factor, P_{cel}. This factor was ignored by the TG-21 protocol but it is included in the k_Q values of the TG-51 protocol. The central electrode effect is quite small for electron beams (<0.2%), but for photon beams it has been shown to be significant. For example, P_{cel} for Farmer-like chambers with an aluminum electrode of 1 mm diameter varies between 0.993 for ${}^{60}Co$ to 0.996 for 24 MV x-rays (42).

From Equations 8.83, 8.84, and 8.85 along with the use of P_{cel} we get the expression for k_Q:

$$k_Q = \frac{\left[\left(\overline{L}/\rho \right)_{air}^w P_{wall} P_{gr} P_{fl} P_{cel} \right]_Q}{\left[\left(\overline{L}/\rho \right)_{air}^w P_{wall} P_{gr} P_{fl} P_{cel} \right]_{{}^{60}Co}} \tag{8.86}$$

1. k_Q for Photon Beams

Using the above relationship, Rogers (33) calculated k_Q values for a variety of commercially available cylindrical ion chambers as a function of photon beam energy from ${}^{60}Co$ to 24 MV. These data comprise Table I of the TG-51 protocol and are reproduced here in Table 8.6. Data for plane-parallel chambers are not included because of insufficient information about P_{wall} in photon beams, other than ${}^{60}Co$ for which $k_Q = 1$ by definition for all chambers.

2. k_Q for Electron Beams

Although Equation 8.76 is general and can be applied for both photon and electron beams (see IAEA Protocol, section 8.7), authors of the TG-51 Protocol felt that for electron beams

TABLE 8.6. k_Q VALUES FOR ACCELERATOR PHOTON-BEAMS AS A FUNCTION OF %DD(10)$_x$ FOR CYLINDRICAL ION CHAMBERS

Ion Chamber	kq					
	%dd(10)$_x$					
	58.0	63.0	66.0	71.0	81.0	93.0
Capintec PR-05/PR-05P	0.999	0.997	0.995	0.990	0.972	0.948
Capintec PR-06C/G 0.6cc Farmer	1.000	0.998	0.994	0.987	0.968	0.944
Exradin A1 Shonka[a]	0.999	0.998	0.996	0.990	0.972	0.948
Exradin A12 Farmer	1.000	0.999	0.996	0.990	0.972	0.948
NE2505/3,3A 0.6cc Farmer	1.000	0.998	0.995	0.988	0.972	0.951
NE2561 0.3cc NPL Sec. Std[b]	1.000	0.998	0.995	0.989	0.974	0.953
NE2571 0.6cc Farmer	1.000	0.998	0.995	0.988	0.972	0.951
NE2577 0.2cc	1.000	0.998	0.995	0.988	0.972	0.951
NE2581 0.6cc robust Farmer	1.000	0.994	0.988	0.979	0.960	0.937
PTW N30001 0.6cc Farmer[c]	1.000	0.996	0.992	0.984	0.967	0.945
PTW N30002 0.6cc all Graphite	1.000	0.997	0.994	0.987	0.970	0.948
PTW N30004 0.6cc Graphite	1.000	0.998	0.995	0.988	0.973	0.952
PTW 31003 0.3cc waterproof[d]	1.000	0.996	0.992	0.984	0.967	0.946
Wellhofer IC-10/IC-5	1.000	0.999	0.996	0.989	0.971	0.946

For ^{60}Co beams, $k_Q = 1.000$ by definition.
[a]The cavity radius of the A1 here is 2 mm although in the past Exradin has designated chambers with another radius as A1.
[b]The NE2611 has replaced the equivalent NE2561.
[c]PTW N30001 is equivalent to the PTW N23333 it replaced.
[d]PTW N31003 is equivalent to the PTW N233641 it replaced.
From AAPM. AAPM's TG-51 protocol for clinical reference dosimetry of high-energy photon and electron beams. Med Phys 1999; 26:1847–1870, with permission.

the P_{gr}^Q factor in Equation (8.86) at the reference point of measurement may vary from one accelerator to another and therefore must be measured in the user's beam. Thus k_Q has been redefined for electron beams by the following equations (43):

$$k_Q = P_{gr}^Q k_{R_{50}} \qquad (8.87)$$

where

$$k_{R_{50}} = \frac{\left[(\overline{L}/\rho)_{air}^w P_{wall} P_{fl} P_{cel}\right]_Q}{\left[(\overline{L}/\rho)_{air}^w P_{wall} P_{fl} P_{cel}\right]_{60_{Co}}} \qquad (8.88)$$

and P_{gr}^Q is the gradient correction at the reference depth of measurement. The reference depth, called d_{ref}, for electron beams is based on recommendation by Burns et al. (44) and is given by:

$$d_{ref} = 0.6 R_{50} - 0.1 \qquad (8.89)$$

The gradient correction at the reference depth is given by:

$$P_{gr}^Q = I(d_{ref} + 0.5 r_{cav})/I(d_{ref}) \qquad \text{[for cylindrical chambers]} \qquad (8.90)$$

$$= 1.0 \quad \text{[for plane-parallel chambers]} \qquad (8.91)$$

where $I(d)$ is the ionization reading of the cylindrical chamber with the cylindrical axis at depth d.

Further, the authors of TG-51 thought that the values of $k_{R_{50}}$ for different ion chambers vary considerably (43) and that there was no provision in this formalism for a future possibility of having chamber calibration factors measured directly for electron beams. These drawbacks could be avoided by arriving at $k_{R_{50}}$ in two steps instead of the one derived directly by quality comparison with ^{60}Co. Thus, $k_{R_{50}}$ is redefined as:

$$k_{R_{50}} = k_{ecal} k'_{R_{50}} \qquad (8.92)$$

where k_{ecal} is the quality conversion factor for a reference electron beam of high energy with an arbitrary beam quality Q_e of $R_{50} = 7.5$ cm, relative to ^{60}Co.

$$k_{ecal} = \frac{N_{D,w}^{Q_e}}{P_{gr}^{Q_e} N_{D,w}^{^{60}Co}} \tag{8.93}$$

or, from Equation 8.88:

$$k_{ecal} = k_{R_{50}}(Q_e) = \frac{\left[(\overline{L}/\rho)_{air}^{w} P_{wall} P_{fl} P_{cel}\right]_{Q_e}}{\left[(\overline{L}/\rho)_{air}^{w} P_{wall} P_{fl} P_{cel}\right]_{^{60}Co}} \tag{8.94}$$

and $k'_{R_{50}}$ is the quality conversion factor for the given electron beam of quality Q relative to the reference electron beam of quality Q_e, that is,

$$k'_{R_{50}} = \frac{\left[(\overline{L}/\rho)_{air}^{w} P_{wall} P_{fl} P_{cel}\right]_{Q}}{\left[(\overline{L}/\rho)_{air}^{w} P_{wall} P_{fl} P_{cel}\right]_{Q_e}} \tag{8.95}$$

Values of k_{ecal} for the plane-parallel and cylindrical ion chambers have been calculated using Equation 8.94 (43) and are presented in Tables II and III of the TG-51 protocol (34). These are reproduced in Tables 8.7 and 8.8 of this chapter. The values of $k'_{R_{50}}$ for Farmer-like cylindrical chambers and plane-parallel chambers are calculated by Rogers (43) using the following equations respectively:

$$k'_{R_{50}}(\text{cyl}) = 0.9905 + 0.0710 e^{(-R_{50}/3.67)} \tag{8.96}$$

and

$$k'_{R_{50}}(\text{pp}) = 1.2239 - 0.145(R_{50})^{0.214} \tag{8.97}$$

C. Calibration Phantom

TG-51 requires that the calibration of photon and electron beams be performed in a water phantom. The recommended dimensions of the phantom are at least $30 \times 30 \times 30$ cm^3. If the beam enters the phantom from the side through a plastic wall, all depths must be scaled to water equivalent depths using a scaling factor of 1 cm acrylic = 1.12 cm H$_2$O.

D. Chamber Waterproofing

A cylindrical ion chamber may be waterproofed using a thin ($\leq$ 1-mm thick) acrylic sleeve. The chamber should slip into the sleeve with little resistance and with minimal air gaps

TABLE 8.7. k_{ecal} **VALUES FOR PLANE-PARALLEL CHAMBERS, ADOPTING A REFERENCE BEAM QUALITY Q$_{ecal}$ OF R$_{50}$ = 7.5 cm**

Chamber	k_{ecal}
Attix	0.883
Capintec	0.921
PTB/Roos	0.901
Extradin	0.888
Holt	0.900
Markus	0.905
NACP	0.888

From AAPM. AAPM's TG-51 protocol for clinical reference dosimetry of high-energy photon and electron beams. Med Phys 1999;26:1847–1970, with permission.

TABLE 8.8. k_{ecal} VALUES FOR CYLINDRICAL CHAMBERS, ADOPTING A REFERENCE ELECTRON BEAM QUALITY Q_{ecal} OF $R_{50} = 7.5$ cm

| Chamber | k_{ecal} | Wall | | | Al Electrode Diameter (mm) |
		Material	Thickness g/cm^2	Cavity Radius r_{cav} (cm)	
Farmer-like					
Exradin A12	0.906	C-552	0.088	0.305	
NE2505/3,3A	0.903	Graphite	0.065	0.315	1.0
NE2561^a	0.904	Graphite	0.090	0.370^e	1.0
NE2571	0.903	Graphite	0.065	0.315	1.0
NE2577	0.903	Graphite	0.065	0.315	1.0
NE2581	0.885	A-150	0.041	0.315	
Capintec PR-06C/G	0.900	C-552	0.050	0.320	
PTW N23331	0.896	Graphite	0.012	0.395^e	1.0
		PMMA	0.048		
PTW N30001^b	0.897	Graphite	0.012	0.305	1.0
		PMMA	0.033		
PTW N30002	0.900	Graphite	0.079	0.305	
PTW N30004	0.905	Graphite	0.079	0.305	1.0
PTW N31003^c	0.898	Graphite	0.012	0.275	1.0^f
		PMMA	0.066		
Other cylindrical					
Exradin A1^d	0.915	C-552	0.176	0.200	
Capintec PR-05/PR-05P	0.916	C-552	0.210	0.200	
Wellhofer IC-10/IC-5	0.904	C-552	0.070	0.300	

^{a}The NE2611 has replaced the equivalent NE2561.
^{b}PTW N30001 is equivalent to the PTW N23333 it replaced.
^{c}PTW N31003 is equivalent to the PTW N233641 it replaced.
^{d}The cavity radius of the A1 here is 2 mm although in the past Exradin has designated chambers with another radius as A1.
^{e}In electron beams there are only data for cavity radii up to 0.35 cm and so 0.35 cm is used rather than the real cavity radius shown here.
^{f}Electrode diameter is actually 1.5 mm, but only data for 1.0 mm is available
From AAPM. AAPM's TG-51 protocol for clinical reference dosimetry of high-energy photon and electron beams. Med Phys 1999;26:1847–1970, with permission.

around the thimble (≤ 0.2 mm). Another option is to use a latex condom but without any talcum powder because the talcum powder could leak into the chamber cavity. Waterproof chambers or chambers with waterproofing kits are also commercially available.

E. Charge Measurement

The fully corrected charge reading, M, from an ion chamber is given by:

$$M = M_{raw} P_{ion} P_{T,P} P_{elec} P_{pol} \qquad (8.98)$$

where M_{raw} is the raw chamber reading in coulombs or the instrument's reading; P_{ion} is the ion recombination correction; $P_{T,P}$ is the air temperature and pressure correction; P_{elec} is the electrometer calibration factor; and P_{pol} is the polarity correction. Rationale for these correction factors has been discussed.

1. P_{ion}

The ion recombination correction has been discussed in section 6.8. In one of the methods, the chamber readings are taken with full voltage and with half-voltage. The ratio of the two readings is related to P_{ion} which is read off from a curve corresponding to the type of beam: pulsed, pulsed scanning or continuous radiation (Fig. 6.17). Alternatively, TG-51 recommends measurements at two voltages: the normal operating voltage, V_H and approximately half-voltage V_L. If the corresponding chamber readings are M_{raw}^H and M_{raw}^L, then P_{ion} at V_H is given by:

$$P_{\text{ion}}(V_H) = \frac{1 - (V_H/V_L)^2}{M_{\text{raw}}^H/M_{\text{raw}}^L - (V_H/V_L)^2}$$

[for a continuous radiation, i.e., ^{60}Co beam] (8.99)

or

$$P_{\text{ion}}(V_H) = \frac{1 - (V_H/V_L)}{M_{\text{raw}}^H/M_{\text{raw}}^L - (V_H/V_L)}$$ [for pulsed or scanning beams] (8.100)

2. $P_{T,P}$

In the United States, the calibration laboratories [National Institute of Standards and Technology (NIST) and Accredited Dose Calibration Laboratories (ADCLs)] provide chamber calibration factors for standard environmental conditions of temperature $T_o = 22°C$ and pressure $P_o = 760$ mm Hg or 101.33 kP$_a$ (1 atmosphere). The temperature and pressure correction, $P_{T,P}$, is given by:

$$P_{T,P} = \left(\frac{760}{P}\right)\left(\frac{273.2 + T}{273.2 + 22.0}\right)$$ [for P in mm of Hg] (8.101)

or

$$P_{T,P} = \left(\frac{101.33}{P}\right)\left(\frac{273.2 + T}{273.2 + 22.0}\right)$$ [for P in kP$_a$] (8.102)

The rationale for the use of temperature and pressure correction for ion chamber readings has been discussed in section 6.10.

3. P_{elec}

The electrometer correction factor, P_{elec}, depends on whether the electrometer is detached or forms an integral unit with the ion chamber. If separate, the electrometer must bear a calibration factor for charge measurement. P_{elec} corrects the electrometer reading to true coulombs. Its unit of measurement is C/C or C/rdg. If the electrometer and ion chamber form a single unit, $P_{\text{elec}} = 1.00$.

4. P_{pol}

Chamber polarity effects depend on the chamber design, cable position, and beam quality (see section 6.9). P_{pol} is the polarity correction factor, which corrects chamber's response for possible polarity effects.

Measurement of P_{pol} involves taking chamber readings with both polarities and determining P_{pol} from:

$$P_{\text{pol}} = \left|\frac{(M_{\text{raw}}^+ - M_{\text{raw}}^-)}{2 M_{\text{raw}}}\right|$$ (8.103)

where M_{raw}^+ is the reading when positive charge is collected and M_{raw}^- is the reading when negative charge is collected, and M_{raw} is the reading corresponding to the polarity used for beam calibration (which is recommended to be the same as used for the chamber calibration). It should be noted that the sign of the charge for M_{raw}^+ and M_{raw}^- (which would normally be opposite) is to be carried in Equation 8.103. Also sufficient time should be given between polarity changes to stabilize the readings.

F. Chamber Calibration Factor, $N_w^{^{60}Co}$

The TG-51 protocol is based on absorbed-dose-to-water calibration factor,

$$N_{D,w}^{^{60}Co} = \frac{D_w^{^{60}Co}}{M} (\text{Gy/C or Gy/rdg}) \qquad (8.104)$$

where $D_w^{^{60}Co}$ is the absorbed dose to water in the calibration laboratory's ^{60}Co beam under reference conditions, at the chamber's point of measurement in the absence of the chamber. As discussed earlier, the calibration factor applies under standard environmental conditions, viz. 22°C, 101.33 kP$_a$, and relative humidity between 20% and 80%. The calibration factor can be obtained from ADCLs in the United States (traceable to NIST).

The NIST's primary standard for the absorbed-dose-to-water calibration of the chamber is currently based on absolute dosimetry with a calorimeter. Transfer ion chambers are used at the ADCLs to provide NIST traceable calibrations.

G. Photon Beam Calibration

The TG-51 provides worksheets to guide the user in a step-by-step implementation of the protocol. These worksheets are highly recommended for the original reference calibration. Simpler forms or worksheets may be designed for routine calibration checks.

The essential equipment for the reference absorbed dose calibration consists of a suitable water phantom, a chamber holder, a waterproof sleeve (if chamber is not waterproof), an ion chamber with calibration factor $N_{D,w}^{^{60}Co}$, electrometer with calibration factor P_{elec}, a calibrated barometer and a calibrated thermometer. One-mm thick lead sheet should be available that can be placed in the beam at a distance of 50 ± 5 cm from the phantom surface. For use at shorter distances such as 30 ± 1 cm, see TG-51 protocol.

Although full details are available in the TG-51 protocol and its worksheets, the calibration steps are summarized below as a quick review:

1. Set up water phantom for calibration.
2. Determine beam quality, i.e. %dd(10)$_x$:
   (a) Set field size at surface, 10×10 cm^2, at SSD = 100 cm.
   (b) Measure %dd(10) with open beam (no lead sheet). For the D_{max} or peak dose measurement, the chambers should be placed where the reading for a set number of monitor units (e.g., 200 MU) is maximum on the central axis. For the dose at 10 cm depth, the center of chamber should be placed at $(10 + 0.6r_{cav})$cm.
   (c) The ratio of ionization at 10 cm depth to that at d_{max} times 100 gives %dd (10). If the beam energy is <10 MV, then %dd(10)$_x$ = %dd(10).
   (d) If the beam energy is ≥10 MV, use 1-mm lead sheet in the beam at a distance of 50 ± 5 cm from the surface. Measure %dd(10)$_{Pb}$ as in (b) above.
   (e) Use Equation 8.79 to determine %dd(10)$_x$ if %dd(10)$_{Pb}$ is ≥73 %; or Equation 8.80 if the lead is not used and %dd(10) is greater than 75% but not exceeding 89%.
   (f) Remove the lead sheet.
3. Depending on the chamber model, determine k_Q corresponding to %dd(10)$_x$ (Table 8.6).
4. Measure temperature and pressure to get $P_{T,P}$ (Eq. 8.101 or 8.102).
5. Measure M_{raw}^+ and M_{raw}^- to determine P_{pol} (Eq. 8.103).
6. Measure M_{raw}^h and M_{raw}^L to determine P_{ion} at V_H (Eq. 8.100).
7. Set 10×10 cm^2 field size at the surface with SSD = 100 cm (SSD-type calibration) or at isocenter with SSD = 90 cm (SAD-type calibration).
8. Position the chamber with its center of cavity at 10 cm depth.
9. Irradiate for a set number of monitor units (e.g., 200 MU). Take an average of at least three consistent ion chamber readings. The fully corrected reading M is given by

Equation 8.98:

$$M = M_{\text{raw}} P_{T,P} P_{\text{ion}} P_{\text{elec}} P_{\text{pol}}$$

10. Dose to water at 10 cm depth:

$$D_w^Q = M k_Q N_{D,w}^{^{60}\text{Co}}$$

11. Dose per monitor unit at reference d_{max}[4]
    (a) For SSD-type calibration,

$$\text{Dose/MU} = \frac{D_w^Q}{MU} \times \frac{100}{\%\text{dd}(10,10 \times 10)}$$

    (b) For SAD-type calibration,

$$\text{Dose/MU} = \frac{D_w^Q}{MU} \times \frac{1}{\text{TMR}(10,10 \times 10)}$$

Note that the gradient correction for shift in the chamber point of measurement is included as part of k_Q. So the measurement depth of 10 cm for calibration is set at the center of chamber cavity. Also, the values of $\%\text{dd}(10,10 \times 10)$ and TMR $(10,10 \times 10)$ used in step 11 above must be derived from data that have been corrected for shift in the chamber's point of measurement if a cylindrical chamber had been used in the acquisition of the data.

H. Electron Beam Calibration

Because of the severe depth dose gradients and increased perturbations caused by chamber cavity in a low energy electron beam, the TG-51 protocol recommends the use of plane-parallel chamber for electrons with $R_{50} \leq 2.6$ cm (incident energies of 6 MeV or less). It offers two methods of obtaining $k_{\text{ecal}} N_{D,w}^{^{60}\text{Co}}$ for plane-parallel chambers: one by cross-calibration against a calibrated cylindrical chamber (preferred method) and the other by using ^{60}Co absorbed-dose calibration factor for the plane-parallel chamber. The reader is referred to TG-51 protocol for details on the use of plane-parallel chamber for calibration.

Although the use of plane-parallel chamber for calibration offers some advantages, for example, absence of gradient correction and minimal fluence perturbation correction, the disadvantages include the lack of absorbed-dose-to-water calibration factor by the ADCLs, the difficulty of waterproofing the chamber, and eliminating water pressure on the thin window of the plane-parallel chamber. Because of these drawbacks, some users ignore the protocol recommendation and use Farmer-type chambers for the whole range of clinically useful energies, for example, from 6 MeV to 20 MeV and higher.

In this section, the calibration steps with cylindrical chambers will be summarized for a quick review.

1. Determine beam quality or R_{50}. This parameter can be determined by point measurements or obtained from the pre-measured depth dose curve, corrected for stopping power ratios and all the perturbation effects as discussed in section 14.3B. A broad beam (e.g., 20×20 cm^2) is used for these measurements.
2. For the given chamber, determine k_{ecal} (Table 8.8).
3. For the given beam energy, determine $k'_{R_{50}}$ (Eq. 8.96).
4. Set up reference conditions for calibration:

   Field size = 10×10 cm^2, SSD = 100 cm, center of chamber cavity at d_{ref}
   $$= 0.6 R_{50} - 0.1$$

---

[4] Reference d_{max} is the fixed d_{max} used for normalizing percent depth dose and TMR data for all field sizes (see Chapter 10).

5. Measure $P_{T,P}$, P_{pol}, and P_{ion}.
6. Irradiate for a set number of monitor units (e.g., 200 MU) and take an average of at least three consistent readings. The fully corrected reading M at d_{ref} is given by:

$$M = M_{raw} P_{ion} P_{T,P} P_{elec} P_{pol}$$

7. Determine gradient correction at d_{ref}:

$$P_{gr}^Q = \frac{M_{raw}(d_{ref} + 0.5r_{cav})}{M_{raw}(d_{ref})}$$

8. Dose to water at d_{ref}:

$$D_w^Q = M P_{gr}^Q k_{ecal} k'_{R_{50}} N_{D,w}^{^{60}Co}$$

9. Dose per monitor unit at $d_{ref} = \frac{D_w^Q}{MU}$
10. Dose per monitor unit at d_{max}

$$= \frac{D_w^Q}{MU} \times \frac{100}{\%dd(d_{ref})}$$

Note that the calibration measurement is made with the center of chamber cavity at d_{ref}. The gradient correction at d_{ref} due to shift in the point of measurement is determined separately and applied explicitly (unlike photons). The $\%dd(d_{ref})$ is obtained from depth dose data which have been corrected for changes in $\left(\overline{L}/\rho\right)_{air}^w$ and perturbation effects if the data were acquired by an ion chamber.

8.7. IAEA TRS 398 PROTOCOL

The IAEA published its most recent calibration protocol, Technical Report Series (TRS) No. 398, in 2000 (36). This protocol supersedes the previous IAEA TRS-277 protocol (45). The development of TRS-398 has paralleled that of the AAPM TG-51 protocol. Consequently, the two protocols are very similar in their formalisms and both are based on absorbed-dose-to-water calibration of the ion chamber in a cobalt-60 beam. Having presented TG-21 and TG-51 in the previous sections, the TRS-398 will be discussed only briefly, primarily to highlight its differences from TG-51. The user of the TRS-398 protocol is advised to follow the protocol document in all its details.

A. Formalism

The basic equation for the determination of absorbed dose to water for a beam of quality Q is the same as the TG-51 equation (Eq. 8.76). Using IAEA's notation,

$$D_{w,Q} = M_Q N_{D,w,Q_0} k_{Q,Q_0} \tag{8.105}$$

where $D_{w,Q}$ is the absorbed dose to water in the user's beam of quality Q, N_{D,w,Q_0} is the chamber calibration factor in terms of absorbed dose to water in the reference beam of quality Q_0 (e.g., ^{60}Co), k_{Q,Q_0} is the factor that corrects for the effects of the difference between the reference beam quality Q_0 and the user quality Q and M_Q is the fully corrected chamber reading. M_Q is given by:

$$M_Q = M_1 h_{pl} k_{TP} k_{elec} k_{pol} K_s \tag{8.106}$$

where M_1 is the dosimeter reading at the normal voltage V_1, h_{pl} is the phantom dependent fluence scaling factor to correct for the difference in electron fluence in plastic (if calibration is performed in a plastic phantom) with that in water at an equivalent depth, k_{TP} is the temperature and pressure correction factor:

$$k_{TP} = \frac{P_0 (273.2 + T)}{P (273.2 + T_0)} \tag{8.107}$$

(noting that many international Primary Standards Laboratories specify reference air temperature of 20°C [instead of 22°C in the United States]), k_{elec} is the electrometer calibration factor, k_{pol} is the chamber polarity correction factor (the same as Eq. 8.103), and k_s is the ion recombination correction.

In the TRS-398, k_s is determined by taking chamber readings M_1 and M_2 at voltages of V_1 (normal operating voltage) and V_2 (half of V_1 or less) and calculating k_s by:

$$k_s = \alpha_0 + \alpha_1 (M_1 / M_2) + \alpha_2 (M_1 / M_2)^2 \tag{8.108}$$

where α_0, α_1, and α_2 are constants that depend on type of beam (pulsed or pulse-scanned). In continuous radiation (e.g., ^{60}Co), the two voltage method may also be used using the relationship:

$$k_s = \frac{(V_1 / V_2)^2 - 1}{(V_1 / V_2)^2 - (M_1 / M_2)} \tag{8.109}$$

For pulsed and pulse-scanned beams, values of α_0, α_1, and α_2 are provided by Table 9 of the protocol.

B. Beam Quality, Q

1. Photon Beams

A major difference between TG-51 and TRS-398 consists of beam quality specification. Whereas, TG-51 recommends %dd(10)$_x$ (see section 8.6A), TRS-398 specifies beam quality by TPR$_{20,10}$. Although the choice of one or the other has been debated in the literature (37,38), this difference has little effect on the end result, namely, the calculation of k_Q or absorbed dose to water. In my opinion, the TPR$_{20,10}$ method is simpler to implement as it avoids the use of a lead filter or dose measurement at d_{max} which is somewhat messy (e.g., width of dose peak relative to chamber cavity diameter and the question of residual electron contamination at d_{max} in spite of the lead filter). In addition, the determination of TPR$_{20,10}$ does not require displacement correction nor is it sensitive to small systematic errors in positioning of the chamber at each depth. However, the user of either protocol is advised to follow the respective method recommended by the protocol.

The experimental setup for the determination of TPR$_{20,10}$ is the same as that for the ionization ratio recommended by the TG-21 protocol (see section 8.6A). The source-to-chamber distance is kept constant at 100 cm and the measurements are made with 10 cm and 20 cm of water over the chamber. The field size at the chamber position is 10×10 cm^2. As previously mentioned, there is no need to use displacement correction. The ratio of ionization at 20cm depth to that at 10cm depth gives the TPR$_{20,10}$.

It has been shown (37) that the restricted stopping power ratio, $(\overline{L}/\rho)_{air}^w$, for all clinical beams decreases with increase in TPR$_{20,10}$ in a sigmoid relationship which has been represented by a cubic polynomial, fitting the data to better than 0.15%. The quality conversion factors, k_{Q,Q_0} (or k_Q in the notation of TG-51) can then be calculated using stopping power ratios and perturbation factors (Eq. 8.86).

2. Electron Beams

The specification of beam quality in the TRS-398 protocol is the same as in the TG-51 protocol, namely, by R_{50} (see section 8.6A.2). A broad beam (e.g., 20×20 cm^2) is recommended for the measurement of R_{50}.

C. Quality Conversion Factor, k_{Q,Q_0}

1. Photon Beams

Using TPR$_{20,10}$ as the index of beam quality, Andreo (46) has calculated k_{Q,Q_0} values for a variety of commercially available ion chambers and photon beams of TPR$_{20,10}$, ranging from 0.5 to 0.84. These values are presented in Table 14 of the TRS-398 protocol.

2. Electron Beams

TRS-398 deviates from the TG-51 methodology in that it directly calculates k_{Q,Q_0} for electrons using relevant stopping power ratios and perturbation factors (see Eq. 8.86) instead of redefining k_{Q,Q_0} in terms of k_{ecal}, $k'_{R_{50}}$ and P_{gr}^Q. In other words, the k_{Q,Q_0} formalism used for electrons is the same as for photons. A table of k_{Q,Q_0} values for electrons is provided by the protocol for various types of ion chambers and beam quality R_{50}. This simplifies the calibration process somewhat since k_{ecal} and P_{gr}^Q do not need to be determined. The gradient correction at d_{ref} (the same as in TG-51) is implicit in the k_{Q,Q_0} factor for electrons as it is for photons.

TRS-398 does provide the option of chamber calibration at a series of electron beam qualities. The calibration laboratories could, in the future, provide N_{D,w,Q_0} for a reference electron beam of quality Q_0 and k_{Q,Q_0} factors corresponding to a number of other beams of quality Q so that the user could determine k_{Q,Q_0} by interpolation. Currently, this option is not available by the Primary Standard Dosimetry Laboratories (PSDLs).

D. Calibration

Reference conditions for the calibration of photon and electron beams in the TRS-398 are the same as in TG-51. TRS-398 also provides worksheets, which guide the user in a step-by-step implementation of the protocol.

Comments: The TG-51 and TRS-398 protocols are similar, except for minor differences in beam quality specification and notation. There is no reason why one protocol could not be followed worldwide. In this day and age, it does not make sense to promote these more or less identical protocols packaged with different names and notations. Although it's too late for these protocols to be merged into one, I hope that the next revision of either of these protocols will be combined and carried out by an internationally constituted panel or a task group.

8.8. EXPOSURE FROM RADIOACTIVE SOURCES

Exposure rate from a radioactive source can be determined from the knowledge of its photon emission spectrum and the relevant mass energy absorption coefficients for air. A relationship between exposure (X) and energy fluence (Ψ) may be derived by comparing Equations 8.19 and 8.21. Under the conditions of changed particle equilibrium,

$$D_{air} = X \cdot \frac{\overline{W}_{air}}{e} = \Psi \cdot \left(\frac{\mu_{en}}{\rho} \right)_{air}$$

Therefore,

$$X = \Psi \cdot \left(\frac{\mu_{en}}{\rho} \right)_{air} \cdot \frac{e}{\overline{W}_{air}} \qquad (8.110)$$

Suppose a radioisotope emits N photons of different energy and with different probability per disintegration. Imagine a sphere of radius 1 m around this point source of activity 1 Ci. Because 1 Ci undergoes 3.7×10^{10} dps, and since area of a sphere of radius 1 m is 4π m^2 and since 1 h = 3,600 sec, we have:

$$\text{Energy fluence/h at 1 m from 1-Ci source} = \frac{3.7 \times 10^{10} \times 3,600}{4\pi} \sum_{i=1}^{N} f_i E_i$$

where f_i is the number of photons emitted/decay of energy E_i. From Equation 8.110,

$$\text{Exposure/h at 1 m from 1-Ci source} = \dot{X}$$

$$= \frac{3.7 \times 10^{10} \times 3,600}{4\pi} \sum_{i=1}^{N} f_i E_i \left(\frac{\mu_{en}}{\rho} \right)_{air,i} \cdot \frac{e}{\overline{W}_{air}}$$

where $\left(\frac{\mu_{en}}{\rho}\right)_{air,i}$ is the mass energy absorption coefficient in air for photon of energy E_i.

Substituting the values $\frac{\overline{W}_{air}}{e} = 0.00876$ J/kg·R, 1 MeV $= 1.602 \times 10^{-13}$ J and expressing mass energy absorption coefficient in square meters per kilogram, the above equation becomes

$$\dot{X} = \frac{3.7 \times 10^{10} \times 3,600}{4\pi \, (m^2)}(h^{-1})\frac{1(R)}{0.00876 \, (J/kg)} \cdot 1.602$$

$$\times 10^{-13} \left(\frac{J}{MeV}\right) \cdot \sum_{i=1}^{N} f_i E_i (MeV) \cdot \left(\frac{\mu_{en}}{\rho}\right)_{air,i} \left(\frac{m^2}{kg}\right)$$

or

$$\dot{X} = 193.8 \sum_{i=1}^{N} f_i E_i \left(\frac{\mu_{en}}{\rho}\right)_{air,i} \quad (Rh^{-1}) \qquad (8.111)$$

A quantity exposure rate constant Γ_δ has been defined (47) as:

$$\Gamma_\delta = \frac{l^2}{A} \cdot (\dot{X})_\delta \qquad (8.112)$$

where $\dot{X}_\delta$ is the exposure rate from photons of energy greater than δ (a suitable cutoff for the energy spectrum) at a distance l from a point source of activity A. If $\dot{X}$ is in R/h, l is in m, and A is in Ci, the dimensions of Γ_δ become $Rm^2h^{-1}Ci^{-1}$. It is also apparent that Γ_δ is numerically equal to $\dot{X}$ in Equation 8.111. Thus the exposure rate constant may be written as:

$$\Gamma_\delta = 193.8 \sum_{i}^{N} f_i E_i \left(\frac{\mu_{en}}{\rho}\right)_{air,i} \quad Rm^2h^{-1}Ci^{-1} \qquad (8.113)$$

where energy E_i is expressed in MeV and $\left(\frac{\mu_{en}}{\rho}\right)_{air,i}$ is in m^2/kg.

Example

Calculate the exposure rate constant for ^{60}Co. Determine the exposure rate in R/min from a 5,000-Ci source of ^{60}Co at a distance of 80 cm.

^{60}Co emits 2 γ-rays of energy 1.17 and 1.33 MeV per disintegration

f_i	E_i(MeV)	$\left(\frac{\mu_{en}}{\rho}\right)_{air,i}$ (m^2/kg)
1.00	1.17	0.00270
1.00	1.33	0.00261

$$\Gamma_\delta = 193.8(1.17 \times 0.00270 + 1.33 \times 0.00261)Rm^2h^{-1}Ci^{-1}$$
$$= 1.29 \, Rm^2h^{-1}Ci^{-1}$$

Exposure rate from 5,000-Ci ^{60}Co source at 1 m $= 1.29 \times 5,000$ R/h

$$= \frac{1.29 \times 5,000}{60}R/min$$

$$= 107.5 \, R/min$$

Exposure rate at 80 cm $= 107.5 \times \left(\frac{100}{80}\right)^2 R/min$

$$= 168 \, R/min$$

The previous calculation applies only very approximately to an actual cobalt teletherapy unit since exposure rate would depend not only on the source activity but also on the collimator scatter, source size, and self-absorption in the source.

8.9. OTHER METHODS OF MEASURING ABSORBED DOSE

A. Calorimetry

Calorimetry is a basic method of determining absorbed dose in a medium. It is based on the principle that the energy absorbed in a medium from radiation appears ultimately as heat energy while a small amount may appear in the form of a chemical change. This results in a small increase in temperature of the absorbing medium which, if measured accurately, can be related to the energy absorbed per unit mass or the absorbed dose.

If a small volume of the medium is thermally isolated from the remainder, the absorbed dose D in this volume is given by:

$$D = \frac{dE_h}{dm} + \frac{dE_s}{dm} \tag{8.114}$$

where dE_h is the energy appearing as heat in the absorber of mass dm and dE_s is the energy absorbed or produced as a result of chemical change, called the heat defect (which may be positive or negative). Neglecting the latter for the moment, one can calculate the rise in temperature of water by the absorption of 1 Gy of dose:

$$1 \text{ Gy} = 1 \text{ J kg}^{-1} = \frac{1}{4.18} \text{ cal kg}^{-1}$$

where 4.18 is the mechanical equivalent of heat (4.18 J of energy = 1 cal of heat). Because the specific heat of water is 1 cal/g/°C or 10^3 cal/kg/°C, the increase in temperature (ΔT) produced by 1 Gy is:

$$\Delta T = \frac{1}{4.18} (\text{cal kg}^{-1}) \cdot \frac{1}{10^3} (\text{kg cal}^{-1} \, ^\circ\text{C})$$
$$= 2.39 \times 10^{-4} \, ^\circ\text{C}$$

To measure such a small temperature rise, thermistors are most commonly used. Thermistors are semiconductors which show a large change in electrical resistance with a small change in temperature (about 5% per 1°C). Thus, by measuring the change in resistance by an apparatus such as a Wheatstone bridge, one can calculate the absorbed dose.

Extensive literature exists on radiation calorimetry to which the reader is referred (48,49). Most of these apparatuses are difficult to construct and, for various reasons, are considered impractical for clinical dosimetry. However, Domen (50) has described a simpler water calorimeter for absolute measurement of absorbed dose. Essential features of this calorimeter are briefly described.

Figure 8.9 is a schematic drawing of Domen's calorimeter. An ultrasmall (0.25-mm diameter) bead thermistor is sandwiched between two 30-μm polyethylene films stretched on polystyrene rings. The thermistors are cemented to one of the films to increase thermal coupling. The films provide the necessary high and stable resistance ($>10^{11}$ Ω) between the thermistor leads and water.

The films held horizontally in a plastic frame are then immersed in an insulated tank of distilled water. Because of the low thermal diffusivity of water and imperviousness of polyethylene film to water, nearly negligible conductive heat transfer occurs at a point in the water medium. Therefore, a thermally isolated volume element of water is not necessary. This apparatus measures dose rates in water of about 4 Gy/min with a precision (for the reproducibility of measurements) of 0.5%.

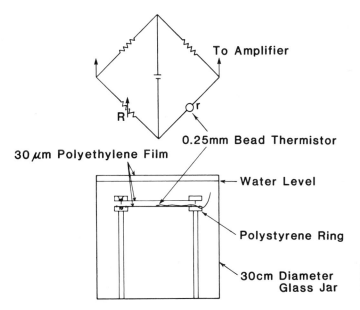

FIG. 8.9. Schematic diagram of Domen's calorimeter. (Redrawn from Domen SR. Absorbed dose water calorimeter. *Med Phys* 1980;7:157.)

B. Chemical Dosimetry

The energy absorbed from ionizing radiation may produce a chemical change, and if this change can be determined, it can be used as a measure of absorbed dose. Many systems of chemical dosimetry have been proposed but the *ferrous sulfate* or the *Fricke dosimeter* is considered to be the most developed system for the precision measurement of absorbed dose. The use of this system has been fully discussed (51). A brief description will be provided.

B.1. Ferrous Sulfate (Fricke) Dosimeter

The dosimeter consists of 1 mmol/l ferrous sulfate (or ferrous ammonium sulfate), 1 mmol/l NaCl, and 0.4 mol/l sulfuric acid. The reason for NaCl in the solution is to counteract the effects of organic impurities present despite all the necessary precautions. When the solution is irradiated, the ferrous ions, Fe^{2+}, are oxidized by radiation to ferric ions, Fe^{3+}. The ferric ion concentration is determined by spectrophotometry of the dosimeter solution, which shows absorption peaks in the ultraviolet light at wavelengths of 224 and 304 nm.

B.2. G Value

The radiation chemical yield may be expressed in terms of the number of molecules produced per 100 eV of energy absorbed. This number is known as the G value. Thus, if the yield of ferric ions can be determined, the energy absorbed can be calculated when the G value is known.

Suppose a ΔM (moles/l) concentration of ferric ions is produced by an absorbed dose of D grays:

$$D(Gy) = D(J/kg) = \frac{D}{1.602 \times 10^{-19}} (eV/kg)$$

Molecules of ferric ions produced $= \Delta M \times 6.02 \times 10^{23}$ molecules/liter

$$\frac{\Delta M \times 6.02 \times 10^{23}}{\rho} \text{molecules/kg}$$

where ρ is the density of the solution in kilograms per liter.

TABLE 8.9. RECOMMENDED *G* VALUES FOR THE FERROUS SULFATE DOSIMETER (0.4 mol/l H_2SO_4 FOR PHOTON BEAMS

Radiation	G Value (No./100 eV)
^{137}Cs	15.3 ± 0.3
2 MV	15.4 ± 0.3
^{60}Co	15.5 ± 0.2
4 MV	15.5 ± 0.3
5–10 MV	15.6 ± 0.4
11–30 MV	15.7 ± 0.6

Data from ICRU. Radiation dosimetry: x rays and gamma rays with maximum photon energies between 0.6 and 50 MeV. Report 14. Bethesda, MD: International Commission on Radiation Units and Measurements, 1969, with permission.

Number of molecules produced per eV of energy absorbed:

$$= \frac{\Delta M \times 6.02 \times 10^{23}}{\rho} \cdot \frac{1.602 \times 10^{-19}}{D}$$

$$= \frac{\Delta M}{\rho D} \cdot 9.64 \times 10^4 \text{ molecules/eV}$$

or

$$G = \frac{\Delta M}{\rho D} \cdot 9.64 \times 10^4 \cdot 100 \text{ molecules/100 eV}$$

$$= \frac{\Delta M}{\rho D} \cdot 9.64 \times 10^6 \text{ molecules/100 eV}$$

Thus,

$$D = \frac{\Delta M}{\rho G} \cdot 9.64 \times 10^6 \text{ (Gy)}$$

The *G* values for the Fricke dosimeter have been determined by many investigators. Table 8.9 gives the values recommended by Nahum (17) for photons from ^{137}Cs to 30 MV. A constant *G* value of $15.7 \pm 0.6/100$ eV is recommended for electrons in the energy range of 1 to 30 MeV for 0.4 mol/liter H_2SO_4 dosimeter solution (29).

C. Solid State Methods

There are several solid state systems available for the dosimetry of ionizing radiation. However, none of the systems is absolute—each needs calibration in a known radiation field before it can be used for the determination of absorbed dose.

There are two types of solid state dosimeters: (a) integrating type dosimeters (thermoluminescent crystals, radiophotoluminescent glasses, optical density type dosimeters such as glass and film), and (b) electrical conductivity dosimeters (semiconductor junction detectors, induced conductivity in insulating materials). Of these, the most widely used systems for the measurement of absorbed dose are the thermoluminescent dosimeter (TLD), diodes, and film, which are described.

C.1. Thermoluminescence Dosimetry

Many crystalline materials exhibit the phenomenon of thermoluminescence. When such a crystal is irradiated, a very minute fraction of the absorbed energy is stored in the crystal lattice. Some of this energy can be recovered later as visible light if the material is

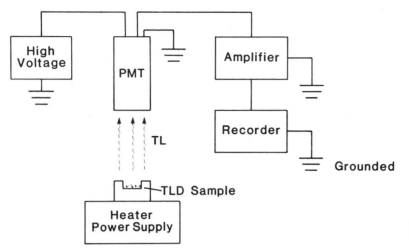

FIG. 8.10. Schematic diagram showing apparatus for measuring thermoluminescence.

heated. This phenomenon of the release of visible photons by thermal means is known as thermoluminescence (TL).

The arrangement for measuring the TL output is shown schematically in Fig. 8.10. The irradiated material is placed in a heater cup or planchet, where it is heated for a reproducible heating cycle. The emitted light is measured by a photomultiplier tube (PMT) which converts light into an electrical current. The current is then amplified and measured by a recorder or a counter.

There are several TL phosphors available but the most noteworthy are lithium fluoride (LiF), lithium borate ($Li_2B_4O_7$), and calcium fluoride (CaF_2). Their dosimetric properties are listed in Table 8.10 (52). Of these phosphors, LiF is most extensively studied and most frequently used for clinical dosimetry. LiF in its purest form exhibits relatively little thermoluminescence. But the presence of a trace amount of impurities (e.g., magnesium)

TABLE 8.10. CHARACTERISTICS OF VARIOUS PHOSPHORS

Characteristic	LiF	Li_2B_{407}:Mn	CaF_2:Mn	CaF_2:nat	$CaSo_4$:Mn
Density (g/cc)	2.64	2.3	3.18	3.18	2.61
Effective atomic no.	8.2	7.4	16.3	16.3	15.3
TL emission spectra (A)					
Range	3,500–6,000	5,300–6,300	4,400–6,000	3,500–5,000	4,500–6,000
Maximum	4,000	6,050	5,000	3,800	5,000
Temperature of main TL glow peak	195°C	200°C	260°C	260°C	110°C
Efficiency at cobalt-60 (relative to LiF)	1.0	0.3	3	23	70
Energy response without added filter (30 keV/cobalt-60)	1.25	0.9	13	13	10
Useful range	Small, <5%/12 wk	mR–10^6 R	mR–3×10^5 R	mR–10^4 R	R–10^4 R
Fading	mR–10^5 R	10% in first mo	10% in first mo	No detectable fading	50–60% in the first 24 hr
Light sensitivity	Essentially none	Essentially none	Essentially none	Yes	Yes
Physical form	Powder, extruded, Teflon-embedded, silicon-embedded, glass capillaries	Powder, Teflon-embedded	Powder, Teflon-embedded, hotpressed chips, glass capillaries	Special dosimeters	Powder, Teflon-embedded

From Cameron JR, Suntharalingam N, Kenney GN. Thermoluminescent dosimetry. Madison: University of Wisconsin Press, 1968, with permission.

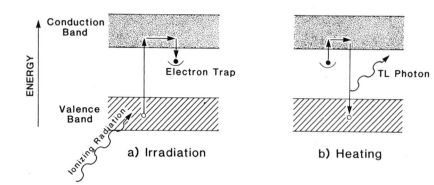

FIG. 8.11. A simplified energy-level diagram to illustrate thermoluminescence process.

provides the radiation-induced TL. These impurities give rise to imperfections in the lattice structure of LiF and appear to be necessary for the appearance of the TL phenomenon.

C.2. Simplified Theory of Thermoluminescent Dosimetry

The chemical and physical theory of TLD is not exactly known, but simple models have been proposed to explain the phenomenon qualitatively. Figure 8.11 shows an energy-level diagram of an inorganic crystal exhibiting TL by ionizing radiation.

In an individual atom, electrons occupy discrete energy levels. In a crystal lattice, on the other hand, electronic energy levels are perturbed by mutual interactions between atoms and give rise to energy bands: the "allowed" energy bands and the forbidden energy bands. In addition, the presence of impurities in the crystal creates energy traps in the forbidden region, providing metastable states for the electrons. When the material is irradiated, some of the electrons in the valence band (ground state) receive sufficient energy to be raised to the conduction band. The vacancy thus created in the valence band is called a positive hole. The electron and the hole move independently through their respective bands until they recombine (electron returning to the ground state) or until they fall into a trap (metastable state). If there is instantaneous emission of light owing to these transitions, the phenomenon is called *fluorescence.* If an electron in the trap requires energy to get out of the trap and fall to the valence band, the emission of light in this case is called *phosphorescence* (delayed fluorescence). If phosphorescence at room temperature is very slow, but can be speeded up significantly with a moderate amount of heating (~300°C), the phenomenon is called *thermoluminescence.*

A plot of thermoluminescence against temperature is called a *glow curve* (Fig. 8.12). As the temperature of the TL material exposed to radiation is increased, the probability of releasing trapped electrons increases. The light emitted (TL) first increases, reaches a maximum value, and falls again to zero. Because most phosphors contain a number of traps at various energy levels in the forbidden band, the glow curve may consist of a number of glow peaks as shown in Fig. 8.12. The different peaks correspond to different "trapped" energy levels.

C.3. Lithium Fluoride

The TL characteristics of LiF have been studied extensively. For details, the reader is referred to Cameron et al. (52).

Lithium fluoride has an effective atomic number of 8.2 compared with 7.4 for soft tissue. This makes this material very suitable for clinical dosimetry. Mass energy absorption coefficients for this material have been given by Greening et al. (53). The dose absorbed in LiF can be converted to dose in muscle by considerations similar to those discussed earlier. For example, under electronic equilibrium conditions, the ratio of absorbed doses in the two media will be the same as the ratio of their mass energy absorption coefficients. If the dimensions of the dosimeter are smaller than the ranges of the electrons crossing the dosimeter, then the Bragg-Gray relationship can also be used. The ratio of absorbed doses in

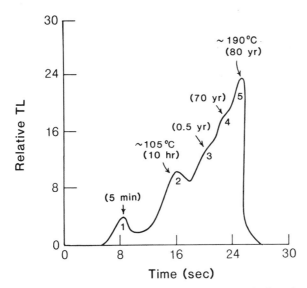

FIG. 8.12. An example of glow curve of LiF (TLD-100) after phosphor has been annealed at 400°C for 1 h and read immediately after irradiation to 100 R. (From Zimmerman DW, Rhyner CR, Cameron JR. Thermal annealing effects on thermoluminescence of LiF. *Health Phys* 1966;12:525, with permission.)

the two media then will be the same as the ratio of mass stopping powers. The applicability of the Bragg-Gray cavity theory to TLD has been discussed by several authors (54,55).

C.4. Practical Considerations

As stated previously, the thermoluminescent dosimeter must be calibrated before it can be used for measuring an unknown dose. Because the response of the TLD materials is affected by their previous radiation history and thermal history, the material must be suitably annealed to remove residual effects. The standard preirradiation annealing procedure for LiF is 1 hour of heating at 400°C and then 24 h at 80°C. The slow heating, namely 24 hours at 80°C, removes peaks 1 and 2 of the glow curve (Fig. 8.12) by decreasing the "trapping efficiency." Peaks 1 and 2 can also be eliminated by postirradiation annealing for 10 minutes at 100°C. The need for eliminating peaks 1 and 2 arises from the fact that the magnitude of these peaks decreases relatively fast with time after irradiation. By removing these peaks by annealing, the glow curve becomes more stable and therefore predictable.

The dose response curve for TLD-100[5] is shown in Fig. 8.13. The curve is generally linear up to 10^3 cGy but beyond this it becomes supralinear. The response curve, however, depends on many conditions that have to be standardized to achieve reasonable accuracy with TLD. The calibration should be done with the same TLD reader, in approximately the same quality beam and to approximately the same absorbed dose level.

The TLD response is defined as TL output per unit absorbed dose in the phosphor. Figure 8.14 gives the energy response curve for LiF (TLD-100) for photon energies below megavoltage range. The studies of energy response for photons above ^{60}Co and high energy electrons have yielded somewhat conflicting results. Whereas the data of Pinkerton et al. (56) and Crosby et al. (57) show some energy dependence, other studies (58) do not show this energy dependence.

When considerable care is used, precision of approximately 3% may be obtained using TLD powder or extruded material. Although not as precise as the ion chamber, TLD's main advantage is in measuring doses in regions where ion chamber cannot be used. For example, TLD is extremely useful for patient dosimetry by direct insertion into tissues or

---

[5] TLD-100 (Harshaw Chemical Co.) contains 7.5% ^{6}Li and 92.5% ^{7}Li.

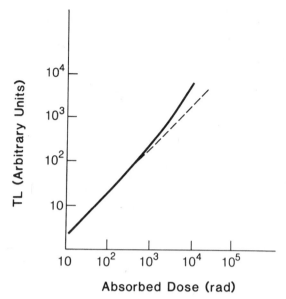

FIG. 8.13. An example of TL versus absorbed dose curve for TLD-100 powder (schematic).

body cavities. Since TLD material is available in many forms and sizes, it can be used for special dosimetry situations such as for measuring dose distribution in the build-up region, around brachytherapy sources, and for personnel dose monitoring.

D. Silicon Diodes

Silicon p-n junction diodes are often used for relative dosimetry. Their higher sensitivity, instantaneous response, small size and ruggedness offer special advantages over ionization chambers. They are particularly well suited for relative measurements in electron beams, output constancy checks and in vivo patient dose monitoring. Their major limitations as dosimeters include energy dependence in photon beams, directional dependence, thermal effects, and radiation-induced damage. Modern diodes for dosimetry have been designed to minimize these effects.

1. Theory

A dosimetry diode consists of a silicon crystal which is mixed or doped with impurities to make p- and n-type silicon. The p-type silicon is made by introducing a small amount of

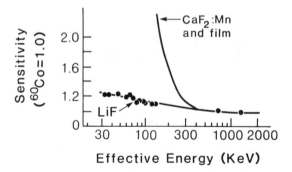

FIG. 8.14. Energy response curve for LiF (TLD-100), CaF_2:Mn and a photographic film. (From Cameron JR, Suntharalingam H, Kenney GN. *Thermoluminescent dosimetry.* Madison: University of Wisconsin Press, 1968, with permission.)

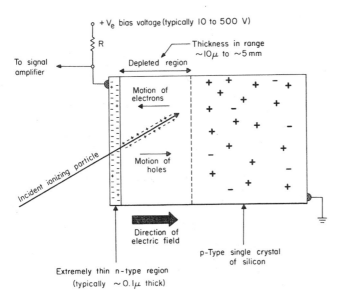

FIG. 8.15. A schematic diagram showing basic design of a silicon p-n junction diode. (From Attix FH. *Introduction to radiological physics and radiation dosimetry.* New York: John Wiley & Sons, 1986, with permission.)

an element from group III of the periodic table (e.g., boron), making it into an electron receptor. When silicon is mixed with a material from group V (e.g., phosphorus) it receives atoms that are carriers of negative charge, thus making it into an electron donor or n-type silicon. A p-n junction diode is designed with one part of a p-silicon disc doped with an n-type material (Fig. 8.15). The p-region of the diode is deficient in electrons (or contains "holes") while the n-region has an excess of electrons.

At the interface between p- and n-type materials, a small region called the depletion zone is created because of initial diffusion of electrons from the n-region and holes from the p-region across the junction, until equilibrium is established. The depletion zone develops an electric field which opposes further diffusion of majority carriers once equilibrium has been achieved.

When a diode is irradiated electron-hole pairs are produced within the depletion zone. They are immediately separated and swept out by the existing electric field in the depletion zone. This gives rise to a radiation-induced current. The current is further augmented by the diffusion of electrons and holes produced outside the depletion zone within a diffusion length. The direction of electronic current flow is from the n- to the p-region (which is opposite to the direction of conventional current).

2. Operation

Figure 8.16A shows schematically a radiation diode detector, which essentially consists of a silicon p-n junction diode connected to a coaxial cable and encased in epoxy potting material. This design is intended for the radiation beam to be incident perpendicularly at the long axis of the detector. Although the collecting or sensitive volume (depletion zone) is not known precisely, it is on the order of 0.2 to 0.3 mm^3. It is located within a depth of 0.5 mm from the front surface of the detector, unless electronic buildup is provided by encasing the diode in a buildup material.

Figure 8.16B shows the diode connected to an operational amplifier with a feedback loop to measure radiation induced current. There is no bias voltage applied. The circuit acts as a current-to-voltage transducer, whereby the voltage readout at point B is directly proportional to the radiation induced current.

Diodes are far more sensitive than ion chambers. Since the energy required to produce an electron-hole pair in Si is 3.5 eV compared to 34eV required to produce an ion-pair in

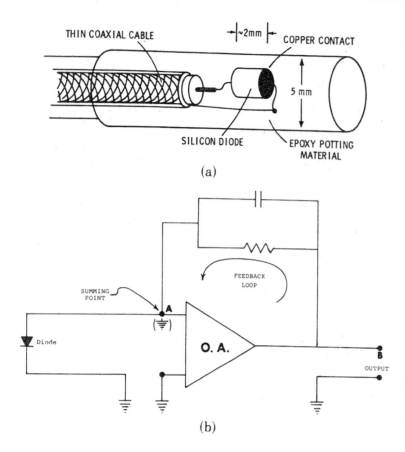

FIG. 8.16. Schematic diagrams showing **(a)** silicon p-n junction diode, and **(b)** basic electronic circuit using operational amplifier with a feedback loop. (From Gager LD, Wright AE, Almond PR. Silicon diode detectors used in radiobiological physics measurements. Part I: Development of an energy compensating shield. *Med Phys* 1977;4:494–498, with permission.)

air and because the density of Si is 1,800 times that of air, the current produced per unit volume is about 18,000 times larger in a diode than in an ion chamber. Thus, a diode, even with a small collecting volume, can provide an adequate signal.

3. Energy Dependence

Because of the relatively high atomic number of silicon (Z = 14) compared to that of water or air, diodes exhibit severe energy dependence in photon beams of non-uniform quality. Although some diodes are designed to provide energy compensation through filtration (59), the issue of energy dependence never goes away and therefore, their use in x-ray beams is limited to relative dosimetry in situations where spectral quality of the beam is not changed significantly, for example, profile measurements in small fields, dose constancy checks. In electron beams, however, the diodes do not show energy dependence as the stopping power ratio of silicon to water does not vary significantly with electron energy or depth. Thus diodes are qualitatively similar to films so far as their energy dependence is concerned.

Some diodes exhibit greater stability and less energy dependence than others. It is therefore incumbent upon the user to establish dosimetric accuracy of a diode by comparative measurements with an ion chamber.

4. Angular Dependence

Diodes exhibit angular dependence, which must be taken into account if the angle of beam incidence is changed significantly. Again these effects should be ascertained in comparative measurements with a detector which does not show angular dependence.

5. Temperature Dependence

Diodes show a small temperature dependence that may be ignored unless the change in temperature during measurements or since the last calibration is drastic. The temperature dependence of diodes is smaller than that of an ion chamber. Moreover, their response is independent of pressure and humidity.

6. Radiation Damage

A diode can suffer permanent damage when irradiated by ultrahigh doses of ionizing radiation. The damage is most probably caused by displacement of silicon atoms from their lattice positions. The extent of damage will depend upon the type of radiation, energy and total dose. Because of the possibility of radiation damage, especially after prolonged use, diode sensitivity should be checked routinely to assure stability and accuracy of calibration.

7. Clinical Applications

As previously mentioned, diodes are useful in electron beam dosimetry and in limited situations in photon beam measurements. Most often their use is dictated by the requirements on the detector size. For example, dose profiles or output factors in a small field may pose difficulties in the use of an ion chamber. So a film or a diode response is checked against an ion chamber under suitable benchmark conditions.

Diodes are becoming increasingly popular with regard to their use in patient dose monitoring. Since diodes do not require high voltage bias, they can be taped directly onto the patient at suitable points to measure dose. The diodes are carefully calibrated to provide a check of patient dose at a reference point (e.g., dose at d_{max}). Different amounts of buildup material can be incorporated to make the diode sample the dose close to the peak dose for a given energy beam. Calibration factors are applied to convert the diode reading into expected dose at the reference point, taking into account source-to-detector distance, field size, and other parameters used in the calculation of monitor units.

For further details on diodes and their clinical applications, the readier is referred to some key articles in the literature (59–62).

E. Radiographic Film

A radiographic film consists of a transparent film base (cellulose acetate or polyester resin) coated with an emulsion containing very small crystals of silver bromide. When the film is exposed to ionizing radiation or visible light, a chemical change takes place within the exposed crystals to form what is referred to as a *latent image*. When the film is developed, the affected crystals are reduced to small grains of metallic silver. The film is then *fixed*. The unaffected granules are removed by the fixing solution, leaving a clear film in their place. The metallic silver, which is not affected by the fixer, causes darkening of the film. Thus the degree of blackening of an area of the film depends on the amount of free silver deposited and, consequently, on the radiation energy absorbed.

The degree of blackening of the film is measured by determining optical density with a densitometer. This instrument consists of a light source, a tiny aperture through which the light is directed and a light detector (photocell) to measure the light intensity transmitted through the film.

The optical density, OD, is defined as:

$$\text{OD} = \log \frac{I_0}{I_t} \tag{8.115}$$

where I_0 is the amount of light collected without film and I_t is the amount of light transmitted through the film. A densitometer gives a direct reading of optical density if it has been calibrated by a standard strip of film having regions of known optical density.

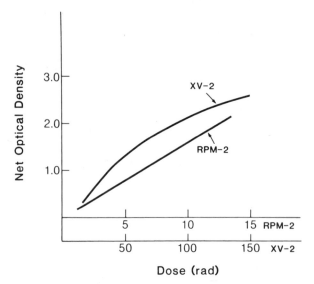

FIG. 8.17. Sensitometric curve of Kodak XV-2 film and Kodak RPM-2 (Type M) film.

In dosimetry, the quantity of interest is usually net optical density which is obtained by subtracting the reading for the base fog (OD of unexposed processed film) from the measured optical density.

A plot of net optical density as a function of radiation exposure or dose is termed the sensitometric curve, or H-D curve.[6] Figure 8.17 shows examples of characteristic curves for two commonly used dosimetry films. Film speed and linearity of the sensitometric curve are the two main characteristics which are considered in selecting a film for dosimetry. If a film is exposed in the nonlinear region, corrections are necessary to convert optical density into dose.

Although film is well-established as a method of measuring electron beam distributions (Chapter 14), its usefulness in photon dosimetry is relatively limited. Because the photoelectric effect depends on the cube of the atomic number, the silver ($Z = 45$) in the film emulsion absorbs radiation below 150 keV very strongly by the photoelectric process. Since most clinical beams contain a scatter component of low-energy photons, the correlation between optical density and dose becomes tenuous. In addition, film suffers from several potential errors such as changes in processing conditions, interfilm emulsion differences, and artifacts caused by air pockets adjacent to the film. For these reasons, absolute dosimetry with film is impractical. However, it is very useful for checking radiation fields, light-field coincidence, field flatness, and symmetry, and obtaining quick qualitative patterns of a radiation distribution.

In the megavoltage range of photon energies, however, film has been used to measure isodose curves with acceptable accuracy ($\pm 3\%$) (63–65). One of the techniques (65) consists of exposing the film packed tightly in a polystyrene phantom, parallel to the central axis of the beam. The film edge is carefully aligned with the phantom surface and air pockets between the film surface and the surrounding jacket are removed by punching holes near the corners. Optical densities are correlated with dose by using a depth-dependent sensitometric curve derived from known central axis depth dose data for a reference field such as 10 × 10 cm. The method is made practical by a computer-controlled densitometer and a computer program that performs the required isodensity-to-isodose curve conversion.

---

[6] The expression *H-D* is derived from the names of Hurter and Driffield, who in 1890 used such curves to characterize the response of photographic film to light.

F. Radiochromic Film

The use of radiochromic films for radiation dosimetry has been evolving since the 1960s (66,67). With the recent improvement in technology associated with the production of these films, their use has become increasingly popular especially in brachytherapy dosimetry. Major advantages of radiochromic film dosimeters include tissue equivalence, high spatial resolution, large dynamic range (10^{-2}-10^6 Gy), relatively low spectral sensitivity variation (or energy dependence), insensitivity to visible light and no need for chemical processing.

Radiochromic film consists of an ultra thin (7- to 23-μm thick), colorless, radiosensitive leuco dye bonded onto a 100-μm thick Mylar base (68). Other varieties include thin layers of radiosensitive dye sandwiched between two pieces of polyester base (69). The unexposed film is colorless and changes to shades of blue as a result of a polymerization process induced by ionizing radiation.

No physical, chemical, or thermal processing is required to bring out or stabilize this color. The degree of coloring is usually measured with a spectrophotometer using a narrow spectral wavelength (nominal 610–670 nm). Commercially available laser scanners and CCD microdensitometer cameras can also be used to scan the films. These measurements are expressed in terms of optical density as defined by Equation 8.115.

Radiochromic films are almost tissue equivalent with effective Z of 6.0 to 6.5. Post irradiation color stability occurs after about 24 hours. Energy dependence is much lower than the silver halide (radiographic) films. Although radiochromic films are insensitive to visible light, they exhibit some sensitivity to ultraviolet light and temperature. They need to be stored in a dry and dark environment at the temperature and humidity not too different from those at which they will be used for dosimetry. Because radiochromic films are sensitive to ultraviolet light, they should not be exposed to fluorescent light or to sunlight. They may be read and handled in normal incandescent light.

Radiochromic films must be calibrated before they can be used for dosimetry. The sensitometric curve shows a linear relationship up to a certain dose level beyond which its response levels off with increase in dose (Fig. 8.18).

The most commonly used radiochromic films for dosimetry that are commercially available are GafChromic HD-810 film (International Specialty Product (ISP), Wayne, NJ) and Double-layer GafChromic MD-55–2 film (ISP or other vendor(s): Nuclear Associates,

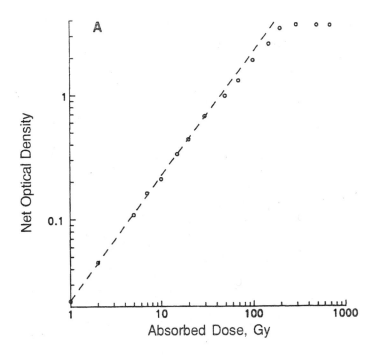

FIG. 8.18. A plot of net optical density as a function of dose for MD-55–2 radiochromic film. (From AAPM. Radiochromic film dosimetry: recommendations of AAPM Radiation Therapy Committee Task Group 55. *Med Phys* 1998;25:2093–2115, with permission.)

Carle Place, NY). Whereas HD-810 films are mainly used in the dose range of 50 to 2,500 Gy, MD-55-2 are useful in the range of 3 to 100 Gy.

For details on radiochromic film and their use in clinical dosimetry, the reader is referred to the AAPM TG-55 report (70).

REFERENCES

1. *ICRU. Radiation quantities and units. Report No. 33.* Washington, DC: International Commission on Radiation Units and Measurements, 1980.
2. Boutillon M, Perroche-Roux AM. Re-evaluation of the W value for electrons in dry air. *Phys Med Biol* 1987;32:213.
3. Loftus TP, Weaver JT. Standardization of ^{60}Co and ^{137}Cs gamma-ray beams in terms of exposure. *J Res Natl Bur Stand* 1974;78A:465.
4. Loevinger R. A formalism for calculation of absorbed dose to a medium from photon and electron beams. *Med Phys* 1981;8:1.
5. Mackie TR, Bielajew AF, Rogers DWO, et al. Generation of photon energy deposition kernels using the EGS Monte Carlo code. *Phys Med Biol* 1988;33:1.
6. American Association of Physicists in Medicine. RTC Task Group 21. A protocol for the determination of absorbed dose from high energy photon and electron beams. *Med Phys* 1983;10:741.
7. Johns HE, Cunningham JR. *The physics of radiology,* 3rd ed. Springfield, IL: Charles C Thomas, 1969.
8. Day MJ, Greene D, Massey JB. Use of a Perspex sheath for ionization chamber measurements in a water phantom. *Phys Med Biol* 1965;10:111.
9. Bragg WH. *Studies in radioactivity.* New York: Macmillan, 1912.
10. Gray LH. An ionization method for the absolute measurement of gamma-ray energy. *Proc R Soc* 1936;A156:578.
11. Spencer LV, Attix FH. A theory of cavity ionization. *Radiat Res* 1955;3:239.
12. Greening JR. An experimental examination of theories of cavity ionization. *Br J Radiol* 1957;30:254.
13. Burlin TE. An experimental examination of theories relating the absorption of gamma-ray energy in medium to the ionization produced in a cavity. *Phys Med Biol* 1961;6:33.
14. Burlin TE. Further examination of theories relating the absorption of gamma-ray energy in a medium to the ionization produced in a cavity. *Phys Med Biol* 1966;11:255.
15. Nahum AE. Dosimetry in radiotherapy. IAEA-SM-298/81. *Proc Symp Int Atomic Energy Agency* 1988;1:87.
16. ICRU. *Stopping powers for electrons and positrons. Report 37.* Bethesda, MD: International Commission on Radiation Units and Measurements, 1984.
17. Nahum AE. Water/air mass stopping power ratios for megavoltage photon and electron beams. *Phys Med Biol* 1978;23:24.
18. Burlin TE. Cavity chamber theory. In: Attix FH, Roesch WC, eds. *Radiation dosimetry, Vol I,* 2nd ed. New York: Academic Press, 1969.
19. ICRU. *Average energy required to produce an ion pair. Report 31.* Washington, DC: ICRU, 1979.
20. Almond PR, Svensson H. Ionization chamber dosimetry for photon and electron beams. *Acta Radiol* 1977;16:177.
21. Lempert GD, Nath R, Schulz RJ. Fraction of ionization from electrons arising in the wall of an ionization chamber. *Med Phys* 1983;10:1.
22. Dutreix J, Dutreix A. Etude comparé d'une série de chambres d'ionization dans des faisceaux d'électrons de 20 et 10 MeV. *Biophysik* 1966;3:249–258.
23. Schulz RJ, Almond PR, Kutcher G, et al. Clarification of the AAPM Task Group 21 protocol. *Med Phys* 1986;13:755.
24. Rogers DWO. *Fundamentals of high energy x-ray and electron dosimetry protocols.* AAPM Summer School, 1990.
25. Khan FM. Replacement correction (P_{repl}) for ion chamber dosimetry. *Med Phys* 1991;18:1244.
26. Cunningham JR, Sontag MC. Displacement correction used in absorbed dose determination. *Med Phys* 1980;7:672–676.
27. Johansson K, Mattsson L, Lindberg L, et al. *Absorbed-dose determination with ionization chambers in electron and photon beams having energies between 1 and 50 MeV. IAEA-SM-222/35.* Vienna: International Atomic Energy Agency, 1977:243–270.
28. AAPM. Clinical electron beam dosimetry. TG-25 Report. *Med Phys* 1991;18:73–109.
29. ICRU. *Radiation dosimetry: electron beams with energies between 1 and 50 MeV. Report 35.* Washington, DC: ICRU, 1984.
30. Nath R, Schulz RJ. Calculated response and wall correction factors for ionization chambers exposed to ^{60}Co gamma-rays. *Med Phys* 1981;8:85.

31. Gastorf R, Humphries L, Rozenfeld M. Cylindrical chamber dimensions and the corresponding values of A_{wall} and $N_{gas}/(N_x A_{ion})$. *Med Phys* 1986;13:751.

32. Bielajew AF. Ionization cavity theory: a formal derivation of perturbation factors for thick walled ion chambers in photon beams. *Phys Med Biol* 1986;31:161.

33. Rogers DWA. Fundamentals of dosimetry based on absorbed dose standards. In: Mackie TR, Palta JR, eds. *Teletherapy: present and future.* Madison, WI: Advanced Medical Publishing, 1996:319–356.

34. AAPM. Protocol for clinical reference dosimetry of high-energy photon and electron beams. *Med Phys* 1999;26:1847–1870.

35. Andreo P, Brahme A. Stopping-power data for high-energy photon beams. *Phys Med Biol* 1986;31:839–858.

36. IAEA. *Absorbed dose determination in external beam radiotherapy. Technical Reports Series No. 398.* Vienna: International Atomic Energy Agency, 2000.

37. Andreo P. On the beam quality specification of high-energy photons for radiotherapy dosimetry. *Med Phys* 2000;27:434–440.

38. Rogers DWO. Comment on "On the beam quality specification of high-energy photons for radiotherapy dosimetry." *Med Phys* 2000;27:441–444.

39. Kosunen A, Rogers DWO. Beam quality specification for photon beam dosimetry. *Med Phys* 1993;20:1181–1188.

40. Li XA, Rogers DWO. Reducing electron contamination for photon-beam quality specification. *Med Phys* 1994;21:791–798.

41. Ding GX, Rogers DWO, Mackie TR. Calculation of stopping-power ratios using realistic clinical electron beams. *Med Phys* 1995;22:489–501.

42. Ma CM, Nahum AE. Effect of size and composition of central electrode on the response of cylindrical ionization chambers in high-energy photon and electron beams. *Phys Med Biol* 1993;38:267–290.

43. Rogers DWO. A new approach to electron-beam reference dosimetry. *Med Phys* 1997;25:310–320.

44. Burns DT, Ding GX, Rogers DWO. R_{50} as a beam quality specifier for selecting stopping-power ratios and reference depths for electron dosimetry. *Med Phys* 1996;23:383–388.

45. IAEA. *Absorbed dose determination in photon and electron beams: an international code of practice. Technical Report Series No. 277.* Vienna: International Atomic Energy Agency, 1987.

46. Andreo P. Absorbed dose beam quality factors for the dosimetry of high-energy photon beams. *Phys Med Biol* 1992;37:2189–2211.

47. ICRU. *Radiation quantities and units. Report No. 19.* Washington, DC: International Commission on Radiation Units and Measurements, 1971.

48. Laughlin JS, Genna S. Calorimetry. In: Attix FH, Roesch WC, eds. *Radiation dosimetry, Vol II.* New York: Academic Press, 1967:389.

49. Gunn SR. Radiometric calorimetry: a review. *Nucl Inst Methods* 1964;29:1; 1970;85:285; 1976;135:251.

50. Domen SR. Absorbed dose water calorimeter. *Med Phys* 1980;7:157.

51. ICRU. *Radiation dosimetry: x-rays generated at potentials of 5 to 150 kV. Report No. 17.* Washington, DC: International Commission on Radiation Units and Measurements, 1970.

52. Cameron JR, Suntharalingam N, Kenney GN. *Thermoluminescent dosimetry.* Madison: University of Wisconsin Press, 1968.

53. Greening JR, Law J, Redpath AT. Mass attenuation and mass energy absorption coefficients for LiF and $Li_2B_4O_7$ for photons from 1 to 150 keV. *Phys Med Biol* 1972;17:585.

54. Paliwal BR, Almond PR. Application of cavity theories for electrons to LiF dosimeters. *Phys Med Biol* 1975;20:547.

55. Holt JG, Edelstein GR, Clark TE. Energy dependence of the response of lithium fluoride TLD rods in high energy electron fields. *Phys Med Biol* 1975;20:559.

56. Pinkerton A, Holt JG, Laughlin JS. Energy dependence of LiF dosimeters at high energies. *Phys Med Biol* 1966;11:129.

57. Crosby EH, Almond PR, Shalek RJ. Energy dependence of LiF dosimeters at high energies. *Phys Med Biol* 1966;11:131.

58. Suntharalingam N, Cameron JR. Thermoluminescent response of lithium fluoride to high-energy electrons [high-energy radiation therapy dosimetry issue]. *Ann NY Acad Sci* 1969;161:77.

59. Gager LD, Wright AE, Almond PR. Silicon diode detectors used in radiobiological physics measurements. Part I: Development of an energy compensating shield. *Med Phys* 1977;4:494–498.

60. Wright AE, Gager LD. Silicon diode detectors used in radiobiological physics measurements. Part II: Measurement of dosimetry data for high-energy photons. *Med Phys* 1977;4:499–502.

61. Dixon RL, Ekstrand KE. Silicon diode dosimetry. *Int J Appl Radiat Isot* 1982;33:1171–1176.

62. Rikner G. Characteristics of a selectively shielded p-Si detector in ^{60}Co and 8 and 16 MV Roentgen radiation. *Acta Radiol Oncol* 1985;24:205–208.

63. Jacobson A. 4 MeV x-ray film dosimetry. *Radiology* 1972;103:703.

64. Patten L, Purdy J, Oliver G. Automated film dosimetry [Abstract]. *Med Phys* 1974;1:110.

65. Williamson JF, Khan FM, Sharma SC. Film dosimetry of megavoltage photon beams: a practical method of isodensity-to-isodose curve conversion. *Med Phys* 1981;8:94.

66. McLaughlin WL, Chalkley L. Low atomic numbered dye systems for ionizing radiation measurements. *Photogr Sci Eng* 1965;9:159–165.
67. McLaughlin WL. Microscopic visualization of dose distribution. *Int J Appl Radiat Isot* 1966;17:85–96.
68. Zhu Y, Kirov AS, Mishra V, et al. Quantitative evaluation of radiochromic film response for two-dimensional dosimetry. *Med Phys* 1997;25:223–231.
69. Soares CG, McLaughlin WL. Measurement of radial dose distributions around small beta-particle emitters using high-resolution radiochromic foil dosimetry. *Radiat Protect Dosim* 1993;47:367–372.
70. AAPM. Radiochromic film dosimetry: recommendations of AAPM Radiation Therapy Committee Task Group 55. *Med Phys* 1998;25:2093–2115.

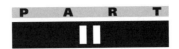

CLASSICAL RADIATION THERAPY

DOSE DISTRIBUTION AND SCATTER ANALYSIS

It is seldom possible to measure dose distribution directly in patients treated with radiation. Data on dose distribution are almost entirely derived from measurements in phantoms—tissue equivalent materials, usually large enough in volume to provide full-scatter conditions for the given beam. These basic data are used in a dose calculation system devised to predict dose distribution in an actual patient. This chapter deals with various quantities and concepts that are useful for this purpose.

9.1. PHANTOMS

Basic dose distribution data are usually measured in a water phantom, which closely approximates the radiation absorption and scattering properties of muscle and other soft tissues. Another reason for the choice of water as a phantom material is that it is universally available with reproducible radiation properties. A water phantom, however, poses some practical problems when used in conjunction with ion chambers and other detectors that are affected by water, unless they are designed to be waterproof. In most cases, however, the detector is encased in a thin plastic (water equivalent) sleeve before immersion into the water phantom.

Since it is not always possible to put radiation detectors in water, solid dry phantoms have been developed as substitutes for water. Ideally, for a given material to be tissue or water equivalent, it must have the same effective atomic number, number of electrons per gram, and mass density. However, since the Compton effect is the most predominant mode of interaction for megavoltage photon beams in the clinical range, the necessary condition for water equivalence for such beams is the same electron density (number of electrons per cubic centimeter) as that of water.

The electron density (ρ_e) of a material may be calculated from its mass density (ρ_m) and its atomic composition according to the formula:

$$\rho_e = \rho_m \cdot N_A \cdot \left(\frac{Z}{A}\right) \qquad (9.1)$$

where

$$\frac{Z}{A} = \sum_i a_i \cdot \left(\frac{Z_i}{A_i}\right) \qquad (9.2)$$

N_A is Avogadro's number and a_i is the fraction by weight of the ith element of atomic number Z_i and atomic weight A_i. Electron densities of various human tissues and body fluids have been calculated according to Equation 9.1 by Shrimpton (1). Values for some tissues of dosimetric interest are listed in Table 5.1.

Table 9.1 gives the properties of various phantoms that have been frequently used for radiation dosimetry. Of the commercially available phantom materials, Lucite and polystyrene are most frequently used as dosimetry phantoms. Although the mass density of these materials may vary depending on a given sample, the atomic composition and the number of electrons per gram of these materials are sufficiently constant to warrant their use for high-energy photon and electron dosimetry.

TABLE 9.1. PHYSICAL PROPERTIES OF VARIOUS PHANTOM MATERIALS

Material	Chemical Composition	Mass Density (g/cm³)	Number of Electrons/g (×10²³)	Z_{eff}[a] (Photoelectric)
Water	H_2O	1	3.34	7.42
Polystyrene	$(C_8H_8)_n$	103–1.05	3.24	5.69
Plexiglas (Perspex, Lucite)	$(C_5O_2H_8)_n$	1.16–1.20	3.24	6.48
Polyethylene	$(CH_2)_n$	0.92	3.44	6.16
Paraffin	C_nH_{2n+2}	0.87–0.91	3.44	5.42
Mix·D	Paraffin: 60.8 Polyethylene: 30.4 MgO: 6.4 TiO₂: 2.4	0.99	3.41	7.05
M 3	Paraffin: 100 MgO: 29.06 CaCO₃: 0.94	1.06	3.34	7.35
Solid water[b]	Expoxy resin-based mixture	1.00	3.34	

[a]Z_{eff} for photoelectric effect is given by Eq. 6.4.
[b]Available from Radiation Measurements, Inc. (Middleton, Wisconsin).
Data are from Tubiana M, Dutreix J, Duterix A, Jocky P. Bases physiques de la radiotherapie et de la radiobiologie. Paris: Masson ET Cie, Éditeurs, 1963:458; and Schulz RJ, Nath R. On the constancy in composition in polystyrene and polymethylmethacrylate plastics. Med Phys 1979;6:153.

In addition to the homogeneous phantoms, anthropomorphic phantoms are frequently used for clinical dosimetry. One such commercially available system, known as Alderson Rando Phantom,[1] incorporates materials to simulate various body tissues—muscle, bone, lung, and air cavities. The phantom is shaped into a human torso (Fig. 9.1) and is sectioned transversely into slices for dosimetric applications.

White et al. (2) have developed extensive recipes for tissue substitutes. The method is based on adding particulate fillers to epoxy resins to form a mixture with radiation properties closely approximating that of a particular tissue. The most important radiation properties in this regard are the mass attenuation coefficient, the mass energy absorption coefficient, electron mass stopping, and angular scattering power ratios. A detailed tabulation of tissue substitutes and their properties for all the body tissues is included in a report by the International Commission on Radiation Units and Measurements (3).

Based on the previous method, Constantinou et al. (4) designed an epoxy resin-based solid substitute for water, called *solid water*. This material could be used as a dosimetric calibration phantom for photon and electron beams in the radiation therapy energy range. Solid water phantoms are now commercially available from Radiation Measurements, Inc. (Middleton, WI).

9.2. DEPTH DOSE DISTRIBUTION

As the beam is incident on a patient (or a phantom), the absorbed dose in the patient varies with depth. This variation depends on many conditions: beam energy, depth, field size, distance from source, and beam collimation system. Thus the calculation of dose in the patient involves considerations in regard to these parameters and others as they affect depth dose distribution.

An essential step in the dose calculation system is to establish depth dose variation along the central axis of the beam. A number of quantities have been defined for this

---

[1] Alderson Research Laboratories, Inc., Stamford, Connecticut.

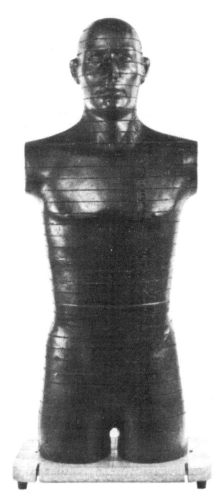

FIG. 9.1. An anthropomorphic phantom (Alderson Rando Phantom) sectioned transversely for dosimetric studies.

purpose, major among these being percentage depth dose (5), tissue-air ratios (6–9), tissue-phantom ratios (10–12), and tissue-maximum ratios (12,13). These quantities are usually derived from measurements made in water phantoms using small ionization chambers. Although other dosimetry systems such as TLD, diodes, and film are occasionally used, ion chambers are preferred because of their better precision and smaller energy dependence.

9.3. PERCENTAGE DEPTH DOSE

One way of characterizing the central axis dose distribution is to normalize dose at depth with respect to dose at a reference depth. The quantity *percentage* (or simply *percent*) *depth dose* may be defined as the quotient, expressed as a percentage, of the absorbed dose at any depth d to the absorbed dose at a fixed reference depth d_0, along the central axis of the beam (Fig. 9.2). Percentage depth dose (P) is thus:

$$P = \frac{D_d}{D_{d_0}} \times 100 \qquad (9.3)$$

For orthovoltage (up to about 400 kVp) and lower-energy x-rays, the reference depth is usually the surface ($d_0 = 0$). For higher energies, the reference depth is taken at the position of the *peak absorbed dose* ($d_0 = d_m$).

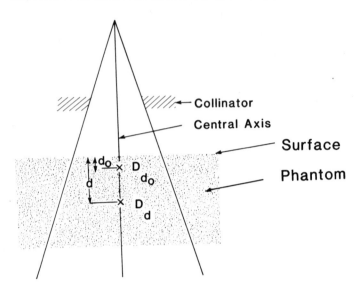

FIG. 9.2. Percentage depth dose is $(D_d/D_{d_0}) \times 100$, where *d* is any depth and d_0 is reference depth of maximum dose.

In clinical practice, the peak absorbed dose on the central axis is sometimes called the *maximum dose*, the *dose maximum*, the *given dose*, or simply the D_{max}. Thus,

$$D_{max} = \frac{D_d}{P} \times 100 \tag{9.4}$$

A number of parameters affect the central axis depth dose distribution. These include beam quality or energy, depth, field size and shape, source to surface distance, and beam collimation. A discussion of these parameters will now be presented.

A. Dependence on Beam Quality and Depth

The percentage depth dose (beyond the depth of maximum dose) increases with beam energy. Higher-energy beams have greater penetrating power and thus deliver a higher percentage depth dose (Fig. 9.3). If the effects of inverse square law and scattering are not considered, the percentage depth-dose variation with depth is governed approximately by exponential attenuation. Thus the beam quality affects the percentage depth dose by virtue of the average attenuation coefficient $\overline{\mu}$.[2] As the $\overline{\mu}$ decreases, the more penetrating the beam becomes, resulting in a higher percentage depth dose at any given depth beyond the build-up region.

A.1. Initial Dose Build-Up

As seen in Fig. 9.3, the percentage depth dose decreases with depth beyond the depth of maximum dose. However, there is an initial buildup of dose which becomes more and more pronounced as the energy is increased. In the case of the orthovoltage or lower-energy x-rays, the dose builds up to a maximum on or very close to the surface. But for higher-energy beams, the point of maximum dose lies deeper into the tissue or phantom. The region between the surface and the point of maximum dose is called the *dose build-up region*.

The dose build-up effect of the higher-energy beams gives rise to what is clinically known as the *skin-sparing effect*. For megavoltage beams such as cobalt-60 and higher energies the surface dose is much smaller than the D_{max}. This offers a distinct advantage over the lower-energy beams for which the D_{max} occurs at the skin surface. Thus, in the case

---

[2] $\overline{\mu}$ is the average attenuation coefficient for the heterogeneous beam.

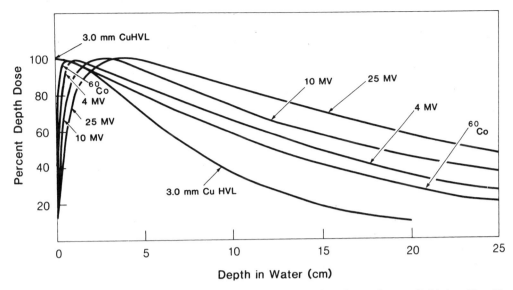

FIG. 9.3. Central axis depth dose distribution for different quality photon beams. Field size, 10 × 10 cm; SSD = 100 cm for all beams except for 3.0 mm Cu HVL, SSD = 50 cm. (Data from Hospital Physicists' Association. Central axis depth dose data for use in radiotherapy. *Br J Radiol* 1978;[suppl 11]; and the Appendix.)

of the higher energy photon beams, higher doses can be delivered to deep-seated tumors without exceeding the tolerance of the skin. This, of course, is possible because of both the higher percent depth dose at the tumor and the lower surface dose at the skin. This topic is discussed in greater detail in Chapter 13.

The physics of dose buildup may be explained as follows: (a) As the high-energy photon beam enters the patient or the phantom, high-speed electrons are ejected from the surface and the subsequent layers; (b) These electrons deposit their energy a significant distance away from their site of origin; (c) Because of (a) and (b), the electron fluence and hence the absorbed dose increase with depth until they reach a maximum. However, the photon energy fluence continuously decreases with depth and, as a result, the production of electrons also decreases with depth. The net effect is that beyond a certain depth the dose eventually begins to decrease with depth.

It may be instructive to explain the buildup phenomenon in terms of absorbed dose and a quantity known as *kerma* (from *k*inetic *e*nergy *r*eleased in the *ma*terial). As discussed in Chapter 8, the kerma (K) may be defined as "the quotient of dE_{tr} by dm, where dE_{tr} is the sum of the initial kinetic energies of all the charged ionizing particles (electrons) liberated by uncharged ionizing particles (photons) in a material of mass dm" (14).

$$K = \frac{dE_{tr}}{dm}$$

Because kerma represents the energy transferred from photons to directly ionizing electrons, the kerma is maximum at the surface and decreases with depth because of the decrease in the photon energy fluence (Fig. 9.4). The absorbed dose, on the other hand, first increases with depth as the high-speed electrons ejected at various depths travel downstream. As a result, there is an electronic build-up with depth. However, as the dose depends on the electron fluence, it reaches a maximum at a depth approximately equal to the range of electrons in the medium. Beyond this depth, the dose decreases as kerma continues to decrease, resulting in a decrease in secondary electron production and hence a net decrease in electron fluence. As seen in Fig. 9.4, the kerma curve is initially higher than the dose curve but falls below the dose curve beyond the build-up region. This effect is explained by the fact that the areas under the two curves taken to infinity must be the same.

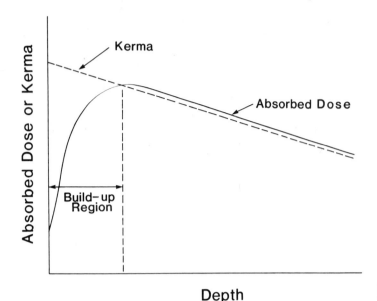

FIG. 9.4. Schematic plot of absorbed dose and kerma as functions of depth.

B. Effect of Field Size and Shape

Field size may be specified either geometrically or dosimetrically. The *geometrical field size* is defined as "the projection, on a plane perpendicular to the beam axis, of the distal end of the collimator as seen from the front center of the source" (15). This definition usually corresponds to the field defined by the light localizer, arranged as if a point source of light were located at the center of the front surface of the radiation source. The *dosimetric,* or the *physical,* field size is the distance intercepted by a given isodose curve (usually 50% isodose) on a plane perpendicular to the beam axis at a stated distance from the source.

Unless stated otherwise, the term *field size* in this book will denote geometric field size. In addition, the field size will be defined at a predetermined distance such as the *source-surface distance* (SSD) or the *source-axis distance* (SAD). The latter term is the distance from the source to axis of gantry rotation known as the *isocenter.*

For a sufficiently small field one may assume that the depth dose at a point is effectively the result of the primary radiation, that is, the photons which have traversed the overlying medium without interacting. The contribution of the scattered photons to the depth dose in this case is negligibly small or 0. But as the field size is increased, the contribution of the scattered radiation to the absorbed dose increases. Because this increase in scattered dose is greater at larger depths than at the depth of D_{max}, the percent depth dose increases with increasing field size.

The increase in percent depth dose caused by increase in field size depends on beam quality. Since the scattering probability or cross-section decreases with energy increase and the higher-energy photons are scattered more predominantly in the forward direction, the field size dependence of percent depth dose is less pronounced for the higher-energy than for the lower-energy beams.

Percent depth dose data for radiation therapy beams are usually tabulated for square fields. Since the majority of the treatments encountered in clinical practice require rectangular and irregularly shaped (blocked) fields, a system of equating square fields to different field shapes is required. Semiempirical methods have been developed to relate central axis depth dose data for square, rectangular, circular, and irregularly shaped fields. Although general methods (based on Clarkson's principle—to be discussed later in this chapter) are available, simpler methods have been developed specifically for interrelating square, rectangular, and circular field data.

Day (16) and others (17,18) have shown that, for central axis depth-dose distribution, a rectangular field may be approximated by an equivalent square or by an equivalent circle.

TABLE 9.2. EQUIVALENT SQUARES OF RECTANGULAR FIELDS

Long Axis (cm)	2	4	6	8	10	12	14	16	18	20	22	24	26	28	30
2	2.0														
4	2.7	4.0													
6	3.1	4.8	6.0												
8	3.4	5.4	6.9	8.0											
10	3.6	5.8	7.5	8.9	10.0										
12	3.7	6.1	8.0	9.6	10.9	12.0									
14	3.8	6.3	8.4	10.1	11.6	12.9	14.0								
16	3.9	6.5	8.6	10.5	12.2	13.7	14.9	16.0							
18	4.0	6.6	8.9	10.8	12.7	14.3	15.7	16.9	18.0						
20	4.0	6.7	9.0	11.1	13.0	14.7	16.3	17.7	18.9	20.0					
22	4.0	6.8	9.1	11.3	13.3	15.1	16.8	18.3	19.7	20.9	22.0				
24	4.1	6.8	9.2	11.5	13.5	15.4	17.2	18.8	20.3	21.7	22.9	24.0			
26	4.1	6.9	9.3	11.6	13.7	15.7	17.5	19.2	20.9	22.4	23.7	24.9	26.0		
28	4.1	6.9	9.4	11.7	13.8	15.9	17.8	19.6	21.3	22.9	24.4	25.7	27.0	28.0	
30	4.1	6.9	9.4	11.7	13.9	16.0	18.0	19.9	21.7	23.3	24.9	26.4	27.7	29.0	30.0

From Hospital Physicists' Association. Central axis depth dose data for use in radiotherapy. Br J Radiol 1978;(suppl 11), with permission.

Data for equivalent squares, taken from Hospital Physicists' Association (5) are given in Table 9.2. As an example, consider a 10 × 20-cm field. From Table 9.2, the equivalent square is 13.0 × 13.0 cm. Thus the percent depth dose data for a 13 × 13-cm field (obtained from standard tables) may be applied as an approximation to the given 10 × 20-cm field.

A simple rule of thumb method has been developed by Sterling et al. (19) for equating rectangular and square fields. According to this rule, a rectangular field is equivalent to a square field if they have the same area/perimeter (A/P). For example, the 10 × 20-cm field has an A/P of 3.33. The square field which has the same A/P is 13.3 × 13.3 cm, a value very close to that given in Table 9.2.

The following formulas are useful for quick calculation of the equivalent field parameters: For rectangular fields,

$$A/P = \frac{a \times b}{2(a + b)} \tag{9.5}$$

where a is field width and b is field length. For square fields, since $a = b$,

$$A/P = \frac{a}{4} \tag{9.6}$$

where a is the side of the square. From Equations 9.5 and 9.6, it is evident that the side of an equivalent square of a rectangular field is $4 \times A/P$. For example, a 10 × 15-cm field has an A/P of 3.0. Its equivalent square is 12 × 12 cm. This agrees closely with the value of 11.9 given in Table 9.2.

Although the concept of A/P is not based on sound physical principles, it is widely used in clinical practice and has been extended as a field parameter to apply to other quantities such as backscatter factors, tissue-air ratios, and even beam output in air or in phantom. The reader may, however, be cautioned against an indiscriminate use of A/P. For example, the A/P parameter, as such, does not apply to circular or irregularly shaped fields, although radii of equivalent circles may be obtained by the relationship:

$$r = \frac{4}{\sqrt{\pi}} \cdot A/P \tag{9.7}$$

Equation 9.7 can be derived by assuming that the equivalent circle is the one that has the same area as the equivalent square. Validity of this approximation has been verified from the table of equivalent circles given in Hospital Physicists' Association (5).

C. Dependence on Source-Surface Distance

Photon fluence emitted by a point source of radiation varies inversely as a square of the distance from the source. Although the clinical source (isotopic source or focal spot) for external beam therapy has a finite size, the source-surface distance is usually chosen to be large ($\geq$80 cm) so that the source dimensions become unimportant in relation to the variation of photon fluence with distance. In other words, the source can be considered as a point at large source-surface distances. Thus the exposure rate or "dose rate in free space" (Chapter 8) from such a source varies inversely as the square of the distance. Of course, the inverse square law dependence of dose rate assumes that we are dealing with a primary beam, without scatter. In a given clinical situation, however, collimation or other scattering material in the beam may cause deviation from the inverse square law.

Percent depth dose increases with SSD because of the effects of the inverse square law. Although the actual dose rate at a point decreases with increase in distance from the source, the percent depth dose, which is a relative dose with respect to a reference point, increases with SSD. This is illustrated in Fig. 9.5 in which relative dose rate from a point source of radiation is plotted as a function of distance from the source, following the inverse square law. The plot shows that the drop in dose rate between two points is much greater at smaller distances from the source than at large distances. This means that the percent depth dose, which represents depth dose relative to a reference point, decreases more rapidly near the source than far away from the source.

In clinical radiation therapy, SSD is a very important parameter. Because percent depth dose determines how much dose can be delivered at depth relative to the surface dose or D_{max}, the SSD needs to be as large as possible. However, because dose rate decreases with distance, the SSD, in practice, is set at a distance which provides a compromise between dose rate and percent depth dose. For the treatment of deep-seated lesions with megavoltage beams, the minimum recommended SSD is 80 cm.

Tables of percent depth dose for clinical use are usually measured at a standard SSD (80 or 100 cm for megavoltage units). In a given clinical situation, however, the SSD set on a patient may be different from the standard SSD. For example, larger SSDs are required for treatment techniques that involve field sizes larger than the ones available at

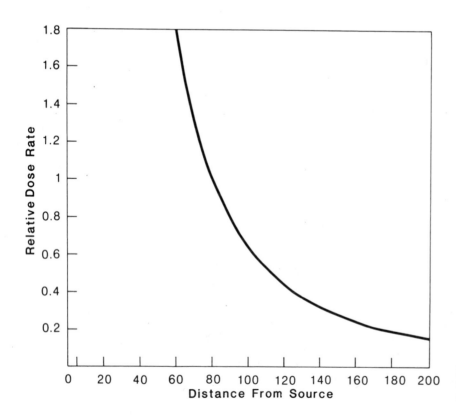

FIG. 9.5. Plot of relative dose rate as inverse square law function of distance from a point source. Reference distance = 80 cm.

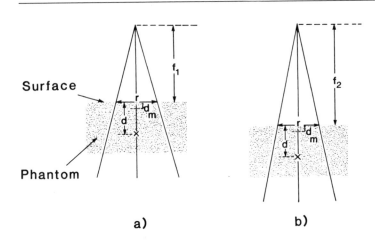

FIG. 9.6. Change of percent depth dose with SSD. Irradiation condition **(a)** has SSD = f_1 and condition **(b)** has SSD = f_2. For both conditions, field size on the phantom surface, $r \times r$, and depth d are the same.

the standard SSDs. Thus the percent depth doses for a standard SSD must be converted to those applicable to the actual treatment SSD. Although more accurate methods are available (to be discussed later in this chapter), we discuss an approximate method in this section: the *Mayneord F Factor* (20). This method is based on a strict application of the inverse square law, without considering changes in scattering, as the SSD is changed.

Figure 9.6 shows two irradiation conditions, which differ only in regard to SSD. Let $P(d,r,f)$ be the percent depth dose at depth d for SSD = f and a field size r (e.g., a square field of dimensions $r \times r$). Since the variation in dose with depth is governed by three effects—inverse square law, exponential attenuation, and scattering—

$$P(d,r,f_1) = 100 \cdot \left(\frac{f_1 + d_m}{f_1 + d} \right)^2 \cdot e^{-\mu(d-d_m)} \cdot K_s \tag{9.8}$$

where μ is the linear attenuation coefficient for the primary and K_s is a function which accounts for the change in scattered dose. Ignoring the change in the value of K_s from one SSD to another,

$$P(d,r,f_2) = 100 \cdot \left(\frac{f_2 + d_m}{f_2 + d} \right)^2 \cdot e^{-\mu(d-d_m)} \cdot K_s \tag{9.9}$$

Dividing Equation 9.9 by 9.8, we have:

$$\frac{P(d,r,f_2)}{P(d,r,f_1)} = \left(\frac{f_2 + d_m}{f_1 + d_m} \right)^2 \cdot \left(\frac{f_1 + d}{f_2 + d} \right)^2 \tag{9.10}$$

The terms on the right-hand side of Equation 9.10 are called the Mayneord F factor. Thus,

$$F = \left(\frac{f_2 + d_m}{f_1 + d_m} \right)^2 \cdot \left(\frac{f_1 + d}{f_2 + d} \right)^2 \tag{9.11}$$

It can be shown that the F factor is greater than 1 for $f_2 > f_1$ and less than 1 for $f_2 < f_1$. Thus it may be restated that the percent depth dose increases with increase in SSD.

Example 1

The percent depth dose for a 15 × 15 field size, 10-cm depth, and 80-cm SSD is 58.4 (^{60}Co beam). Find the percent depth dose for the same field size and depth for a 100-cm SSD.

From Equation 9.11, assuming $d_m = 0.5$ cm for ^{60}Co γ rays:

$$F = \left(\frac{100 + 0.5}{80 + 0.5} \right)^2 \left(\frac{80 + 10}{100 + 10} \right)^2$$

$$= 1.043$$

From Equation 9.10,

$$\frac{P(10,15,100)}{P(10,15,80)} = 1.043$$

Thus, the desired percent depth dose is:

$$P(10,15,100) = P(10,15,80) \times 1.043$$
$$= 58.4 \times 1.043$$
$$= 60.9$$

More accurate methods that take scattering change into account would yield a value close to 60.6.

The Mayneord F factor method works reasonably well for small fields since the scattering is minimal under these conditions. However, the method can give rise to significant errors under extreme conditions such as lower energy, large field, large depth, and large SSD change. For example, the error in dose at a 20-cm depth for a 30×30-cm field and 160-cm SSD (^{60}Co beam) will be about 3% if the percent depth dose is calculated from the 80-cm SSD tables.

In general, the Mayneord F factor overestimates the increase in percent depth dose with increase in SSD. For example, for large fields and lower energy radiation where the proportion of scattered radiation is relatively greater, the factor $(1 + F)/2$ applies more accurately. Factors intermediate between F and $(1 + F)/2$ have also been used for certain conditions (20).

9.4. TISSUE-AIR RATIO

Tissue-air ratio (TAR) was first introduced by Johns et al. (6) in 1953 and was originally called the "tumor-air ratio." At that time, this quantity was intended specifically for rotation therapy calculations. In rotation therapy, the radiation source moves in a circle around the axis of rotation which is usually placed in the tumor. Although the SSD may vary depending on the shape of the surface contour, the source-axis distance remains constant.

Since the percent depth dose depends on the SSD (section 9.3C), the SSD correction to the percent depth dose will have to be applied to correct for the varying SSD—a procedure that becomes cumbersome to apply routinely in clinical practice. A simpler quantity—namely, TAR—has been defined to remove the SSD dependence. Since the time of its introduction, the concept of TAR has been refined to facilitate calculations not only for rotation therapy but also for stationary isocentric techniques as well as irregular fields.

Tissue-air ratio may be defined as the ratio of the dose (D_d) at a given point in the phantom to the dose in free space (D_{fs}) at the same point. This is illustrated in Fig. 9.7.

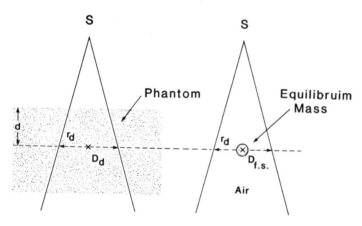

FIG. 9.7. Illustration of the definition of tissue-air ratio. TAR $(d, r_d) = D_d/D_{fs}$.

For a given quality beam, TAR depends on depth d and field size r_d at that depth:

$$\text{TAR}(d, r_d) = \frac{D_d}{D_{fs}} \tag{9.12}$$

A. Effect of Distance

One of the most important properties attributed to TAR is that it is independent of the distance from the source. This, however, is an approximation which is usually valid to an accuracy of better than 2% over the range of distances used clinically. This useful result can be deduced as follows.

Because TAR is the ratio of the two doses (D_d and D_{fs}) at the same point, the distance dependence of the photon fluence is removed. Thus the TAR represents modification of the dose at a point owing only to attenuation and scattering of the beam in the phantom compared with the dose at the same point in the miniphantom (or equilibrium phantom) placed in free air. Since the primary beam is attenuated exponentially with depth, the TAR for the primary beam is only a function of depth, not of SSD. The case of the scatter component, however, is not obvious. Nevertheless, Johns et al. (21) have shown that the fractional scatter contribution to the depth dose is almost independent of the divergence of the beam and depends only on the depth and the field size at that depth. Hence the tissue-air ratio, which involves both the primary and scatter component of the depth dose, is independent of the source distance.

B. Variation with Energy, Depth, and Field Size

Tissue-air ratio varies with energy, depth, and field size very much like the percent depth dose. For the megavoltage beams, the tissue-air ratio builds up to a maximum at the depth of maximum dose (d_m) and then decreases with depth more or less exponentially. For a narrow beam or a 0×0 field size[3] in which scatter contribution to the dose is neglected, the TAR beyond d_m varies approximately exponentially with depth

$$\text{TAR}(d, 0) = e^{-\bar{\mu}(d - d_m)} \tag{9.13}$$

where $\bar{\mu}$ is the average attenuation coefficient of the beam for the given phantom. As the field size is increased, the scattered component of the dose increases and the variation of TAR with depth becomes more complex. However, for high-energy megavoltage beams, for which the scatter is minimal and is directed more or less in the forward direction, the TAR variation with depth can still be approximated by an exponential function, provided an effective attenuation coefficient (μ_{eff}) for the given field size is used.

B.1. Backscatter Factor

The term backscatter factor (BSF) is simply the tissue-air ratio at the depth of maximum dose on central axis of the beam. It may be defined as the ratio of the dose on central axis at the depth of maximum dose to the dose at the same point in free space. Mathematically,

$$\text{BSF} = \frac{D_{\max}}{D_{fs}} \tag{9.14}$$

or

$$\text{BSF} = \text{TAR}(d_m, r_{d_m}) \tag{9.15}$$

where r_{d_m} is the field size at the depth d_m of maximum dose.

---

[3] A 0×0 field is a hypothetical field in which the depth dose is entirely due to primary photons.

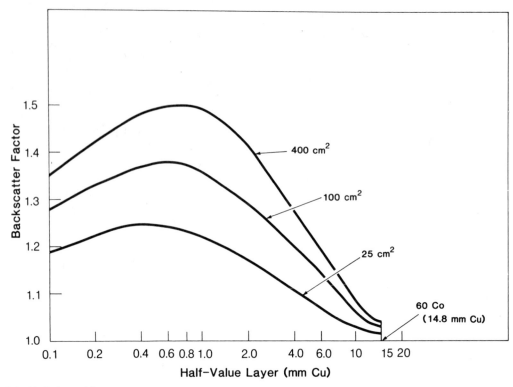

FIG. 9.8. Variation of backscatter factors with beam quality (half-value layer). Data are for circular fields. (Data from Hospital Physicists' Association. Central axis depth dose data for use in radiotherapy. *Br J Radiol* 1978;[suppl 11]; and Johns HE, Hunt JW, Fedoruk SO. Surface back-scatter in the 100 kV to 400 kV range. *Br J Radiol* 1954;27:443.)

The backscatter factor, like the tissue-air ratio, is independent of distance from the source and depends only on the beam quality and field size. Figure 9.8 shows backscatter factors for various quality beams and field areas. Whereas BSF increases with field size, its maximum value occurs for beams having a half-value layer between 0.6 and 0.8 mm Cu, depending on field size. Thus, for the orthovoltage beams with usual filtration, the backscatter factor can be as high as 1.5 for large field sizes. This amounts to a 50% increase in dose near the surface compared with the dose in free space or, in terms of exposure, 50% increase in exposure on the skin compared with the exposure in air.

For megavoltage beams (^{60}Co and higher energies), the backscatter factor is much smaller. For example, BSF for a 10×10-cm field for ^{60}Co is 1.036. This means that the D_{max} will be 3.6% higher than the dose in free space. This increase in dose is the result of radiation scatter reaching the point of D_{max} from the overlying and underlying tissues. As the beam energy is increased, the scatter is further reduced and so is the backscatter factor. Above about 8 MV, the scatter at the depth of D_{max} becomes negligibly small and the backscatter factor approaches its minimum value of unity.

C. Relationship between TAR and Percent Depth Dose

Tissue-air ratio and percent depth dose are interrelated. The relationship can be derived as follows: Considering Fig. 9.9A, let TAR(d,r_d) be the tissue-air ratio at point Q for a field size r_d at depth d. Let r be the field size at the surface, f be the SSD, and d_m be the reference depth of maximum dose at point P. Let $D_{fs}(P)$ and $D_{fs}(Q)$ be the doses in free space at points P and Q, respectively (Fig. 9.9B,C). $D_{fs}(P)$ and $D_{fs}(Q)$ are related by inverse square law.

$$\frac{D_{fs}(Q)}{D_{fs}(P)} = \left(\frac{f + d_m}{f + d} \right)^2 \tag{9.16}$$

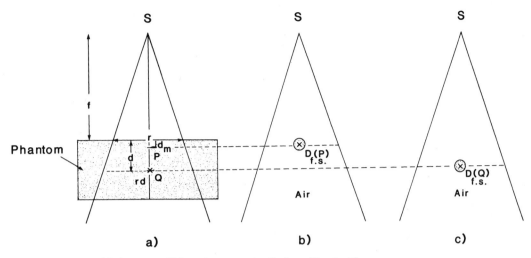

FIG. 9.9. Relationship between TAR and percent depth dose. (See text.)

The field sizes r and r_d are related by:

$$r_d = r \cdot \frac{f + d}{f} \tag{9.17}$$

By definition of TAR,

$$\text{TAR}(d, r_d) = \frac{D_d(Q)}{D_{fs}(Q)} \tag{9.18}$$

or

$$D_d(Q) = \text{TAR}(d, r_d) \cdot D_{fs}(Q) \tag{9.19}$$

Since

$$D_{\max}(P) = D_{fs}(P) \cdot \text{BSF}(r) \tag{9.20}$$

and, by definition, the percent depth dose $P(d, r, f)$ is given by:

$$P(d, r, f) = \frac{D_d(Q)}{D_{\max}(P)} \cdot 100 \tag{9.21}$$

we have, from Equations 9.19, 9.20, and 9.21,

$$P(d, r, f) = \text{TAR}(d, r_d) \cdot \frac{1}{\text{BSF}(r)} \cdot \frac{D_{fs}(Q)}{D_{fs}(P)} \cdot 100 \tag{9.22}$$

From Equations 9.16 and 9.22,

$$P(d, r, f) = \text{TAR}(d, r_d) \cdot \frac{1}{\text{BSF}(r)} \cdot \left(\frac{f + d_m}{f + d} \right)^2 \cdot 100 \tag{9.23}$$

C.1. Conversion of Percent Depth Dose from One SSD to Another—the TAR Method

In section 9.3C, we discussed a method of converting percent depth dose from one SSD to another. That method used the Mayneord F factor which is derived solely from inverse square law considerations. A more accurate method is based on the interrelationship between percent depth dose and TAR. This TAR method can be derived from Equation 9.23 as follows.

Suppose f_1 is the SSD for which the percent depth dose is known and f_2 is the SSD for which the percent depth dose is to be determined. Let r be the field size at the surface and *d* be the depth, for both cases. Referring to Fig. 9.6, let r_{d,f_1} and r_{d,f_2} be the field sizes projected at depth *d* in Fig. 9.6A,B, respectively.

$$r_{d,f_1} = r \cdot \frac{f_1 + d}{f_1} \tag{9.24}$$

$$r_{d,f_2} = r \cdot \frac{f_2 + d}{f_2} \tag{9.25}$$

From Equation 9.23,

$$P(d,r,f_1) = \text{TAR}(d,r_{d,f_1}) \cdot \frac{1}{\text{BSF}(r)} \cdot \left(\frac{f_1 + d_m}{f_1 + d}\right)^2 \cdot 100 \tag{9.26}$$

and

$$P(d,r,f_2) = \text{TAR}(d,r_{d,f_2}) \cdot \frac{1}{\text{BSF}(r)} \cdot \left(\frac{f_2 + d_m}{f_2 + d}\right)^2 \cdot 100 \tag{9.27}$$

From Equations 9.26 and 9.27, the conversion factor is given by:

$$\frac{P(d,r,f_2)}{P(d,r,f_1)} = \frac{\text{TAR}(d,r_{d,f_2})}{\text{TAR}(d,r_{d,f_1})} \cdot \left[\left(\frac{f_1 + d}{f_2 + d}\right)^2 \cdot \left(\frac{f_2 + d_m}{f_1 + d_m}\right)^2\right] \tag{9.28}$$

The last term in the brackets is the Mayneord factor. Thus the TAR method corrects the Mayneord *F* factor by the ratio of TARs for the fields projected at depth for the two SSDs.

Burns (22) has developed the following equation to convert percent depth dose from one SSD to another:

$$P(d,r,f_2) = P\left(d,\frac{r}{\sqrt{F}},f_1\right) \cdot \frac{\text{BSF}(r/\sqrt{F})}{\text{BSF}(r)} \cdot F \tag{9.29}$$

where *F* is the Mayneord *F* factor given by

$$\left(\frac{f_1 + d}{f_2 + d}\right)^2 \cdot \left(\frac{f_2 + d_m}{f_1 + d_m}\right)^2$$

Equation 9.29 is based on the concept that TARs are independent of the source distance. Burns's equation may be used in a situation where TARs are not available but instead a percent depth dose table is available at a standard SSD along with the backscatter factors for various field sizes.

As mentioned earlier, for high-energy x-rays, that is, above 8 MV, the variation of percent depth dose with field size is small and the backscatter is negligible. Equations 9.28 and 9.29 then simplify to a use of Mayneord *F* factor.

Practical Examples

In this section, I will present examples of typical treatment calculations using the concepts of percent depth dose, backscatter factor, and tissue-air ratio. Although a more general system of dosimetric calculations will be presented in the next chapter, these examples are presented here to illustrate the concepts presented thus far.

Example 2

A patient is to be treated with an orthovoltage beam having a half-value layer of 3 mm Cu. Supposing that the machine is calibrated in terms of exposure rate in air, find the time required to deliver 200 cGy (rad) at 5 cm depth, given the following data: exposure rate = 100 R/min at 50 cm, field size = 8 × 8 cm, SSD = 50 cm, percent depth dose = 64.8, backscatter factor = 1.20, and rad/R = 0.95 (check these data in reference 5).

$$\text{Dose rate in free space} = \text{exposure rate} \times \text{rad/R factor} \times A_{eq}$$
$$= 100 \times 0.95 \times 1.00$$
$$= 95 \text{ cGy/min}$$
$$D_{max} \text{ rate} = \text{dose rate free space} \times \text{BSF}$$
$$= 95 \times 1.20$$
$$= 114 \text{ cGy/min}$$
$$\text{Tumor dose to be delivered} = 200 \text{ cGy}$$
$$D_{max} \text{ to be delivered} = \frac{\text{tumor dose}}{\text{percent depth dose}} \times 100$$
$$= \frac{200}{64.8} \times 100$$
$$= 308.6 \text{ cGy}$$
$$\text{Treatment time} = \frac{D_{max} \text{ to be delivered}}{D_{max} \text{ rate}}$$
$$= \frac{308.6}{114}$$
$$= 2.71 \text{ min}$$

Example 3

A patient is to be treated with ^{60}Co radiation. Supposing that the machine is calibrated in air in terms of dose rate free space, find the treatment time to deliver 200 cGy (rad) at a depth of 8 cm, given the following data: dose rate free space = 150 cGy/min at 80.5 cm for a field size of 10 × 10 cm, SSD = 80 cm, percent depth dose = 64.1, and backscatter factor = 1.036.

$$D_{max} \text{ rate} = 150 \times 1.036 = 155.4 \text{ cGy/min}$$
$$D_{max} = \frac{200}{64.1} \times 100 = 312 \text{ cGy}$$
$$\text{Treatment time} = \frac{312}{155.4} = 2.01 \text{ min}$$

Example 4

Determine the time required to deliver 200 cGy (rad) with a ^{60}Co γ ray beam at the *isocenter* (a point of intersection of the collimator axis and the gantry axis of rotation) which is placed at a 10 cm depth in a patient, given the following data: SAD = 80 cm, field size = 6 × 12 cm (at the isocenter), dose rate free space at the SAD for this field = 120 cGy/min and TAR = 0.681.

$$A/P \text{ for } 6 \times 12 \text{ cm field} = \frac{6 \times 12}{2(6 \times 12)} = 2$$
$$\text{Side of equivalent square field} = 4 \times A/P = 8 \text{ cm}$$
$$\text{TAR}(10, 8 \times 8) = 0.681 \text{ (given)}$$
$$D_d = 200 \text{ cGy (given)}$$
$$\text{Since TAR} = D_d/D_{fs}$$
$$D_{fs} = \frac{200}{0.681} = 293.7 \text{ cGy}$$

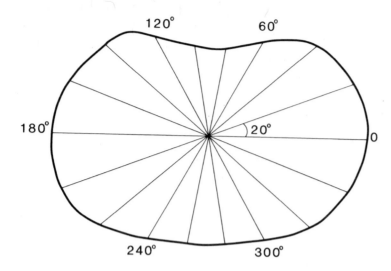

FIG. 9.10. Contour of patient with radii drawn from the isocenter of rotation at 20-degree intervals. Length of each radius represents a depth for which TAR is determined for the field size at the isocenter. (See Table 9.3.)

$$D_{fs} \text{ rate} = 120 \text{ cGy/min (given)}$$

$$\text{Treatment time} = \frac{293.7}{120} = 2.45 \text{ min}$$

D. Calculation of Dose in Rotation Therapy

The concept of tissue-air ratios is most useful for calculations involving isocentric techniques of irradiation. Rotation or arc therapy is a type of isocentric irradiation in which the source moves continuously around the axis of rotation.

The calculation of depth dose in rotation therapy involves the determination of average TAR at the isocenter. The contour of the patient is drawn in a plane containing the axis of rotation. The isocenter is then placed within the contour (usually in the middle of the tumor or a few centimeters beyond it) and radii are drawn from this point at selected angular intervals (e.g., 20 degrees) (Fig. 9.10). Each radius represents a depth for which TAR can be obtained from the TAR table, for the given beam energy and field size defined at the isocenter. The TARs are then summed and averaged to determine $\overline{\text{TAR}}$, as illustrated in Table 9.3.

Example 5

For the data given in Table 9.3, determine the treatment time to deliver 200 cGy (rad) at the center of rotation, given the data: dose rate free space for 6 × 6-cm field at the SAD

TABLE 9.3. DETERMINATION OF AVERAGE *TAR* AT THE CENTER OF ROTATION[a]

Angle	Depth along Radius	TAR	Angle	Depth along Radius	TAR
0	16.6	0.444	180	16.2	0.450
20	16.0	0.456	200	16.2	0.450
40	14.6	0.499	220	14.6	0.499
60	11.0	0.614	240	12.4	0.563
80	9.0	0.691	260	11.2	0.606
100	9.4	0.681	280	11.0	0.614
120	11.4	0.597	300	12.0	0.580
140	14.0	0.515	320	14.2	0.507
160	15.6	0.470	340	16.0	0.456

[a] ^{60}Co beam, field size at the isocenter = 6 × 6 cm. Average tissue-air ratio $(\overline{\text{TAR}})$ = 9.692/18 = 0.538.

is 86.5 cGy/min.

$$\overline{\text{TAR}} = 0.538 \text{ (as calculated in Table 9.3)}$$

Dose to be delivered at isocenter $= 200$ cGy (given)

Dose free space to be delivered at isocenter $= \dfrac{200}{0.538} = 371.8$ cGy

Dose rate free space at isocenter $= 86.5$ cGy/min (given)

Treatment time $= \dfrac{371.8}{86.5} = 4.30$ min

9.5. SCATTER-AIR RATIO

Scatter-air ratios are used for the purpose of calculating scattered dose in the medium. The computation of the primary and the scattered dose separately is particularly useful in the dosimetry of irregular fields.

Scatter-air ratio may be defined as the ratio of the scattered dose at a given point in the phantom to the dose in free space at the same point. The scatter-air ratio like the tissue-air ratio is independent of the source-to-surface distance but depends on the beam energy, depth, and field size.

Because the scattered dose at a point in the phantom is equal to the total dose minus the primary dose at that point, scatter-air ratio is mathematically given by the difference between the TAR for the given field and the TAR for the 0×0 field.

$$\text{SAR}(d, r_d) = \text{TAR}(d, r_d) - \text{TAR}(d, 0) \tag{9.30}$$

Here TAR(d,0) represents the primary component of the beam.

Because SARs are primarily used in calculating scatter in a field of any shape, SARs are tabulated as functions of depth and radius of a circular field at that depth. Also, because SAR data are derived from TAR data for rectangular or square fields, radii of equivalent circles may be obtained from the table in reference 5 or by Equation 9.7.

A. Dose Calculation in Irregular Fields—Clarkson's Method

Any field other than the rectangular, square, or circular field may be termed irregular. Irregularly shaped fields are encountered in radiation therapy when radiation sensitive structures are shielded from the primary beam or when the field extends beyond the irregularly shaped patient body contour. Examples of such fields are the mantle and inverted Y fields used for the treatment of Hodgkin's disease. Since the basic data (percent depth dose, tissue-air ratios, or tissue-maximum ratios—to be discussed later) are available usually for rectangular fields, methods are required to use these data for general cases of irregularly shaped fields. One such method, originally proposed by Clarkson (23) and later developed by Cunningham (24,25), has proved to be the most general in its application.

Clarkson's method is based on the principle that the scattered component of the depth dose, which depends on the field size and shape, can be calculated separately from the primary component which is independent of the field size and shape. A special quantity, SAR, is used to calculate the scattered dose. This method has been discussed in detail in the literature (26,27) and only a brief discussion will be presented here.

Let us consider an irregularly shaped field as shown in Fig. 9.11. Assume this field cross-section to be at depth d and perpendicular to the beam axis. Let Q be the point of calculation in the plane of the field cross-section. Radii are drawn from Q to divide the field into elementary sectors. Each sector is characterized by its radius and can be considered as part of a circular field of that radius. If we suppose the sector angle is 10 degrees, then the scatter contribution from this sector will be $10°/360° = 1/36$ of that contributed by a

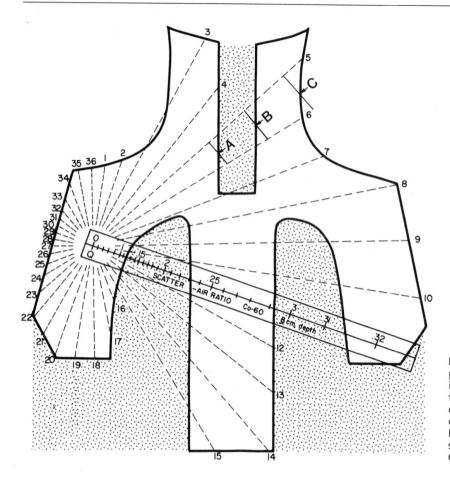

FIG. 9.11. Outline of mantle field in a plane perpendicular to the beam axis and at a specified depth. Radii are drawn from point Q, the point of calculation. Sector angle = 10 degrees. (Redrawn from American Association of Physicists in Medicine. Dosimetry workshop: Hodgkin's disease. Chicago, IL, M.D. Anderson Hospital, Houston, TX, Radiological Physics Center, 1970.)

circular field of that radius and centered at Q. Thus the scatter contribution from all the sectors can be calculated and summed by considering each sector to be a part of its own circle the scatter-air ratio of which is already known and tabulated.

Using an SAR table for circular fields, the SAR values for the sectors are calculated and then summed to give the average scatter-air ratio $(\overline{SAR})$ for the irregular field at point Q. For sectors passing through a blocked area, the net SAR is determined by subtracting the scatter contribution by the blocked part of sector. For example, net $(SAR)_{QC} = (SAR)_{QC} - (SAR)_{QB} + (SAR)_{QA}$.

The computed $\overline{SAR}$ is converted to average tissue-air ratio $(\overline{TAR})$ by the equation:

$$\overline{TAR} = TAR(0) + \overline{SAR} \tag{9.31}$$

where TAR(0) is the tissue-air ratio for 0×0 field, that is,

$$TAR(0) = e^{-\overline{\mu}(d-d_m)}$$

where $\overline{\mu}$ is the average linear attenuation coefficient for the beam and d is the depth of point Q.

The percent depth dose (%DD) at Q may be calculated relative to D_{max} on the central axis using Equation 9.23.

$$\%DD = 100 \times \overline{TAR} \times \left(\frac{f + d_m}{f + d}\right)^2 \Big/ BSF \tag{9.32}$$

where BSF is the backscatter factor for the irregular field and can be calculated by Clarkson's method. This involves determining *TAR* at the depth d_m on the central axis, using the field contour or radii projected at the depth d_m.

In clinical practice, additional corrections are usually necessary such as for the variation of SSD within the field and the primary beam profile. The details of these corrections will be discussed in the next chapter.

REFERENCES

1. Shrimpton PC. Electron density values of various human tissues: in vitro Compton scatter measurements and calculated ranges. *Phys Med Biol* 1981;26:907.
2. White DR, Martin RJ, Darlison R. Epoxy resin based tissue substitutes. *Br J Radiol* 1977;50:814.
3. International Commission on Radiation Units and Measurements. *Tissue substitutes in radiation dosimetry and measurement. Report No. 44.* Bethesda, MD: International Commission on Radiation Units and Measurements, 1989.
4. Constantinou C, Attix FH, Paliwal BR. A solid phantom material for radiation therapy x-ray and γ-ray beam calibrations. *Med Phys* 1982;9:436.
5. Hospital Physicists' Association. Central axis depth dose data for use in radiotherapy. *Br J Radiol* 1978;[suppl 11].
6. Johns HE, Whitmore GF, Watson TA, et al. A system of dosimetry for rotation therapy with typical rotation distributions. *J Can Assoc Radiol* 1953;4:1.
7. Johns HE. Physical aspects of rotation therapy. *AJR* 1958;79:373.
8. Cunningham JR, Johns HE, Gupta SK. An examination of the definition and the magnitude of back-scatter factor for cobalt 60 gamma rays. *Br J Radiol* 1965;38:637.
9. Gupta SK, Cunningham JR. Measurement of tissue-air ratios and scatter functions for large field sizes for cobalt 60 gamma radiation. *Br J Radiol* 1966;39:7.
10. Karzmark CJ, Dewbert A, Loevinger R. Tissue-phantom ratios—an aid to treatment planning. *Br J Radiol* 1965;38:158.
11. Saunders JE, Price RH, Horsley RJ. Central axis depth doses for a constant source-tumor distance. *Br J Radiol* 1968;41:464.
12. Holt JG, Laughlin JS, Moroney JP. Extension of concept of tissue-air ratios (TAR) to high energy x-ray beams. *Radiology* 1970;96:437.
13. Khan FM, Sewchand W, Lee J, et al. Revision of tissue-maximum ratio and scatter-maximum ratio concepts for cobalt 60 and higher energy x-ray beams. *Med Phys* 1980;7:230.
14. International Commission on Radiation Units and Measurements. *Radiation quantities and units. Report No. 33.* Washington, DC: U.S. National Bureau of Standards, 1980.
15. International Commission on Radiation Units and Measurements. *Determination of absorbed dose in a patient irradiated by beams of x or gamma rays in radiotherapy procedures. Report No. 24.* Washington, DC: U.S. National Bureau of Standards, 1976.
16. Day MJ. A note on the calculation of dose in x-ray fields. *Br J Radiol* 1950;23:368.
17. Jones DEA. A note on back-scatter and depth doses for elongated rectangular x-ray fields. *Br J Radiol* 1949;22:342.
18. Batho HF, Theimer O, Theimer R. A consideration of equivalent circle method of calculating depth doses for rectangular x-ray fields. *J Can Assoc Radiol* 1956;7:51.
19. Sterling TD, Perry H, Katz I. Derivation of a mathematical expression for the percent depth dose surface of cobalt 60 beams and visualization of multiple field dose distributions. *Br J Radiol* 1964;37:544.
20. Mayneord WV, Lamerton LF. A survey of depth dose data. *Br J Radiol* 1944;14:255.
21. Johns HE, Bruce WR, Reid WB. The dependence of depth dose on focal skin distance. *Br J Radiol* 1958;31:254.
22. Burns JE. Conversion of depth doses from one FSD to another. *Br J Radiol* 1958;31:643.
23. Clarkson JR. A note on depth doses in fields of irregular shape. *Br J Radiol* 1941;14:265.
24. Johns HE, Cunningham JR. *The physics of radiology,* 3rd ed. Springfield, IL: Charles C Thomas, 1969.
25. Cunningham JR. Scatter-air ratios. *Phys Med Biol* 1972;17:42.
26. American Association of Physicists in Medicine. Dosimetry workshop: Hodgkin's disease. Chicago, IL, MD Anderson Hospital, Houston, TX, Radiological Physics Center, 1970.
27. Khan FM, Levitt SH, Moore VC, et al. Computer and approximation methods of calculating depth dose in irregularly shaped fields. *Radiology* 1973;106:433.

A SYSTEM OF DOSIMETRIC CALCULATIONS

Several methods are available for calculating absorbed dose in a patient. Two of these methods using percent depth doses and *tissue-air ratios* (TARs) were discussed in Chapter 9. However, there are some limitations to these methods. For example, the dependence of percent depth dose on source-to-surface distance (SSD) makes this quantity unsuitable for isocentric techniques. Although tissue-air ratios (TAR) and scatter-air ratios (SAR) eliminate that problem, their application to beams of energy higher than those of ^{60}Co has been seriously questioned (1–3) as they require measurement of dose in free space. As the beam energy increases, the size of the chamber build-up cap for in-air measurements has to be increased and it becomes increasingly difficult to calculate the dose in free space from such measurements. In addition, the material of the build-up cap is usually different from that of the phantom and this introduces a bias or uncertainty in the TAR measurements.

In order to overcome the limitations of the TAR, Karzmark et al. (1) introduced the concept of *tissue-phantom ratio* (TPR). This quantity retains the properties of the TAR but limits the measurements to the phantom rather than in air. A few years later, Holt et al. (4) introduced yet another quantity, *tissue-maximum ratio* (TMR), which also limits the measurements to the phantom.

In this chapter, I develop a dosimetric system based on the TMR concept, although a similar system can also be derived from the TPR concept (5).

10.1. DOSE CALCULATION PARAMETERS

The dose to a point in a medium may be analyzed into primary and scattered components. The primary dose is contributed by the initial or original photons emitted from the source and the scattered dose is the result of the scattered photons. The scattered dose can be further analyzed into collimator and phantom components, because the two can be varied independently by blocking. For example, blocking a portion of the field does not significantly change the output or exposure in the open portion of the beam (6,7) but may substantially reduce the phantom scatter.

The above analysis presents one practical difficulty, namely, the determination of primary dose in a phantom which excludes both the collimator and phantom scatter. However, for megavoltage photon beams, it is reasonably accurate to consider collimator scatter as part of the primary beam so that the phantom scatter could be calculated separately. We, therefore, define an *effective primary dose* as the dose due to the primary photons as well as those scattered from the collimating system. The effective primary in a phantom may be thought of as the dose at depth minus the phantom scatter. Alternatively, the effective primary dose may be defined as the depth dose expected in the field when scattering volume is reduced to zero while keeping the collimator opening constant.

Representation of primary dose by the dose in a 0×0 field poses conceptual problems because of the lack of lateral electronic equilibrium in narrow fields in megavoltage photon beams. This issue has been debated in the literature (8–10), but practical solutions are still not agreed on. Systems that use electron transport in the calculation of primary and scattered components of dose would be appropriate but are not as yet fully developed and

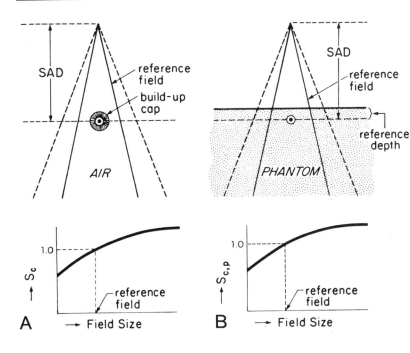

FIG. 10.1. Arrangement for measuring S_c and $S_{c,p}$. **A:** Chamber with build-up cap in air to measure output relative to a reference field, for determining S_c versus field size. **B:** Measurements in a phantom at a fixed depth for determining $S_{c,p}$ versus field size. (From Khan FM, Sewchand W, Lee J, et al. Revision of tissue-maximum ratio and scatter-maximum ratio concepts for cobalt 60 and higher energy x-ray beams. *Med Phys* 1980;7:230, with permission.)

implemented. Until then, the concept of 0×0 field to represent primary beams with the implicit assumption that lateral electronic equilibrium exists at all points will continue to be used for routine dosimetry.

A. Collimator Scatter Factor

The beam output (exposure rate, dose rate in free space, or energy fluence rate) measured in air depends on the field size. As the field size is increased, the output increases because of the increased collimator scatter,[1] which is added to the primary beam.

The *collimator scatter factor* (S_c) is commonly called the *output factor* and may be defined as the ratio of the output in air for a given field to that for a reference field (e.g., 10×10 cm). S_c may be measured with an ion chamber with a build-up cap of a size large enough to provide maximum dose build-up for the given energy beam. The measurement setup is shown in Fig. 10.1A. Readings are plotted against field size (side of equivalent square or area/perimeter [A/P]) and the values are normalized to the reference field (10×10 cm).

In the measurement of S_c, the field must fully cover the build-up cap for all field sizes if measurements are to reflect relative photon fluences. For small fields, one may take the measurements at large distances from the source so that the smallest field covers build-up cap. Normally, the collimator scatter factors are measured at the source-to-axis distance (SAD). However, larger distances can be used provided the field sizes are all defined at the SAD.

B. Phantom Scatter Factor

The *phantom scatter factor* (S_p) takes into account the change in scatter radiation originating in the phantom at a reference depth as the field size is changed. S_p may be defined as the ratio of the dose rate for a given field at a reference depth (e.g., depth of maximum dose) to the dose rate at the same depth for the reference field size (e.g., 10×10 cm), with the same collimator opening. In this definition, it should be noted that S_p is related to the changes in the volume of the phantom irradiated for a fixed collimator opening. Thus one

---

[1] Collimator scatter includes photons scattered by all components of the machine head in the path of the beam.

could determine S_p, at least in concept, by using a large field incident on phantoms of various cross-sectional sizes.

For photon beams for which backscatter factors can be accurately measured (e.g., ^{60}Co and 4 MV), S_p factor at the depth of maximum dose may be defined simply as the ratio of backscatter factor (BSF) for the given field to that for the reference field (see Appendix, section A). Mathematically,

$$S_p(r) = \frac{\text{BSF}(r)}{\text{BSF}(r_0)}$$

(10.1)

where r_0 is the side of the reference field size (10×10 cm).

A more practical method of measuring S_p, which can be used for all beam energies, consists of indirect determination from the following equation (for derivation, see Appendix, section A):

$$S_p(r) = \frac{S_{c,p}(r)}{S_c(r)}$$

(10.2)

where $S_{c,p}(r)$ is the *total scatter factor* defined as the dose rate at a reference depth for a given field size r divided by the dose rate at the same point and depth for the reference field size (10×10 cm) (Fig. 10.1B). Thus $S_{c,p}(r)$ contains both the collimator and phantom scatter and when divided by $S_c(r)$ yields $S_p(r)$.

Since S_p and $S_{c,p}$ are defined at the reference depth of D_{max}, actual measurement of these factors at this depth may create problems because of the possible influence of contaminant electrons incident on the phantom. This can be avoided by making measurements at a greater depth (e.g., 10 cm) and converting the readings to the reference depth of D_{max} by using percent depth dose data, presumably measured with a small-diameter chamber. The rationale for this procedure is the same as for the recommended depths of calibration (11).

C. Tissue-Phantom and Tissue-Maximum Ratios

The TPR is defined as the ratio of the dose at a given point in phantom to the dose at the same point at a fixed reference depth, usually 5 cm. This is illustrated in Fig. 10.2. The corresponding quantity for the scattered dose calculation is called the scatter-phantom ratio (SPR), which is analogous in use to the scatter-air ratio discussed in the previous chapter. Details of the TPR and SPR concepts have been discussed in the literature (1,3,5).

TPR is a general function which may be normalized to any reference depth. But there is no general agreement concerning the depth to be used for this quantity, although a 5-cm depth is the usual choice for most beam energies. On the other hand, the point of central axis D_{max} has a simplicity that is very desirable in dose computations. If adopted as a fixed

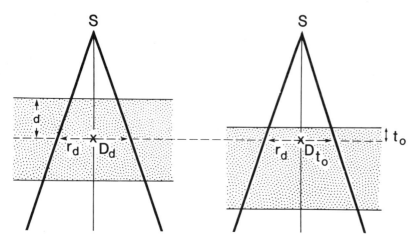

FIG. 10.2. Diagram illustrating the definitions of tissue-phantom ratio (TPR) and tissue-maximum ratio (TMR). TPR(d, r_d) = D_d /D_{t0}, where t_0 is a reference depth. If t_0 is the reference depth of maximum dose, then TMR(d, r_d) = TPR(d, r_d).

reference depth, the quantity TPR gives rise to the TMR. Thus TMR is a special case of TPR and may be defined as the ratio of the dose at a given point in phantom to the dose at the same point at the reference depth of maximum dose (Fig. 10.2).

For megavoltage beams in the range of 20 to 45 MV, the depth of maximum dose (d_m) has been found to depend significantly on field size (12,13) as well as on SSD (14,15). For the calculative functions to be independent of machine parameters, they should not involve measurements in the build-up region. Therefore, the reference depth must be equal to or greater than the largest d_m. Since d_m tends to decrease with field size (12) and increase with SSD (14), one should choose (d_m) for the smallest field and the largest SSD. In practice, one may plot $[(\%DD) \times (SSD + d)^2]$ as a function of depth d to find d_m (15). This eliminates dependence on SSD. The maximum d_m can then be obtained by plotting d_m as a function of field size and extrapolating to 0×0 field size.

The *reference depth of maximum dose* (t_0), as determined above, should be used for percent depth dose, TMR, and S_p factors, irrespective of field size and SSD.

C.1. Properties of TMR

The concept of tissue-maximum ratio is based on the assumption that the fractional scatter contribution to the depth dose at a point is independent of the divergence of the beam and depends only on the field size at the point and the depth of the overlying tissue. This has been shown to be essentially true by Johns et al. (16). This principle, which also underlies TAR and TPR, makes all these functions practically independent of source-surface distance. Thus a single table of TMRs can be used for all SSDs for each radiation quality.

Figure 10.3 shows TMR data for for 10-MV x-ray beams as an example. The curve for 0×0 field size shows the steepest drop with depth and is caused entirely by the primary beam. For megavoltage beams, the primary beam attenuation can be approximately represented by:

$$\mathrm{TMR}(d, 0) = e^{-\mu(d-t_0)} \tag{10.3}$$

where μ is the effective linear attenuation coefficient and t_0 is the reference depth of maximum dose. μ can be determined from TMR data by plotting μ as a function of field size (side of equivalent square) and extrapolating it back to 0×0 field.

TMR and percent depth dose P are interrelated by the following equation (see Appendix, section B, for derivation).

$$\mathrm{TMR}(d, r_d) = \left(\frac{P(d, r, f)}{100} \right) \left(\frac{f + d}{f + t_0} \right)^2 \left(\frac{S_p(r_{t_0})}{S_p(r_d)} \right) \tag{10.4}$$

where

$$f = \mathrm{SSD}, r_d = r \cdot \left(\frac{f + d}{f} \right)$$

$$r_{t_0} = r \cdot \left(\frac{f + t_0}{f} \right)$$

Here the percent depth dose is referenced against the dose at depth t_0 so that $P(t_0, r, f) = 100$ for all field sizes and SSDs.

Although TMRs can be measured directly, they can also be calculated from percent depth doses, as shown by Equation 10.4. For ^{60}Co, Equations 10.2 and 10.4 can be used to calculate TMRs. In addition, TMRs can be derived from TAR data in those cases, such as ^{60}Co, where TARs are accurately known:

$$\mathrm{TMR}(d, r_d) = \frac{\mathrm{TAR}(d, r_d)}{\mathrm{BSF}(r_d)} \tag{10.5}$$

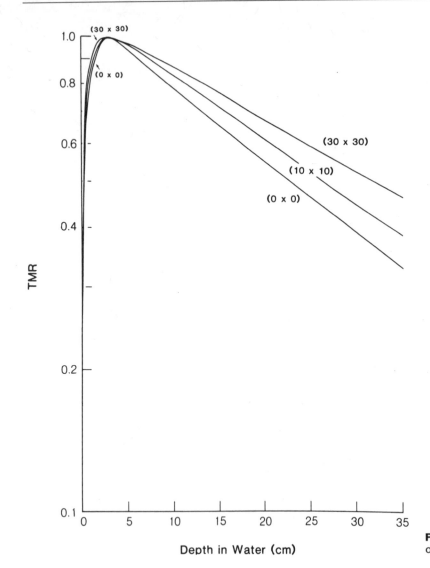

FIG. 10.3. Plot of TMR for 10-MV x-rays as a function of depth for a selection of field sizes.

D. Scatter-Maximum Ratio

The scatter-maximum ratio (SMR), like the SAR, is a quantity designed specifically for the calculation of scattered dose in a medium. It may be defined as the ratio of the scattered dose at a given point in phantom to the effective primary dose at the same point at the reference depth of maximum dose (5). Mathematically,

$$\text{SMR}(d, r_d) = \text{TMR}(d, r_d) \left(\frac{S_p(r_d)}{S_p(0)} \right) - \text{TMR}(d, 0) \tag{10.6}$$

For derivation of the above equation, see Appendix, section C.

From Equations 10.1, 10.5, and 10.6, it can be shown that for ^{60}Co γ rays, SMRs are approximately the same as SARs. However, for higher energies, SMRs should be calculated from TMRs by using Equations 9.7 and 10.6.

Another interesting relationship can be obtained at the reference depth of maximum dose (t_0). Since TMR at depth t_0 is unity by definition, Equation 10.6 becomes:

$$\text{SMR}(t_0, r_{t_0}) = \frac{S_p(r_{t_0})}{S_p(0)} - 1 \tag{10.7}$$

This equation will be used in section 10.2C.

10.2. PRACTICAL APPLICATIONS

Radiotherapy institutions vary in their treatment techniques and calibration practices. For example, some rely exclusively on the SSD or the SAD (isocentric) type techniques, while others use both. Accordingly, units are calibrated in air or in phantom at a suitable reference depth. In addition, clinical fields, although basically rectangular or square, are often shaped irregularly to protect critical or normal regions of the body. Thus a calculation system must be generally applicable to the above practices, with acceptable accuracy and simplicity for routine use.

A. Accelerator Calculations

A.1. SSD Technique

Percent depth dose is a suitable quantity for calculations involving SSD techniques. Machines are usually calibrated to deliver 1 rad (10^{-2} Gy) per monitor unit (MU) at the reference depth t_0, for a reference field size 10×10 cm and a source-to-calibration point distance of SCD. Assuming that the S_c factors relate to collimator field sizes defined at the SAD, the monitor units necessary to deliver a certain tumor dose (TD) at depth d for a field size r at the surface at any SSD are given by:

$$MU = \frac{TD \times 100}{K \times (\%DD)_d \times S_c(r_c) \times S_p(r) \times (SSD\ factor)} \tag{10.8}$$

where K is 1 rad per MU, r_c is the collimator field size, given by:

$$r_c = r \cdot \frac{SAD}{SSD}$$

and:

$$SSD\ factor = \left(\frac{SCD}{SSD + t_0} \right)^2$$

It must be remembered that, whereas the field size for the S_c is defined at the SAD, S_p relates to the field irradiating the patient.

Example 1

A 4-MV linear accelerator is calibrated to give 1 rad (10^{-2} Gy) per MU in phantom at a reference depth of maximum dose of 1 cm, 100-cm SSD, and 10×10 cm field size. Determine the MU values to deliver 200 rads to a patient at 100-cm SSD, 10-cm depth, and 15×15 cm field size, given $S_c(15 \times 15) = 1.020$, $S_p(15 \times 15) = 1.010$, %DD = 65.1. From Equation 10.8,

$$MU = \frac{200 \times 100}{65.1 \times 1.020 \times 1.010 \times 1} = 298$$

A form for treatment calculations is shown in Fig. 10.4 with the above calculations filled in.

Example 2

Determine the MU for the treatment conditions given in Example 1 except that the treatment SSD is 120 cm, given $S_c(12.5 \times 12.5) = 1.010$ and %DD for the new SSD is 66.7.

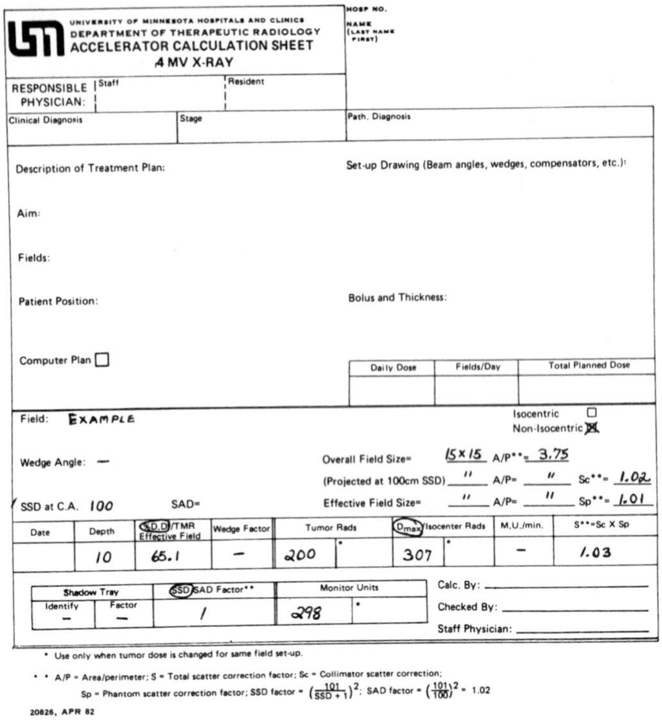

UNIVERSITY OF MINNESOTA HOSPITALS AND CLINICS
DEPARTMENT OF THERAPEUTIC RADIOLOGY
ACCELERATOR CALCULATION SHEET
4 MV X-RAY

HOSP NO.
NAME (LAST NAME FIRST)

RESPONSIBLE PHYSICIAN: Staff | Resident

Clinical Diagnosis | Stage | Path. Diagnosis

Description of Treatment Plan:

Set-up Drawing (Beam angles, wedges, compensators, etc.):

Aim:

Fields:

Patient Position:

Bolus and Thickness:

Computer Plan ☐

Daily Dose	Fields/Day	Total Planned Dose

Field: EXAMPLE

Isocentric ☐
Non-Isocentric ☒

Wedge Angle: —

Overall Field Size= 15×15 A/P**= 3.75
(Projected at 100cm SSD) " A/P= " Sc**= 1.02
SSD at C.A. 100 SAD= Effective Field Size= " A/P= " Sp**= 1.01

Date	Depth	SSD, D/TMR Effective Field	Wedge Factor	Tumor Rads	*	Dmax/Isocenter Rads	*	M.U./min.	S**=Sc X Sp
	10	65.1	—	200		307		—	1.03

Shadow Tray: Identify	Shadow Tray: Factor	SSD/SAD Factor**	Monitor Units	*
—	—	1	298	

Calc. By: ______
Checked By: ______
Staff Physician: ______

* Use only when tumor dose is changed for same field set-up.

** A/P = Area/perimeter; S = Total scatter correction factor; Sc = Collimator scatter correction; Sp = Phantom scatter correction factor; SSD factor = $\left(\frac{101}{SSD+1}\right)^2$; SAD factor = $\left(\frac{101}{100}\right)^2$ = 1.02

20826, APR 82

FIG. 10.4. Accelerator calculation sheet.

$$\text{Field size projected at SAD}(= 100\text{ cm}) = 15 \times \frac{100}{120} = 12.5\text{ cm}$$

$S_c(12.5 \times 12.5)$ is given as 1.010 and $S_p(15 \times 15) = 1.010$

$$\text{SSD factor} = \left(\frac{100+1}{120+1}\right)^2 = 0.697$$

From Equation 10.8,

$$\text{MU} = \frac{200 \times 100}{66.7 \times 1.010 \times 1.010 \times 0.697} = 442$$

A.2. Isocentric Technique

TMR is the quantity of choice for dosimetric calculations involving isocentric techniques. Since the unit is calibrated to give 1 rad (10^{-2} Gy)/MU at the reference depth t_0, calibration distance SCD, and for the reference field (10 × 10 cm), then the monitor units necessary to deliver isocenter dose (ID) at depth d are given by:

$$\text{MU} = \frac{\text{ID}}{\text{K} \times \text{TMR}(d, r_d) \times S_c(r_c) \times S_p(r_d) \times \text{SAD factor}} \tag{10.9}$$

where

$$\text{SAD factor} = \left(\frac{\text{SCD}}{\text{SAD}}\right)^2$$

Example 3

A tumor dose of 200 rads is to be delivered at the isocenter which is located at a depth of 8 cm, given 4-MV x-ray beam, field size at the isocenter = 6 × 6 cm, $S_c(6 \times 6) = 0.970$,

$S_p(6 \times 6) = 0.990$, machine calibrated at SCD = 100 cm, TMR(8, 6 × 6) = 0.787. Since the calibration point is at the SAD, SAD factor = 1. Thus, using Equation 10.9,

$$MU = \frac{200}{0.787 \times 0.970 \times 0.990 \times 1} = 265$$

Example 4

Calculate MU values for the case in Example 3, if the unit is calibrated nonisocentrically, i.e., source to calibration point distance = 101 cm.

$$SAD \ factor = \left(\frac{101}{100}\right)^2 = 1.020$$

Thus,

$$MU = \frac{200}{0.787 \times 0.970 \times 0.99 \times 1.02} = 260$$

B. Cobalt-60 Calculations

The above calculation system is sufficiently general that is can be applied to any radiation generator, including ^{60}Co. In the latter case, the machine can be calibrated either in air or in phantom provided the following information is available: (*a*) dose rate $D_0(t_0, r_0, f_0)$ in phantom at depth t_0 of maximum dose for a reference field size r_0 and standard SSD f_0; (*b*) S_c; (*c*) S_p; (*d*) percent depth doses; and (*e*) TMR values. If universal depth dose data for ^{60}Co (16) are used, then the S_p and TMRs can be obtained by using Equations 10.1 and 10.5. In addition, the SSD used in these calculations should be confined to a range for which the output in air obeys an inverse square law for a constant collimator opening.

A form for cobalt calculations is presented in Fig. 10.5.

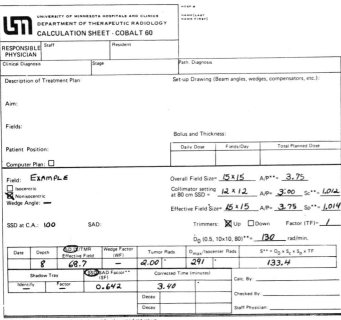

FIG. 10.5. Calculation sheet—cobalt-60.

Example 5

A tumor dose of 200 rads is to be delivered at a 8-cm depth, using 15×15-cm field size, 100-cm SSD, and penumbra trimmers up. The unit is calibrated to give 130 rads/min in phantom at a 0.5-cm depth for a 10×10-cm field with trimmers up and SSD = 80 cm. Determine the time of irradiation, given $S_c(12 \times 12) = 1.012$, $S_p(15 \times 15) = 1.014$, and %DD $(8, 15 \times 15, 100) = 68.7$.

$$\text{Field size projected at SAD}(= 80 \text{ cm})$$

$$= 15 \times \frac{80}{100} = 12 \text{ cm} \times 12 \text{ cm}$$

$$\text{SSD factor} = \left(\frac{80 + 0.5}{100 + 0.5} \right)^2 = 0.642$$

$$\text{Time} = (\text{TD} \times 100)/[D_0(0.5, 10 \times 10, 80)$$
$$\times \text{\%DD}(8, 15 \times 15, 100) \times S_c(12 \times 12)$$
$$\times S_p(15 \times 15) \times \text{SSD factor}]$$
$$= \frac{200 \times 100}{130 \times 68.7 \times 1.012 \times 1.014 \times 0.642}$$
$$= 3.40 \text{ min}$$

C. Irregular Fields

Dosimetry of irregular fields using TMRs and SMRs is analogous to the method using TARs and SARs (section 9.5). Since the mathematical rationale of the method has been discussed in detail in the literature (5), only a brief outline will be presented here to illustrate the procedure.

An irregular field at depth d may be divided into n elementary sectors with radii emanating from point Q of calculation (Fig. 9.10). A Clarkson type integration (Chapter 9) may be performed to give averaged scatter-maximum ratio ($\overline{\text{SMR}}(d, r_d)$) for the irregular field r_d:

$$\overline{\text{SMR}}(d, r_d) = \frac{1}{n} \sum_{i=1}^{n} \text{SMR}(d, r_i) \tag{10.10}$$

where r_i is the radius of the ith sector at depth d and n is the total number of sectors ($n = 2\pi/\Delta\theta$, where $\Delta\theta$ is the sector angle).

The computed $\overline{\text{SMR}}(d, r_d)$ is then converted to $\overline{\text{TMR}}(d, r_d)$ by using Equation 10.6.

$$\overline{\text{TMR}}(d, r_d) = [\text{TMR}(d, 0) + \overline{\text{SMR}}(d, r_d)] \times \frac{S_p(0)}{\overline{S}_p(r_d)} \tag{10.11}$$

where $\overline{S}_p, (r_d)$ is the averaged S_p for the irregular field and $S_p(0)$ is the S_p for the 0×0 area field. The above equation is strictly valid only for points along the central axis of a beam that is normally incident on an infinite phantom with flat surface. For off-axis points in a beam with nonuniform primary dose profile, one should write

$$\overline{\text{TMR}}(d, r_d) = [K_p \cdot \text{TMR}(d, 0) + \overline{\text{SMR}}(d, r_d)] \times \frac{S_p(0)}{\overline{S}_p(r_d)} \tag{10.12}$$

where K_p is the off-axis ratio representing primary dose at point Q relative to that at the central axis.

$\overline{\text{TMR}}(d, r_d)$ may be converted into percent depth dose $P(d, r, f)$ by using Equation 10.4.

$$P(d, r, f) = 100[K_p \cdot \text{TMR}(d, 0) + \overline{\text{SMR}}(d, r_d)]$$

$$\times \frac{S_p(0)}{\overline{S}_p(r_d)} \times \frac{\overline{S}_p(r_d)}{\overline{S}_p(r_{t_0})} \times \left(\frac{f + t_0}{f + d}\right)^2 \quad (10.13)$$

From Equations 10.7 and 10.13 we get the final expression:

$$P(d, r, f) = 100[K_p \cdot \text{TMR}(d, 0) + \overline{\text{SMR}}(d, r_d)]$$

$$\times \frac{1}{1 + \overline{\text{SMR}}(t_0, r_{t_0})} \times \left(\frac{f + t_0}{f + d}\right)^2 \quad (10.14)$$

Thus the calculation of percent depth dose for an irregular field requires a Clarkson integration over the function SMR both at the point of calculation Q as well as at the reference depth (t_0) at central axis.

C.1. SSD Variation Within the Field

The percent depth dose at Q is normalized with respect to the D_{max} on the central axis at depth t_0. Let f_0 be the nominal SSD along the central axis, g be the vertical gap distance, i.e., "gap" between skin surface over Q and the nominal SSD plane, and d be the depth of Q from skin surface. The percent depth dose is then given by:

$$\%\text{DD} = 100 \times [K_p \cdot \text{TMR}(d, 0) + \overline{\text{SMR}}(d, r_d)]$$

$$\times \frac{1}{1 + \overline{\text{SMR}}(t_0, r_{t_0})} \times \left(\frac{f + t_0}{f + g + d}\right)^2 \quad (10.15)$$

The sign of g should be set positive or negative, depending on if the SSD over Q is larger or smaller than the nominal SSD.

C.2. Computer Program

A computer algorithm embodying the Clarkson's principle and scatter-air ratios was developed by Cunningham et al. (17) at the Princess Margaret Hospital, Toronto, and was published in 1970. Another program, based on the same principle, was developed by Khan (18) at the University of Minnesota. It was originally written for the CDC-3300 computer using SARs and later rewritten for the Artronix PC-12 and PDP 11/34 computers. The latter versions use SMRs instead of SARs.

The following data are permanently stored in this computer program: (a) a table of SMRs as functions of radii of circular fields and (b) the off-axis ratios K_p, derived from dose profiles at selected depths. These data are then stored in the form of a table of K_p as a function of l/L where l is the lateral distance of a point from the central axis and L is the distance along the same line to the geometric edge of the beam. Usually large fields are used for these measurements.

The following data are provided for a particular patient:

1. Contour points: the outline of the irregular field can be drawn from the port (field) film with actual blocks or markers in place to define the field. The field contour is then digitized and the coordinates stored in the computer.
2. The coordinates *(x, y)* of the points of calculation are also entered, including the reference point, usually on the central axis, against which the percent depth doses are calculated.
3. Patient measurements: patient thickness at various points of interest, SSDs, and source-to-film distance are measured and recorded as shown in Fig. 10.6 for a mantle field as an example.

Figure 10.7 shows a daily table calculated by the computer for a typical mantle field. Such a table is useful in programming treatments so that the dose to various regions of the

University of Minnesota
Mantle Field Measurement Sheet

DATE:
NAME:

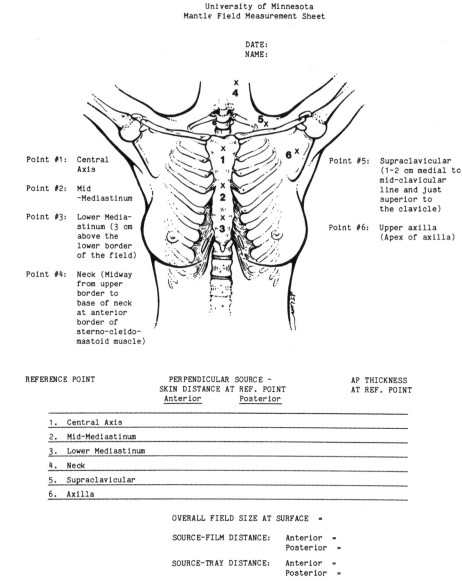

Point #1: Central
Axis

Point #2: Mid
-Mediastinum

Point #3: Lower Media-
stinum (3 cm
above the
lower border
of the field)

Point #4: Neck (Midway
from upper
border to
base of neck
at anterior
border of
sterno-cleido-
mastoid muscle)

Point #5: Supraclavicular
(1-2 cm medial to
mid-clavicular
line and just
superior to
the clavicle)

Point #6: Upper axilla
(Apex of axilla)

REFERENCE POINT	PERPENDICULAR SOURCE – SKIN DISTANCE AT REF. POINT		AP THICKNESS AT REF. POINT
	Anterior	Posterior	
1. Central Axis			
2. Mid-Mediastinum			
3. Lower Mediastinum			
4. Neck			
5. Supraclavicular			
6. Axilla			

OVERALL FIELD SIZE AT SURFACE =

SOURCE-FILM DISTANCE: Anterior =
Posterior =

SOURCE-TRAY DISTANCE: Anterior =
Posterior =

FIG. 10.6. Form for recording patient and dosimetric data for mantle field. Note that the measurement points are standardized by anatomic landmarks.

field can be adjusted. The areas that receive the prescribed dose after a certain number of treatments are shielded for the remaining sessions.

D. Asymmetric Fields

Many of the modern linear accelerators are equipped with x-ray collimators (or jaws) that can be moved independently to allow asymmetric fields with field centers positioned away from the true central axis of the beam. For example, an independent jaw can be moved to block off half of the field along central axis to eliminate beam divergence. This feature is useful for matching adjacent fields. Although this function can also be performed by beam splitters or secondary blocking on a shadow tray, an independent jaw feature reduces the setup time and spares the therapist from handling heavy blocks.

The effect of asymmetric beam collimation on dose distribution has been discussed in the literature (19,20). When a field is collimated asymmetrically, one needs to take into account changes in the collimator scatter, phantom scatter, and off-axis beam quality. The

C

TREATMENT NO.	DMAX ANT	DMAX POST	TUMOR DOSE CA 1	2	3	4	5	6 UAX	7 LAX
1	157		150	147	142	169	173	157	157
2		187	300	294	284	338	346	314	314
3	374		450	442	426	507	519	470	471
4		374	600	589	568	676	692	627	629
5	562		750	736	710	845	865	784	786
5		562	900	883	851	1014	1038	941	943
7	749		1050	1030	993	1183	1211	1098	1100
8		749	1200	1177	1135	1352	1385	1254	1257
9	936		1350	1325	1277	1520	1558	1411	1414
10		936	1500	1472	1419	1689	1731	1568	1571
11	1123		1650	1619	1561	1858	1904	1725	1729
12		1123	1800	1766	1703	2027	2077	1881	1886
13	1310		1950	1913	1845	2196	2250	2038	2043
14		1310	2100	2060	1987	2365	2423	2195	2200
15	1498		2250	2208	2129	2534	2596	2352	2357
16		1498	2400	2355	2271	2703	2769	2509	2514
17	1685		2550	2502	2412	2872	2942	2665	2671
18		1685	2700	2649	2554	3041	3115	2822	2829
19	1872		2850	2796	2696	3210	3288	2979	2986
20		1872	3000	2943	2838	3379	3461	3136	3143
21	2059		3150	3091	2980	3548	3634	3293	3300
22		2059	3300	3238	3122	3717	3807	3449	3457
23	2247		3450	3385	3264	3886	3981	3606	3614
24		2247	3600	3532	3406	4055	4154	3763	3771
25	2434		3750	3679	3548	4224	4327	3920	3928
26		2434	3900	3826	3690	4392	4500	4077	4086 R+
27	2621		4050	3974	3832	4561	4673	4233	4243
28		2621	4200	4121	3974	4730	4846	4390	4400
29	2808		4350	4268	4115	4899	5019	4547	4557 L+
30		2808	4500	4415	4257	5068	5192	4704	4714
31	2995		4650	4562	4399	5237	5365	4860	4871
32		2995	4800	4709	4541	5406	5538	5017	5028
33	3183		4950	4857	4683	5575	5711	5174	5186
34		3183	5100	5004	4825	5744	5884	5331	5343
35	3370		5250	5151	4967	5913	6057	5488	5500

FIG. 10.7. Computer output sheet showing cumulative midthickness doses for a mantle field. Total dose to various points is programmed by a line drawn through the table. As soon as a given area reaches its prescribed dose, it is shielded during subsequent treatments. It is not necessary to recalculate the table with this change in blocking since only a few treatments are affected.

latter effect arises as a consequence of using beam-flattening filters (thicker in the middle and thinner in the periphery), which results in greater beam hardening close to the central axis compared with the periphery of the beam (21,22).

A dose calculation formalism for asymmetric fields has been developed which is described below.

For a point at the center of an asymmetric field and a lateral distance x away from the beam central axis, the collimator scatter factor may be approximated to a symmetric field of the same collimator opening as that of the given asymmetric field. In other words, the S_c will depend on the actual collimator opening, ignoring small changes in the scattered photon fluence that may result owing to the change in the angle of the asymmetric jaws relative to the beam. This approximation is reasonable as long as the point of dose calculation is centrally located, that is, away from field edges.

The phantom scatter can also be assumed to be the same for an asymmetric field as for a symmetric field of the same dimension and shape, provided the point of calculation is located away from the field edges to avoid penumbral effects.

The primary dose distribution has been shown to vary with lateral distance from central axis because of the change in beam quality, as mentioned earlier. Therefore, the percent depth dose or TMR distribution along the *central ray* of an asymmetric field is not the same as along the central axis of a symmetric field of the same size and shape. In addition, the incident primary beam fluence at off-axis points varies as a function of distance from the central axis, depending on the flattening filter design. These effects are not emphasized in the dosimetry of symmetric fields, because target doses are usually specified at the beam central axis and the off-axis dose distributions are viewed from the isodose curves. In asymmetric fields, however, the target or the point of interest does not lie on the beam central axis; therefore, an off-axis dose correction may be required in the calculation of target dose. This correction will depend on the depth and the distance from the central axis of the point of interest.

Since beam flatness within the central 80% of the maximum field size is specified within ±3% at a 10-cm depth, ignoring off-axis dose correction in asymmetric fields will introduce errors of that magnitude under these conditions. Thus the off-axis dose correction will follow changes in the primary beam flatness as a function of depth and distance from central axis.

In view of the above discussion, the following equations are proposed for the calculation of monitor units for asymmetric fields.

For SSD type of treatments, Equation 10.8 is modified to:

$$MU = \frac{TD \times 100}{K \times (\%DD)_d \times S_c(r_c) \times S_p(r) \times (SSD\ factor) \times OAR_d(x)} \tag{10.16}$$

where $OAR_d(x)$ is the primary off-axis ratio at depth d, that is, ratio of primary dose at the off-axis point of interest to the primary dose at the central axis at the same depth for a symmetrically wide open field. Primary off-axis ratios may be extracted from depth dose profiles of the largest field available by subtracting scatter. A direct method consists of measuring transmitted dose profiles through different thicknesses of an absorber under "good geometry" conditions (a narrow beam and a large detector-to-absorber distance) (23). Another direct but approximate method is to measure profiles as a function of depth for a narrow elongated field (e.g., 5 × 40 cm). Since the primary dose profile is created by the flattening filter, which has a radial symmetry, primary OAR data can be tabulated as a function of depth and radial distance from central axis.

For isocentric type of treatments, Equation 10.9 is modified to:

$$MU = \frac{ID}{K \times TMR(d, r_d) \times S_c(r_c) \times S_p(r_d) \times (SAD\ factor) \times OAR_d(x)} \tag{10.17}$$

The above formalism is general and can be used for an off-axis point dose calculation in symmetric or asymmetric fields generated by blocks or collimators, including multileaf collimators. For irregularly shaped fields the parameter r_d is the equivalent field size determined by Clarkson's technique or geometric approximation (section 10.3). The parameter r_c is the collimator opening size projected at the standard SSD.

10.3. OTHER PRACTICAL METHODS OF CALCULATING DEPTH DOSE DISTRIBUTION

A. Irregular Fields

Clarkson's technique is a general method of calculating depth dose distribution in an irregularly shaped field, but it is not practical for routine manual calculations. Even when computerized, it is time-consuming since a considerable amount of input data is required by the computer program. However, with the exception of mantle, inverted *Y*, and a few other complex fields, reasonably accurate calculations can be made for most blocked fields using an approximate method (18), to be discussed.

Figure 10.8 shows a number of blocked fields encountered in radiotherapy. Approximate rectangles may be drawn containing the point of calculation to include most of the irradiated area surrounding the point and exclude only those areas that are remote to the point. In so doing, a blocked area may be included in the rectangle, provided this area is small and is remotely located relative to that point. The rectangle thus formed may be called the *effective field,* while the unblocked field, defined by the collimator, may be called the *collimator field.*

Once the effective field has been determined, one may proceed with the usual calculations as discussed in section 10.2. However, it is important to remember that, whereas the S_c is related to the collimator field, the percent depth dose, TMR, or S_p corresponds to the effective field.

B. Point Off-Axis

It is possible to calculate depth dose distributions at any point within the field or outside the field using Clarkson's technique. However, as stated earlier, it is not practical for manual calculations. Day (24) has proposed a particularly simple calculation method for

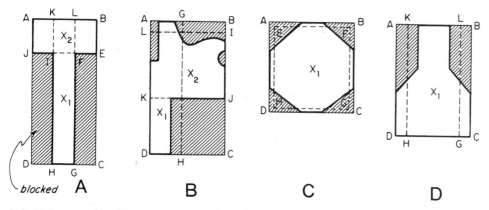

FIG. 10.8. Examples of irregularly shaped fields. Equivalent rectangles for dose at points of interest are shown by dashed lines. Points versus equivalent rectangles are **(A)** 1, *GHKL;* 2, *ABEJ;* **(B)** 1, *AGHD;* 2, *LIJK;* **(C)** 1, *EFGH;* **(D)** 1, *KLGH.* From Levitt SH, Khan FM, Potish RA, eds. *Technological basis of radiation therapy: practical and clinical applications,* 2nd ed. Philadelphia: Lea & Febiger, 1992:73, with permission.

rectangular fields. In this method, percent depth dose can be calculated at any point within the medium using the central axis data.

To calculate dose at any point Q, the field is imagined to be divided into four sections (Fig. 10.9) and their contribution is computed separately. Thus the dose at depth d along the axis through Q is given by $1/4$(sum of central axis dose at depth d for fields $2a \times 2b$, $2a \times 2c$, $2d \times 2b$, and $2d \times 2c$).

Suppose the dose in free space on the central axis through P at SSD $+ d_m$ is 100 cGy (rad) and its value at a corresponding point over Q is $K_Q \times 100$, where K_Q is the off-axis ratio determined in air from the primary beam profile. If the BSF and central axis %DD for rectangular fields are available, the dose at depth d along the axis through Q will be given by:

$$\frac{K_Q \times 100}{4}(\text{sum of BSF} \times \text{\%DD at depth } d \text{ for fields } 2a$$

$$\times 2b, 2a \times 2c, 2d \times 2b, \text{ and } 2d \times 2c)$$

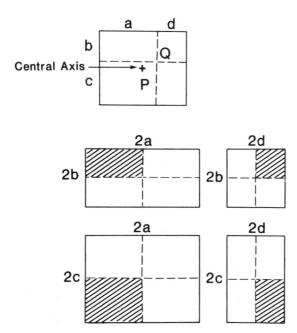

FIG. 10.9. Day's method of calculating dose at any point Q in a rectangular field. (See text.)

Since the D_{max} at P is $100 \times BSF[(a+d) \times (b+c)]$, the percent depth dose at depth d along the axis through Q, relative to D_{max} at P, will be given by:

$$\frac{K_Q}{4 \times BSF[(a+d) \times (b+c)]} \quad \text{(sum of BSF}$$

$$\times \text{ %DD at depth } d \text{ for fields } 2a \times 2b, 2a \times 2c, 2d \times 2b, \text{ and } 2d \times 2c)$$

Example 6

Suppose in Fig. 10.9 that the overall field size is 15×15 cm. Find the percent depth dose at point Q at 10 cm depth, given $a = 10$, $b = 5$, $c = 10$, and $d = 5$. Assume ^{60}Co beam with $K_Q = 0.98$ and SSD = 80 cm.

Using the above procedure and consulting Table A.9.1 in the Appendix to the book, the required percent depth dose is given by:

$$\frac{K_Q}{4 \times BSF(15 \times 15)}[BSF(20 \times 10) \times \text{%DD}(20 \times 10) + BSF(20 \times 20)$$

$$\times \text{%DD}(20 \times 20) + BSF(10 \times 10) \times \text{%DD}(10 \times 10) + BSF(10 \times 20)$$

$$\times \text{%DD}(10 \times 20)]$$

or

$$\frac{0.98}{4 \times 1.052}[(1.043 \times 56.3) + (1.061 \times 60.2)$$

$$+ (1.036 \times 55.6) + (1.043 \times 56.3)] = 55.8$$

In the above example, if the primary beam profile were flat, that is, $K_Q = 1$, the percent depth dose at Q would be 56.9, which is still less than 58.4, the percent depth dose at P. This off-axis decrease in dose is due to the reduced scatter at point Q compared with point P. Similarly, it can be shown that the magnitude of the reduction in scatter depends on the distance of Q from P as well as depth. Thus the depth dose profile across the field is a function not only of the beam flatness in air but also the depth in the phantom.

For higher-energy beams (≥ 8 MV), the above procedure may be further simplified by assuming BSF = 1 for all field sizes. Also, Day's procedure can be adopted using S_p values instead of BSF, since the two quantities are related by Equation 10.1.

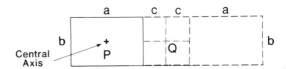

FIG. 10.10. Calculation of depth dose outside a rectangular field. (See text.)

C. Point Outside the Field

Day's method can be extended also to the case of determining dose distribution at points outside the field limits. In Fig. 10.10, a rectangular field of dimensions $a \times b$ is shown with the central axis passing through P. Suppose Q is a point outside the field at a distance c from the field border. Imagine a rectangle adjacent to the field such that it contains point Q and has dimensions $2c \times b$. Place another rectangle of dimensions $a \times b$ on the other side of Q such that the field on the right of Q is a mirror image of the field on the left, as shown in the figure. The dose at point Q at depth d is then given by subtracting the depth dose at Q for field $2c \times b$ from that for field $(2a + 2c) \times b$ and dividing by 2. The procedure is illustrated by the following example.

Example 7

Suppose it is required to determine percent depth dose at Q (relative to D_{max} at P) outside a 15×10-cm field at a distance of 5 cm from the field border. In Fig. 10.10, then, $a = 15$, $b = 10$, and $c = 5$. Suppose Q is at the center of the middle rectangle of dimensions $2c \times b$. Then the dose D_Q at 10-cm depth is given by:

$$\tfrac{1}{2}[D_Q(40 \times 10) - D_Q(10 \times 10)]$$

If D_Q is normalized to D_{max} at P, one gets the percent depth dose at Q or %D_Q.

$$\%D_Q = \frac{1}{\text{BSF}(15 \times 15)} \cdot \tfrac{1}{2}[\text{BSF}(40 \times 10)$$
$$\times \%\text{DD}(40 \times 10) - \text{BSF}(10 \times 10) \times \%\text{DD}(10 \times 10)]$$

Thus for a ^{60}Co beam at SSD $= 80$ cm,

$$\%D_Q = \frac{1}{1.052} \cdot \tfrac{1}{2}[1.054 \times 58.8 - 1.036 \times 55.6] = 2.1$$

Again for higher-energy beams, the above procedure is simplified by assuming BSF $= 1$. Also, if S_p values are known instead of BSF, the above calculation can be performed by substituting S_p for BSF.

D. Point Under the Block

As discussed earlier, the dose distribution in a blocked field is best determined by Clarkson's method of irregular field dosimetry. However, if the blocked portion of the field is approximated to a rectangle, a simpler method known as negative field method may be used. The concept of negative field has been described in the literature (25,26). In this method, the dose at any point is equal to the dose from the overall (unblocked) field minus the dose expected if the entire field were blocked, leaving the shielded volume open. In other words, the blocked portion of the field is considered a negative field and its contribution is subtracted from the overall field dose distribution.

A computerized negative field method not only is a fast method of calculating isodose distribution in blocked fields but is very convenient for manual point dose calculation. Its practical usefulness is illustrated by Example 8.

Example 8

A patient is treated with a split field of overall size 15×15 cm, blocked in the middle to shield a region of size 4×15 cm on the surface (Fig. 10.11). Calculate (a) the treatment time to deliver 200 cGy (rad) at a 10-cm depth at point P in the open portion of the field

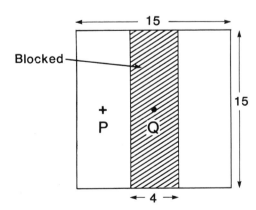

FIG. 10.11. Example of calculating depth dose under a block.

and (b) what percentage of that dose is received at point Q in the middle of the blocked area, given ^{60}Co beam, SSD = 80 cm, dose rate free space for a 15 × 15-cm field at 80.5 cm = 120 rads/min, lead block thickness = 5 cm with primary beam transmission of 5%, and shadow tray (or block tray) transmission = 0.97.

(a) Approximate equivalent field at point $P \simeq 5.5 \times 15$, assuming negligible scatter contribution to P from the other open portion of the field across the blocked area.

$A/P(5.5 \times 15) = 2.01$
Equivalent square = $4 \times A/P = 8 \times 8$ cm
%DD(10, 8 × 8, 80) = 54.0
BSF = 1.029

$$\text{Treatment time} = \frac{200 \times 100}{120 \times 1.029 \times 54.0 \times 0.97}$$
$$= 3.09 \, \text{min}$$

(b) $$D_Q = D_Q(15 \times 15) - D_Q(4 \times 15) \times (1 - T)$$

where T is the transmission factor for the lead block.

$D_Q(15 \times 15) = (\text{dose rate free space} \times \text{time}) \times \text{BSF} \times \%DD$

$$= 120 \times 3.09 \times 1.052 \times \frac{58.4}{100}$$
$$= 227.8 \, \text{cGy}$$

$D_Q(4 \times 15) = 120 \times 3.09 \times 1.023 \times \dfrac{52.3}{100} [A/P(4 \times 15) = 1.58.$

$$\text{Equivalent square} = 6.3 \times 6.3 \, \text{cm}]$$

$$= 198.4 \, \text{cGy}$$

Thus,

$$D_Q = 227.8 - 198.4(1 - 0.05)$$
$$= 39.3 \, \text{cGy}$$

Since $D_p = 200$ cGy (given)

$$D_Q \text{ as a percentage of } D_p = \frac{D_Q}{D_p} \times 100 = \frac{39.3}{200} \times 100$$
$$= 20\%$$

Alternative

Let us project all fields at depth = 10 cm.

$$\text{Magnification} = \frac{80 + 10}{80} = 1.125$$

Projected fields.

(15 × 15) cm × 1.125 = 17 × 17 cm
(4 × 15) cm × 1.125 = 4.5 × 17 cm = 7 × 7 cm equivalent square
(5.5 × 15) cm × 1.125 = 6.2 × 17 cm = 9 × 9 cm equivalent square

$$\frac{D_Q}{D_p} = \frac{\text{TAR}(10, 17 \times 17) - [\text{TAR}(10, 7 \times 7)](1 - T)}{\text{TAR}(10, 9 \times 9)}$$

$$= \frac{0.771 - 0.667(1 - 0.05)}{0.694}$$

$$= 0.20 \text{ or } 20\%$$

Alternative

Since

$$\text{TAR}(d, r_d) = \text{TMR}(d, r_d) \cdot S_p(r_d) \text{ (from Equation 10.5)}$$

$$\frac{D_Q}{D_p} = \frac{\text{TMR}(10, 17 \times 17) \cdot S_p(17 \times 17) - \text{TMR}(10, 7 \times 7) \cdot S_p(7 \times 7)(1 - T)}{\text{TMR}(10, 9 \times 9) \cdot S_p(9 \times 9)}$$

Substituting values from Table A.9.2 in the Appendix to the book

$$\frac{D_Q}{D_p} = \frac{0.733 \times 1.02 - 0.651 \times 0.989(1 - 0.05)}{0.672 \times 0.997}$$

$$= 0.20 \text{ or } 20\%$$

Although the primary transmission through the lead block is only 5%, the dose at a 10-cm depth under the block in the middle is about 20% of the dose in the open portion. This increase in dose is a result of the internal scatter contributed by the open areas of the field to point Q. Of course, the dose under the block depends on the extent of the blocked area, overall field size, block thickness, depth, and location of point Q.

APPENDIX TO CHAPTER

A. Derivation of *Sp*

$S_p(r)$, as defined in section 10.1B, is the ratio of dose rate for the given field (r) at a reference depth to the dose rate at the same point for the reference field size (r_0), with the same collimator opening. This is illustrated in Fig. 10.12. The given field in Fig. 10.12A is blocked down to the size of the reference field in Fig. 10.12B without changing the collimator opening. Thus both arrangements have the same collimator scatter factor, $S_c(r)$,

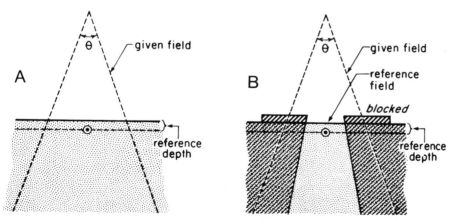

FIG. 10.12. Diagrams to illustrate definition of S_p. **A:** Dose in phantom at reference depth for a given field. **B:** Dose at the same point for a reference field with the same collimator opening. (From Khan FM, Sewchand W, Lee J, et al. Revision of tissue-maximum ratio and scatter-maximum ratio concepts for cobalt 60 and higher energy x-ray beams. *Med Phys* 1980;7:230, with permission.)

but different phantom scatter. Let D_{fs} and D_{max} be the free space dose rate and D_{max} dose rate, respectively. Then, at the reference depth of maximum dose,

$$S_p(r) = \frac{D_{max} \text{ in arrangement A}}{D_{max} \text{ in arrangement B}} \tag{A1}$$

$$= \frac{D_{fs}(r_0) \cdot S_c(r) \cdot \text{BSF}(r)}{D_{fs}(r_0) \cdot S_c(r) \cdot \text{BSF}(r_0)}$$

$$= \frac{\text{BSF}(r)}{\text{BSF}(r_0)} \tag{A2}$$

which is the same as Equation 10.1.

Equation A1 can also be written as:

$$S_p(r) = \frac{D_{fs}(r) \cdot \text{BSF}(r)}{D_{fs}(r_0) \cdot \text{BSF}(r_0) \cdot S_c(r)} \tag{A3}$$

$$= \frac{D_{max}(r)}{D_{max}(r_0) \cdot S_c(r)}$$

$$= \frac{S_{c,p}(r)}{S_c(r)}$$

where $S_{c,p}(r)$ is the total scatter correction factor defined as the ratio of D_{max} dose rate for a given field to the D_{max} dose rate for the reference field (Fig. 10.1B).

B. Derivation of TMR

In Fig. 10.2, let D_1 and D_2 be the doses at depths d and t_0 (reference depth of maximum dose), respectively. Let r, r_{t0}, and r_d be the field sizes at distances f, $f + t_0$, and $f + d$ from the source, respectively. Then, by definition:

$$\text{TMR}(d, r_d) = \frac{D_1}{D_2} \tag{A4}$$

and

$$\frac{D_1}{D(t_0, r_{t0}, f)} = \frac{P(d, r, f)}{100} \tag{A5}$$

where $D(t_0, r_{t0}, f)$ is the dose at depth t_0, field size r_{t0} and SSD $= f$.

$$\frac{D_2}{D(t_0, r_{t0}, f)} = \frac{S_p(r_d)}{S_p(r_{t0})} \cdot \left(\frac{f + t_0}{f + d}\right)^2 \tag{A6}$$

Combining Equations A4, A5, and A6,

$$\text{TMR}(d, r_d) = \frac{P(d, r, f)}{100}\left(\frac{f + d}{f + t_0}\right)^2 \left(\frac{S_p(r_{t0})}{S_p(r_d)}\right) \tag{A7}$$

C. Derivation of SMR

Referring to Fig. 10.2, let $D_1(d, r_d)$ be the dose at point 1 and $D_2(t_0, r_d)$ be the dose at point 2 for field size r_d. Let $D_1(d, 0)$ and $D_2(t_0, 0)$ be the corresponding doses for 0×0 field with the same collimator opening. Then:

$$\text{SMR}(d, r_d) = \frac{D_1(d, r_d) - D_1(d, 0)}{D_2(t_0, 0)} \tag{A8}$$

or

$$\text{SMR}(d, r_d) = \frac{D_1(d, r_d)}{D_2(t_0, r_d)} \times \frac{D_2(t_0, r_d)}{D_2(t_0, r_0)} \times \frac{D_2(t_0, r_0)}{D_2(t_0, 0)} - \frac{D_1(d, 0)}{D_2(t_0, 0)} \qquad \text{(A9)}$$

where r_0 is the reference field (10×10 cm) for normalizing S_p. Since:

$$\text{TMR}(d, r_d) = \frac{D_1(d, r_d)}{D_2(t_0, r_d)}$$

$$\text{TMR}(d, 0) = \frac{D_1(d, 0)}{D_2(t_0, 0)}$$

$$S_p(r_d) = \frac{D_2(t_0, r_d)}{D_2(t_0, r_0)} \qquad \text{(same collimator opening)}$$

and

$$S_p(0) = \frac{D_2(t_0, 0)}{D_2(t_0, r_0)} \qquad \text{(same collimator opening)}$$

Equation A9 becomes:

$$\text{SMR}(d, r_d) = \text{TMR}(d, r_d) \cdot \frac{S_p(r_d)}{S_p(0)} - \text{TMR}(d, 0) \qquad \text{(A10)}$$

REFERENCES

1. Karzmark CJ, Deubert A, Loevinger R. Tissue-phantom ratios—an aid to treatment planning. *Br J Radiol* 1965;38:158.
2. Holt JG. Letter to the editor. *Am Assoc Phys Med Q Bull* 1972;6:127.
3. Saunders JE, Price RH, Horsley RJ. Central axis depth doses for a constant source-tumor distance. *Br J Radiol* 1968;41:464.
4. Holt JG, Laughlin JS, Moroney JP. The extension of the concept of tissue-air ratios (TAR) to high energy x-ray beams. *Radiology* 1970;96:437.
5. Khan FM, Sewchand W, Lee J, et al. Revision of tissue-maximum ratio and scatter-maximum ratio concepts for cobalt 60 and higher energy x-ray beams. *Med Phys* 1980;7:230.
6. Khan FM. *Dose distribution problems in cobalt teletherapy [Thesis].* University of Minnesota, 1969:106.
7. Cundiff JH, Cunningham JR, Golden R, et al. In: RPC/AAPM, compiler. *Dosimetry workshop on Hodgkin's disease.* Houston, TX: MD Anderson Hospital, 1970.
8. Mohan R, Chui C. Validity of the concept of separating primary and scatter dose. *Med Phys* 1985;12:726.
9. Bjarngard BE, Cunningham JR. Comments on "Validity of the concept of separating primary and scatter dose." *Med Phys* 1986;13:760.
10. Mohan R, Chui C. Reply to comments by Bjarngard and Cunningham. *Med Phys* 1986;13:761.
11. American Association of Physicists in Medicine. A protocol for the determination of absorbed dose from high energy photon and electron beams. *Med Phys* 1983;10:741.
12. Almond P, Roosenbeek EV, Browne R, et al. Variation in the position of the central axis maximum build-up point with field size for high-energy photon beams [Letter to the Editor]. *Br J Radiol* 1970;43:911.
13. Dawson DJ. Percentage depth doses for high energy x-rays. *Phys Med Biol* 1976;21:226.
14. Bagne F. Physical aspects of supervoltage x-ray therapy. *Med Phys* 1974;1:266.
15. Suntharalingam N, Steben DJ. Physical characterization of 45-MV photon beams for use in treatment planning. *Med Phys* 1977;4:134.
16. Johns HE, Bruce WR, Reid WB. The dependence of depth dose on focal skin distance. *Br J Radiol* 1958;31:254.
17. Cunningham JR, Shrivastava PN, Wilkinson JM. Computer calculation of dose within an irregularly shaped beam. In: RPC/AAPM, compiler. *Dosimetry workshop on Hodgkin's disease.* Houston, TX: MD Anderson Hospital, 1970.
18. Khan FM, Levitt SH, Moore VC, et al. Computer and approximation methods of calculating depth dose in irregularly shaped fields. *Radiology* 1973;106:433.
19. Khan FM, Gerbi BJ, Deibel FC. Dosimetry of asymmetric x-ray collimators. *Med Phys* 1986;13:936.
20. Loshek DD. Analysis of tissue-maximum ratio/scatter-maximum ratio model relative to the prediction of tissue-maximum ratio in asymmetrically collimated fields. *Med Phys* 1988;15:672.

21. Hanson WF, Berkley LW. Off-axis beam quality change in linear accelerator x-ray beams. *Med Phys* 1980;7:145.
22. Kepka AG, Johnson PM, David J. The effect of off-axis quality changes on zero area TAR for megavoltage beams. *Phys Med Biol* 1985;30:589.
23. Gibbons JP, Khan FM. Calculation of dose in asymmetric x-ray collimators. *Med Phys* 1995;22:1451–1457.
24. Day MJ. A note on the calculation of dose in x-ray fields. *Br J Radiol* 1950;23:368.
25. Sundbom L. Method of dose planning on application of shielding filters in cobalt 60 teletherapy. *Acta Radiol Ther Phys Biol* 1965;3:210.
26. Khan FM. Computer dosimetry of partially blocked fields in cobalt teletherapy. *Radiology* 1970;97:405.

TREATMENT PLANNING I: ISODOSE DISTRIBUTIONS

The central axis depth dose distribution by itself is not sufficient to characterize a radiation beam that produces a dose distribution in a three-dimensional volume. In order to represent volumetric or planar variation in absorbed dose, distributions are depicted by means of *isodose curves,* which are lines passing through points of equal dose. The curves are usually drawn at regular intervals of absorbed dose and expressed as a percentage of the dose at a reference point. Thus the isodose curves represent levels of absorbed dose in the same manner that isotherms are used for heat and isobars, for pressure.

11.1. ISODOSE CHART

An *isodose chart* for a given beam consists of a family of isodose curves usually drawn at equal increments of percent depth dose, representing the variation in dose as a function of depth and transverse distance from the central axis. The depth-dose values of the curves are normalized either at the point of maximum dose on the central axis or at a fixed distance along the central axis in the irradiated medium. The charts in the first category are applicable when the patient is treated at a constant source-to-surface distance (SSD) irrespective of beam direction. In the second category, the isodose curves are normalized at a certain depth beyond the depth of maximum dose, corresponding to the axis of rotation of an isocentric therapy unit. This type of representation is especially useful in rotation therapy but can also be used for stationary isocentric treatments. Figure 11.1 shows both types of isodose charts for a ^{60}Co γ ray beam.

   Examination of isodose charts reveals some general properties of x- and γ-ray dose distributions.

1. The dose at any depth is greatest on the central axis of the beam and gradually decreases toward the edges of the beam, with the exception of some Linac x-ray beams, which exhibit areas of high dose or "horns" near the surface in the periphery of the field. These horns are created by the flattening filter, which is usually designed to overcompensate near the surface in order to obtain flat isodose curves at greater depths.
2. Near the edges of the beam (the penumbra region), the dose rate decreases rapidly as a function of lateral distance from the beam axis. As discussed in Chapter 4, the width of geometric penumbra, which exists both inside and outside the geometrical boundaries of the beam, depends on source size, distance from the source, and source-to-diaphragm distance.
3. Near the beam edge, falloff of the beam is caused not only by the geometric penumbra but also by the reduced side scatter. Therefore, the geometric penumbra is not the best measure of beam sharpness near the edges. Instead the term *physical penumbra* may be used. The *physical penumbra* width is defined as the lateral distance between two specified isodose curves at a specified depth (e.g., lateral distance between 90% and 20% isodose lines at the depth of D_{max}).

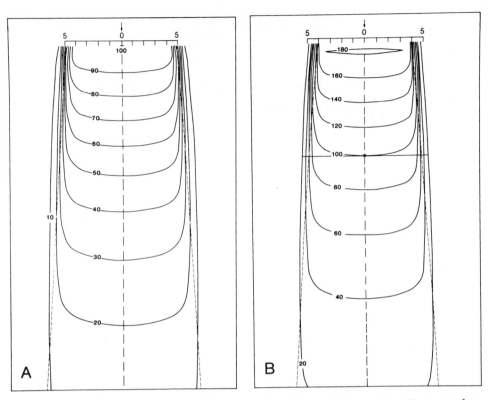

FIG. 11.1. Example of an isodose chart. **A:** SSD type, ^{60}Co beam, SSD = 80 cm, field size = 10 × 10 cm at surface. **B:** SAD type, ^{60}Co beam, SAD = 100 cm, depth of isocenter = 10 cm, field size at isocenter = 10 × 10 cm. (Data from University of Minnesota Hospitals, Eldorado 8 Cobalt Unit, source size = 2 cm.)

4. Outside the geometric limits of the beam and the penumbra, the dose variation is the result of side scatter from the field and both leakage and scatter from the collimator system. Beyond this collimator zone, the dose distribution is governed by the lateral scatter from the medium and leakage from the head of the machine (often called *therapeutic housing* or *source housing*).

Figure 11.2 shows the dose variation across the field at a specified depth. Such a representation of the beam is known as the *beam profile*. It may be noted that the field

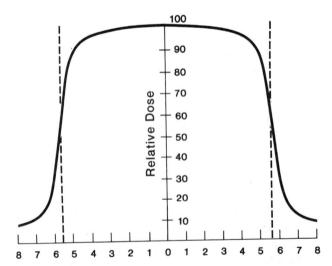

FIG. 11.2. Depth dose profile showing variation of dose across the field. ^{60}Co beam, SSD = 80 cm, depth = 10 cm, field size at surface = 10 × 10 cm. Dotted line indicates geometric field boundary at a 10-cm depth.

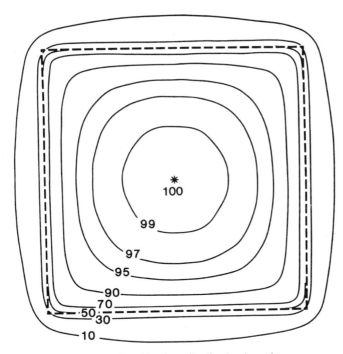

FIG. 11.3. Cross-sectional isodose distribution in a plane perpendicular to the central axis of the beam. Isodose values are normalized to 100% at the center of the field.

size is defined as the lateral distance between the 50% isodose lines at a reference depth. This definition is practically achieved by a procedure called the beam *alignment* in which the field-defining light is made to coincide with the 50% isodose lines of the radiation beam projected on a plane perpendicular to the beam axis and at the standard SSD or source-to-axis distance (SAD).

Another way of depicting the dose variation across the field is to plot isodose curves in a plane perpendicular to the central axis of the beam (Fig. 11.3). Such a representation is useful for treatment planning in which the field sizes are determined on the basis of an isodose curve (e.g., 90%) that adequately covers the target volume.

11.2. MEASUREMENT OF ISODOSE CURVES

Isodose charts can be measured by means of ion chambers, solid state detectors, or radiographic films (Chapter 8). Of these, the ion chamber is the most reliable method, mainly because of its relatively flat energy response and precision. Although any of the phantoms described in Chapter 9 may be used for isodose measurements, water is the medium of choice for ionometric measurements. The chamber can be made waterproof by a thin plastic sleeve that covers the chamber as well as the portion of the cable immersed in the water.

As measurement of isodose charts has been discussed in some detail in the International Commission on Radiation Units and Measurements (ICRU) (1), only a few important points will be discussed here. The ionization chamber used for isodose measurements should be small so that measurements can be made in regions of high dose gradient, such as near the edges of the beam. It is recommended that the sensitive volume of the chamber be less than 15 mm long and have an inside diameter of 5 mm or less. Energy independence of the chamber is another important requirement. Because the x-ray beam spectrum changes with position in the phantom owing to scatter, the energy response of the chamber should be as flat as possible. This can be checked by obtaining the exposure calibration of the chamber for orthovoltage (1 to 4 mm Cu) and ^{60}Co beams. A variation of approximately 5% in response throughout this energy range is acceptable.

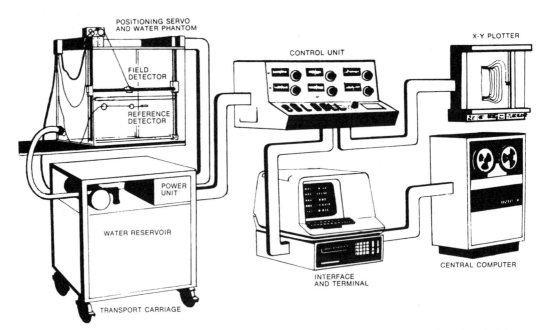

FIG. 11.4. Schematic diagram of an automatic isodose plotter system, Therados RFA-3. (Reprinted with permission from Instrument AB Therados, Uppsala, Sweden.)

Automatic devices for measuring isodose curves have been developed for rapid mapping of the isodose curves. These systems are designed to be either stand alone or computer driven. Basically, the apparatus (Fig. 11.4) consists of two ionization chambers, referred to as the detector A (or probe) and the monitor B. Whereas the probe is arranged to move in the tank of water to sample the dose rate at various points, the monitor is fixed at some point in the field to monitor the beam intensity with time. The ratio of the detector to the monitor response *(A/B)* is recorded as the probe is moved in the phantom. Thus the final response *A/B* is independent of fluctuations in output. In the stand-alone system, the probe searches for points at which *A/B* is equal to a preset percentage value of *A/B* measured at a reference depth or the depth of maximum dose. The motion of the probe is transmitted to the plotter which records its path, the isodose curve.

In the computer-driven models, the chamber movement of the probe is controlled by a computer program. The probe-to-monitor ratio is sampled as the probe moves across the field at preset increments. These beam profiles are measured at a number of depths, determined by computer program. The data thus measured are stored in the computer in the form of a matrix that can then be transformed into isodose curves or other formats allowed by the computer program.

A. Sources of Isodose Charts

Acquisition of isodose charts has been discussed (1). Atlases of premeasured isodose charts for a wide range of radiation therapy equipment are available from the sources listed in the literature (2–4). In addition, isodose distributions may also be obtained from manufacturers of radiation generators or from other institutions having the same unit. However, the user is cautioned against accepting isodose charts from any source and using them as basis for patient treatment without adequate verification. The first and most important check to be performed is to verify that the central axis depth-dose data correspond with percent depth-dose data measured independently in a water phantom. A deviation of 2% or less in local dose is acceptable up to depths of 20 cm. The edges of the distribution should be checked by measuring beam profiles for selected field sizes and depths. An agreement within 2 mm in the penumbra region is acceptable.

Besides direct measurements, isodose charts can also be generated by calculations using various algorithms for treatment planning (5–9). More current algorithms are discussed in

Part III of this book. Some of these programs are commercially available with treatment planning computers. Again, the applicability of the computer-generated isodose curves to the user's machine must be carefully checked.

11.3. PARAMETERS OF ISODOSE CURVES

Among the parameters that affect the single-beam isodose distribution are beam quality, source size, beam collimation, field size, SSD, and the source-to-diaphragm distance (SDD). A discussion of these parameters will be presented in the context of treatment planning.

A. Beam Quality

As discussed previously, the central axis depth dose distribution depends on the beam energy. As a result, the depth of a given isodose curve increases with beam quality. Beam energy also influences isodose curve shape near the field borders. Greater lateral scatter associated with lower-energy beams causes the isodose curves outside the field to bulge out. In other words, the absorbed dose in the medium outside the primary beam is greater for low-energy beams than for those of higher energy.

Physical penumbra depends on beam quality as illustrated in Fig. 11.5. As expected, the isodose curves outside the primary beam (e.g., 10% and 5%) are greatly distended in the case of orthovoltage radiation. Thus one disadvantage of the orthovoltage beams is the increased scattered dose to tissue outside the treatment region. For megavoltage beams, on the other hand, the scatter outside the field is minimized as a result of predominantly forward scattering and becomes more a function of collimation than energy.

B. Source Size, Source-to-Surface Distance, and Source-to-Diaphragm Distance—The Penumbra Effect

Source size, SSD, and SDD affect the shape of isodose curves by virtue of the geometric penumbra, discussed in Chapter 4. In addition, the SSD affects the percent depth dose and therefore the depth of the isodose curves.

As discussed previously, the dose variation across the field border is a complex function of geometric penumbra, lateral scatter, and collimation. Therefore, the field sharpness at depth is not simply determined by the source or focal spot size. For example, by using penumbra trimmers or secondary blocking, the isodose sharpness at depth for ^{60}Co beams with a source size less than 2 cm in diameter can be made comparable with higher-energy Linac beams, although the focal spot size of these beams is usually less than 2 mm. Comparison of isodose curves for ^{60}Co, 4 and 10 MV in Fig. 11.5 illustrates the point that the physical penumbra width for these beams is more or less similar.

C. Collimation and Flattening Filter

The term *collimation* is used here to designate not only the collimator blocks that give shape and size to the beam but also the flattening filter and other absorbers or scatterers in the beam between the target and the patient. Of these, the flattening filter, which is used for megavoltage x-ray beams, has the greatest influence in determining the shape of the isodose curves. Without this filter, the isodose curves will be conical in shape, showing markedly increased x-ray intensity along the central axis and a rapid reduction transversely. The function of the flattening filter is to make the beam intensity distribution relatively uniform across the field (i.e., "flat"). Therefore, the filter is thickest in the middle and tapers off toward the edges.

The cross-sectional variation of the filter thickness also causes variation in the photon spectrum or beam quality across the field owing to selective hardening of the beam by the filter. In general, the average energy of the beam is somewhat lower for the peripheral areas

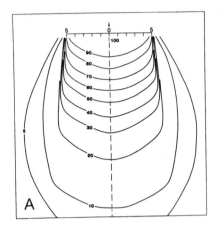

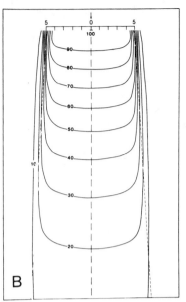

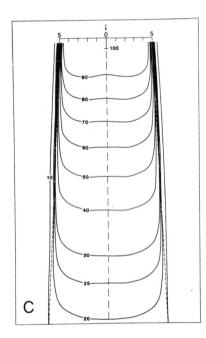

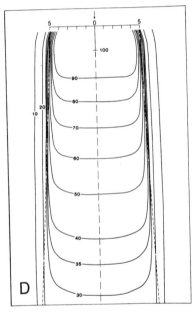

FIG. 11.5. Isodose distributions for different quality radiations. **A:** 200 kVp, SSD = 50 cm, HVL = 1 mm Cu, field size = 10 × 10 cm. **B:** ⁶⁰Co, SSD = 80 cm, field size = 10 × 10 cm. **C:** 4-MV x-rays, SSD = 100 cm, field size = 10 × 10 cm. **D:** 10-MV x-rays, SSD = 100 cm, field size = 10 × 10 cm.

compared with the central part of the beam. This change in quality across the beam causes the flatness to change with depth. However, the change in flatness with depth is caused by not only the selective hardening of the beam across the field but also the changes in the distribution of radiation scatter as the depth increases.

Beam flatness is usually specified at a 10-cm depth with the maximum limits set at the depth of maximum dose. By careful design of the filter and accurate placement in the beam, it is possible to achieve flatness to within ± 3% of the central axis dose value at a 10-cm depth. This degree of flatness should extend over the central area bounded by at least 80% of the field dimensions at the specified depth or 1 cm from the edge of the field. The above specification is satisfactory for the precision required in radiation therapy.

To obtain acceptable flatness at 10-cm depth, an area of high dose near the surface may have to be accepted. Although the extent of the high dose regions, or horns, varies with the design of the filter, lower-energy beams exhibit a larger variation than higher-energy beams. In practice, it is acceptable to have these "superflat" isodose curves near the surface provided no point in any plane parallel to the surface receives a dose greater than 107% of the central axis value (10).

D. Field Size

Field size is one of the most important parameters in treatment planing. Adequate dosimetric coverage of the tumor requires a determination of appropriate field size. This determination must always be made dosimetrically rather than geometrically. In other words, a certain isodose curve (e.g., 90%) enclosing the treatment volume should be the guide in choosing a field size rather than the geometric dimensions of the field.

Great caution should also be exercised in using field sizes smaller than 6 cm in which a relatively large part of the field is in the penumbra region. Depending on the source size, collimation, and design of the flattening filter, the isodose curves for small field sizes, in general, tend to be bell-shaped. Thus treatment planning with isodose curves should be mandatory for small field sizes.

The isodose curvature for ^{60}Co increases as the field size becomes overly large unless the beam is flattened by a flattening filter. The reason for this effect is the progressive reduction of scattered radiation with increasing distance from the central axis as well as the obliquity of the primary rays. The effect becomes particularly severe with elongated fields such as cranial spinal fields used in the treatment of medulloblastoma. In these cases, one needs to calculate doses at several off-axis points or use a beam-flattening compensator.

11.4. WEDGE FILTERS

Frequently, special filters or absorbing blocks are placed in the path of a beam to modify its isodose distribution. The most commonly used beam-modifying device is the *wedge filter*. This is a wedge-shaped absorber that causes a progressive decrease in the intensity across the beam, resulting in a tilt of the isodose curves from their normal positions. As shown in Fig. 11.6, the isodose curves are tilted toward the thin end, the degree of tilt depends

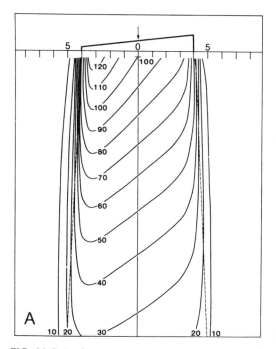
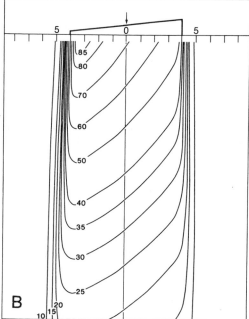

FIG. 11.6. Isodose curves for a wedge filter. **A:** normalized to D_{max}. **B:** normalized to D_{max} without the wedge. ^{60}Co, wedge angle = 45 degrees, field size = 8 × 10 cm, SSD = 80 cm.

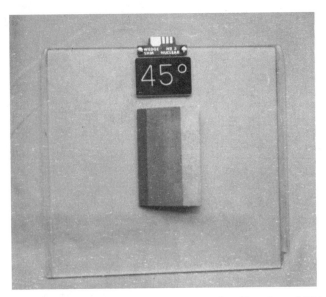

FIG. 11.7. Photograph of a 45 degree wedge filter for a 4-MV x-ray Linac (ATC 400).

on the slope of the wedge filter. In actual wedge filter design, the sloping surface is made either straight or sigmoid in shape; the latter design is used to produce straighter isodose curves.

The wedge is usually made of a dense material, such as lead or steel, and is mounted on a transparent plastic tray which can be inserted in the beam at a specified distance from the source (Fig. 11.7). This distance is arranged such that the wedge tray is always at a distance of at least 15 cm from the skin surface, so as to avoid destroying the skin-sparing effect of the megavoltage beam.

Another class of wedges (not discussed here) are the dynamic wedges. These wedges are generated electronically by creating wedged beam profiles through dynamic motion of an independent jaw within the treatment beam. Dynamic wedges do not offer significant clinical advantages over the traditional metal wedges. Moreover, all wedges and compensators are now superseded by the new technology using dynamic multileaf collimators in conjunction with the intensity-modulated radiation therapy (IMRT).

A. Wedge Isodose Angle

The term *wedge isodose angle* (or simply *wedge angle*) refers to "the angle through which an isodose curve is titled at the central ray of a beam at a specified depth" (11). In this definition, one should note that the wedge angle is the angle between the isodose curve and the normal to the central axis, as shown in Fig. 11.6. In addition, the specification of depth is important since, in general, the presence of scattered radiation causes the angle of isodose tilt to decrease with increasing depth in the phantom. However, there is no general agreement as to the choice of reference depth. Some choose depth as a function of field size (e.g., 1/2 or 2/3 of the beam width) while others define wedge angle as the angle between the 50% isodose curve and the normal to the central axis. The latter choice, however, becomes impractical when higher-energy beams are used. For example, the central axis depth of the 50% isodose curve for a 10-MV beam lies at about 18 cm for a 10 × 10-cm field and 100-cm SSD. This depth is too large in the context of most wedge filter applications. As will be discussed in section 11.7, the wedge filters are mostly used for treating superficial tumors, for example, not more than 10 cm deep. Therefore, the current recommendation is to use a single reference depth of 10 cm for wedge angle specification (11).

B. Wedge Transmission Factor

The presence of a wedge filter decreases the output of the machine, which must be taken into account in treatment calculations. This effect is characterized by the *wedge transmission factor* (or simply *wedge factor*), defined as the ratio of doses with and without the wedge, at a point in phantom along the central axis of the beam. This factor should be measured in phantom at a suitable depth beyond the depth of maximum dose (e.g., 10 cm).

In cobalt-60 teletherapy, the wedge factor is sometimes incorporated into the isodose curves, as shown in Fig. 11.6B. In this case, the depth dose distribution is normalized relative to the D_{max} without the wedge. For example, the isodose curve at depth of D_{max} is 72%, indicating that the wedge factor is already taken into account in the isodose distribution. If such a chart is used for isodose planning, no further correction should be applied to the output. In other words, the machine output corresponding to the open beam should be used.

A more common approach is to normalize the isodose curves relative to the central axis D_{max} with the wedge in the beam. As see in Fig. 11.6A, the 100% dose is indicated at the depth of D_{max}. With this approach, the output of the beam must be corrected using the wedge factor.

C. Wedge Systems

Wedge filters are of two main types. The first may be called the *individualized wedge system,* which requires a separate wedge for each beam width, optimally designed to minimize the loss of beam output. A mechanism is provided to align the thin end of the wedge with the border of the light field (Fig. 11.8A). The second system uses a *universal wedge,* that is, a single wedge serves for all beam widths. Such a filter is fixed centrally in the beam while the field can be opened to any size. As illustrated in Fig. 11.8B, only a small part of this wedge, i.e., *ABC,* is effective in producing the given wedge angle. The rest *(ACDE),* being unwedged, does not contribute to the isodose tilt but unnecessarily reduces the beam intensity. Since the individualized system economizes on the beam output, it is preferred for use in cobalt teletherapy. The universal wedge, on the other hand, is useful for linear accelerator beams where the output is plentiful. From the set-up and treatment planning points of view, the universal wedge is simpler to use than the individualized filter.

D. Effect on Beam Quality

In general, the wedge filter alters the beam quality by preferentially attenuating the lower-energy photons (beam hardening) and, to a lesser extent, by Compton scattering, which results in energy degradation (beam softening). For the ^{60}Co beam, because the primary beam is essentially monoenergetic, the presence of the wedge filter does not significantly alter the central axis percent depth dose distribution. For x-rays, on the other hand, there can be some beam hardening (12), and consequently, the depth dose distribution can be somewhat altered, especially at large depths.

Although the wedge filters produce some change in beam quality, as noted above, the effect is not large enough to alter other calculation parameters such as the backscatter factor or the equivalent square, which may be assumed to be the same as for the corresponding open beams. Even central axis percent depth doses, tissue-air ratios or tissue maximal ratios may be assumed unchanged for small depths (e.g., less than 10 cm). The error caused by this assumption is minimized if the wedge transmission factor has been measured at a reference depth close to the point of interest.

E. Design of Wedge Filters

The design of wedge filters for megavoltage beams has been described by many authors (13–16). Here I will briefly present the design of a universal wedge filter following the

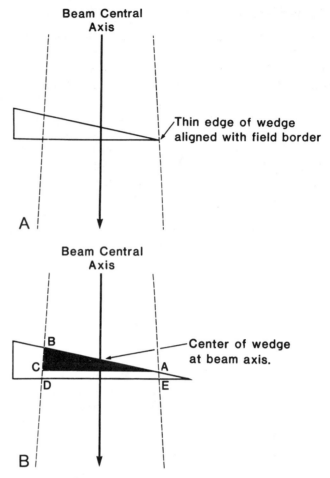

FIG. 11.8. Schematic representation of **(A)** an individualized wedge for a specific field width in which the thin end of the wedge is always aligned with the field border and **(B)** a universal wedge in which the center of the wedge filter is fixed at the beam axis and the field can be opened to any width.

technique of Aron and Scapicchio (16). The principle of this method is to determine the ratio of percent depth doses at various points for wedged and nonwedged fields. The thickness of the wedge filter material at these points is then determined from these ratios and the knowledge of the half-value layer or the attenuation coefficient of the given beam for the filter material.

Figure 11.9 illustrates the design of a wedge filter. A line is drawn at a selected depth across the nonwedged field at right angles to the central axis. This depth should correspond to the reference depth used for the wedge angle definition. Fan lines, representing rays from the source, are drawn at fixed intervals (e.g., 1 cm) on both sides of the central axis. A series of parallel lines is drawn making an angle with the central axis equal to the complement of the given wedge angle and intersecting the central axis at the same points of intersection as the nonwedged isodose lines. A table is constructed that includes the percentage depth doses at the points of intersection of the fan lines and the reference depth line for the nonwedged isodose curves and the wedged isodose lines (sloping lines). The ratio of the wedged to nonwedged values is calculated as shown in Table 11.1. These ratios are normalized to the highest value within the field (excluding the penumbra region) to give the relative transmission ratio along the designated fan lines. A wedge filter of a given material can then be designed to provide these transmission ratios.

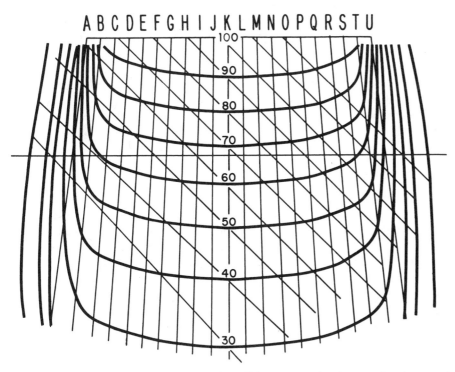

FIG. 11.9. New 45 degree lines constructed parallel to one another, intersecting the central axis at same points of intersection as nonwedge isodose lines. (Redrawn from Aron BS, Scapicchio M. Design of universal wedge filter system for a cobalt 60 unit. *Am J Roentgenol* 1966;96:70.)

11.5. COMBINATION OF RADIATION FIELDS

Treatment by a single photon beam is seldom used except in some cases in which the tumor is superficial. The following criteria of acceptability may be used for a single field treatment: (a) the dose distribution within the tumor volume is reasonably uniform (e.g., within ±5%); (b) the maximum dose to the tissues in the beam is not excessive (e.g., not more than 110% of the prescribed dose); and (c) normal critical structures in the beam do not receive doses near or beyond tolerance. Whereas single fields of superficial x-rays are routinely used for treating skin cancers which are confined to a depth of a few millimeters, single megavoltage beams are used only in rare cases for which a combination of beams is either technically difficult or results in unnecessary or excessive irradiation of the normal tissues. Examples of a few treatments that use single megavoltage beams include the supraclavicular region, internal mammary nodes (anterior field), and the spinal

TABLE 11.1. TRANSMISSION RATIOS FOR THE CONSTRUCTION OF WEDGE FILTER

	A	B	C	E	G	I	K	M	O	Q	S	T	U
Nonwedge isodose	40	55	62	65	67	68	68	68	67	65	62	55	40
Wedge isodose	35	39	41	47	53	60	68	76	86	95	105	110	115
Ratio (wedge/nonwedge)	0.875	0.710	0.660	0.720	0.790	0.880	1.00	1.12	1.28	1.46	1.70	1.20	2.88
Transmission ratio	—	—	0.387	0.425	0.462	0.515	0.59	0.66	0.75	0.86	1.0	—	—
mm Pb	—	—	15.2	13.6	12.2	10.5	8.3	6.5	4.5	2.3	0	—	—

From Aron BS, Scapicchio M. Design of universal wedge filter system for a cobalt 60 unit. *AJR* 1966;96:70, with permission.

cord (posterior field). Although the dose distribution is not ideal, the single-field technique in these cases results in simplicity of set-up without violating the above criteria of acceptability.

For treatment of most tumors, however, a combination of two or more beams is required for an acceptable distribution of dose within the tumor and the surrounding normal tissues. Although radiation fields may be combined in many ways, the discussion here will be confined to the basic principles that are useful in treating tumors involving different sites.

A. Parallel Opposed Fields

The simplest combination of two fields is a pair of fields directed along the same axis from opposite sides of the treatment volume. The advantages of the parallel opposed fields are the simplicity and reproducibility of set-up, homogeneous dose to the tumor, and less chances of geometrical miss (compared with angled beams), given that the field size is large enough to provide adequate lateral coverage of the tumor volume. A disadvantage is the excessive dose to normal tissues and critical organs above and below the tumor.

A composite isodose distribution for a pair of parallel opposed fields may be obtained by adding the depth dose contribution of each field (Fig. 11.10). The manual procedure consists of joining the points of intersection of isodose curves for the individual fields which sum to the same total dose value. The resultant distribution shows the combined isodose

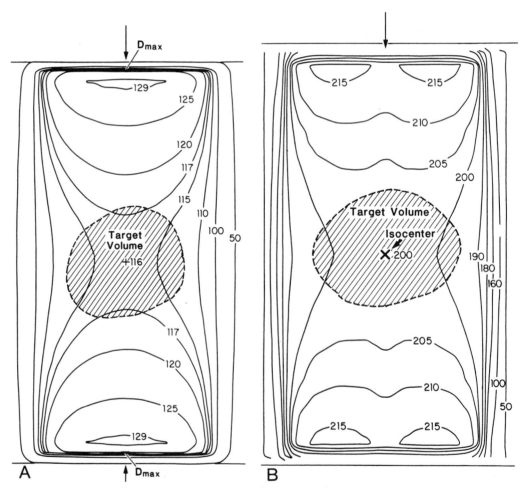

FIG. 11.10. Composite isodose distribution for a pair of parallel opposed fields. **A:** Each beam is given a weight of 100 at the depth of D_{max}. **B:** Isocentric plan with each beam weighted 100 at the isocenter.

distribution normalized to the individual beam weights. The beams are usually weighted in dose units of 100 at the depth of D_{max} in the case of SSD techniques or at the isocenter for the isocentric techniques. For the example shown in Fig. 11.10A, the minimum percent isodose surrounding the tumor is 110. This means that the minimum dose to the tumor (with a generous margin) is 110 rads if 100 rads are delivered at the depth of D_{max} by each field. Thus, if the tumor dose were to be specified at this isodose level, one could calculate the D_{max} dose and the treatment time for each field. For the isocentric plan shown in Fig. 11.10B, the beam weights refer to doses delivered to the isocenter. Thus the 190% isodose curve represents the specified minimum dosage level if each beam delivered 100 rads to its isocenter. Once the isocenter dose is calculated, one can determine the treatment time or monitor units as described in section 10.2.

A.1. Patient Thickness Versus Dose Uniformity

One advantage of equally weighted parallel opposed beams is that the dose distribution within the irradiated volume can be made uniform. However, the uniformity of distribution depends on the patient thickness, beam energy, and beam flatness. In general, as the patient thickness increases or the beam energy decreases, the central axis maximum dose near the surface increases relative to the midpoint dose. This effect, called *tissue lateral effect,* is shown in Fig. 11.11 in which two opposing beams are placed 25 cm apart with the midpoint dose normalized to 100. The curves for cobalt-60 and 4 MV show that for a patient of this thickness parallel opposed beams would give rise to an excessively higher dose to the subcutaneous tissues compared with the tumor dose at the midpoint. As the energy is increased to 10 MV, the distribution becomes almost uniform and at 25 MV it shows significant sparing of the superficial tissues relative to the midline structures.

The ratio of maximum *peripheral dose* to midpoint dose is plotted in Fig. 11.12 as a function of patient thickness for a number of beam energies. Such data are useful in choosing the appropriate beam energy for a given patient thickness when using parallel opposed fields. For example, acceptable uniformity of dose, that is, within ± 5%, is achievable with cobalt-60 or 4- to 6-MV beams for thicknesses of about 15 cm or less (e.g., head, neck, and extremities). However, for thicknesses of 20 cm or greater (e.g., thorax, abdomen, and pelvis), 10-MV or higher energies must be used to spare the normal subcutaneous tissues.

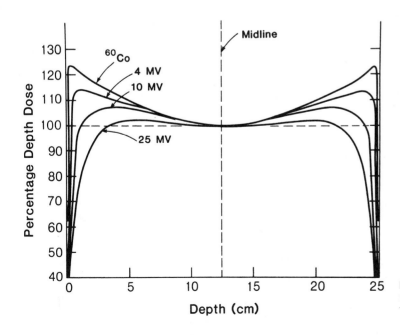

FIG. 11.11. Depth dose curves for parallel opposed field normalized to midpoint value. Patient thickness = 25 cm, field size = 10 × 10 cm, SSD = 100 cm.

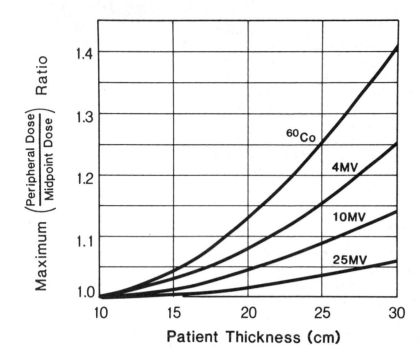

FIG. 11.12. Ratio of maximum peripheral dose to the midpoint dose plotted as a function of patient thickness for different beam qualities. Parallel opposed fields, field size = 10 × 10 cm SSD = 100 cm.

A.2. Edge Effect (Lateral Tissue Damage)

When treating with multiple beams, the question arises whether one should treat one field per day or all fields per day. Wilson and Hall (17) have discussed this problem in terms of cell survival curves and Ellis's time-dose-fractionation formula (18,19). For parallel opposed beams, they have shown that treating with one field per day produces greater biologic damage to normal subcutaneous tissue than treating with two fields per day, despite the fact that the total dose is the same. Apparently, the biologic effect in the normal tissue is greater if it receives alternating high- and low-dose fractions compared with the equal but medium-size dose fractions resulting from treating both fields daily. This phenomenon has been called *the edge effect,* or *the tissue lateral damage* (20). The problem becomes more severe when larger thicknesses (e.g., ≥20 cm) are treated with one field per day using a lower-energy beam (e.g., ≤6 MV). In such cases, the dose per fraction to the subcutaneous tissues, although delivered on alternate days, becomes prohibitively high.

A.3. Integral Dose

One way of comparing dose distributions for different quality beams is to calculate the *integral dose* for a given tumor dose. Integral dose is a measure of the total energy absorbed in the treated volume. If a mass of tissue receives a uniform dose, then the integral dose is simply the product of mass and dose. However, in practice, the absorbed dose in the tissue is nonuniform so rather complex mathematical formulas are required to calculate it.

For a single beam of x- or γ radiation, Mayneord (21) formulated the following expression:

$$\sum = 1.44 D_0 \, A d_{1/2}(1 - e^{-0.693d/d_{1/2}})\left(1 + \frac{2.88 d_{1/2}}{\text{SSD}}\right) \tag{11.1}$$

where $\sum$ is the integral dose, D_0 is the peak dose along the central axis, A is the geometric area of the field, d is the total thickness of patient in the path of the beam, $d_{1/2}$ is the half-value depth or the depth of 50% depth dose and SSD is the source-surface distance. The term $\left(1 + \frac{2.88 d_{1/2}}{\text{SSD}}\right)$ is a correction for geometric divergence of the beam.

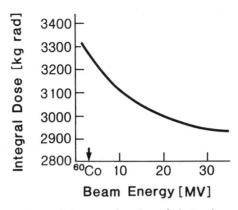

FIG. 11.13. Integral dose as a function of photon beam energy, when 1,000 rad are delivered at a midpoint of a 25-cm–thick patient. Field size, 10-cm diameter at an SSD of 100 cm. (Redrawn from Podgorsak EB, Rawlinson JA, Johns HE. X-ray depth doses for linear accelerators in the energy range from 10 to 32 MeV. *Am J Roentgenol* 1975;123:182.)

Because integral dose is basically the product of mass and dose, its unit is the gram-rad or kilogram-gray or simply joule (since 1 Gy = 1 J/kg). Figure 11.13 shows the integral dose as a function of the energy of radiation for a tumor dose of 1,000 rad (1 rad = 10^{-2} Gy) at a depth of 12.5 cm in the patient of 25-cm thickness treated with parallel opposed beams (22). The curve shows a useful result, namely, the higher the photon energy the lower the integral dose.

Although it is generally believed that the probability of damage to normal tissue increases with the increase in the integral dose, this quantity is seldom used clinically to plan dosages or predict treatment outcome. However, it does provide qualitative guidelines for treatment planning for selecting beam energy, field sizes, and multiplicity of fields. As a general rule, one should keep the integral dose to a minimum, provided the adequacy of tumor irradiation and the sparing of critical organs are not compromised.

B. Multiple Fields

One of the most important objectives of treatment planing is to deliver maximum dose to the tumor and minimum dose to the surrounding tissues. In addition, dose uniformity within the tumor volume and sparing of critical organs are important considerations in judging a plan. Some of the strategies useful in achieving these goals are (a) using fields of appropriate size; (b) increasing the number of fields or *portals;* (c) selecting appropriate beam directions; (d) adjusting beam weights (dose contribution from individual fields); (e) using appropriate beam energy; and (f) using beam modifiers such as wedge filters and compensators. Although obtaining a combination of these parameters that yields an optimal plan is time-consuming if done manually, treatment-planning computers are now available that can do the job quickly and accurately. Some of these systems are highly interactive so that the user can almost instantly modify, calculate, and examine various plans to select one that is clinically superior.

In section 11.5A, I discussed the case of two parallel opposed fields. Although the technique results in uniform irradiation of the tumor, there is little sparing of the surrounding normal tissue. In fact, the dose to the peripheral tissues can be significantly higher than the midline dose. Reduction of dose to subcutaneous tissue and normal tissue surrounding the tumor can be achieved by using a combination of three or more fields. Figure 11.14 illustrates various multiple-field arrangements in which the beam enters the patient from various directions, always directed at the tumor. Thus, by using multiple fields, the ratio of the tumor dose to the normal tissue dose is increased. Figure 11.15A,B shows typical examples of multiple fields, one used for treatment of the esophagus and the other, for the prostate gland. Figure 11.15C illustrates a fixed SSD-type technique in which the beam

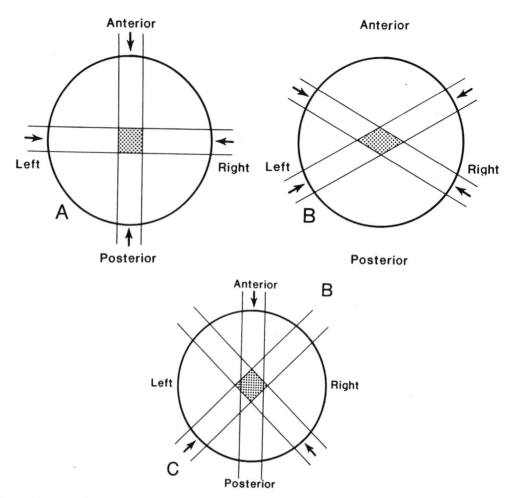

FIG. 11.14. Schematic diagram showing examples of multiple fields. **A:** Two opposing pairs at right angles. **B:** Two opposing pairs at 120 degrees. **C:** Three fields: one anterior and two posterior oblique, at 45 degrees with the vertical.

weights are delivered to D_{max} points. In actual practice, one may use a combination of parallel opposed fields and multiple fields to achieve the desired dose distribution.

Although multiple fields can provide good distribution, there are some clinical and technical limitations to these methods. For example, certain beam angles are prohibited because of the presence of critical organs in those directions. Also, the set-up accuracy of a treatment may be better with parallel opposed than with the multiple angled beam arrangement. It is, therefore, important to realize that the acceptability of a treatment plan depends not only on the dose distribution on paper but also on the practical feasibility, set-up accuracy, and reproducibility of the treatment technique.

11.6. ISOCENTRIC TECHNIQUES

Most modern machines are constructed so that the source of radiation can rotate about a horizontal axis. The gantry of the machine is capable of rotating through 360 degrees with the collimator axis moving in a vertical plane. The *isocenter* is the point of intersection of the collimator axis and the gantry axis of rotation.

A. Stationary Beams

The isocentric technique of irradiation consists of placing the isocenter of the machine at a depth within the patient and directing the beams from different directions. The distance

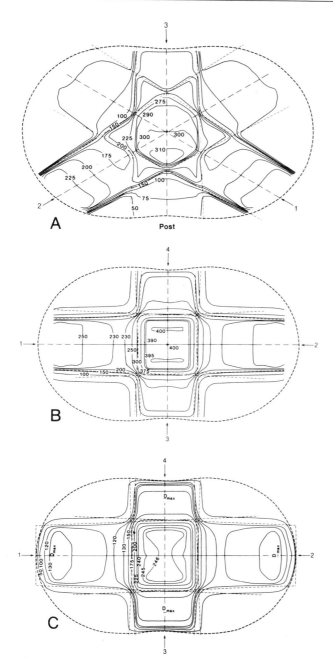

FIG. 11.15. Examples of multiple field plans. **A:** Three-field isocentric technique. Each beam delivers 100 units of dose at the isocenter; 4 MV, field size = 8 × 8 cm at isocenter, SAD = 100 cm. **B:** Four-field isocentric technique. Each beam delivers 100 units of dose at the isocenter; 10 MV, field size = 8 × 8 cm at isocenter, SAD = 100 cm. **C:** Four-field SSD technique in which all beams are weighted 100 units at their respective points of D_{max}; 10 MV, field size = 8 × 8 cm at surface, SSD = 100 cm.

of the source from the isocenter, or the SAD, remains constant irrespective of the beam direction. However, the SSD in this case may change, depending on the beam direction and the shape of the patient contour. For any beam direction, the following relationship holds:

$$SSD = SAD - d \qquad (11.2)$$

where d is the depth of the isocenter. Knowing the depth and position of isocenter from one direction such as the anterior posterior, the SSD can be calculated according to Equation

11.2 and set up from that direction. Then the positioning of subsequent fields simply requires moving the gantry and not the patient.

Although all techniques for which SSD ≤ SAD can be carried out isocentrically, the major advantage of this method is the ease with which multiple field set-ups (three or more) can be treated when all fields are treated the same day. This technique not only dispenses with the setting up of SSD for each beam direction but relies primarily on the accuracy of machine isocentricity and not on the skin marks which are unreliable points of reference in most cases.

The treatment calculations for isocentric treatments have been presented in section 10.2A.2. Figure 11.15A,B shows examples of isodose distribution for isocentric techniques.

B. Rotation Therapy

Rotation therapy is a special case of the isocentric technique in which the beam moves continuously about the patient, or the patient is rotated while the beam is held fixed. Although this technique has been used for treating tumors of the esophagus, bladder, prostate gland, cervix, and brain, the technique offers little advantage over the isocentric technique using multiple stationary beams. For example, the esophagus can be treated equally well with three fields; the prostate gland and bladder, with four fields (sometimes combined with parallel opposed fields); and the brain, with two or three fields or with wedges, depending on the size and location of the tumor. Many times it is a matter of individual preference, although one technique may offer particular advantages over the other in regard to patient positioning, blocking, and the size of volume to be irradiated. Especially when intricate blocking is required, rotation therapy should not be attempted.

Rotation therapy is best suited for small, deep-seated tumors. If the tumor is confined within a region extending not more than halfway from the center of the contour cross-section, rotation therapy may be a proper choice. However, rotation therapy is not indicated if (a) volume to be irradiated is too large, (b) the external surface differs markedly from a cylinder, and (c) the tumor is too far off center.

Calculation for rotation therapy can be made in the same way as for the stationary isocentric beams, except that a reasonably large number of beams should be positioned around the patient contour at fixed angular intervals. The dose rate at the isocenter is given by:

$$\dot{D}_{\text{iso}} = \dot{D}_{\text{ref}} \times \overline{T} \qquad (11.3)$$

where $\dot{D}_{\text{ref}}$ is the reference dose rate related to the quantity $\overline{T}$ which may be average tissue-to-air ratio (TAR) or tissue maximal ratio (TMR) (averaged over all depths at the selected angles). In the case of TARs, $\dot{D}_{\text{ref}}$ is the dose rate in free space for the given field at the isocenter. A method of manual calculations based on this system was discussed in section 9.4D. If the TMRs are used, $\dot{D}_{\text{ref}}$ is the D_{max} dose rate for the given field at the SAD. Using the TMR system discussed in Chapter 10,

$$\dot{D}_{\text{iso}} = \dot{D}_0 \times S_c \times S_p \times \overline{\text{TMR}} \qquad (11.4)$$

where $\dot{D}_0$ is the D_{max} dose rate for a 10 × 10-cm field at the SAD, and S_c and S_p are the collimator and phantom scatter correction factors for the given field size at the isocenter. In the case of a linear accelerator, $\dot{D}_0$ is the monitor unit (MU) rate (assuming 1 MU = 1 rad (cGy) at the isocenter for a depth of D_{max} for a 10 × 10-cm field).

Example

A patient is to receive 250 rad at the isocenter by rotation therapy, using 4-MV x-rays, 6 × 10-cm field at the isocenter, and a SAD of 100 cm. If $\overline{\text{TMR}}$ calculated according to the procedure in section 9.4D is 0.746, calculate the number of monitor units to be set on the machine if the machine output is set at 200 MU/min and given S_c (6 × 10) = 0.98 and S_p (6 × 10) = 0.99. From Equation 11.4,

$$\dot{D}_{\text{iso}} = \dot{D}_0 \times S_c \times S_p \times \overline{\text{TMR}}$$

or

$$\dot{D}_{\text{iso}} = 200 \times 0.98 \times 0.99 \times 0.746$$

$$= 144.8 \,\text{rad/min}$$

$$\text{Treatment time} = \frac{250 \,\text{rad}}{144.8 \,\text{rad/min}} = 1.73 \,\text{min}$$

$$\text{Total MU to be set} = 200 \,(\text{MU/min}) \times 1.73 \,\text{min}$$

$$= 345 \,\text{MU}$$

Gantry rotation speed is set so that 345 MU are delivered at the conclusion of the rotation. Some machines perform only one rotation, whereas others can perform a specified number of arcs or rotations in a pendulum manner. Most modern machines allow for automatic adjustment of rotation speed to deliver a preset number of monitor units by the end of a single rotation.

The determination of complete isodose curves for rotation therapy by manual means is very time-consuming. It is essentially the same procedure as used in multiple fixed beams, but with a large number of beams. The isocentric isodose chart (Fig. 11.1B) in which isodoses are normalized to a point at depth on the central axis is used with the isocenter placed at the point of normalization. By summing the isodose values at selected points while the chart is placed at different angles, the dose distribution can be determined relative to the isocenter. Because of the tedium involved in the procedure, this task is ideally suited for computer application. Such programs are available with commercial treatment planning computers.

Figure 11.16 shows three examples of isodose distribution for rotation therapy: (a) 100 degree arc rotation; (b) 180 degree arc rotation; and (c) full 360 degree rotation. It should be noted that whereas the maximum dose for the 360-degree rotation occurs at the isocenter, for the partial arcs it is displaced toward the irradiated sector. This illustrates an important principle that in arc therapy or when oblique fields are directed through one side of a patient, they should be aimed a suitable distance beyond the tumor area. This is sometimes referred to as *past pointing*. The extent of past pointing required to bring the maximum dose to the tumor site depends on the arc angle and should be determined for an individual case by actual isodose planning.

11.7. WEDGE FIELD TECHNIQUES

Relatively superficial tumors, extending from the surface to a depth of several centimeters, can be irradiated by two "wedged" beams directed from the same side of the patient. Figure 11.17A shows isodose distribution of two angled beams with no wedge in the beams. It is seen that in the region of overlap of the beams, the dose distribution is quite nonuniform. The dose is highest in the superficial or proximal region of overlap and falls off to lower values toward the deeper areas. By inserting appropriate wedge filters in the beam and positioning them with the thick ends adjacent to each other, the angled field distribution can be made fairly uniform (Fig. 11.17B). Each wedged beam in this case has a reduced dose in the superficial region relative to the deeper region so that the dose gradient in the overlap region is minimized. The dose falls off rapidly beyond the region of overlap or the "plateau" region, which is clinically a desirable feature.

There are three parameters that affect the plateau region in terms of its depth, shape, and dose distribution: θ, ϕ, and S, where θ is the wedge angle (section 11.4A), ϕ is the hinge angle, and S is the separation. These parameters are illustrated in Fig. 11.18. The hinge angle

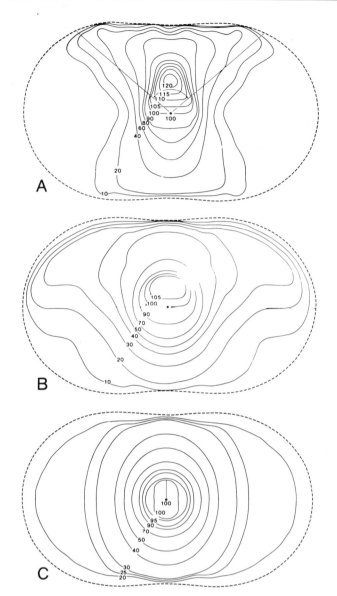

FIG. 11.16. Examples of isodose distribution for rotation therapy. **A:** Arc angle = 100 degrees. **B:** Arc angle = 180 degrees. **C:** Full 360 degree rotation; 4 MV, field size = 7 × 12 cm at isocenter, SAD = 100 cm.

is the angle between the central axes of the two beams and the separation S is the distance between the thick ends of the wedge filters as projected on the surface. Cohen and Martin (3) have discussed in detail how θ, ϕ, and S can be adjusted to achieve a desired plateau.

There is an optimum relationship between the wedge angle θ and the hinge angle ϕ which provides the most uniform distribution of radiation dose in the plateau:

$$\theta = 90° - \phi/2 \qquad (11.5)$$

This equation is based on the principle that for a given hinge angle the wedge angle should be such that the isodose curves from each field are parallel to the bisector of the hinge angle (Fig. 11.18). Under these conditions, when the isodoses are combined, the resultant distribution is uniform.

The Equation 11.5, although helpful in treatment planning, may not yield an optimum plan for a given patient contour. The relationship assumes that the wedge isodose curves are not modified by the surface contour. In practice, however, contours are usually curved

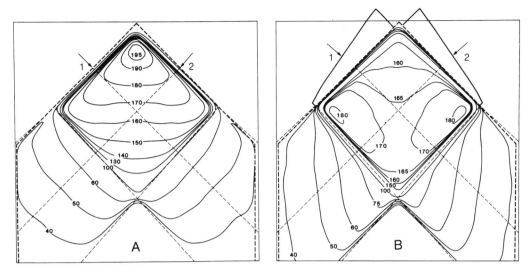

FIG. 11.17. Isodose distribution for two angle beams. **A:** Without wedges. **B:** With wedges; 4 MV, field size = 10 × 10 cm, SSD = 100 cm, wedge angle = 45 degrees.

or irregular in shape and thus modify the isodose distribution for the wedged beams. As a result, the isodose curves for the individual fields are no longer parallel to the bisector of the hinge angle, thus giving rise to a nonuniform distribution in the overlap region. This problem can be solved by using *compensators* (discussed in Chapter 12), which make the skin surface effectively flat and perpendicular to each beam. An alternative approach is to modify the wedge angle (using a different wedge angle filter from that given by Equation 11.5) so that a part of the wedge angle acts as a compensator and the rest as a true wedge filter. The main objective is to make the isodose curves parallel to the hinge angle bisector. Although the latter approach obviates the need for a compensator, the determination of an

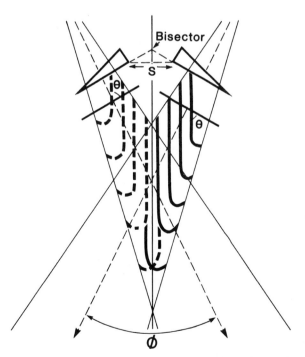

FIG. 11.18. Parameters of the wedge beams, θ is wedge angle, ϕ is hinge angle, and S is separation. Isodose curves for each wedge field are parallel to the bisector.

optimum wedge angle may not be easy if planning is done manually. The former method, on the other hand, is well-suited for manual calculations since all you need is a compensator and an atlas of precalculated isodose distributions for a variety of θ, ϕ, and S values. This method, however, becomes technically difficult to implement if complicated secondary blocking is required in addition to the compensator and the wedge filter.

Equation 11.5 suggests that for each hinge angle one should use a different wedge angle. However, in practice, selected wedge angles, i.e., 15 degrees, 30 degrees, 45 degrees, and 60 degrees, are adequate over a wide range of hinge angles.

In modern radiation therapy, complex treatment techniques are frequently used, which may involve wedge filters, compensators, field blocking, and field reductions, all for the same patient. Manual treatment planning is difficult for such cases. For this reason, in many institutions, all complex treatments, including wedged fields, are planned by computer as a matter of standard practice.

A. Uniformity of Dose Distribution

Because wedge pair techniques are normally used for treating small, superficial tumor volumes, a high-dose region *(hot spot)* of up to $+10\%$ within the treatment volume is usually acceptable. These hot spots occur under the thin ends of the wedges and their magnitude increases with field size and wedge angle. This effect is related to the differential attenuation of the beam under the thick end relative to the thin end.

Generally, the wedge filter technique is suitable when the tumor is approximately from 0 to 7 cm deep and when it is necessary to irradiate from one side of the skin surface. The most desirable feature of this technique is the rapid dose falloff beyond the region of overlap. This falloff can be exploited to protect a critical organ such as the spinal cord. Although wedge filters are invaluable in radiotherapy, some of these techniques are being replaced by electron beam techniques (Chapter 14).

B. Open and Wedged Field Combinations

Although wedge filters were originally designed for use in conjunction with the wedge-pair arrangement, it is possible to combine open and wedged beams to obtain a particular dose distribution. One such arrangement which uses an open field anteriorly and wedged field laterally in the treatment of some tumors is shown in Fig. 11.19A. The anterior field is weighted to deliver 100 units to the lateral 15 units to the isocenter (these beams could be weighted in terms of D_{max} in the SSD technique). The weights and wedge angle are usually adjusted for an individual case to obtain an acceptable distribution. The principle of this technique is that as the dose contribution from the anterior field decreases with depth, the lateral beam provides a boost to offset this decrease. As seen in Fig. 11.19A, a wedged beam with the thick end positioned superiorly provides the desired compensation for the dose dropoff. Thus such a combination of open and wedged beams gives rise to a distribution which remains constant with depth within certain limits.

Figure 11.19B shows another technique in which the anterior open beam is combined with the two lateral wedged beams. Again, the beam weights and wedge angles are chosen to make the open beam distribution remain constant throughout the tumor volume.

11.8. TUMOR DOSE SPECIFICATION FOR EXTERNAL PHOTON BEAMS

The results of treatments can be meaningfully interpreted only if sufficient information is provided regarding the irradiation technique and the distribution of dose in space and time. In the absence of this information, recording of only the so-called tumor dose serves little purpose. Unfortunately, this important problem is often ignored. More often than not, treatment summaries and records are ambiguous and even incomprehensible

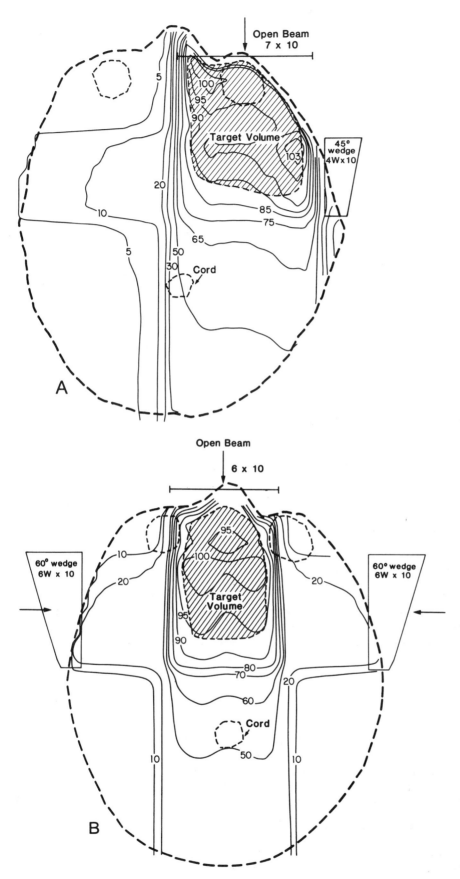

FIG. 11.19. Treatment plans using open and wedged field combinations. **A:** Isocentric plan with anterior open field weighted 100 and lateral wedged field weighted 15 at the isocenter. **B:** A combination of anterior open beam and two lateral wedged beams; 4 MV x-ray beam from ATC-400 Linac.

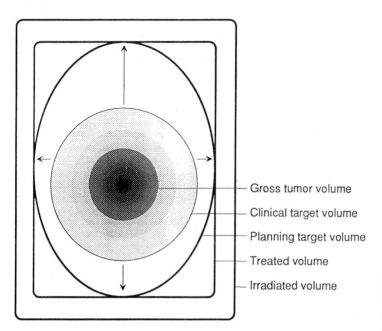

- Gross tumor volume
- Clinical target volume
- Planning target volume
- Treated volume
- Irradiated volume

FIG. 11.20. Schematic illustration of ICRU volumes. (From ICRU. Prescribing, recording, and reporting photon beam therapy. ICRU Report 50. Bethesda, Maryland. International Commission of Radiation Units and Measurements, 1993.)

to other people. Therefore, one cannot overemphasize the need for a dose recording system which is sufficiently explicit and detailed to enable other centers to reproduce the treatment.

In 1978, the ICRU (23) recognized the need for a general dose-specification system which could be adopted universally. Although the system proposed by the ICRU has not been universally implemented, there is a substantial advantage in adopting a common method of dose specification. In this section, I present the highlights of the ICRU proposal. For details, the reader is referred to current documents: Report No. 50 and 62 (24,25).

Figure 11.20 is a schematic representation of various volumes that the ICRU Report no. 50 (24) recommends to be identified in a treatment plan. Delineation of these volumes is greatly facilitated by 3-D imaging but the concept is independent of the methodology used for their determination.

A.1. Gross Tumor Volume

The gross tumor volume (GTV) is the gross demonstrable extent and location of the tumor. It may consist of primary tumor, metastatic lymphadenopathy, or other metastases. Delineation of GTV is possible if the tumor is visible, palpable or demonstrable through imaging. GTV cannot be defined if the tumor has been surgically removed, although an outline of the tumor bed may be substituted by examining preoperative and postoperative images.

A.2. Clinical Target Volume

The CTV consists of the demonstrated tumor(s) if present and any other tissue with presumed tumor. It represents, therefore, the true extent and location of the tumor. Delineation of CTV assumes that there are no tumor cells outside this volume. The CTV must receive adequate dose to achieve the therapeutic aim.

A.3. Internal Target Volume

ICRU Report no. 62 (25) recommends that an internal margin (IM) be added to CTV to compensate for internal physiological movements and variation in size, shape, and position of the CTV during therapy in relation to an internal reference point and its corresponding coordinate system. The volume that includes CTV with these margins is called the *internal target volume* (ITV).

A.4. Planning Target Volume

The volume that includes CTV with an IM as well as a set-up margin (SM) for patient movement and set-up uncertainties is called the *planning target volume* (PTV). To delineate the PTV, the IM and SM are not added linearly but are combined rather subjectively. The margin around CTV in any direction must be large enough to compensate for internal movements as well as patient-motion and set-up uncertainties.

A.5. Planning Organ at Risk Volume

The organ(s) at risk (OR) needs adequate protection just as CTV needs adequate treatment. Once the OR is identified, margins need to be added to compensate for its movements, internal as well as set-up. Thus, in analogy to the PTV, one needs to outline planning organ at risk volume (PRV) to protect OR effectively.

Figure 11.21 schematically illustrates the process of outlining PTV and PRV. This process is intended to make the radiation oncologist think methodically and analytically when outlining targets and organs at risk instead of taking a wild guess. Although absolute accuracy in either case cannot be assured, the objective of this approach is to minimize errors by paying attention to details.

It is also important to point out that there is a common tendency among practitioners to draw target volumes based on GTV with little margins to account for subclinical

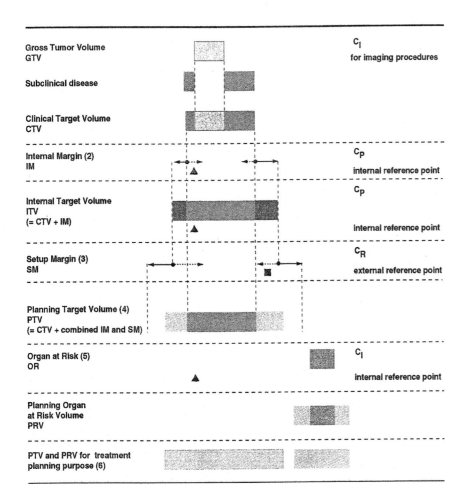

FIG. 11.21. Schematic representation of ICRU volumes and margins. (From ICRU. Prescribing, recording and reporting photon beam therapy [supplement to ICRU Report 50]. ICRU Report 62. Bethesda, Maryland. International Commission on Radiation Units and Measurements, 1999.)

disease, organ motion, or set-up uncertainties. The so-called conformal radiation therapy is a double-edged sword—a high degree of plan conformity can create a high probability of geographical miss. Thus great caution must be exercised in designing PTV and PRV. It is just as important to know the limitations of the system as it is to know its capabilities.

A.6. Treated Volume

Additional margins must be provided around the target volume to allow for limitations of the treatment technique. Thus the minimum target dose should be represented by an isodose surface which adequately covers the PTV to provide that margin. The volume enclosed by this isodose surface is called the *treated volume*. The treated volume is, in general, larger than the planning target volume and depends on a particular treatment technique.

A.7. Irradiated Volume

The volume of tissue receiving a significant dose (e.g., $\geq 50\%$ of the specified target dose) is called the *irradiated volume*. The irradiated volume is larger than the treated volume and depends on the treatment technique used.

A.8. Maximum Target Dose

The highest dose in the target area is called the *maximum target dose,* provided this dose covers a minimum area of 2 cm^2. Higher dose areas of less than 2 cm^2 may be ignored in designating the value of maximum target dose.

A.9. Minimum Target Dose

The *minimum target dose* is the lowest absorbed dose in the target area.

A.10. Mean Target Dose

If the dose is calculated at a large number of discrete points uniformly distributed in the target area, the *mean target dose* is the mean of the absorbed dose values at these points. Mathematically:

$$\text{Mean target dose} = \frac{1}{N} \sum_{A_T} D_{i,j}$$

where N is the number of points in the matrix and $D_{i,j}$ is the dose at lattice point i,j located inside the target area (A_T).

A.11. Median Target Dose

The *median target dose* is simply the value between the maximum and the minimum absorbed dose values within the target.

A.12. Modal Target Dose

The *modal target dose* is the absorbed dose that occurs most frequently within the target area. If the dose distribution over a grid of points covering the target area is plotted as a frequency histogram, the dose value showing the highest frequency is called the modal dose. In Fig. 11.22 the modal dose corresponds to the peak of the frequency curve.

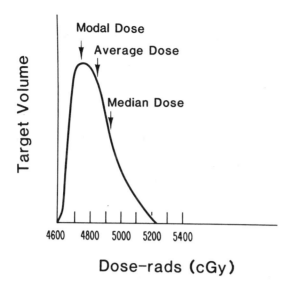

FIG. 11.22. Target volume-dose frequency curve. (Reprinted with permission from Ellis F, Oliver R. The specification of tumor dose. *Br J Radiol* 1961;34:258.)

A.13. Hot Spots

A *hot spot* is an area outside the target that receives a higher dose than the specified target dose. Like the maximum target dose, a hot spot is considered clinically meaningful only if it covers an area of at least 2 cm².

B. Specification of Target Dose

The absorbed dose distribution in the target volume is usually not uniform. Although a complete dosimetric specification is not possible without the entire dose distribution, there is value in having one figure as the main statement of *target dose*. The use of the term *tumor dose* is not recommended (23).

The quantity maximum target dose alone cannot be used for reporting, since it can conceal serious underdosages in some parts of the target volume. Although local tumor control depends on the minimum target dose, this quantity alone is not recommended by the ICRU (23), because it is difficult to determine the extent of the tumor, and therefore, the selection of the minimum target dose becomes difficult if not arbitrary. Moreover, if most of the target volume receives a dose that is appreciably different from the minimum, this may also reduce its clinical significance. A statement of both the maximum and minimum values is useful, but it is not always representative of the dose distribution. Furthermore, this would do away with the simplicity of having one quantity for reporting target dose.

The mean, median, and modal doses are not generally recommended, because they usually require elaborate calculations for their accurate determination and may not be feasible by institutions having limited computation facilities.

B.1. The ICRU Reference Point

The target dose should be specified and recorded at what is called the ICRU reference point. This point should satisfy the following general criteria (25):

1. The point should be selected so that the dose at this point is clinically relevant and representative of the dose throughout the PTV;
2. The point should be easy to define in a clear and unambiguous way;
3. The point should be selected where the dose can be accurately calculated;
4. The point should not lie in the penumbra region or where there is a steep dose gradient.

In most cases the ICRU reference point should lie well within the PTV, provided it generally meets the above mentioned criteria. Recommendations for simple beam arrangements are discussed below as examples.

B.1.1. Stationary Photon Beams

1. For a single beam, the target absorbed dose should be specified on the central axis of the beam placed within the PTV.
2. For parallel opposed, equally weighted beams, the point of target dose specification should be on the central axis midway between the beam entrances.
3. For parallel opposed, unequally weighted beams, the target dose should be specified on the central axis placed within the PTV.
4. For any other arrangement of two or more intersecting beams, the point of target dose specification should be at the intersection of the central axes of the beams placed within the PTV.

B.1.2. Rotation Therapy

For full rotation or arcs of at least 270 degrees, the target dose should be specified at the center of rotation in the principal plane. For smaller arcs, the target dose should be stated in the principal plane, first, at the center of rotation and, second, at the center of the target volume. This dual-point specification is required because in a small arc therapy, *past-pointing* techniques are used that give maximum absorbed dose close to the center of the target area. The dose at the isocenter in these cases, although important to specify, is somewhat less.

B.2. Additional Information

The specification of target dose is meaningful only if sufficient information is provided regarding the irradiation technique. The description of technique should include radiation quality, SSD or SAD, field sizes, beam-modification devices (wedges and shielding blocks, etc.), beam weighting, correction for tissue heterogeneities, dose fractionation, and patient positioning. Many of the above treatment parameters are listed with the treatment plan (isodose pattern) and can be attached to the patient chart. In vivo absorbed dose measurements can also provide useful information and should be recorded in the chart.

Finally, the main objectives of a dose specification and reporting system are to achieve uniformity of dose reporting among institutions, to provide meaningful data for assessing the results of treatments, and to enable the treatment to be repeated elsewhere without having recourse to the original institution for further information.

REFERENCES

1. International Commission on Radiation Units and Measurements. Measurement of absorbed dose in a phantom irradiated by a single beam of x or gamma rays. Report No. 23. Washington, DC: National Bureau of Standards, 1973.
2. Webster EW, Tsien KC, eds. *Atlas of radiation dose distributions*. Vol. I of Single-field isodose charts. Vienna: International Atomic Energy Agency, 1965.
3. Cohen M, Martin SM, eds. *Atlas of radiation dose distributions*. Vol. II of Multiple-field isodose charts. Vienna: International Atomic Energy Agency, 1966.
4. Tsien KC, Cunningham JR, Wright DJ, et al., eds. *Atlas of radiation dose distributions*. Vol. III of Moving field isodose charts. Vienna: International Atomic Energy Agency, 1967.
5. Sterling TD, Perry H, Katz I. Automation of radiation treatment planning. IV. Derivation of a mathematical expression for the percent depth dose surface of cobalt 60 beams and visualization of multiple field dose distributions. *Br J Radiol* 1964;37:544.
6. Khan FM. Computer dosimetry of partially blocked fields in cobalt teletherapy. *Radiology* 1970;97:405.
7. Van de Geijn J. A computer program for 3-D planning in external beam radiation therapy, EXTD ϕ T S. *Comput Prog Biomed* 1970;1:47.

8. Cunningham JR, Shrivastava PN, Wilkinson JM. Program IRREG—calculation of dose from irregularly shaped radiation beams. *Comput Prog Biomed* 1972;2:192.

9. Weinkam JJ, Kolde RA, Sterling TD. Extending the general field equation to fit the dose distributions of a variety of therapy units. *Br J Radiol* 1973;46:983.

10. Nordic Association of Clinical Physics. Procedures in external beam radiation therapy dosimetry with electron and photon beams with maximum energies between 1 and 50 MeV. *Acta Radiol Oncol* 1980;19:58.

11. International Commission on Radiation Units and Measurements. Determination of absorbed dose in a patient irradiated by beams of x or gamma rays in radiotherapy procedures. Report No. 24. Washington, DC: National Bureau of Standards, 1976.

12. Sewchand W, Khan FM, Williamson J. Variation in depth dose data between open and wedge fields for 4 MV X-rays. *Radiology* 1978;127:789.

13. Cohen M, Burns JE, Sears R. Physical aspects of cobalt 60 teletherapy using wedge filters. I. Physical investigation. *Acta Radiol* 1960;53:401. II. Dosimetric considerations. *Acta Radiol* 1960;53:486.

14. Tranter FW. Design of wedge filters for use with 4 MeV linear accelerator. *Br J Radiol* 1957;30:329.

15. Van de Geijn J. A simple wedge filter technique for cobalt 60 teletherapy. *Br J Radiol* 1962;35:710.

16. Aron BS, Scapicchio M. Design of universal wedge filter system for a cobalt 60 unit. *Am J Roentgenol* 1966;96:70.

17. Wilson CS, Hall EJ. On the advisability of treating all fields at each radiotherapy session. *Radiology* 1971;98:419.

18. Ellis F. Nominal standard dose and the ret. *Br J Radiol* 1971;44:101.

19. Orton CG, Ellis F. A simplification in the use of the NSD concept in practical radiotherapy. *Br J Radiol* 1973;46:529.

20. Tapley N. Parallel opposing portals technique. In: Fletcher GH, ed. *Text book of radiotherapy,* 3rd ed. Philadelphia: Lea & Febiger, 1980:60.

21. Mayneord WV. The measurement of radiation for medical purposes. *Proc Phys Soc* 1942;54:405.

22. Podgorsak EB, Rawlinson JA, Johns HE. X-ray depth doses for linear accelerators in the energy range from 10 to 32 MeV. *Am J Roentgenol* 1975;123:182.

23. International Commission on Radiation Units and Measurements. Dose specification for reporting external beam therapy with photons and electrons. Report No. 29. Washington, DC: National Bureau of Standards, 1978.

24. ICRU. Prescribing, recording, and reporting photon beam therapy. ICRU Report 50. Bethesda, Maryland. International Commission on Radiation Units and Measurements, 1993.

25. ICRU. Prescribing, recording, and reporting photon beam therapy (supplement to ICRU Report 50). ICRU Report 62. Bethesda, Maryland. International Commission of Radiation Units and Measurements, 1999.

TREATMENT PLANNING II: PATIENT DATA, CORRECTIONS, AND SET-UP

Basic depth-dose data and isodose curves are usually measured in a cubic water phantom having dimensions much larger than the field sizes used clinically. Phantom irradiations for this purpose are carried out under standard conditions, for example, beams incident normally on the flat surface at specified distances. The patient's body, however, is neither homogeneous nor flat in surface contour. Thus the dose distribution in a patient may differ significantly from the standard distribution. This chapter discusses several aspects of treatment planning, including acquisition of patient data, correction for contour curvature, and tissue inhomogeneities and patient positioning.

12.1. ACQUISITION OF PATIENT DATA

Accurate patient dosimetry is only possible when sufficiently accurate patient data are available. Such data include body contour, outline, and density of relevant internal structures, location, and extent of the target volume. Acquisition of these data is necessary whether the dosimetric calculations are performed manually or with a computer. However, this important aspect of treatment planning is often executed poorly. For example, in a busy department there may be an inordinate amount of pressure to begin the patient's treatment without adequate dosimetric planning. In other cases, lack of sufficient physics support and/or equipment is the cause of this problem. In such a case, it must be realized that the final accuracy of the treatment plan is strongly dependent on the availability of the patient data and that great effort is needed to improve its quality.

A. Body Contours

Acquisition of body contours and internal structures is best accomplished by imaging (computed tomography [CT] and magnetic resonance imaging, etc.). The scans are performed specifically for treatment planning purposes, with the patient positioned the same way as for actual treatment. In 3-D treatment planning (Chapter 19) these data are all image-based and are acquired as part of the treatment planning process. However, for cases in which 3-D treatment planning is not considered necessary or if body contours are obtained manually for verification of the image-based contours, mechanical or electromechanical methods are used for contouring.

A number of devices have been made to obtain patient contours. Some of these are commercially available while others can be fabricated in the department machine shop. The most common and the simplest of the devices is a solder wire or a lead wire embedded in plastic. Because the wire may not faithfully retain the contour dimensions when transferring it from the patient to the paper, one must independently measure anteroposterior and/or lateral diameters of the contour with a caliper.

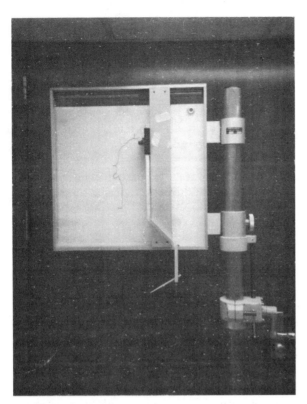

FIG. 12.1. Photograph of a contour plotter. (Courtesy of Radiation Products Design, Buffalo, MN.)

Another kind of simple device (1) consists of an array of rods, the tips of which are made to touch the patient's skin and then placed on a sheet of paper for contour drawing. Perhaps the most accurate of the mechanical devices is a pantograph type apparatus (Fig. 12.1) in which a rod can be moved laterally as well as up and down. When the rod is moved over the patient contour, its motion is followed by a pen that records the outline on paper.

Clarke (2) has described an electromechanical device in which motion of the rod over the patient contour is read by a sensing device and transferred to an X-Y recorder. Such a device can be used for digitizing the patient contour for direct input to the treatment planning computer. Optical (3) and ultrasonic (4) methods have also been devised to obtain the contour information.

Although any of the above methods can be used with sufficient accuracy if carefully used, some important points must be considered in regard to manual contour making.

(a) The patient contour must be obtained with the patient in the same position as used in the actual treatment. For this reason, probably the best place for obtaining the contour information is with the patient properly positioned on the treatment simulator couch.

(b) A line representing the tabletop must be indicated in the contour so that this horizontal line can be used as a reference for beam angles.

(c) Important bony landmarks as well as beam entry points, if available, must be indicated on the contour.

(d) Checks of body contour are recommended during the treatment course if the contour is expected to change due to a reduction of tumor volume or a change in patient weight.

(e) If body thickness varies significantly within the treatment field, contours should be determined in more than one plane.

B. Internal Structures

Localization of internal structures for treatment planning should provide quantitative information in regard to the size and location of critical organs or inhomogeneities. Although qualitative information can be obtained from diagnostic radiographs or atlases of cross-sectional anatomy, they cannot be used directly for precise localization of organs relative to the external contour. In order for the contour and the internal structure data to be realistic for a given patient, the localization must be obtained under conditions similar to those of the actual treatment position and on a couch similar to the treatment couch.

The following devices are used for the localization of internal structures and the target volume. A brief discussion regarding their operation and function will be presented.

B.1. Transverse Tomography

Conventional tomography pre-dates the introduction of CT. A transverse tomography unit (Fig. 12.2) consists of a diagnostic x-ray tube and a film cassette that rotates simultaneously with the x-ray tube. The tube is set in such a position that the central axis of the beam makes an angle of about 20 degrees with the film surface. The patient is positioned on the table so that the x-ray beam can pass through a desired body cross-section. As the gantry rotates, structures in only one transverse plane are "in focus." The structures in regions other than that plane are blurred because of the motion of the x-ray tube and the film cassette.

The difference between conventional tomography and transverse tomography is the orientation of the plane in focus. Whereas a conventional tomographic image is parallel to the long axis of the patient, the transverse tomogram provides a cross-sectional image perpendicular to the body axis.

Transverse tomograms have been used in radiation therapy to provide cross-sectional information of internal structures in relation to the external contour (5,6). Although the

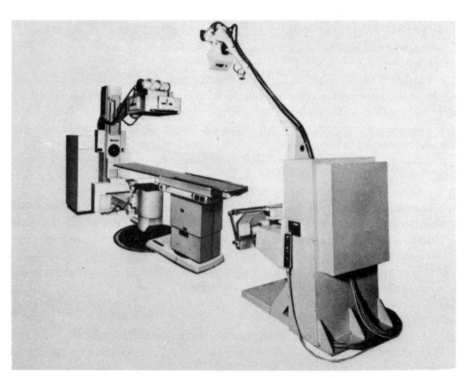

FIG. 12.2. Photograph of a conventional transverse tomography unit (*right*) in combination with a treatment simulator. (Courtesy of Toshiba Medical Systems, Chicago, IL.)

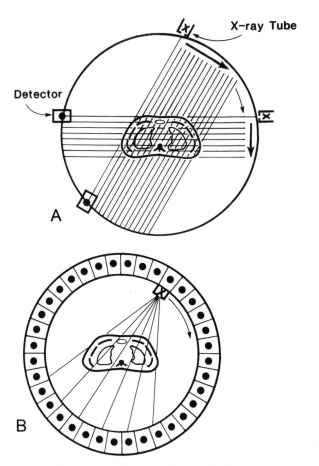

FIG. 12.3. Illustration of scan motions in CT. **A:** An early design in which the x-ray source and the detector performed a combination of translational and rotational motion. **B:** A modern scanner in which the x-ray tube rotates within a stationary circular array of detectors.

method can be used for localizing bone, lung, air cavities, and organs with contrast media, the tomograms have poor contrast and spatial resolution. In addition, the images are marred by artifacts and require interpretation.

B.2. Computed Tomography

The main disadvantage of conventional transverse tomography is the presence of blurred images resulting from structures outside the plane of interest. In CT, the x-rays used for reconstructing the image enter only the layer under examination, so that unwanted planes are completely omitted. Basically, a narrow beam of x-rays scans across a patient in synchrony with a radiation detector on the opposite side of the patient. If a sufficient number of transmission measurements are taken at different orientations of the x-ray source and detector (Fig. 12.3A), the distribution of attenuation coefficients within the layer may be determined. By assigning different levels to different attenuation coefficients, an image can be reconstructed that represents various structures with different attenuation properties. Such a representation of attenuation coefficients constitutes a CT image.

Since CT scanning was introduced about 30 years ago, there has been a rapid development in both the software and hardware. Most of the improvements in hardware had to do with the scanner motion and the multiplicity of detectors to decrease the scan time. Figure 12.3B shows a modern scanner in which the x-ray tube rotates within a circular

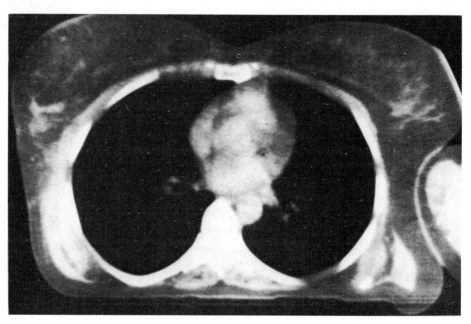

FIG. 12.4. Typical CT image.

array of 1,000 or more detectors. With such scanners, scan times as fast as 1 sec or less are achievable. Figure 12.4 shows a typical CT image.

Spiral or helical CT scanners were introduced in the early 1990s in which the x-ray tube rotates continuously as the patient is slowly translated through the CT aperture. Helical CTs are faster and provide better visualization of anatomy and target volumes.

The reconstruction of an image by CT is a mathematical process of considerable complexity, generally performed by a computer. For a review of various mathematical approaches for image reconstruction, the reader is referred to a paper by Brooks and Di Chiro (7). The reconstruction algorithm generates what is known as *CT numbers,* which are related to attenuation coefficients. The CT numbers range from −1,000 for air to +1,000 for bone, with that for water set at 0. The CT numbers normalized in this manner are called Hounsfield numbers (*H*).

$$H = \frac{\mu_{\text{tissue}} - \mu_{\text{water}}}{\mu_{\text{water}}} \times 1,000 \tag{12.1}$$

where μ is the linear attenuation coefficient. Thus a Hounsfield unit represents a change of 0.1% in the attenuation coefficient of water.

Because the CT numbers bear a linear relationship with the attenuation coefficients, it is possible to infer electron density (electrons cm^{-3}) as shown in Fig. 12.5. Although CT numbers can be correlated with electron density, the relationship is not linear in the entire range of tissue densities. The nonlinearity is caused by the change in atomic number of tissues, which affects the proportion of beam attenuation by Compton versus photoelectric interactions. Figure 12.5 shows a relationship that is linear between lung and soft tissue but nonlinear between soft tissue and bone.

Atomic number information can also be obtained if attenuation coefficients are measured at two different x-ray energies (8). It is possible to transform the attenuation coefficients measured by CT at diagnostic energies to therapeutic energies (9). However, for low atomic number materials such as fat, air, lung, and muscle, this transformation is not necessary for the purpose of calculating dose distributions and inhomogeneity corrections (9).

Application of CT in radiation therapy treatment planning has been the subject of many papers (9–21). The CT information is useful in two aspects of treatment planning: (a) delineation of target volume and the surrounding structures in relation to the external contour; and (b) providing quantitative data (in the form of CT numbers) for tissue

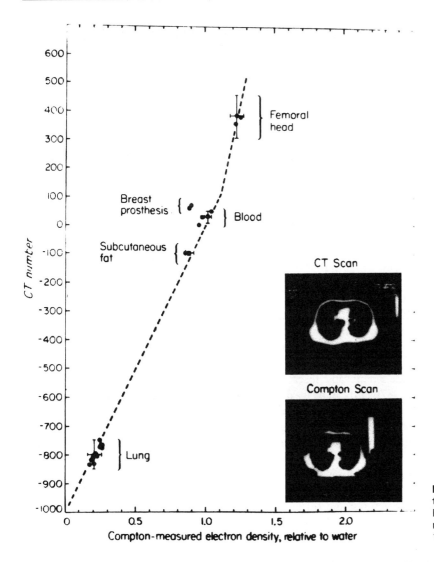

FIG. 12.5. CT numbers plotted as a function of electron density relative to water. (From Battista JJ, Rider WD, Van Dyk J. Computed tomography for radiotherapy planning. *Int J Radiat Oncol Biol Phys* 1980;6:99, with permission.)

heterogeneity corrections. From a practical point of view, the first aspect is more important than the second. Accurate delineation of surface contour, internal structures, and target volume is not only crucial for optimizing a treatment technique but also necessary for accurate calculation of dose distribution. Even the tissue heterogeneity corrections for megavoltage photon beams can be made with acceptable accuracy by using the CT cross-sectional image to determine the extent of the inhomogeneity and employing published values of electron density. To quote Sontag et al. (12), "The most severe errors in computing the dose distribution are caused by inaccurate delineation of the geometric outlines of tissue inhomogeneities. Less severe errors in the dose calculation are caused by using an inaccurate relative electron density for the inhomogeneity, provided the outline is accurate." Similar observations were also made by Geise and McCullough (11).

From these investigations, it seems that more sophisticated inhomogeneity correction algorithms such as those using "pixel-by-pixel" CT data produce only small improvements in dose accuracy compared with the traditional methods using equivalent depth, provided the extent of the inhomogeneity is accurately known. However, greater precision in the inhomogeneity outline and electron density may be required in regions where severe dose gradients exist in the direction of the beam. For example, the electron density information may be critical for some cases of electron beam therapy and, for high energy photons, in regions where electronic equilibrium is not established. In such instances, methods using pixel-by-pixel correction methods may be required (16,22,23).

There are several commercially available computer treatment planning systems that allow display and use of CT images for treatment planning. Once the CT image has been produced, the data can be transferred to the treatment-planning computer either directly or the outlines of the contour and internal structures can be traced by hand and then entered into the computer. In direct systems, the CT scan is displayed in gray-scale mode on the computer monitor of the treatment planning system and relevant structures can be outlined on the basis of CT number distribution. After the treatment plan is finalized, it can be superimposed on the CT image for visual display.

The use of CT scans in treatment planning is now an established procedure. Comparative studies of treatment planning with and without CT have demonstrated significantly improved accuracy of target delineation, field shaping and normal tissue exclusion from the field when treatments are designed with the aid of CT scans. A review of CT applications in radiotherapy is presented in a book edited by Ling et al. (24). More current applications are discussed in part III of this book.

Although external contour and internal structures are well-delineated by CT, their use in treatment planning requires that they be localized accurately with respect to the treatment geometry. Diagnostic CT scans obtained typically on a curved tabletop with patient position different from that to be used in treatment have limited usefulness in designing technique and dose distribution. Special treatment planning CT scans are required with full attention to patient positioning and other details affecting treatment parameters.

Some of the common considerations in obtaining treatment planning CT scans are the following: (a) a flat tabletop should be used, usually a flat wooden board can be designed to provide a removable insert for the diagnostic CT couch; (b) a large diameter CT aperture (e.g., ≥ 70 cm) can be used to accommodate unusual arm positions and other body configurations encountered in radiation therapy; (c) care should be taken to use patient-positioning or immobilization devices that do not cause image artifacts; (d) patient-positioning, leveling, and immobilization should be done in accordance with the expected treatment technique or simulation if done before CT; (e) external contour landmarks can be delineated, using radiopaque markers such as plastic catheters; (f) sufficiently magnified images for digitization can be obtained if radiographs on film are to be used for drawing target and other structures; and (g) image scale should be accurate both in the X and Y directions.

Three-dimensional Treatment Planning

Additional considerations go into CT scanning for 3-D treatment planning. Because the 3-D anatomy is derived from individual transverse scans (which are imaged in 2-D), the interslice distance must be sufficiently small to reconstruct the image in three dimensions. Depending on the tumor site or the extent of contemplated treatment volume, contiguous scans are taken with slice thickness ranging from 2 to 10 mm. The total number of slices may range from 30 to 80 mm. This requires fast scan capability to avoid patient movement or discomfort.

Delineation of target and critical organs on each of the scans is necessary for the 3-D reconstruction of these structures. This is an extremely time-consuming procedure, which has been a deterrent to the adoption of 3-D treatment planning on a routine basis. Efforts have been directed toward making this process less cumbersome such as automatic contouring, pattern recognition, and other computer manipulations. However, the basic problem remains that target delineation is inherently a manual process. Although radiographically visible tumor boundaries can be recognized by appropriate computer software, the extent of target volume depends on grade, stage, and patterns of tumor spread to the surrounding structures. Clinical judgment is required in defining the target volume. Obviously, a computer cannot replace the radiation oncologist! At least, not yet.

Besides the time-consuming process of target localization, 3-D computation of dose distribution and display requires much more powerful computers in terms of speed and storage capacity than the conventional treatment-planning systems. However, with the phenomenal growth of computer technology this is not perceived to be a significant barrier to the adoption of routine 3-D planning. The biggest deterrent, however, is going to be the cost of treatment, including equipment and personnel.

Whereas 3-D planning for every patient may not be presently realistic, it has already been found to be quite useful and practical for certain tumors or tumor sites (head and neck, lung, prostrate). Treatment of well-localized small lesions (e.g., less than 4 cm in diameter) in the brain by *stereotactic radiosurgery* has greatly benefited by 3-D planning. In this procedure, the target volume is usually based on the extent of radiographically visible tumor (with contrast), thus obviating the need for manual target delineation on each CT slice. The 3-D display of dose distribution to assess coverage of the target volume confined to a relatively small number of slices is both useful and practical. Similarly, brachytherapy is amenable to 3-D planning because of the limited number of slices involving the target.

The next best thing to full-fledged 3-D planning (e.g., 3-D computation and display) is to do 2-D planning, using a limited number of CT scans, selected to obtain a reasonably adequate perspective of the dose distribution in three dimensions. For example, targets and other critical structures may be drawn on 5 to 10 CT cuts, spanning the volume of interest. This can be done either by drawing targets and structures on the CT films or directly on the computer screen by using a cursor or a light pen. Treatment-planning software is available whereby margins around the target volume can be specified to set the field boundaries. After optimizing field margins, beam angles, and other plan parameters relative to the central CT cut, the dose distributions can be viewed in other slices either individually or simultaneously by serial display on the screen. *Beam's eye view* (BEV) display in which the plan is viewed from the vantage point of the radiation source (in a plane perpendicular to the central axis) is useful in providing the same perspective as a simulator or port film. In addition, a BEV outline of the field can be obtained to aid in the drawing of custom blocks on the simulator film. More discussion on CT-based treatment planning is provided in Chapter 19.

B.3. Magnetic Resonance Imaging

Magnetic resonance imaging (MRI) has developed, in parallel to CT, into a powerful imaging modality. Like CT, it provides anatomic images in multiple planes. Whereas CT provides basically transverse axial images (which can be further processed to reconstruct images in other planes or in three dimensions) MRI can be used to scan directly in axial, sagittal, coronal, or oblique planes. This makes it possible to obtain optimal views to enhance diagnostic interpretation or target delineation for radiotherapy. Other advantages over CT include not involving the use of ionizing radiation, higher contrast, and better imaging of soft tissue tumors. Some disadvantages compared with CT include lower spatial resolution; inability to image bone or calcifications; longer scan acquisition time, thereby increasing the possibility of motion artifacts; technical difficulties due to small hole of the magnet and magnetic interference with metallic objects; and current unavailability of many approved MRI contrast agents.

The previous cursory comparison between CT and MRI shows that the two types of imaging are complementary.

Basic physics of MRI involves a phenomenon known as nuclear magnetic resonance (NMR). It is a resonance transition between nuclear spin states of certain atomic nuclei when subjected to a radiofrequency (RF) signal of a specific frequency in the presence of an external magnetic field. The nuclei that participate in this phenomenon are the ones that intrinsically possess spinning motion, i.e., have angular momentum. These rotating charges act as tiny magnets with associated magnetic dipole moment, a property that gives a measure of how quickly the magnet will align itself along an external magnetic field. Because of the spinning motion or the magnetic dipole moment, nuclei align their spin axes along the external magnetic field (H) as well as orbit or precess around it (Fig. 12.6).

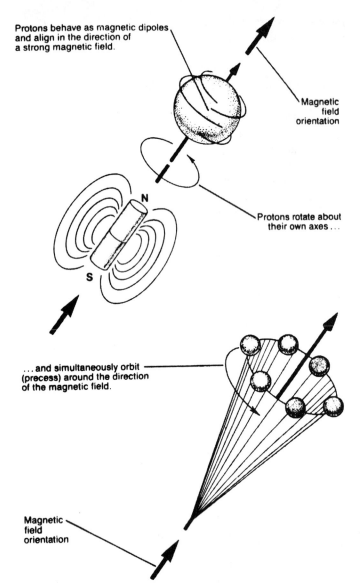

Protons behave as magnetic dipoles and align in the direction of a strong magnetic field.

Magnetic field orientation

Protons rotate about their own axes...

...and simultaneously orbit (precess) around the direction of the magnetic field.

Magnetic field orientation

FIG. 12.6. Alignment and precession of protons in a strong magnetic field. (From Halverson RA, Griffiths HJ, Lee BCP, et al. Magnetic resonance imaging and computed tomography in the determination of tumor and treatment volume. In: Levitt SH, Khan FM, Potish RA, eds. *Technological basis of radiation therapy*, 2nd ed. Philadelphia: Lea & Febiger, 1992:38, with permission.)

The frequency of precession is called the Larmor frequency. A second alternating field is generated by applying an alternating voltage (at the Larmor frequency) to an RF coil. This field is applied perpendicular to H and rotates around H at the Larmor frequency. This causes the nuclei to precess around the new field in the transverse direction. When the RF signal is turned off, the nuclei return to their original alignment around H. This transition is called *relaxation*. It induces a signal in the receiving RF coil (tuned to the Larmor frequency) which constitutes the NMR signal.

The turning off of the transverse RF field causes nuclei to relax in the transverse direction (T_2 relaxation) as well as to return to the original longitudinal direction of the magnetic field (T_1 relaxation). This is schematically illustrated in Fig. 12.7. The relaxation times, T_1 and T_2, are actually time constants (like the decay constant in radioactive decay) for the exponential function that governs the two transitions.

The signal source in MRI can be any nucleus with nonzero spin or angular momentum. However, certain nuclei give larger signal than the others. Hydrogen nuclei (protons), because of their high intrinsic sensitivity and high concentration in tissues, produce signals of sufficient strength for imaging. Work with other possible candidates, ^{31}P, ^{23}Na, ^{19}F,

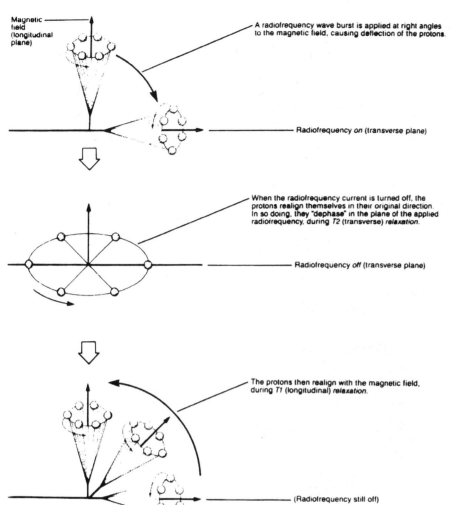

Magnetic field (longitudinal plane)

A radiofrequency wave burst is applied at right angles to the magnetic field, causing deflection of the protons.

Radiofrequency *on* (transverse plane)

When the radiofrequency current is turned off, the protons realign themselves in their original direction. In so doing, they "dephase" in the plane of the applied radiofrequency, during *T2* (transverse) *relaxation.*

Radiofrequency *off* (transverse plane)

The protons then realign with the magnetic field, during *T1* (longitudinal) *relaxation.*

(Radiofrequency still off)

FIG. 12.7. Effects of radiofrequency applied at right angles to the magnetic field. (From Halverson RA, Griffiths HJ, Lee BCP, et al. Magnetic resonance imaging and computed tomography in the determination of tumor and treatment volume. In: Levitt SH, Khan FM, Potish RA, eds. *Technological basis of radiation therapy,* 2nd ed. Philadelphia: Lea & Febiger, 1992:38, with permission.)

^{13}C, and ^{2}H is continuing. Currently, routine MRI is based exclusively on proton density and proton relaxation characteristics of different tissues.

Localization of protons in a 3-D space is achieved by applying magnetic field gradients produced by gradient RF coils in three orthogonal planes. This changes the precession frequency of protons spatially, because the MR frequency is linearly proportional to field strength. Thus by the appropriate interplay of the external magnetic field and the RF field gradients, proton distribution can be localized. A body slice is imaged by applying field gradient along the axis of the slice and selecting a frequency range for a readout. The strength of the field gradient determines the thickness of the slice (the greater the gradient, thinner the slice). Localization within the slice is accomplished by phase encoding (using back-to-front Y-gradient) and frequency encoding (using transverse X-gradient). In the process, the computer stores phase (angle of precession of the proton at a particular time) and frequency information and reconstructs the image by mathematical manipulation of the data.

Most MR imaging uses a spin echo technique in which a 180-degree RF pulse is applied after the initial 90-degree pulse, and the resulting signal is received at a time that is equal to twice the interval between the two pulses. This time is called the *echo time* (TE). The time between each 90-degree pulse in an imaging sequence is called the *repetition time* (TR). By adjusting TR and TE, image contrast can be affected. For example, a long TR and short TE produces a proton (spin) density-weighted image, a short TR and a short TE produces a T_1-weighted image, and a long TR and a long TE produces a T_2-weighted

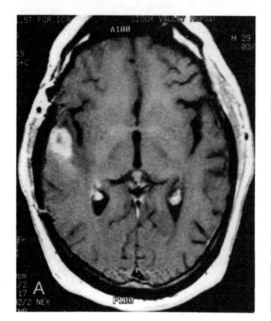
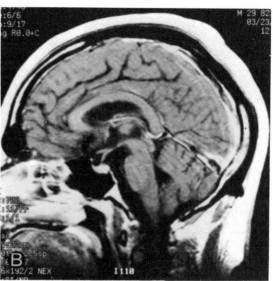
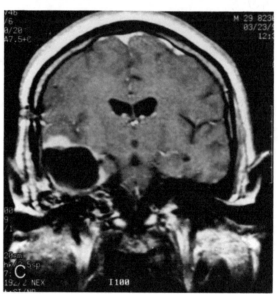

FIG. 12.8. Examples of MR images of the head. **A:** Transverse plane. **B:** Sagittal plane. **C:** Coronal plane.

image. Thus differences in proton density, T_1, and T_2 between different tissues can be enhanced by a manipulation of TE and TR in the spin echo technique.

Figure 12.8 shows examples of MR images obtained in the axial, sagittal, and coronal planes. By convention, a strong MR signal is displayed as white and a weak signal is displayed as dark on the cathode ray tube or film.

B.4. Ultrasound

Ultrasonic imaging for delineating patient contours and internal structure is becoming widely recognized as an important tool in radiation therapy. Tomographic views provide cross-sectional information that is always helpful for treatment planning. Although in most cases the image quality or clinical reliability is not as good as that of the CT, ultrasonic procedure does not involve ionizing radiation, is less expensive, and in some cases, yields data of comparable usefulness.

Ultrasound can provide useful information in localizing many malignancy-prone structures in the lower pelvis, retroperitoneum, upper abdomen, breast, and chest wall (25). A detailed review of these techniques in the context of radiation therapy planning has been presented by Carson et al. (25,26).

An ultrasound (or ultrasonic) wave is a sound wave having a frequency greater than 20,000 cycles per sec or hertz (Hz). At this frequency, the sound is inaudible to the human ear. Ultrasound waves of frequencies 1 to 20 MHz are used in diagnostic radiology.

Ultrasound may be used to produce images either by means of transmission or reflection. However, in most clinical applications, use is made of ultrasonic waves reflected from different tissue interfaces. These reflections or echoes are caused by variations in *acoustic impedance* of materials on opposite sides of the interfaces. The acoustic impedance (Z) of a medium is defined as the product of the density of the medium and the velocity of ultrasound in the medium. The larger the difference in Z between the two media, the greater is the fraction of ultrasound energy reflected at the interface. For example, strong reflections of ultrasound occur at the air-tissue, tissue-bone, and chest wall-lung interfaces due to high impedance mismatch. However, because lung contains millions of air-tissue interfaces, strong reflections at the numerous interfaces prevents its use in lung imaging.

Attenuation of the ultrasound by the medium also plays an important role in ultrasound imaging. This attenuation takes place as the energy is removed from the beam by absorption, scattering, and reflection. The energy remaining in the beam decreases approximately exponentially with the depth of penetration into the medium, allowing attenuation in different media to be characterized by attenuation coefficients. As the attenuation coefficient of ultrasound is very high for bone compared with soft tissue, together with the large reflection coefficient of a tissue-bone interface, it is difficult to visualize structures lying beyond bone. On the other hand, water, blood, fat, and muscle are very good transmitters of ultrasound energy.

Ultrasonic waves are generated as well as detected by an *ultrasonic probe* or *transducer.* A transducer is a device that converts one form of energy into another. An ultrasonic transducer converts electrical energy into ultrasound energy, and vice versa. This is accomplished by a process known as the *piezoelectric effect.* This effect is exhibited by certain crystals in which a variation of an electric field across the crystal causes it to oscillate mechanically, thus generating acoustic waves. Conversely, pressure variations across a piezoelectric material (in response to an incident ultrasound wave) result in a varying electrical potential across opposite surfaces of the crystal.

Although the piezoelectric effect is exhibited by a number of naturally occurring crystals, most common crystals used clinically are made artificially such as barium titanate, lead zirconium titanate, and lead metaniobate. The piezoelectric effect produced by these materials is mediated by their electric dipole moment, the magnitude of which can be varied by addition of suitable impurities.

As the ultrasound wave reflected from tissue interfaces is received by the transducer, voltage pulses are produced that are processed and displayed on the cathode ray tube (CRT), usually in one of three display modes: A (amplitude) mode, B (brightness) mode, and M (motion) mode. A mode consists of displaying the signal amplitude on the ordinate and time on the abscissa. The time, in this case, is related to distance or tissue depth, given the speed of sound in the medium. In the B mode, a signal from a point in the medium is displayed by an echo dot on the CRT. The (x, y) position of the dot on the CRT indicates the location of the reflecting point at the interface and its proportional brightness reveals the amplitude of the echo. By scanning across the patient, the B-mode viewer sees an apparent cross-section through the patient. Such cross-sectional images are called *ultrasonic tomograms.*

In the M mode of presentation, the ultrasound images display the motion of internal structures of the patient's anatomy. The most frequent application of M mode scanning is echocardiography. In radiotherapy, the cross-sectional information used for treatment planning is exclusively derived from the B scan images (Fig. 12.9). The use of ultrasound in brachytherapy (e.g., ultrasound-guided prostate implants) is discussed in Chapter 23.

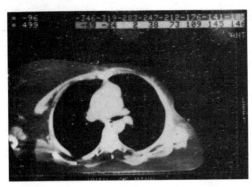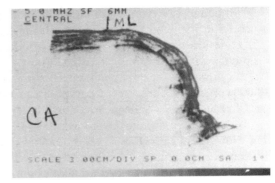

FIG. 12.9. Ultrasonic tomogram showing chest wall thickness (*right*) compared with the CT image (*left*).

12.2. TREATMENT SIMULATION

A treatment simulator (Fig. 12.10) is an apparatus that uses a diagnostic x-ray tube but duplicates a radiation treatment unit in terms of its geometrical, mechanical, and optical properties. The main function of a simulator is to display the treatment fields so that the target volume may be accurately encompassed without delivering excessive irradiation to surrounding normal tissues. By radiographic visualization of internal organs, correct positioning of fields and shielding blocks can be obtained in relation to external landmarks. Most commercially available simulators have fluoroscopic capability by dynamic visualization before a hard copy is obtained in terms of the simulator radiography.

Specifications of a treatment simulator must closely match those of the treatment unit. Several authors (27–31) have discussed these aspects. For a comprehensive discussion, the reader is referred to the paper by McCullough and Earl (31).

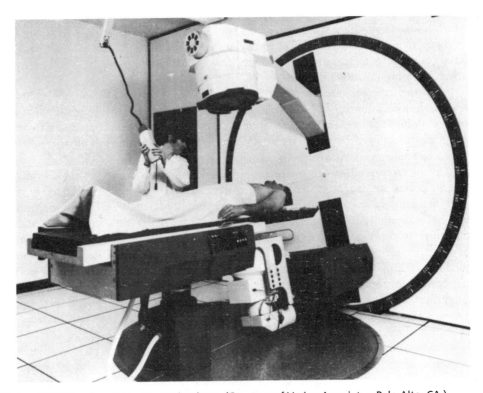

FIG. 12.10. Varian (TEM) Ximatron 5 treatment simulator. (Courtesy of Varian Associates, Palo Alto, CA.)

The need for simulators arises from four facts: (a) geometrical relationship between the radiation beam and the external and internal anatomy of the patient cannot be duplicated by an ordinary diagnostic x-ray unit; (b) although field localization can be achieved directly with a therapy machine by taking a port film, the radiographic quality is poor because of very high beam energy, and for cobalt-60, a large source size as well; (c) field localization is a time-consuming process which, if carried out in the treatment room, could engage a therapy machine for a prohibitive length of time; (d) unforeseen problems with a patient set-up or treatment technique can be solved during simulation, thus conserving time within the treatment room.

Although the practical use of simulators varies widely from institution to institution, the simulator room is increasingly assuming the role of a treatment-planning room. Besides localizing treatment volume and setting up fields, other necessary data can also be obtained at the time of simulation. Because the simulator table is supposed to be similar to the treatment table, various patient measurements such as contours and thicknesses, including those related to compensator or bolus design, can be obtained under appropriate set-up conditions. Fabrication and testing of individualized shielding blocks can also be accomplished with a simulator. To facilitate such measurements, modern simulators are equipped with accessories such as laser lights, contour maker, and shadow tray.

Some simulators have a tomography attachment in which the image from the image intensifier is analyzed and reconstructed using either analogue[1] or digital[2] processing. Because of the poor image quality, this technology cannot compete with CT-based virtual simulation.

An exciting development in the area of simulation is that of converting a CT scanner into a simulator. A commercial device[3] known as CT-SIM uses a CT scanner to localize the treatment fields on the basis of the patient's CT scans. A computer program, specifically written for simulation, automatically positions the patient couch and the laser cross hairs to define the scans and the treatment fields. The software provides automatic outlining of external contours and critical structures, interactive portal displays and placement, display of isodose distribution, and review of multiple treatment plans. Such an integrated approach to treatment planning has the potential of becoming the simulator cum treatment-planning system of the future.

12.3. TREATMENT VERIFICATION

A. Port Films

The primary purpose of port filming is to verify the treatment volume under actual conditions of treatment. Although the image quality with the megavoltage x-ray beam is poorer than with the diagnostic or the simulator film, a port film is considered mandatory not only as a good clinical practice but as a legal record.

As a treatment record, a port film must be of sufficiently good quality so that the field boundaries can be described anatomically. However, this may not always be possible due to either very high beam energy (10 MV or higher), large source size (cobalt-60), large patient thickness (>20 cm), or poor radiographic technique. In such a case, the availability of a simulator film and/or a treatment diagram with adequate anatomic description of the field is helpful. Anatomic interpretation of a port film is helped by obtaining a full-field exposure on top of the treatment port exposure.

---

[1] Oldelft Corporation of America, Fairfax, Virginia.
[2] Varian Associates, Palo Alto, California.
[3] Theratronics International Ltd., Kanata, Ontario, Canada. Also, Picker International, Inc., St. Davids, Pennsylvania.

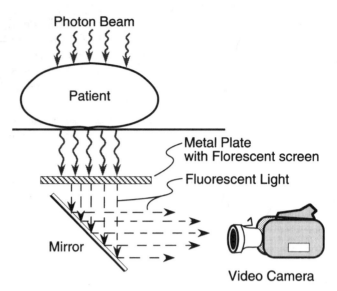

FIG. 12.11. Schematic diagram of video-based electronic portal imaging device.

Radiographic technique significantly influences image quality of a port film. The choice of film and screen as well as the exposure technique is important in this regard. Droege and Bjärngard (32) have analyzed the film screen combinations commonly used for port filming at megavoltage x-ray energies. Their investigation shows that the use of a single emulsion film with the emulsion adjacent to a single lead screen[4] between the film and the patient is preferable to a double emulsion film or a film with more than one screen. Thus, for optimum resolution, one needs a single emulsion film with a front lead screen and no rear screen. Conventional nonmetallic screens are not recommended at megavoltage energies. Although thicker metallic screens produce a better response, an increase in thickness beyond the maximum electron range produces no further changes in resolution (32).

Certain slow-speed films, ready packed but without a screen, can be exposed during the entire treatment duration. A therapy verification film such as Kodak XV-2 is sufficiently slow to allow an exposure of up to 200 cGy without reaching saturation. In addition, such films can be used to construct compensators for both the contours and tissue heterogeneity (33).

B. Electronic Portal Imaging

Major limitations of port films are (a) viewing is delayed because of the time required for processing; (b) it is impractical to do port films before each treatment; and (c) film image is of poor quality especially for photon energies greater than 6 MV. Electronic portal imaging overcomes the first two problems by making it possible to view the portal images instantaneously, i.e., images can be displayed on computer screen before initiating a treatment or in real-time during the treatment. Portal images can also be stored on computer discs for later viewing or archiving.

On-line electronic portal imaging devices (EPIDs) are currently being clinically used in several institutions, and some of them are commercially available. Many of the systems are video based; the beam transmitted through the patient excites a metal fluorescent screen, which is viewed by a video camera using a 45 degree mirror (34–37) (Fig. 12.11).

---

[4] Such a sheet of lead acts as an intensifying screen by means of electrons ejected from the screen by photon interactions. These electrons provide an image on the film which reflects the variation of beam intensity transmitted through the patient.

The camera is interfaced to a microcomputer through a frame-grabber board for digitizing the video image. The images are acquired and digitized at the video rate of 30 frames per second. An appropriate number of frames is averaged to produce a final image. Depending on the computer software, the image data can be further manipulated to improve the image quality or perform a special study.

One problem with mirror-based EPIDs is the large size of the mirror, which can pose practical problems. Wong et al. (38) have developed a system that replaces the mirror with a fiberoptics system to direct the fluorescent light to the video camera. The fiberoptics channels consist of thin clear polystyrene columns encased by a thin acrylic cladding. Because of the difference in the refractive indices of the two plastics, it is possible to conduct light without significant loss of intensity. This "light piping" is accomplished by the process of total internal reflection at the cladding interface.

Another class of EPIDs consists of a matrix of liquid ion chambers used as detectors (39, 40). These devices are much more compact than the video-based systems and are comparable in size to a film cassette, albeit a little heavier. Figure 12.12 shows a system developed at The Nederlands Kanker Institute. The system consists of a matrix of 256 × 256 ion chambers containing an organic fluid and a microcomputer for image processing. Figure 12.13 shows an image obtained with such a device. Besides imaging, another potential use of this device is on-line patient dose monitoring. Further work is needed to develop this application.

Yet another type of EPID uses solid-state detectors. One approach employs a scanning linear array of silicon diodes. Another uses a linear array of zinc tungstate (Zn WO$_4$) scintillating crystals attached to photodiodes. An excellent review of these developments is provided by Boyer et al. (41).

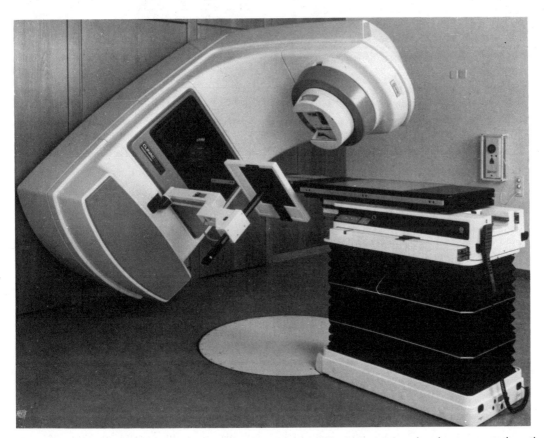

FIG. 12.12. Varian Portalvision system containing a matrix of liquid ionization chambers, mounted on the accelerator gantry. The mounting arm swings into position for imaging and out of the way when not needed. (Courtesy of Varian Associates, Palo Alto, CA.)

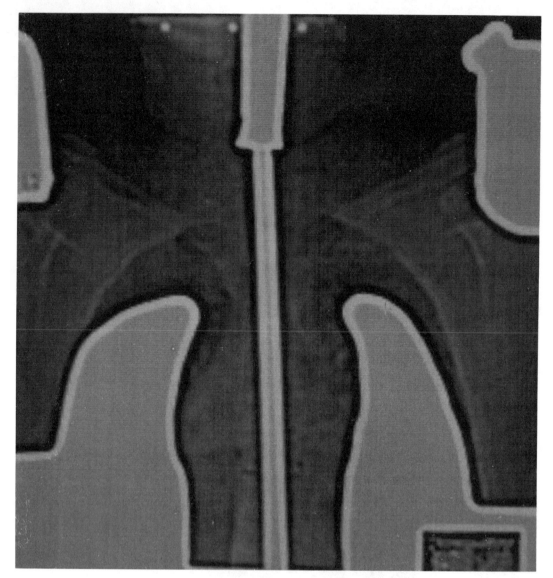

FIG. 12.13. Example of a portal image. (Courtesy of Varian Associates, Palo Alto, CA.)

A variety of technologies are being explored to develop new EPIDS or refine the existing ones. For example, Varian Medical Systems has recently introduced PortalVision aS500 featuring an array of image detectors based on Amorphous Silicon (a-Si) technology. Within this unit a scintillator converts the radiation beam into visible photons. The light is detected by an array of photodiodes implanted on an amorphous silicon panel. The photodiodes integrate the light into charge captures. The sensitive area of the EPID is 40 × 30 cm^2 with 512 × 384 pixels, spatial resolution is 0.78 mm and the read-out image has about 200,000 pixels. This system offers better image quality than the previous system using liquid ion chambers.

12.4. CORRECTIONS FOR CONTOUR IRREGULARITIES

As mentioned at the beginning of this chapter, basic dose distribution data are obtained under standard conditions, which include homogeneous unit density phantom, perpendicular beam incidence, and flat surface. During treatment, however, the beam may be obliquely incident with respect to the surface and, in addition, the surface may be curved or irregular in shape. Under such conditions, the standard dose distributions cannot be applied without proper modifications or corrections.

Contour corrections may be avoided by using a bolus or a compensator (to be discussed in section 12.4) but under some circumstances, it is permissible or even desirable, to determine the actual dose distribution by calculation. The following three methods are recommended for angles of incidence of up to 45 degree for megavoltage beams and of up to 30 degree from the surface normal for orthovoltage x-rays (42). Although all computer treatment-planning algorithms are capable of correcting for contour irregularities, these methods are discussed below to illustrate the basic principles.

A. Effective Source-to-Surface Distance Method

Consider Fig. 12.14 in which source-to-surface is an irregularly shaped patient contour. It is desired to calculate the percent depth dose at point A (i.e., dose at A as a percentage of D_{max} dose at point Q). The diagram shows that the tissue deficit above point A is h cm and the depth of D_{max} is d_m. If we note that the percent depth dose does not change rapidly with SSD (provided that the SSD is large), the relative depth dose distribution along the line joining the source with point A is unchanged when the isodose chart is moved down by the distance h and positioned with its surface line at $S'–S'$. Suppose D_A is the dose at point A. Assuming beam to be incident on a flat surface located at: $S'–S'$,

$$D_A = D'_{max} \cdot P' \qquad (12.2)$$

where P' is percent depth dose at A relative to D'_{max} at point Q'. Suppose P_{corr} is the correct percent depth dose at A relative to D_{max} at point Q. Then,

$$D_A = D_{max} \cdot P_{corr} \qquad (12.3)$$

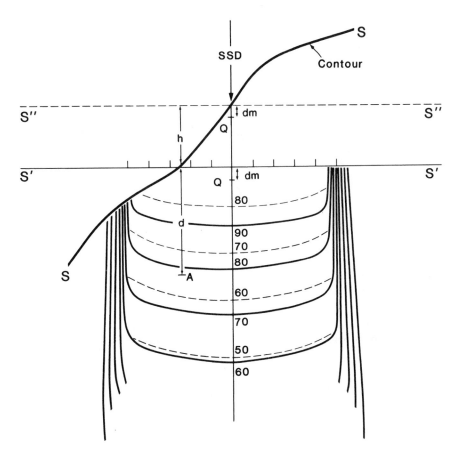

FIG. 12.14. Diagram illustrating methods of correcting dose distribution under an irregular surface such as *S–S*. The solid isodose curves are from an isodose chart which assumes a flat surface located at *S′-S′*. The dashed isodose curves assume a flat surface at *S″–S″* without any air gap.

From Equation 12.2 and 12.3,

$$P_{corr} = P' \cdot \left(\frac{D'_{max}}{D_{max}} \right) \qquad (12.4)$$

Because, when the distribution is moved, the SSD is increased by a distance h, we have:

$$\frac{D'_{max}}{D_{max}} = \left(\frac{SSD + d_m}{SSD + h + d_m} \right)^2 \qquad (12.5)$$

Therefore,

$$P_{corr} = P' \cdot \left(\frac{SSD + d_m}{SSD + h + d_m} \right)^2 \qquad (12.6)$$

Thus the effective SSD method consists of sliding the isodose chart down so that its surface line is at S'–S', reading off the percent dose value at A and multiplying it by the inverse square law factor to give the corrected percent depth dose value.

The above method applies the same way when there is excess tissue above A instead of tissue deficit. In such a case, the isodose chart is moved up so that its surface line passes through the point of intersection of the contour line and the ray line through A. The value of h is assigned a negative value in this case.

B. Tissue-air (or Tissue-maximum) Ratio Method

This method depends on the principle that the tissue-air, or tissue-maximum, ratio does not depend on the SSD and is a function only of the depth and the field size at that depth. Suppose, in Fig. 12.14, the surface is located at S''–S'' and the air space between S–S and S''–S'' is filled with tissue-like material. Now, if a standard isodose chart for the given beam and SSD is placed with its surface at S''–S'', the percent depth dose value at A will correspond to the depth $d + h$. But the actual value at A is greater than this as there is a tissue deficit. The correction factor can be obtained by the ratio of tissue-air or tissue-maximum ratios for depths d and $d + h$.

$$\text{Correction factor } (CF) = \frac{T(d, \, r_A)}{T(d + h, \, r_A)} \qquad (12.7)$$

where T stands for tissue-air ratio or tissue-maximum ratio and r_A is the field size projected at point A (i.e., at a distance of $SSD + d + h$ from the source).

Thus if the uncorrected value of percent depth dose at A with the surface line of the isodose chart at S''–S'' is P'', then the corrected value P_{corr} is given:

$$P_{corr} = P'' \cdot CF$$

C. Isodose Shift Method

The preceding methods are useful for making individual point dose calculations. However, for manual treatment planning, it is convenient to correct the entire isodose chart for contour irregularities. This can be done by an empirical method, known as the isodose shift method. The procedure is illustrated in Fig. 12.15. Suppose S–S is the patient contour drawn on a transparent paper and S'–S' is a flat surface line passing through the point of intersection of the central axis with the contour. From the line S'–S', draw vertical grid lines, parallel to the central axis and spaced about 1 cm apart, to cover the full field width. Place the standard isodose chart underneath this paper and align the central line of the chart with that of the grid. Mark the percent depth dose values on the central axis. For each grid line, slide the isodose chart up or down, depending on whether there is tissue

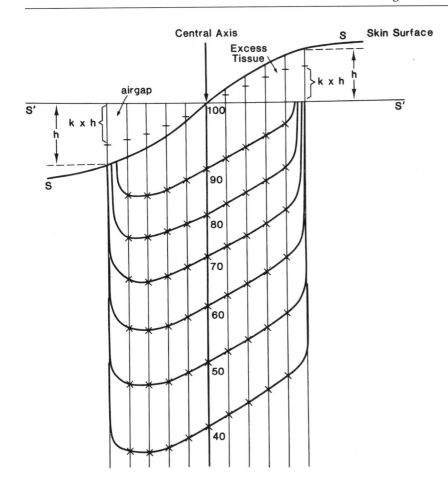

FIG. 12.15. Diagram illustrating isodose shift method of correcting isodose curves for surface contour irregularity.

excess or deficit along that line, by an amount $k \times h$ where k is a factor less than 1 (given in Table 12.1). Then mark the isodose values at points of intersection of the given grid line and the shifted isodose curves. After all the isodose positions along all the grid lines have been marked, new isodose curves are drawn by joining the marked points having the same isodose values.

The factor k depends on the radiation quality, field size, depth of interest, and SSD. Table 12.1 gives approximate values recommended for clinical use when manual corrections are needed.

Of the three methods discussed above, the tissue-air or tissue-maximum ratio method gives the most accurate results. The first two methods are especially useful in computer treatment planning.

TABLE 12.1. ISODOSE SHIFT FACTORS FOR DIFFERENT BEAM ENERGIES

Photon Energy (MV)	Approximate Factor k
Up to 1	0.8
^{60}Co-5	0.7
5–15	0.6
15–30	0.5
Above 30	0.4

Data from Giessen PH. A method of calculating the isodose shift in correcting for oblique incidence in radiotherapy. *Br J Radiol* 1973;46:978.

Example 1

For point A in Fig. 12.14, $h = 3$ cm and $d = 5$ cm. Calculate the percent depth dose at point A using (a) the effective SSD method and (b) the tissue-air ratio method.

Given ^{60}Co beam, TAR(5, 11 × 11) = 0.910 and TAR(8, 11 × 11) = 0.795 and SSD = 80 cm:

(a) using solid isodose curve lines in Fig. 12.14,

Percent depth dose at $A = 78.1$

$$\text{Inverse square law factor} = \left(\frac{80 + 0.5}{80 + 3 + 0.5} \right)^2$$

$$= 0.929$$

Corrected percent depth dose at $A = 78.1 \times 0.929$

$$= 72.6$$

(b) Field dimension projected at $A = 10 \times \dfrac{88}{80} = 11$ cm. Thus field size at $A = 11 \times 11$ cm:

$$CF = \frac{\text{TAR}(5, 11 \times 11)}{\text{TAR}(8, 11 \times 11)} = \frac{0.910}{0.795} = 1.145$$

Using dashed isodose lines in Fig. 12.14, uncorrected percent depth dose = 65.2.

Corrected percent depth dose = 65.2×1.145

$$= 74.6$$

Comparing the results for (a) and (b), the agreement between the two methods is within 3%.

12.5. CORRECTIONS FOR TISSUE INHOMOGENEITIES

Applications of standard isodose charts and depth dose tables assume homogeneous unit density medium. In a patient however, the beam may transverse layers of fat, bone, muscle, lung, and air. The presence of these inhomogeneities will produce changes in the dose distribution, depending on the amount and type of material present and on the quality of radiation.

The effects of tissue inhomogeneities may be classified into two general categories: (a) changes in the absorption of the primary beam and the associated pattern of scattered photons and (b) changes in the secondary electron fluence. The relative importance of these effects depends on the region of interest where alterations in absorbed dose are considered. For points that lie beyond the inhomogeneity, the predominant effect is the attenuation of the primary beam. Changes in the associated photon scatter distribution alters the dose distribution more strongly near the inhomogeneity than farther beyond it. The changes in the secondary electron fluence, on the other hand, affects the tissues within the inhomogeneity and at the boundaries.

For x-ray beams in the megavoltage range, where Compton effect is a predominant mode of interaction, the attenuation of the beam in any medium is governed by electron density (number of electrons per cm^3). Thus an effective depth can be used for calculating transmission through nonwater-equivalent materials. However, close to the boundary or interface, the distribution is more complex. For example, for megavoltage beams, there may be loss of electronic equilibrium close to the boundaries of low-density materials or air cavities. For orthovoltage and superficial x-rays, the major problem is the bone. Absorbed dose within the bone or in the immediate vicinity of it may be several times higher than the dose in the soft tissue in the absence of bone. This increased energy absorption is caused

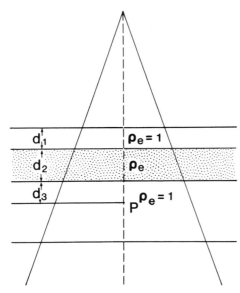

FIG. 12.16. Schematic diagram showing a water equivalent phantom containing an inhomogeneity of electron density ρ_e relative to that of water. *P* is the point of dose calculation.

by the increase in the electron fluence arising from the photoelectric absorption in the mineral contents of the bone.

A. Corrections for Beam Attenuation and Scattering

Figure 12.16 is a schematic diagram showing an inhomogeneity of electron density ρ_e relative to that of water. The material preceding and following the inhomogeneity is water equivalent (relative $\rho_e = 1$). Lateral dimensions of this composite phantom are assumed infinite or much larger than the field size. Calculation is to be made at point *P*, which is located at a distance d_3 from the lower boundary, distance $(d_2 + d_3)$ from the front boundary of the inhomogeneity, and distance $d = d_1 + d_2 + d_3$ from the surface.

Three methods of correcting for inhomogeneities are illustrated with reference to Fig. 12.16.

A.1. Tissue-air Ratio Method

The following *CF* applies to the dose at *P* if the entire phantom was water equivalent:

$$CF = \frac{T(d', r_d)}{T(d, r_d)} \tag{12.8}$$

where d' is the equivalent water depth, i.e., $d' = d_1 + \rho_e\, d_2 + d_3$, and d is the actual depth of *P* from the surface; r_d is the field size projected at point *P*.

The above correction method does not take into account the position of the inhomogeneity relative to point *P*. In other words, the correction factor will not change with d_3 as long as d and d' remain constant.

A.2. Power Law Tissue-air Ratio Method

Batho (43) and Young and Gaylord (44) have proposed a method in which the ratio of the tissue-air ratios is raised to a power. Referring again to Fig. 12.16, the correction factor at point P is:

$$CF = \left[\frac{T(d_2 + d_3, r_d)}{T(d_3, r_d)} \right]^{\rho_e - 1} \tag{12.9}$$

Here ρ_e is the electron density (number of electrons/cm^3) of the heterogeneity relative to that of water.

As seen in Equation 12.9, the correction factor does depend on the location of the inhomogeneity relative to point P but not relative to the surface. This formulation is based on theoretical considerations assuming Compton interactions only. It does not apply to points inside the inhomogeneity or in the build-up region. Experimental verification of the model has been provided for ^{60}Co γ beams (43,44).

A more general form of the power law method is provided by Sontag and Cunningham (45) that allows for correction of the dose to points within an inhomogeneity as well as below it. This is given by:

$$CF = \frac{T(d_3, r_d)^{\rho_3 - \rho_2}}{T(d_2 + d_3, r_d)^{1 - \rho_2}} \tag{12.10}$$

where ρ_3 is the density of the material in which point P lies and d_3 is its depth within this material. ρ_2 is the density of the overlying material, and $(d_2 + d_3)$ is the depth below the upper surface of it. It may be pointed out that Equation 12.10 reduces to Equation 12.9 if P lies in a unit density medium as shown in Fig. 12.16.

A.3. Equivalent Tissue-air Ratio Method

The use of water equivalent depth in Equation 12.8 appropriately corrects for the primary component of dose. However, the change in scattered dose is not correctly predicted because the effect of scattering structures depends on their geometric arrangement with respect to point P. Sontag and Cunningham (21) accounted for these geometric factors through the scaling of the field size parameter. Their method using "equivalent" tissue-air ratios (ETARs) is given by:

$$CF = \frac{T(d', r')}{T(d, r)} \tag{12.11}$$

where d' is the water equivalent depth, d is the actual depth, r is the beam dimension at depth d, $r' = r \cdot \bar{\rho}$ = scaled field size dimension, and $\bar{\rho}$ is the weighted density of the irradiated volume.

The weighted density $\bar{\rho}$ can be determined by the averaging procedure:

$$\bar{\rho} = \frac{\sum_i \sum_j \sum_k \rho_{ijk} \cdot W_{ijk}}{\sum_i \sum_j \sum_k W_{ijk}} \tag{12.12}$$

where ρ_{ijk} are the relative electron densities of scatter elements (e.g., pixels in a series of CT images of the irradiated volume) and W_{ijk} are the weighting factors assigned to these elements in terms of their relative contribution to the scattered dose at the point of calculation.

The weighting factors are calculated using Compton scatter cross-sections and integrating scatter over the entire irradiated volume for each point of dose calculation. A more practical approach is to "coalesce" all of the density information from individual slices into a single "equivalent" slice, thus reducing the volume integration to an integration over a plane. Details of this procedure are discussed by Sontag and Cunningham (21).

An alternative approach to the ETAR method is to calculate scattered dose separately from the primary dose by summation of the scatter contribution from individual scatter elements in the irradiated heterogeneous volume. This method is known as the differential scatter-air ratio (DSAR) method (46,47). More advanced computer-based methods such

TABLE 12.2. ISODOSE SHIFT FACTORS[a] FOR INHOMOGENEITIES

Inhomogeneity	Shift Factor n^a
Air cavity	−0.6
Lung	−0.4
Hard bone	0.5
Spongy bone	0.25

[a]Approximate factors, determined empirically for ^{60}Co and 4-MV x-rays.
From Greene D, Stewart JR. Isodose curves in non-uniform phantoms. *Br J Radiol* 1965;38:378; Sundblom L. Dose planning for irradiation of thorax with cobalt in fixed beam therapy. *Acta Radiol* 1965;3:342; with permission.

as delta volume (DV) (47,48), dose spread array (DSA) (49) and differential pencil beam (DPB) (50) methods have been proposed to take into account multiple scattering of photons and electron transport to predict dose more accurately as well as in the regions where electronic equilibrium does not exist. A discussion of model-based algorithms using dose kernels (e.g., convolution/superposition algorithms) and Monte Carlo techniques is presented in Chapter 19.

A.4. Isodose Shift Method

This method, proposed by Greene and Stewart (51) and Sundblom (52), is convenient for manually correcting isodose charts for the presence of inhomogeneities. The isodose curves beyond the inhomogeneity are moved by an amount equal to n times the thickness of the inhomogeneity as measured along a line parallel to the central axis and passing through the point of interest. The shift is toward the skin for bone and away from the skin for lung or air cavities. Table 12.2 gives experimentally determined values of n which apply to ^{60}Co radiation and 4-MV x-rays. The factors are believed to be independent of field size.

A.5. Typical Correction Factors

None of the methods discussed above can claim an accuracy of ±5% for all irradiation conditions encountered in radiotherapy. The new generation of algorithms that take account of the 3-D shape of the irradiated volume and the electron transport are expected to achieve that goal but are still under development. Most commercial systems use one-dimensional methods in which bulk density-based inhomogeneity corrections are applied along ray lines, disregarding the extent of inhomogeneities in the other dimensions.

Tang et al. (53) have compared a few commonly used methods, namely, the TAR, the ETAR, and the generalized Batho against measured data using a heterogeneous phantom containing layers of polystyrene and cork. Their results show that for the geometries considered (a) the TAR method overestimates the dose for all energies, (b) the ETAR is best suited for the lower-energy beams (≤ 6 MV), and (c) the generalized Batho method is the best in the high-energy range (≥ 10 MV). Thus the accuracy of different methods depend on the irradiation conditions, e.g., energy, field size, location and extent of inhomogeneity, and location of point of calculation.

Table 12.3 gives some examples of increase in dose beyond healthy lung for various beam energies. These correction factors have been calculated by using Equation 12.10, assuming $d_1 = 6$ cm, $d_2 = 8$ cm, and $d_3 = 3$ cm, relative ρ_e for lung = 0.25, and field size = 10×10 cm. The values were rounded off to represent approximate factors for typical lung corrections. More detailed tables of the beyond-lung and in-lung correction factors have been calculated by McDonald et al. (54) for several representative beam energies and field sizes.

TABLE 12.3. INCREASE IN DOSE TO TISSUES BEYOND HEALTHY LUNG[a]

Beam Quality	Correction Factor
Orthovoltage	+10%/cm of lung
^{60}Co γ rays	+4%/cm of lung
4-MV x-rays	+3%/cm of lung
10-MV x-rays	+2%/cm of lung
20-MV x-rays	+1%/cm of lung

[a]Approximate values calculated with Equation 12.10 for typical clinical situations.

Table 12.4 gives the decrease in dose beyond bone that might be expected with beams of different energies. These are approximate values because the shielding effect of bone depends on the size of the bone, field size, and other parameters that affect scattering. The shielding effect of bone diminishes quite rapidly as the beam energy increases. The shielding effect of bone for x-rays generated between 500 kV and 4 MV is entirely due to its greater electron density (electrons per cm^3), as all the attenuation is due to the Compton process. In the megavoltage range, the corrections for bone attenuation in most clinical situations are small and are usually neglected. However, as the x-ray energy increases beyond 10 MV, the shielding effect begins to increase because pair production becomes significant. Recall that the absorption of radiation as a result of pair production depends on the atomic number.

B. Absorbed Dose within an Inhomogeneity

As mentioned earlier, the absorbed dose within an inhomogeneity or in the soft tissues adjacent to it is strongly influenced by alterations in the secondary electron fluence. For example, for x-rays generated at potentials less than 250 kVp, there is a substantial increase in absorbed dose inside bone because of increased electron fluence arising from photoelectric absorption. Spiers (55,56) has made a comprehensive study of absorbed dose within mineral bone as well as within soft tissue components of bone. The interested reader is referred to the original work or to Johns and Cunningham (57) for details. Some practical aspects of the problem will be discussed in this section.

B.1. Bone Mineral

Under the conditions of electronic equilibrium, the ratio of absorbed doses in different media, for a given photon energy fluence, is given by the ratio of their energy absorption coefficients (see Chapter 8). Because the rad/R or the f factor is proportional to the energy

TABLE 12.4. REDUCTION IN DOSE BEYOND 1 CM OF HARD BONE[a]

Beam Quality	Correction Factor (%)
1 mm Cu HVL	−15[b]
3 mm Cu HVL	−7
^{60}Co	−3.5
4 MV	−3
10 MV	−2

[a]Approximate values calculated with Equation 12.8 for typical clinical situations. Assumed electron density of bone relative to water = 1.65.
[b]Estimated from measured data by Haas LL, Sandberg GH. Modification of the depth dose curves of various radiations by interposed bone. *Br J Radiol* 1957;30:19.

absorption coefficient relative to air, the ratio of f factors also reflects the relative absorbed dose. Thus, for a given quality radiation and the energy fluence, the absorbed dose in bone mineral relative to absorbed dose in muscle is the ratio:

$$\frac{f_{bone}}{f_{muscle}} \quad \text{or} \quad \left(\frac{\mu_{en}}{\rho}\right)^{bone}_{muscle}$$

under electronic equilibrium conditions.

Figure 12.17A shows a plot of absorbed dose as a function of depth for an orthovoltage beam incident on a composite phantom containing 2-cm thick bone. Because for this quality radiation $f_{bone}/f_{muscle} = 1.9/0.94 = 2.0$, the dose in the first layer of bone will be about twice as much as in soft tissue. In the subsequent layers, the dose will drop from this value due to increased attenuation by bone (Table 12.4). Figure 12.17B compares the

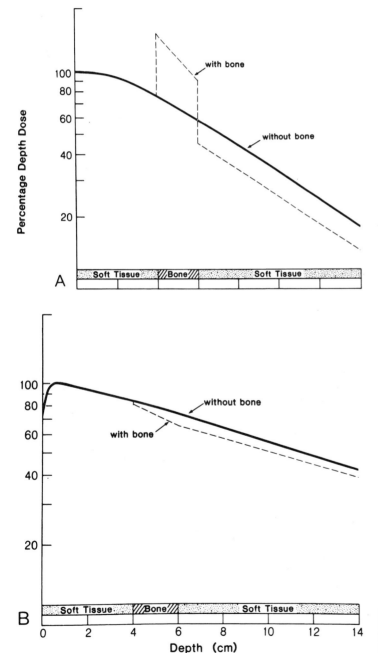

FIG. 12.17. Percentage depth dose as a function of depth in a phantom containing 2 cm of bone. **A:** HVL = 1 mm Cu; SSD = 50 cm; field size = 10 × 10 cm. **B:** ^{60}Co γ ray beam; SSD = 80 cm; field size = 10 × 10 cm.

TABLE 12.5. ABSORBED DOSE TO BONE RELATIVE TO SOFT TISSUE FOR DIFFERENT ENERGY BEAMS

	Radiation Quality		
HVL[a]	Approximate Effective Energy	Bone Mineral[b]	Soft Tissue in Bone
1 mm Al	20 keV	4.6	5.0
3 mm Al	30 keV	4.8	5.3
1 mm Cu	80 keV	2.1	3.8
2 mm Cu	110 keV	1.4	2.4
3 mm Cu	135 keV	1.2	1.6
10.4 mm Pb (^{60}Co γ rays)	1.25 MeV	0.96	1.03
11.8 mm Pb (4-MV x-rays)	1.5 MeV	0.96	1.03
14.7 mm Pb (10-MV x-rays)	4 MeV	0.98	1.05
13.7 mm Pb (20-MV x-rays)	8 MeV	1.02	1.09
12.3 mm Pb (40-MV x-rays)	10 MeV	1.04	1.11

HVL, half-value layer.
[a]HVL and approximate effective energies calculated using attenuation coefficients (chapter 7).
[b]Derived from data given in Johns HE, Cunningham JP. *The physics of radiology.* 4th ed. Springfield, IL: Charles C Thomas, 1983.

situation with ^{60}Co beam. Since $f_{bone}/f_{muscle} = 0.955/0.957 = 0.96$ for this energy, the dose to bone mineral for a ^{60}Co beam is slightly less than that expected in the soft tissue. Beyond the bone, the dose is reduced due to the shielding effect of bone because the electron density of bone is higher than that of the muscle tissue.

Table 12.5, column 3, gives the change in dose expected in the bone mineral for different energy beams. These calculations are made on the basis of the f factor ratios of bone to muscle or the ratio of energy absorption coefficients. For orthovoltage beams, these values represent the maximal enhancement in dose occurring just inside bone on the entrance side of the beam.

B.2. Bone-tissue Interface

Soft Tissue in Bone

The bone discussed in section B.1 is the inorganic bone (bone mineral). Of greater importance biologically, however, is the dose to soft tissue embedded in bone or adjacent to bone. The soft tissue elements in bone may include blood vessels (the Haversian canals), living cells called osteocytes and bone marrow. These structures may have very small thicknesses, ranging from a few microns to a millimeter. When the thickness of a soft tissue structure in bone is small compared with the range of the electrons traversing it, it may be considered as a Bragg-Gray cavity (see Chapter 8), containing soft tissue embedded in the bone medium. Under these conditions photon interactions in the cavity can be ignored and the ionization in the cavity is considered entirely due to electrons (photo-, Compton-, or pair-production electrons) originating from the surrounding material. The dose D_{STB} to a very small volume of soft tissue embedded in bone, assuming no perturbation of the photon or electron fluences, is given by:

$$D_{STB} = D_B \cdot (\overline{S}/\rho)_B^{ST} \tag{12.13}$$

where D_B is the dose to the surrounding bone matrix and $(\overline{S}/\rho)_B^{ST}$ is the ratio of average mass collision stopping power of soft tissue to bone for the electrons.

As discussed earlier in section B.1, the dose at a point in the bone mineral is related to the dose (D_{ST}) at the same point if the bone is replaced by a homogeneous medium of soft tissue:

$$D_B = D_{ST} \cdot (\overline{\mu}_{en}/\rho)_{ST}^B \tag{12.14}$$

From equations 12.13 and 12.14, we get:

$$D_B = D_{ST} \cdot (\overline{\mu}_{en}/\rho)_{ST}^B \cdot (\overline{S}/\rho)_B^{ST} \tag{12.15}$$

The ratio γ of dose to a soft tissue element embedded in bone to the dose in a homogeneous medium of soft tissue, for the same photon energy fluence, is given by:

$$\gamma = D_{STB}/D_{ST} = (\overline{\mu}_{en}/\rho)_{ST}^B \cdot (\overline{S}/\rho)_B^{ST} \tag{12.16}$$

Calculated values of γ for different energy beams are given in column 4 of Table 12.5. These data show that for the same photon energy fluence, soft tissue structures inside the bone will receive higher dose than the dose to the bone mineral or the dose to soft tissue in the absence of bone. There are two reasons for this increase in dose: (a) $\overline{\mu}_{en}/\rho$ is greater for bone than soft tissue in the very low energy range because of the photoelectric process and in the very high energy range because of the pair production. However, in the Compton range of energies, $\overline{\mu}_{en}/\rho$ for bone is slightly less than that for soft tissue; (b) $\overline{S}/\rho$ is greater for soft tissue at all energies because it contains greater number of electrons per unit mass than the bone (Table 5.1). The combined effect of (a) and (b) gives rise to a higher dose to the soft tissue embedded in bone than the surrounding bone mineral or the homogeneous soft tissue in the absence of bone.

In a clinical situation, the dose to a small tissue cavity inside a bone may be calculated by the following equation:

$$D_{STB} = D_{ST} \cdot \gamma \cdot TMR(t_{ST} + \rho_B \cdot t_B)/TMR(t_{ST} + t_B) \tag{12.17}$$

where t_{ST} and t_B are thicknesses of soft tissue and bone, respectively, traversed by the beam before reaching the point of interest; ρ_B is the relative electron density of bone; and TMR is the tissue-maximum ratio (or similar attenuation function) for the given field size.

Soft Tissue Surrounding Bone

On the entrance side of the photon beam, there is a dose enhancement in the soft tissue adjacent to the bone. In the megavoltage range of energies, this increase in dose is primarily due to the electron backscattering. Das and Khan (58) have shown that the magnitude of the backscatter is nearly the same for all photon energies from ^{60}Co to 24 MV. For bone, the dose enhancement due to backscatter is approximately 8% in the above energy range. Because of the very short range of the backscattered electrons, the enhancement effect is limited only to a few millimeters (Fig. 12.18). For instance the dose enhancement drops from 8% to less than 2% within 2 mm upstream from the interface.

On the transmission side of the beam, the forward scatter of electrons from bone and the buildup of electrons in soft tissue give rise to a dose perturbation effect which depends on photon energy (59). Figure 12.19 shows this energy dependence. For energies up to 10 MV, the dose at the interface is initially less than the dose in a homogeneous soft tissue medium but then builds up to a dose that is slightly greater than that in the homogeneous case. For higher energies, there is an enhancement of dose at the interface because of the increased electron fluence in bone due to pair production. The effect decreases with distance and lasts up to the range of the electrons.

Most patients are treated with parallel-opposed beams. Also dose distributions are normally not corrected for the presence of bone when using megavoltage photon beams. The following discussion analyzes the bone dosage problem in a practical clinical situation.

Figure 12.20 shows examples of depth dose distributions expected in a patient treated with parallel-opposed beams. Doses are normalized to the midpoint dose expected in a homogeneous soft tissue medium. The distribution corrected for increased bone attenuation (shielding effect) alone shows dose reduction throughout. The magnitude of this reduction depends on bone thickness relative to the soft tissue thickness, bone density and beam energy. The actual distribution in the presence of bone includes both bone attenuation and bone-tissue interface effects discussed earlier. These effects in the megavoltage range of

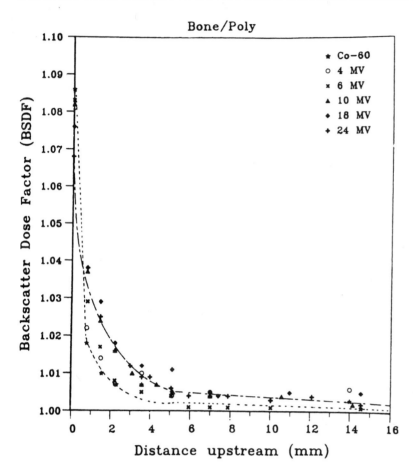

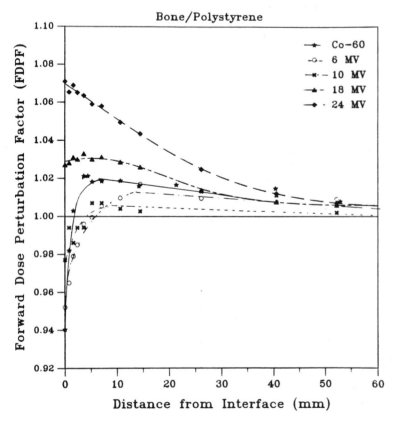

FIG. 12.18. Backscatter dose factor (BSDF) for various energy photon beams plotted as a function of distance, toward the source, from the bone-polystyrene interface. BSDF is the ratio of dose at the interface with bone to that without bone. (From Das IJ, Khan FM. Backscatter dose perturbation at high atomic number interfaces in megavoltage photon beams. *Med Phys* 1989;16:367, with permission.)

FIG. 12.19. Forward dose perturbation factor (FDPF) for various energy photon beams plotted as a function of distance, away from the source, from bone-polystyrene interface. FDPF is the ratio of dose at the interface with bone to that without bone for the same photon energy fluence. (From Das IJ. Study of dose perturbation at bone-tissue interfaces in megavoltage photon beam therapy. [Dissertation.] University of Minnesota, 1988:119, with permission.)

6-MV Beam

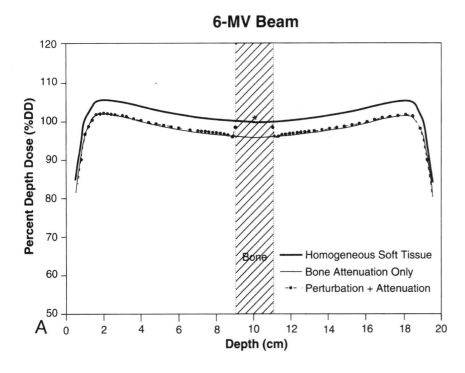

24-MV Beam

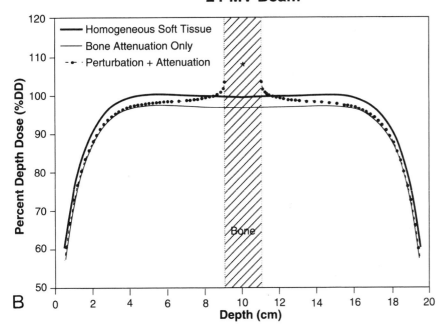

FIG. 12.20. Percent depth dose distribution in a 20-cm–thick polystyrene phantom containing a bone substitute material. Doses are normalized to midpoint dose in the homogeneous polystyrene phantom of the same thickness. Parallel-opposed beams, field size = 10 × 10 cm, SSD = 100 cm. The symbol * signifies dose to a small tissue cavity in bone. **A:** 6 MV photon beam. **B:** 24 MV photon beam. (From Das IJ, Khan FM, Kase KR. Dose perturbation at high atomic number interfaces in parallel opposed megavoltage photon beam irradiation [abst.]. *Phys Med Biol* 1988;33[suppl 1]:121, with permission.)

energies cause an increase in dose to soft tissue adjacent to bone, but the net increase is not significant at lower energies (≤10 MV). However, as the pair production process becomes significant at higher energies and the electron range increases, appreciable enhancement in dose occurs at the bone tissue interfaces. This is seen in Fig. 12.20 and Table 12.6.

B.3. Lung Tissue

Dose within the lung tissue is primarily governed by its density. As discussed in section 12.5A, lower lung density gives rise to higher dose within and beyond the lung. Figure 12.21

TABLE 12.6. DOSE ENHANCEMENT AT BONE-TISSUE INTERFACE FOR PARALLEL-OPPOSED BEAMS[a]

Thickness of Bone (cm)	6 MV	10 MV	18 MV	24 MV
0.5	1.01	1.02	1.03	1.04
1.0	1.01	1.02	1.03	1.05
2.0	1.00	1.01	1.03	1.05
3.0	0.99	1.00	1.03	1.05

[a]Dose to soft tissue adjacent to bone relative to midpoint dose in a homogeneous soft tissue; total thickness = 20 cm; field size = 10 × 10 cm; SSD = 100 cm.
From Das IJ, Khan FM, Kase KR. Dose perturbation at high atomic number interfaces in parallel opposed megavoltage photon beam irradiation [abstract]. *Phys Med Biol* 1988;33[Suppl 1]:121, with permission.

gives the increase in lung dose as a function of depth in the lung for selected energies using a 10 × 10 cm field. But in the first layers of soft tissue beyond a large thickness of lung, there is some loss of secondary electrons (60). This gives rise to a slight decrease in dose relative to that calculated on the basis of lung transmission.

Kornelson and Young (61) have discussed the problem of loss of lateral electronic equilibrium when a high-energy photon beam traverses the lung. Because of the lower density of lung, an increasing number of electrons travel outside the geometrical limits of the beam. This causes the dose profile to become less sharp. For the same reason there is a greater loss of laterally scattered electrons, causing a reduction in dose on the beam axis. The effect is significant for small field sizes (<6 × 6 cm) and higher energies (>6 MV). Clinically, when treating a tumor in the lung there is a possibility of underdosage in the periphery of the tumor if small fields and high-energy beams are used. However, considering the fact that most protocols in this country require no lung correction in dose prescription, consideration of this effect in dosimetry becomes rather academic.

B.4. Air Cavity

The most important effect of air cavities in megavoltage beam dosimetry is the partial loss of electronic equilibrium at the cavity surface. The actual dose to tissue beyond and in front of the cavity may be appreciably lower than expected. This phenomenon of dose buildup at the air cavities has been extensively studied by Epp et al. (62,63). The most significant decrease in dose occurs at the surface beyond the cavity, for large cavities (4 cm deep) and the smallest field (4 × 4 cm). Epp et al. (62) have estimated that in the case of ^{60}Co the reduction in dose in practical cases, such as the lesions located in the upper

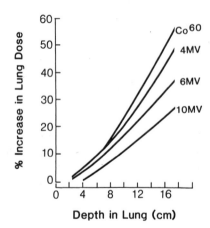

FIG. 12.21. Percentage increase in lung dose as a function of depth in the lung for selected energies. Field size = 10 × 10 cm. (From McDonald SC, Keller BE, Rubin P. Method for calculating dose when lung tissue lies in the treatment field. *Med Phys* 1976;3:210, with permission.)

respiratory air passages, will not be greater than 10% unless field sizes smaller than 4 × 4 cm are used. The underdosage is expected to be greater for higher-energy radiation (63).

12.6. TISSUE COMPENSATION

A radiation beam incident on an irregular or sloping surface produces skewing of the isodose curves. Corrections for this effect were discussed in section 12.2. In certain treatment situations, however, the surface irregularity gives rise to unacceptable nonuniformity of dose within the target volume or causes excessive irradiation of sensitive structures such as the spinal cord. Many techniques have been devised to overcome this problem, including the use of wedged fields or multiple fields and the addition of bolus material or compensators. Areas having a smaller thickness of tissue can also be blocked for the last few treatments to reduce the dose in these areas.

Bolus is a tissue-equivalent material placed directly on the skin surface to even out the irregular contours of a patient to present a flat surface normal to the beam. This use of bolus should be distinguished from that of a bolus layer, which is thick enough to provide adequate dose buildup over the skin surface. The latter should be termed the *build-up bolus*.

Placing bolus directly on the skin surface is satisfactory for orthovoltage radiation, but for higher-energy beams results in the loss of the *skin sparing* advantage. For such radiations, a *compensating filter* should be used, which approximates the effect of the bolus as well as preserves the skin-sparing effect. To preserve the skin-sparing properties of the megavoltage photon beams, the compensator is placed a suitable distance (≥20 cm) away from the patient's skin. Yet the compensator is so designed that its introduction in the beam gives rise to isodose curves within the patient that duplicate, as closely as possible, those for the bolus.

A. Design of Compensators

Figure 12.22 illustrates schematically the use of a compensator to provide the required beam attenuation that would otherwise occur in the "missing" tissue when the body surface is

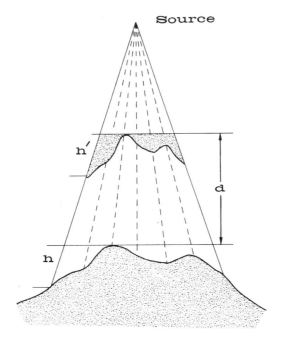

FIG. 12.22. Schematic representation of a compensator designed for an irregular surface. (From Khan FM, Moore VC, Burns DJ. The construction of compensators for cobalt teletherapy. *Radiology* 1970;96:187, with permission.)

irregular or curved. Because the compensator is designed to be positioned at a distance from the surface, the dimensions and shape of the compensator must be adjusted because of (a) the beam divergence, (b) the relative linear attenuation coefficients of the filter material and soft tissues, and (c) the reduction in scatter at various depths when the compensator is placed at a distance from the skin rather than in contact with it. To compensate for this scatter, the compensator is designed such that the attenuation of the filter is less than that required for primary radiation only. These considerations and others have been discussed in the literature (64–70).

Minification of the compensating material for geometric divergence of the beam has been achieved in many ways. One method (64,66–68) constructs the compensator out of aluminum or brass blocks, using a matrix of square columns corresponding to the irregular surface. The dimension of each column is minified according to the geometric divergence correction, which is calculated from the SSD and the filter-surface distance. Khan et al. (71) described an apparatus that uses thin rods duplicating the diverging rays of the therapy beam (Fig. 12.23). The rods move freely in rigid shafts along the diverging paths and can be locked or released by a locking device. The apparatus is positioned over the patient so that the lower ends of the rods touch the skin surface. When the rods are locked, the upper ends of the rods generate a surface that is similar to the skin surface but corrected for divergence. A plastic compensator can then be built over this surface (69). Beck et al. (72) and Boge et al. (73) have described Styrofoam cutters (Fig. 12.24) that work on a pantographic principle and use a heating element or a routing tool mechanism for the hollowing of the Styrofoam. The cavity thus produced is a minified version of the patient surface, which can be filled with the compensator material.

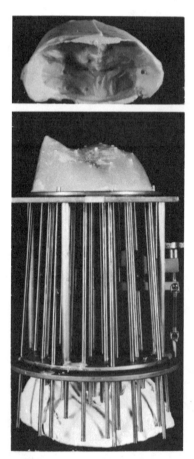

FIG. 12.23. An apparatus for the construction of 3-D compensator in one piece. (From Khan FM, Moore VC, Burns DJ. An apparatus for the construction of irregular surface compensators for use in radiotherapy. *Radiology* 1968;90:593, with permission.)

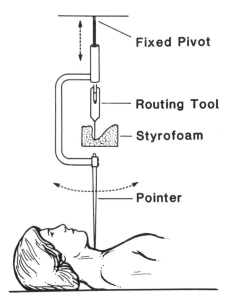

FIG. 12.24. Schematic diagram of a Styrofoam cutter fitted with a routing tool for constructing compensators. (Redrawn from Boge RJ, Edland RW, Mathes DC. Tissue compensators for megavoltage radiotherapy fabricated from hollowed Styrofoam filled with wax. *Radiology* 1974;111:193, with permission.)

A tissue equivalent compensator designed with the same thickness as that of the missing tissue will overcompensate, i.e., the dose to the underlying tissues will be less than that indicated by the standard isodose chart. This decrease in depth dose, which is due to the reduction in scatter reaching a point at depth, depends on the distance of the compensator from the patient, field size, depth, and beam quality. To compensate for this decrease in scatter, one may reduce the thickness of the compensator to increase the primary beam transmission. The compensator thickness should be such that the dose at a given depth is the same whether the missing tissue is replaced with the bolus in contact or with the compensator at the given distance from the skin surface. The required thickness of a tissue-equivalent compensator along a ray divided by the missing tissue thickness along the same ray may be called the *density ratio* or *thickness ratio* (69) (h'/h in Fig. 12.22). Figure 12.25

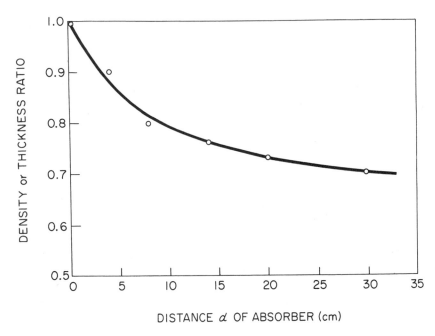

FIG. 12.25. A plot of density ratio or thickness ratio as a function of compensator distance for a uniformly thick compensator. ^{60}Co γ rays, field size = 10 × 10 cm, SSD = 80 cm, compensation depth = 7 cm, and tissue deficit = 5.0 cm. (From Khan FM, Moore VC, Burns DJ. The construction of compensators for cobalt teletherapy. *Radiology* 1970;96:187, with permission.)

gives a plot of thickness ratio, τ, as a function of compensator-surface distance, d. τ is unity at the surface and decreases as d increases.

Thickness ratio depends, in a complex way, on compensator-surface distance, thickness of missing tissue, field size, depth, and beam quality. However, a detailed study of this parameter has shown that τ is primarily a function of d (for $d \leq 20$ cm) and that its dependence on other parameters is relatively less critical (69,74). Thus a fixed value of τ, based on a given d (usually 20 cm), 10×10 cm field, 7-cm depth, and a tissue deficit of 5 cm can be used for most compensator work.

The concept of thickness ratios also reveals that a compensator cannot be designed to provide absorbed dose compensation exactly at all depths. If, for given irradiation conditions, τ is chosen for a certain compensation depth, the compensator overcompensates at shallower depths and undercompensates at greater depths. Considering the limitations of the theory and too many variables affecting τ, we have found that an average value of 0.7 for τ may be used for all irradiation conditions provided $d \geq 20$ cm. The same value has been tested to yield satisfactory results (errors in depth dose within $\pm 5\%$) for ^{60}Co, 4-MV and 10-MV x-rays (74).

In the actual design of the compensator, the thickness ratio is used to calculate compensator thickness (t_c) at a given point in the field:

$$t_c = \text{TD} \cdot (\tau/\rho_c) \tag{12.18}$$

where TD is the tissue deficit at the point considered and ρ_c is the density of the compensator material.

A direct determination of thickness (τ/ρ_c) for a compensator system may be made by measuring dose at an appropriate depth and field size in a tissue equivalent phantom (e.g., polystyrene) with a slab of compensator material placed in the beam at the position of the compensator tray. Pieces of phantom material are removed from the surface until the dose equals that measured in the intact phantom, without the compensator. The ratio of compensator thickness to the tissue deficit gives the thickness ratio.

It may be mentioned that a term *compensator ratio* (CR) has also been used in the literature to relate tissue deficit to the required compensator thickness (75). It is defined as the ratio of the missing tissue thickness to the compensator thickness necessary to give the dose for a particular field size and depth. The concepts of compensator ratio and the thickness ratio are the same, except that the two quantities are inverse of each other, i.e., $\text{CR} = \text{TD}/t_c = \rho_c/\tau$.

B. Two-dimensional Compensators

Designing a 3-D compensator is a time-consuming procedure. In a well-equipped mold or machine shop, a trained technician can probably construct such compensators routinely with a reasonable expenditure of time. In the absence of such facilities and personnel, however, most situations requiring compensation can be handled satisfactorily with simple 2-D compensators. In many treatment situations, the contour varies significantly in only one direction: along the field width or length. In such cases, a compensator can be constructed in which the thickness varies only along this dimension. For example, if anterior and posterior fields are incident on a sloping mediastinum, compensation is usually not changed in the lateral direction but only in the craniocaudal direction.

One simple way of constructing a two-dimensional compensator is to use thin sheets of lead (with known thickness ratio or effective attenuation coefficient) and gluing them together in a stepwise fashion to form a laminated filter. The total thickness of the filter at any point is calculated to compensate for the air gap at the point below it. Another method, used routinely at the University of Minnesota, is to construct the compensator in one piece from a block of Lucite. The patient contour is taken showing body thickness at at least three reference points: central axis, inferior margin, and superior margin of the field. Tissue deficits, Δt, are calculated by subtracting thicknesses at the reference points from the maximum thickness. A thickness minification factor is calculated by dividing the thickness ratio τ by the electron density (e^- per cm^3) of Lucite relative to that of tissue. The geometric minification factor is calculated by $(f - d)/f$ where f is the SSD at the point of maximum thickness and d is the filter-surface distance. The compensator dimensions can now be drawn by multiplying the Δt values with the thickness minification factor and the spacing between the reference points with the geometric minification factor. A Lucite block is then machined and glued on a thin Lucite plate for placement in the beam. The same method may be used to construct a compensator by stacking Lucite plates in a stepwise fashion and attaching them together firmly with pieces of Scotch tape.

C. Three-dimensional Compensators

Early 3-D compensator systems were mechanical devices to measure tissue deficits within the field in both the transverse and the longitudinal body cross-sections. Examples of these systems include Ellis type filters (64,66), rod boxes (68,69) and pantographic devices (72,73). More recent devices include Moiré camera, 3-D magnetic digitizers, CT-based compensator programs and electronic compensation using Multileaf collimators (Chapter 20).

C.1. Moiré Camera

A specially designed camera system allows topographic mapping of the patient body surface and provides tissue deficit data necessary for the design of a 3-D compensator. The principle of operation of the camera has been discussed by Boyer and Goitein (76). The camera can be mounted on a simulator without interfering with the simulator's normal use. Moiré fringes observed on the patient's surface represent iso-SSD lines from which the tissue deficit data can be deduced. The data can be used to drive a pantographic cutting unit. A commercial version of this system is manufactured by DCD, S&S PAR Scientific (Brooklyn, NY).

C.2. Magnetic Digitizer

A handheld stylus containing a magnetic field sensor is used to digitize the position of the sensor as it is scanned over the patient's surface in the presence of a low-strength, low-frequency magnetic field. Tissue deficit data are calculated by the computer from the sensor coordinates and used to drive a Styrofoam cutter. Cavities corresponding to the tissue deficit are then filled with an appropriate compensator material to design a compensator. A commercially available system, known as Compuformer is manufactured by Huestis Corporation (Bristol, RI).

C.3. Computed Tomography–based Compensator Systems

Three-dimensional radiotherapy treatment planning systems that use multilevel CT scans have sufficient data available to provide compensation not only for the irregular surface contours but also for the tissue inhomogeneities. There are two commercial systems that provide software for the design of compensating filters: the Target (G.E. Medical Systems, Milwaukee, WI) and the Theracomp/HEK (Theratronics Ltd., Ontario, Canada). These systems extract the tissue deficit data from the CT scans, which are then used to cut the Styrofoam mold using a drill bit or a heated wire loop. Although any compensator material of known compensator ratio may be cast into the filter molds, it is desirable to use medium-density materials rather than heavier materials such as Cerrobend. The main reason for this is to minimize error in dose distribution when small errors are made in cutting the mold.

There are several other compensator systems that have not been discussed here. For a detailed review of this topic the reader is referred to Reinstein (77).

D. Compensating Wedges

For oblique beam incidence or curved surfaces for which the contour can be approximated with a straight line, standard compensating wedges are very convenient (69,70). Compensating wedges (C-wedges) are fabricated from a metal such as copper, brass, or lead. They are designed to compensate for a "missing" wedge of tissue, using the same design principles as discussed in section 12.4B.

Distinction needs to be made between a wedge filter and a compensating wedge. Although a wedge filter can be used effectively as a compensator, it is primarily designed to tilt the standard isodose curves through a certain wedge angle in conjunction with the wedge-pair technique (Chapter 11). The wedge filter isodose curves must be available and used to obtain the composite isodose curves before the filter is used in a treatment set-up. The C-wedge, on the other hand, is used just as a compensator, so that the standard isodose charts can be used without modification. In addition, no wedge transmission factors are required for the C-wedges.

An important advantage of C-wedges over wedge filters used as compensators is that the C-wedges can be used for partial field compensation, that is, the C-wedge is used to compensate only a part of the contour, which is irregular in shape. A wedge filter, in this case, could not be used as a compensator because it is designed to be placed in the field in a fixed position.

E. Other Applications

Compensating filters can be designed to compensate for tissue heterogeneity. Most of this work was done by Ellis and his coworkers (33) in which compensators were designed from the knowledge of cross-sectional anatomy using transaxial tomography or a photographic film. More recently, Khan et al. (78) have described compensators for total body irradiation including compensation for lungs.

Compensators have also been used to improve dose uniformity in the fields where nonuniformity of the dose distribution arises from sources other than contour irregularity: reduced scatter near the field edges and unacceptable high dose regions or "horns" in the beam profile. Leung et al. (79) have discussed the design of filters for the mantle technique in which the compensator is designed on the basis of calculated dose distribution in the absence of a compensator. Boge et al. (80) have described a special compensator filter to reduce the horns present in large fields of a 4-MV linear accelerator.

F. Compensator Set-up

As mentioned earlier, the compensator should be placed at a distance of 20 cm or more away from the skin surface to preserve the skin-sparing properties of the megavoltage beams. Because the dimensions of the compensator are reduced (compared to the bolus) in the plane perpendicular to the beam axis to allow for beam divergence, the filter must be placed at the filter-surface distance for which it is designed. In addition, the nominal SSD should be measured from the plane perpendicular to the beam axis, containing the most elevated point on the contour included in the field (Fig. 12.22). For isocentric treatments, it is most convenient to use field dimensions projected at the isocenter in compensator design. Accordingly, the depth of the isocenter is measured from the level of the most elevated point on the contour to be compensated.

12.7. PATIENT POSITIONING

Availability of isocentric treatment machines, simulators, CT scanners, and computers has made it possible to achieve a high degree of precision in radiation therapy. However, one of the weakest links in the treatment-planning process is the problem of patient positioning

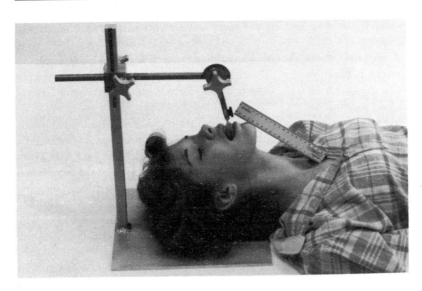

FIG. 12.26. Bite block system for head and neck immobilization. (Courtesy of Radiation Products Design, Buffalo, MN.)

and immobilization. It is frequently observed that some of the treatment techniques in current practice are outdated or do not take advantage of the accuracy available with the modern equipment. For example, the patients are treated in less than a stable position, are moved between different fields, and set up primarily by marks inked or tattooed on the skin surface. But, as any experienced observer knows, such practices are prone to serious errors. Skin marks are vulnerable to variation in skin sag and body position on the treatment table.

The problem of precise patient positioning and immobilization has been addressed by a number of investigators (81–86), including a recent review by Reinstein (87). But this problem still remains the area of greatest variance in actual treatment. The following ideas are presented to focus attention on this important area and offer some guidelines for precise patient positioning.

A. General Guidelines

1. Treatments should be set up isocentrically. The principal advantage of isocentric technique over SSD technique is that the patient is not moved between fields. Once the isocenter is positioned accurately within the patient, the remaining fields are arranged simply by gantry rotation or couch movement, not by displacing the patient relative to the couch.

2. Isocenter position within the patient can be established using the treatment simulator. This is usually accomplished by anterior and lateral radiographs, using the radiographically visible structures to define the target volume.

3. To accurately define the patient's position, thick pads or mattresses should not be used on the simulator table or the treatment table. This is essential for accurate measurement of set-up parameters as well as reproducibility.

4. For head and neck treatments, flexible head rests, such as pillows or sponges, should be avoided. The head should rest on a rigid surface such as a block of hard Styrofoam or a plastic "head-neck" support (Fig. 12.26).

5. Many methods of head immobilization are available such as partial body casts (85), bite block system (88),[5] nose bridges,[5] head clamps,[5] or simple masking tape. Choice of any of the above will depend on the location of the treatment fields.

6. As far as possible, the patient should be treated in the supine position. An overhead

---

[5] Such devices are commercially available, for example, from Radiation Products Design, Inc., Buffalo, Minnesota and Med-Tec, Orange City, Iowa.

sagittal laser line is useful in aligning the sagittal axis of the patient with the axis of gantry rotation.

7. For head and neck treatments, the chin extension should be defined anatomically, for example, distance between the sternal notch and the chin bone. This measurement should be accurately made after the head position has been established on the basis of stability and field localization.

8. During simulation as well as treatment, the depth of isocenter should be defined by either the set-up SSD (usually measured anteriorly or posteriorly) or by setting the distance between the tabletop distance and lateral beam axis. Side laser lights may also be used for this purpose. In the latter case, the laser lights should be checked frequently for alignment accuracy, because these lights are known to drift presumably by expansion and contraction of the walls on which they are mounted.

9. Skin marks should not be relied on for daily localization of the treatment field. The field boundaries should be defined relative to the bony landmarks established during simulation. Do not force the field to fit the skin marks!

10. For lateral portals, the Mylar section of the couch or tennis racket should be removed and the patient placed on a solid surface to avoid sag. These should be used only for anteroposterior (AP) treatments for which skin sparing is to be achieved. For example, if the four-field pelvis technique is used, one can use two fields a day in which case AP treatments are given isocentrically on a Mylar window using anterior or posterior set-up SSD, and lateral fields are treated on a flat tabletop section using the tabletop distance to lateral beam axis. Or if four fields are treated the same day, the posterior field can be treated through the rigid Plexiglas section of the couch instead of the Mylar window. Or AP treatments can be given on the Mylar window and then the window can be replaced by the Plexiglas section for the lateral treatments. The last alternative involves two separate set-ups, one for the AP and the other for the lateral fields. It should be used only when skin dose from the posterior fields is to be reduced to a minimum.

11. For isocentric techniques, field sizes must be defined at the isocenter which will, in most cases, be at the center of the treatment volume and not on the skin surface. Physicians who are accustomed to using standard field sizes (e.g., pelvic fields) defined at the skin surface should make adjustments in field sizes so that the fields encompass the same irradiated volume.

Some institutions have developed elaborate casting techniques to immobilize patients during treatments. This requires a well-equipped mold room as well as personnel trained in mold technology. Some of these techniques have been shown to be quite effective in minimizing patient motion (85,87). However, patients are known to move within a cast especially if the fit is not good or if there is a change in the surfaces contour due to regression of the tumor or weight loss.

Detection of patient motion is possible by using small dots of reflective tape on the patient with a pencil light ray and photocell device. Laser localization lights can also be used for this purpose. The signal received from the photocell can be further processed to activate an interlock to interrupt treatment or sound an alarm if pertinent motion exceeds a preset limit. Thus a good motion detection system can complement patient positioning and immobilization techniques by monitoring the stability of patient position as well as the effectiveness of immobilization.

B. The XYZ Method of Isocenter Set-up

In the isocentric technique, the isocenter is placed inside the patient, usually at the center of the target volume. Once this point has been localized by simulation, a good treatment set-up should reproduce it quickly and accurately. The following steps outline a procedure, hereby called the XYZ method, for the localization of this important point.

B.1. Simulation Procedure

1. The patient is positioned on the simulator couch following the general guidelines discussed in section 12.7A.
2. The patient is leveled using the side lasers (or a bubble level) and the sagittal laser beam to define the sagittal axis of the patient. The patient is then constrained from movement by a suitable immobilization device. For head and neck positioning, chin extension (distance between chin bone and the sternal notch) should be accurately measured.
3. The treatment fields are simulated using anterior and lateral radiographs and the isocenter is established according to the treatment plan.
4. A *reference anatomic point* is chosen on the sagittal axis, somewhere in the neighborhood of the treatment area, to represent a stable anatomic landmark. For example, nasion for head and neck, sternal notch for neck and thorax, tip of xiphoid for thorax and abdomen, and bottom of pubic ramus or tip of coccyx for pelvis, can be chosen as reasonably stable reference points.
5. The coordinates of the treatment isocenter are represented by (X, Y, Z) where X is the lateral distance and Y is the longitudinal distance (along patient axis) of the isocenter from the reference point and Z is the tabletop to isocenter distance (Fig. 12.27). Beam angle θ is recorded.

B.2. Treatment Set-up

1. Position and level the patient on the treatment couch as in simulation.
2. With the gantry vertical, place the central axis at the reference anatomic point and mark it with ink.
3. Move the couch: up or down to obtain Z using the side laser; laterally through X and

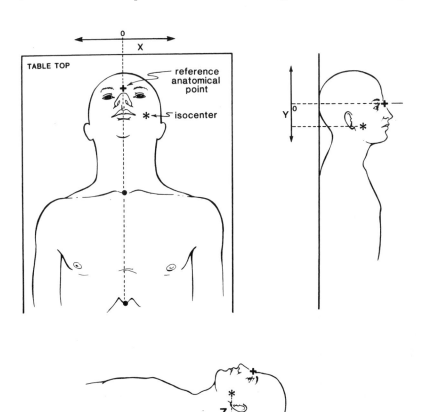

FIG. 12.27. A diagram to illustrate X, Y, Z coordinates to a patient set-up.

longitudinally through distance Y. Rotate the gantry through angle θ. This gives the required central axis of the field and the isocenter location.

4. Make secondary checks according to the field diagram such as SSD, location of field borders, etc.

5. For isocentric set-up, other fields are positioned by simply rotating the gantry and positioning it at predetermined angles.

One potential advantage of this method is that the set-up parameters X, Y, Z, and θ could be computer controlled, thereby decreasing the set-up time and minimizing human errors. The therapist, in this case, will position the patient as usual and place the central axis vertically at the reference point. Then, with a switch on the hand pendant, the computer control could be initiated to move the couch and the gantry to the X, Y, Z, and θ coordinates. Such a method could be adopted by some of the existing treatment monitoring systems that are capable of moving the couch and the gantry.

Even manually, the XYZ method can greatly economize set-up time as well as enhance set-up precision. Most modern couches are motor driven and equipped with motion-sensing devices. Videographic display of the couch motions could be conveniently used to position the couch. A reset switch for the X, Y, and Z coordinates would make it easier to move the couch through the X, Y, and Z distances.

REFERENCES

1. Kuisk H. "Contour maker" eliminating body casting in radiotherapy planning. *Radiology* 1971; 101:203.
2. Clarke HC. A contouring device for use in radiation treatment planning. *Br J Radiol* 1969;42: 858.
3. Clayton C, Thompson D. An optical apparatus for reproducing surface outlines of body cross-sections. *Br J Radiol* 1970;43:489.
4. Carson PL, Wenzel WW, Avery P, et al. Ultrasound imaging as an aid to cancer therapy—part I. *Int J Radiat Oncol Biol Phys* 1975;1:119. Part II. *Int J Radiat Oncol Biol Phys* 1976;2:335.
5. Takahashi S, Matsuda T. Axial transverse laminography applied to rotation therapy. *Radiology* 1960;74:61.
6. Pierquin B. La tomographie transversale: technique de routine en radiotherapie. *J Radiol Electrol* 1961;42:131.
7. Brooks RA, Di Chiro G. Principles of computer assisted tomography (CAT) in radiographic and radioisotopic imaging. *Phys Med Biol* 1976;21:689.
8. Rutherford RA, Pullan BR, Isherwood I. Measurement of effective atomic number and electron density using an EMI scanner. *Neuroradiology* 1976;11:15.
9. Kijewski PK, Bjärngard BE. The use of computed tomography data for radiotherapy dose calculations. *Int J Radiat Oncol Biol Phys* 1978;4:429.
10. Munzenrider JE, Pilepich M, Ferrero JBR, et al. Use of body scanners in radiotherapy treatment planning. *Cancer* 1977;40:170.
11. Geise RA, McCullough EC. The use of CT scanners in megavoltage photon-beam therapy planning. *Radiology* 1977;124:133.
12. Sontag MR, Battista JJ, Bronskill MJ, et al. Implications of computed tomography for inhomogeneity corrections in photon beam dose calculations. *Radiology* 1977;124:143.
13. Chernak ES, Antunez RA, Jelden GL, et al. The use of computed tomography for radiation therapy treatment planning. *Radiology* 1975;117:613.
14. Sternick ES, Lane FW, Curran B. Comparison of computed tomography and conventional transverse axial tomography in radiotherapy treatment planning. *Radiology* 1977;124:835.
15. Fullerton GD, Sewchand W, Payne JT, et al. CT determination of parameters for inhomogeneity corrections in radiation therapy of the esophagus. *Radiology* 1978;124:167.
16. Parker RP, Hobday PA, Cassell KJ. The direct use of CT numbers in radiotherapy dosage calculations for inhomogeneous media. *Phys Med Biol* 1979;24:802.
17. Hobday P, Hodson NJ, Husband J, et al. Computed tomography applied to radiotherapy treatment planning: techniques and results. *Radiology* 1979;133:477.
18. Ragan DP, Perez CA. Efficacy of CT-assisted two-dimensional treatment planning: analysis of 45 patients. *Am J Roentgenol* 1978;131:75.
19. Goitein M. The utility of computed tomography in radiation therapy: an estimate of outcome. *Int J Radiat Oncol Biol Phys* 1979;5:1799.

20. Goitein M. Computed tomography in planning radiation therapy. *Int J Radiat Oncol Biol Phys* 1979;5:445.
21. Sontag MR, Cunningham JR. The equivalent tissue-air ratio method for making absorbed dose calculations in a heterogeneous medium. *Radiology* 1978;129:787.
22. Hogstrom KR, Mills MD, Almond PR. Electron beam dose calculations. *Phys Med Biol* 1981;26:445.
23. Cassell KJ, Hobday PA, Parker RP. The implementation of a generalized Batho inhomogeneity correction for radiotherapy planning with direct use of CT numbers. *Phys Med Biol* 1981;26:825.
24. Ling CC, Rogers CC, Morton RJ, eds. *Computed tomography in radiation therapy.* New York: Raven Press, 1983.
25. Carson PL, Wenzel WW, Hendee WR. Ultrasound imaging as an aid to cancer therapy—I. *Int J Radiat Oncol Biol Phys* 1975;1:119.
26. Carson PL, Wenzel WW, Avery P, et al. Ultrasound imaging as an aid to cancer therapy—II. *Int J Radiat Oncol Biol Phys* 1976;1:335.
27. Green D, Nelson KA, Gibb R. The use of a linear accelerator "simulator" in radiotherapy. *Br J Radiol* 1964;37:394.
28. Ovadia J, Karzmark CJ, Hendrickson FR. *Radiation therapy simulation and transverse tomography: apparatus bibliography and tumor localization.* Houston: American Association of Physicists in Medicine Radiological Physics Center, 1971.
29. Karzmark CJ, Rust DC. Radiotherapy simulators and automation. *Radiology* 1972;105:157.
30. Bomford CK, Craig LM, Hanna FA, et al. Treatment simulators. Report no. 10. London: British Institute of Radiology, 1976.
31. McCullough EC, Earl JD. The selection, acceptance testing, and quality control of radiotherapy treatment simulators. *Radiology* 1979;131:221.
32. Droege RT, Bjärngard BE. Metal screen-film detector MTF at megavoltage x-ray energies. *Med Phys* 1979;6:515.
33. Ellis F, Lescrenier C. Combined compensation for contours and heterogeneity. *Radiology* 1973;106:191.
34. Baily NA, Horn RA, Kampp TD. Fluoroscopic visualization of megavoltage therapeutic x-ray beams. *Int J Radiat Oncol Biol Phys* 1980;6:935.
35. Leong J. Use of digital fluoroscopy as an on-line verification device in radiation therapy. *Phys Med Biol* 1986;31:985.
36. Shalev S, Lee T, Leszczynski K, et al. Video techniques for on-line portal imaging. *Comput Med Imaging Graph* 1989;13:217.
37. Visser AG, Huizenga H, Althof VGM, et al. Performance of a prototype fluoroscopic imaging system. *Int J Radiat Oncol Biol Phys* 1990;18:43.
38. Wong JW, Binns WR, Cheng AY, et al. On-line radiotherapy imaging with an array of fiber-optic image reducers. *Int J Radiat Oncol Biol Phys* 1990;18:1477.
39. Van Herk M, Meertens H. A matrix ionization chamber imaging device for on-line patient set up verification during radiotherapy. *Radiother Oncol* 1988;11:369.
40. Meertens H, Van Herk M, Bijhold J, et al. First clinical experience with a newly developed electronic portal imaging device. *Int J Radiat Oncol Biol Phys* 1990;18:1173.
41. Boyer AL, Antnuk L, Fenster A, et al. A review of electronic portal imaging devices (EPIDs). *Med Phys* 1992;19:1.
42. International Commission on Radiation Units and Measurements (ICRU). Determination of absorbed dose in a patient irradiated by beams of x or gamma rays in radiotherapy procedures. Report No. 24. Washington, DC: United States National Bureau of Standards, 1976.
43. Batho HF. Lung corrections in cobalt 60 beam therapy. *J Can Assn Radiol* 1964;15:79.
44. Young MEJ, Gaylord JD. Experimental tests of corrections for tissue inhomogeneities in radiotherapy. *Br J Radiol* 1970;43:349.
45. Sontag MR, Cunningham JR. Corrections to absorbed dose calculations for tissue inhomogeneities. *Med Phys* 1977;4:431.
46. Cunningham JR. Scatter-air ratios. *Phys Med Biol* 1972;17:42.
47. Wong JW, Henkelman RM. A new approach to CT pixel-based photon dose calculation in heterogeneous media. *Med Phys* 1983;10:199.
48. Krippner K, Wong JW, Harms WB, et al. The use of an array processor for the delta volume dose computation algorithm. In: Proceedings of the 9th international conference on the use of computers in radiation therapy, Scheveningen, The Netherlands. North Holland: The Netherlands, 1987:533.
49. Mackie TR, Scrimger JW, Battista JJ. A convolution method of calculating dose for 15-MV x-rays. *Med Phys* 1985;12:188.
50. Mohan R, Chui C, Lidofsky L. Differential pencil beam dose computation model for photons. *Med Phys* 1986;13:64.
51. Greene D, Stewart JR. Isodose curves in non-uniform phantoms. *Br J Radiol* 1965;38:378.
52. Sundblom I. Dose planning for irradiation of thorax with cobalt in fixed beam therapy. *Acta Radiol* 1965;3:342.

53. Tang WL, Khan FM, Gerbi BJ. Validity of lung correction algorithms. *Med Phys* 1986;13:683.

54. McDonald SC, Keller BE, Rubin P. Method for calculating dose when lung tissue lies in the treatment field. *Med Phys* 1976;3:210.

55. Spires SW. Dosage in irradiated soft tissue and bone. *Br J Radiol* 1951;24:365.

56. International Commission on Radiation Units and Measurements (ICRU). Clinical dosimetry. Report No. 10d. Washington, DC: United States Bureau of Standards, 1963.

57. Johns HE, Cunningham JR. *The physics of radiology,* 2nd ed. Springfield, IL: Charles C Thomas, 1969:455.

58. Das IJ, Khan FM. Backscatter dose perturbation at high atomic number interfaces in megavoltage photon beams. *Med Phys* 1989;16:367.

59. Werner BL, Das IJ, Khan FM, et al. Dose perturbation at interfaces in photon beams. *Med Phys* 1987;14:585.

60. Leung PMK, Seaman B, Robinson P. Low-density inhomogeneity corrections for 22-MeV x-ray therapy. *Radiology* 1970;94:449.

61. Kornelson RO, Young MEJ. Changes in the dose-profile of a 10 MV x-ray beam within and beyond low density material. *Med Phys* 1982;9:114.

62. Epp ER, Lougheed MN, McKay JW. Ionization buildup in upper respiratory air passages during teletherapy units with cobalt 60 radiation. *Br J Radiol* 1958;31:361.

63. Epp ER, Boyer AL, Doppke KP. Underdosing of lesions resulting from lack of electronic equilibrium in upper respiratory air cavities irradiated by 10 MV x-ray beam. *Int J Radiat Oncol Biol Phys* 1977;2:613.

64. Ellis F, Hall EJ, Oliver R. A compensator for variations in tissue thickness for high energy beam. *Br J Radiol* 1959;32:421.

65. Cohen M, Burns JE, Sear R. Physical aspects of cobalt 60 teletherapy using wedge filters. II. Dosimetric considerations. *Acta Radiol* 1960;53:486.

66. Hall EJ, Oliver R. The use of standard isodose distributions with high energy radiation beams—the accuracy of a compensator technique in correcting for body contours. *Br J Radiol* 1961;34:43.

67. Sundblom I. Individually designed filters in cobalt-60 teletherapy. *Acta Radiol Ther Phys Biol* 1964;2:189.

68. Van De Geijn J. The construction of individualized intensity modifying filters in cobalt 60 teletherapy. *Br J Radiol* 1965;38:865.

69. Khan FM, Moore VC, Burns DJ. The construction of compensators for cobalt teletherapy. *Radiology* 1970;96:187.

70. Sewchand W, Bautro N, Scott RM. Basic data of tissue-equivalent compensators for 4 MV x-rays. *Int J Radiat Oncol Biol Phys* 1980;6:327.

71. Khan FM, Moore VC, Burns DJ. An apparatus for the construction of irregular surface compensators for use in radiotherapy. *Radiology* 1968;90:593.

72. Beck GG, McGonnagle WJ, Sullivan CA. Use of Styrofoam block cutter to make tissue-equivalent compensators. *Radiology* 1971;100:694.

73. Boge RJ, Edland RW, Matthes DC. Tissue compensators for megavoltage radiotherapy fabricated from hollowed Styrofoam filled with wax. *Radiology* 1974;111:193.

74. Khan FM, Sewchand W, Williamson JF. Unpublished data.

75. Henderson SD, Purdy JA, Gerber RL, et al. Dosimetry considerations for a Lipowitz metal tissue compensator system. *Int J Radiat Oncol Biol Phys* 1987;13:1107.

76. Boyer AL, Goitein M. Simulator mounted Moiré topography camera for constructing compensator filters. *Med Phys* 1980;7:19.

77. Reinstein LE. New approaches to tissue compensation in radiation oncology. In: Purdy JA, ed. *Advances in radiation oncology physics.* Medical Physics Monograph No. 19. Woodbury, NY: American Institute of Physics, Inc., 1992:535.

78. Khan FM, Williamson JF, Sewchand W, et al. Basic data for dosage calculation and compensation. *Int J Radiat Oncol Biol Phys* 1980;6:745.

79. Leung PMK, Van Dyke J, Robins J. A method for large irregular field compensation. *Br J Radiol* 1974;47:805.

80. Boge RJ, Tolbert DD, Edland RW. Accessory beam flattening filter for the Varian Clinac-4 linear accelerator. *Radiology* 1975;115:475.

81. Chung-Bin A, Kartha P, Wachtor T, et al. Development and experience in computer monitoring and the verification of daily patient treatment parameters. In: Sternick ES, ed. Proceedings of the 5th international conference on use of computers in radiation therapy. Hanover, NH: University Press of New England, 1976:551.

82. Haus A, Marks J. Detection and evaluation of localization errors in patient radiation therapy. *Invest Radiol* 1973;8:384.

83. Kartha PKI, Chung-Bin A, Wachtor T, et al. Accuracy in patient set-up and its consequence in dosimetry. *Med Phys* 1975;2:331.

84. Williamson TJ. Improving the reproducibility of lateral therapy portal placement. *Int J Radiat Oncol Biol Phys* 1979;5:407.

85. Verhey LJ, Goitein M, McNulty P, et al. Precise positioning of patients for radiation therapy. *Int J Radiat Oncol Biol Phys* 1982;8:289.
86. Hendrickson FR. Precision in radiation oncology. *Int J Radiat Oncol Biol Phys* 1981;8:311.
87. Reinstein LE. Patient positioning and immobilization. In: Khan FM, Potish RA eds. *Treatment planning in radiation oncology.* Baltimore: Williams & Wilkins, 1998:55–88.
88. Huaskins LA, Thomson RW. Patient positioning device for external-beam radiation therapy of the head and neck. *Radiology* 1973;106:706.

TREATMENT PLANNING III: FIELD SHAPING, SKIN DOSE, AND FIELD SEPARATION

Shielding of vital organs within a radiation field is one of the major concerns of radiation therapy. Considerable time and effort are spent in shaping fields not only to protect critical organs but also to avoid unnecessary irradiation of the surrounding normal tissue. Attendant to this problem is its effect on skin dose and the buildup of dose in the subcutaneous tissue. Skin sparing is an important property of megavoltage photon beams, and every effort should be directed to maintaining this effect when irradiating normal skin.

Another problem frequently encountered in radiation therapy is the matching of adjacent fields. This situation arises when radiation fields available with the equipment are not large enough to encompass the entire target volume. In some cases, the target volume is divided into two parts so treatment to the second part does not commence until the treatment course to the first part has been completed. Such a scheme is designed to avoid toxicity due to irradiating an excessive volume of tissue. Multiple adjacent fields are also used when tumor distribution or patient anatomy does not allow coplanar fields (fields with central axes in the same plane). The main problem with these techniques is the possibility of extreme dose inhomogeneity in the junctional region. Because radiation beams are divergent, adjacent fields can overlap at depth and give rise to regions of excessive dose or hot spots. Overlaps can be avoided by separating the fields, but this in turn can give rise to areas of reduced dose or "cold spots."

This chapter on treatment planning focuses on the above problems and discusses their possible solutions.

13.1. FIELD BLOCKS

The shaping of treatment fields is primarily dictated by tumor distribution—local extensions as well as regional metastases. Not only should the dose to vital organs not exceed their tolerance but the dose to normal tissue, in general, should be minimized. As long as the target volume includes, with adequate margins, the demonstrated tumor as well as its presumed occult spread, significant irradiation of the normal tissue outside this volume must be avoided as much as possible. These restrictions can give rise to complex field shapes, which require intricate blocking.

The frequency and complexity of field shaping vary from institution to institution. However, if complex techniques involving elaborate blocking are used often, it is necessary to establish a rational system of field shaping.

A. Block Thickness

Shielding blocks are most commonly made of lead. The thickness of lead required to provide adequate protection of the shielded areas depends on the beam quality and the allowed transmission through the block. A primary beam transmission of 5% through the block is considered acceptable for most clinical situations. If n is the number of half-value layers to achieve this transmission,

$$\frac{1}{2^n} = 0.05$$

or

$$2^n = \frac{1}{0.05} = 20$$

or

$$n \log 2 = \log 20$$

or

$$n = \frac{\log 20}{\log 2} = 4.32$$

Thus a thickness of lead between 4.5 and 5.0 half-value layers would give less than 5% primary beam transmission and is, therefore, recommended for most clinical shielding.

Shielding against primary radiation for superficial and orthovoltage beams is readily accomplished by thin sheets of lead that can be placed or molded on to the skin surface. However, as the beam energy increases to the megavoltage range, the thickness of lead required for shielding increases substantially. The lead blocks are then placed above the patient supported in the beam on a transparent plastic tray, called the *shadow tray*. Table 13.1 gives the recommended lead shield thicknesses for various quality beams.

Although the primary beam transmission can be reduced further by using extra thick blocks, the reduction in dose in the shielded region may not be that significant due to the predominance of scattered radiation from the adjoining open areas of the field.

B. Block Divergence

Ideally, the blocks should be shaped or tapered so that their sides follow the geometric divergence of the beam. This minimizes the block transmission penumbra (partial transmission of the beam at the edges of the block). However, divergent blocks offer little advantage for beams with large geometric penumbra. For example, in the case of ^{60}Co, the sharpness of the beam cutoff at the block edge is not significantly improved by using divergent blocks. Also, for some clinical situations this sharpness is not critical or worth the time required for making divergent blocks, which have to be invariably custom designed for a given treatment set-up. Therefore, most institutions keep a stock of straight-cut blocks of various shapes and dimensions.

TABLE 13.1. RECOMMENDED MINIMUM THICKNESS OF LEAD FOR SHIELDING[a]

Beam Quality	Required Lead Thickness
1.0 mm Al HVL	0.2 mm
2.0 mm Al HVL	0.3 mm
3.0 mm Al HVL	0.4 mm
1.0 mm Cu HVL	1.0 mm
3.0 mm Cu HVL	2.0 mm
4.0 mm Cu HVL	2.5 mm
^{137}Cs	3.0 cm
^{60}Co	5.0 cm
4 MV	6.0 cm
6 MV	6.5 cm
10 MV	7.0 cm
25 MV	7.0 cm

HVL, half-value layer.
[a]Approximate values to give ≤5% primary transmission.

Divergent blocks are most suited for beams having small focal spots. Because the sides of these blocks follow beam divergence, one can reduce the lateral dimensions by designing the shields for smaller source-to-block distances without increasing the block transmission penumbra.

13.2. FIELD SHAPING

A. Custom Blocking

Although a number of systems have been used for field shaping (1–8), the one introduced by Powers et al. (1) is most commonly used in radiation therapy. This system uses a low melting point alloy, Lipowitz metal (brand name, Cerrobend), which has a density of 9.4 g/cm^3 at 20°C (~83% of lead density). This material consists of 50.0% bismuth, 26.7% lead, 13.3% tin, and 10.0% cadmium (1). The main advantage of Cerrobend over lead is that it melts at about 70°C (compared with 327°C for lead) and, therefore, can be easily cast into any shape. At room temperature, it is harder than lead.

The minimum thickness of Cerrobend blocks required for blocking may be calculated from Table 13.1 using its density ratio relative to lead (e.g., multiply lead thickness by 1.21). In the megavoltage range of photon beams, the most commonly used thickness is 7.5 cm, which is equivalent to about 6 cm of pure lead.

The procedure for constructing Cerrobend blocks starts with a simulator radiograph or a port film on which the radiotherapist draws the outline of the treatment field indicating areas to be shielded. The film is then used to construct divergent cavities in a Styrofoam block that are used to cast Cerrobend blocks. Figure 13.1 shows a Styrofoam-cutting device that consists of an electrically heated wire which pivots about a point simulating the source or the x-ray target. The film, the Styrofoam block, and the wire apparatus are so adjusted

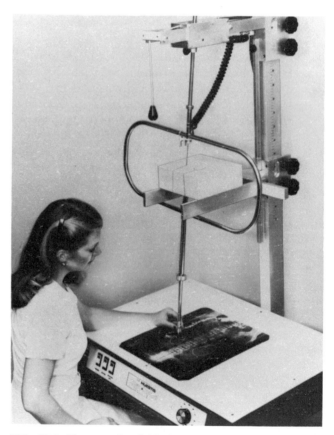

FIG. 13.1. Photograph of block cutter. (Courtesy of Huestis Machine Corp., Bristol, RI.)

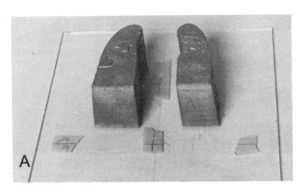

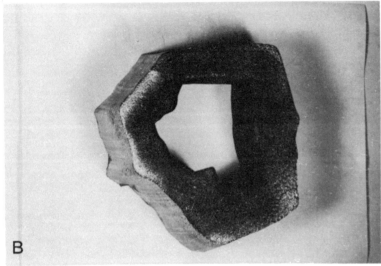

FIG. 13.2. A: Cerrobend blocks for lung shielding. **B:** Custom blocks for head and neck.

that the actual treatment geometry (same source to film and source to block distances) is obtained. The lower end of the wire traces the outline on the film.

If "positive" blocks such as lung blocks are to be made, cavities are cut in the Styrofoam with the heated segment of the wire and subsequently filled with melted Cerrobend. If a "negative" block with central area open and peripheral areas blocked is desired, an inner cut is first made to outline the field opening. An outer rectangular cut is then made to define the collimator field with 1- to 2-cm margin. The three Styrofoam pieces thus made are placed on a Lucite plate and carefully aligned relative to the central axis. The intermediate piece, corresponding to the areas to be shielded, is then removed and Cerrobend is poured into the cavity.

It is important that the Cerrobend is poured slowly to prevent formation of air bubbles. Also, the Styrofoam block should be pressed tightly against a rubber pad at the bottom to avoid leakage of the liquid metal. The inside walls of the cavity may be sprayed with silicone for easy release of the Styrofoam pieces from the block.

The blocks can be mounted on a Lucite plate or blocking tray, which is premarked with the central axis cross hairs. Blocks can also be placed on a template made on a clear film by tracing the outline of the field at the shadow tray position while the port film outline is placed at the distance at which the radiograph was taken.

Figure 13.2 shows examples of Cerrobend blocks, one constructed for shielding lungs and the other for a head and neck field.

B. Independent Jaws

Asymmetric fields are sometimes used to block off a part of the field without changing the position of the isocenter. Although blocking is often used to generate irregular field shapes, rectangular blocking can be easily done by independently movable collimators, or jaws. This feature is very convenient when matching fields or *beam splitting*. In the latter case, the beam is blocked off at the central axis to remove divergence. Whereas half-beam blocks have been used as beam splitters in the past, this can now be done simply by moving in the independent jaws.

Most modern machines are equipped with independently movable jaws. Some machines have one independent jaw, others have two independent pairs, and some have all four jaws as independent. Operationally, the independent jaw option is interlocked to avoid errors in the setting of symmetric fields, in which case the opposite jaws open or close symmetrically.

One of the effects of asymmetric collimation is the change in the physical penumbra (defined in section 11.1) and the tilt of the isodose curves toward the blocked edge (Fig. 13.3). This effect is simply the result of blocking, which eliminates photon and electron scatter from the blocked portion of the field, thereby reducing the dose near the edge. The same effect would occur on the isodose curves if the blocking were done with a lead or Cerrobend block on a tray.

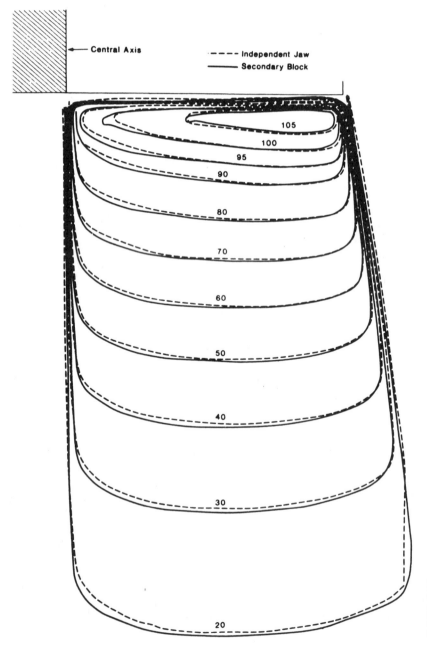

FIG. 13.3. Comparison of isodose distribution with half the beam blocked by an independent jaw versus a block on a tray. Notice close agreement as well as the tilt of the isodose curves toward the blocked edge.

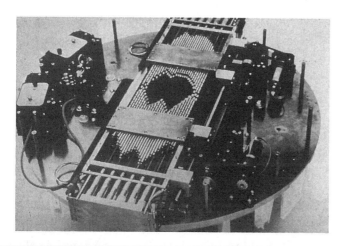

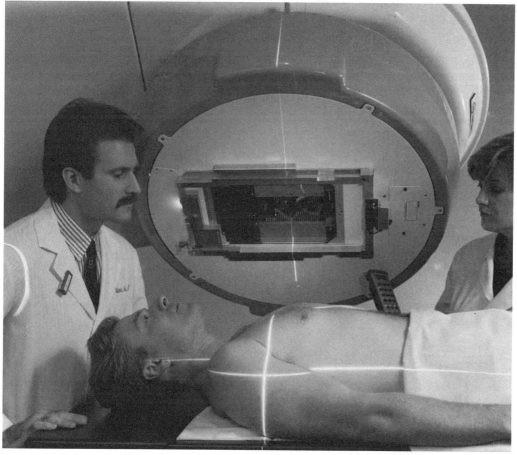

FIG. 13.4. Varian multileaf collimator: (*top*) attached to accelerator and (*bottom*) with an end-on view. (Courtesy of Varian Associates, Palo Alto, CA.)

When asymmetric fields are used, special considerations must be given to the beam flatness and the dosimetric parameters used to calculate monitor units. Khan et al. (9) have proposed a system of dose calculation for fields generated by asymmetric collimators, which was discussed in Chapter 10.

C. Multileaf Collimators

A multileaf collimator (MLC) for photon beams consists of a large number of collimating blocks or leaves that can be driven automatically, independent of each other, to generate a field of any shape (Fig. 13.4). Typical MLC systems consist of 80 leaves (40 pairs) or more. The individual leaf has a width of 1cm or less as projected at the isocenter. The leaves are made of tungsten alloy ($\rho = 17.0$ to 18.5 g/cm^3) and have thickness along the beam direction ranging from 6 cm to 7.5 cm, depending on the type of accelerator. The leaf thickness is sufficient to provide primary x-ray transmission through the leaves of less than 2% (compared with about 1% for jaws and 3.5% for Cerrobend blocks). The interleaf (between sides) transmission is usually less than 3%. The primary beam transmission may be further minimized by combining jaws with the MLC in shielding areas outside the MLC field opening.

Some MLC systems have double-focused leaves, that is, the leaves form a cone of irregular cross-section diverging from the source position and move on a spherical shell centered at the source. The rationale behind a double-focused MLC is to provide a sharp beam cutoff at the edge. However, for high-energy beams this objective is achieved only to a limited extent, because the dose falloff at the edge is largely determined by scattered photons and electrons. Because double-focused MLCs are difficult to manufacture, some systems have been designed with rounded leaf edges and directions of travel perpendicular to the central ray. The purpose of rounded edges is to provide constant beam transmission through a leaf edge, regardless of its position in the field.

An important consideration in the use of MLCs for stationary fields is the conformity between the planned field boundary, which is continuous, and the jagged stepwise boundary created by the MLC. The degree of conformity between the two depends not only on the projected leaf width but also on the shape of the target volume and the angle of rotation of the collimator. Optimization of MLC rotation and setting has been discussed by Brahme (10). His analysis shows that the best orientation of the collimator is when the direction of motion of the leaves is parallel with the direction in which the target volume has the smallest cross-section.

The physical penumbra (section 11.1) with MLC is larger than that produced by the collimator jaws or the Cerrobend blocks (Fig. 13.5). This is usually not a serious drawback except for the treatment of small fields or when blocking is required close to critical structures. Also, jaggedness of the field edges makes it difficult to match adjacent fields.

The use of MLC in blocking and field shaping is ideally suited for treatments requiring large numbers of multiple fields because of automation of the procedure thus resulting in a significant reduction of set-up time. MLC can practically eliminate the use of Cerrobend blocking except for shaping small fields or "island" blocking in which an area within the open portion of the fields needs to be blocked.

The importance of MLC is not just the replacement of Cerrobend blocking. The greater impact of this technology is in the automation of field shaping and modulation of beam intensity. Modern radiotherapy techniques such as 3-D conformal radiation therapy (Chapter 19) and intensity-modulated radiation therapy (Chapter 20) are dependent on the dynamically controlled MLC. Other applications include dynamic wedges and electronic compensation. For further details on MLC designs and applications, the reader is referred to a review by Boyer (11).

13.3. SKIN DOSE

When a patient is treated with a megavoltage beam, the surface dose or skin dose can be substantially lower than the maximum dose that occurs in the subcutaneous tissues. In contrast to lower energy beams (e.g., superficial and orthovoltage x-rays), which give rise to maximum ionization at or close to the skin surface, the megavoltage beams produce an initial electronic buildup with depth, resulting in a reduced dose at the surface and maximum dose at the equilibrium depth. This phenomenon of dose buildup was discussed in Chapter 9.

Skin sparing is one of the most desirable features of high-energy photon beams. However, this effect may be reduced or even lost if the beam is excessively contaminated

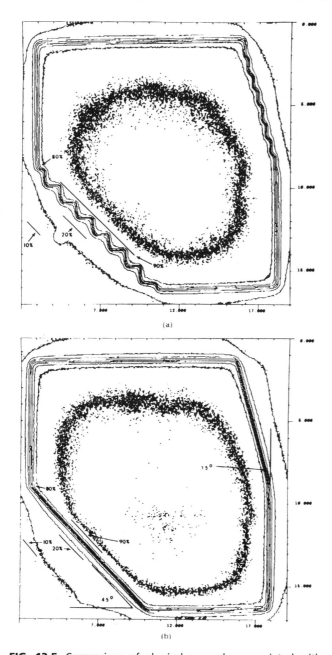

FIG. 13.5. Comparison of physical penumbra associated with MLC **(A)** and cerrobend blocks **(B)**. Field size 15 × 15, depth 10 cm, and energy 6MV. Dose distribution normalized to 100% at central axis. (From Galvin JM, et al. Evaluation of multileaf collimator design for a photon beam. *Int J Radiat Oncol Biol Phys* 1992;23:789–801, with permission.)

with secondary electrons. In the following sections, the sources of this contamination and the methods used to reduce it will be discussed.

A. Electron Contamination of Photon Beams

Surface dose is the result of electron contamination of the incident beam as well as the backscattered radiation (both electrons and photons) from the medium. It is well-known that all x-ray and γ ray beams used in radiation therapy are contaminated with secondary electrons. These electrons arise from photon interactions in the air, in the collimator, and in any other scattering material in the path of the beam. If a shadow tray is used to support beam-shaping blocks, secondary electrons produced by photon interactions in the tray and the air column between the tray and the skin surface significantly increase skin dose. The shadow tray is usually thick enough to absorb most of the electrons incident on the tray.

There has been a controversy as to the relative contribution of secondary electrons vs. low energy scattered photons to the dose in the build-up region. It is well known that as the field size increases, the depth dose in the build-up region increases resulting in a shift in the depth of maximum dose, d_{max}, to increasingly shallower depths (12–14). Specifically, the cause of the d_{max} shift with field size has been studied by several investigators (15–17). Current evidence favors the hypothesis that the effect is predominantly caused by the secondary electrons.

B. Measurement of Dose Distribution in the Build-up Region

Because of the steep dose gradient in the build-up region, the size of the dosimeter along the beam direction should be as small as possible. Extrapolation chambers (see Chapter 6) are the instruments of choice for these measurements. However, few institutions have these instruments available. Instead, fixed-separation plane-parallel ionization chambers are most commonly used for this purpose. Although these chambers are very suitable for measurements in regions of severe dose gradients, their response is dependent, in a complex manner, on their design. Several papers have discussed the inaccuracies in the measurement of dose in the build-up region when using fixed-separation plane-parallel chambers. These inaccuracies arise primarily as a result of electron scattering from the side walls of the chamber (18–20). These may be minimized by using a smaller plate separation and wider guard ring in the design of the chamber. Furthermore, the chambers may exhibit a significant polarity effect in the build-up region, which may be corrected by averaging the readings obtained with the positive and negative polarities. Gerbi and Khan (21) have studied several commercially available plane-parallel chambers and found that they overrespond in the build-up region. The errors were more severe at the surface and for the lower beam energies (e.g., ^{60}Co). The magnitude of overresponse at the surface for a ^{60}Co beam ranged from 9% to 20% for the chambers studied.

Thin layers (<0.5 mm) of thermoluminescent dosimeter (TLD) material can also be used for measuring dose distribution in the build-up region. The TLD phosphor (e.g., LiF) can be in the form of chips, crystals embedded in plastic, or powder layers (18,22,23). The surface dose may be obtained by extrapolating the depth dose distribution curve to zero depth. In vivo measurements of surface dose can also be made by placing thin TLD chips directly on the skin surface. Such measurements are useful in checking dosimetry if an unacceptable degree of skin reaction develops.

C. Skin Sparing as a Function of Photon Energy

Studies have shown that the dose distribution in the build-up region depends on many variables such as beam energy, SSD, field size, and configuration of secondary blocking tray (18,22–26). Table 13.2 gives values for different energies. These data are presented here as an example and should not be considered universal for all machines, especially for depths less than 2 mm. Reasonable agreement between different machines has been shown to exist for greater depths.

Examination of Table 13.2 would also indicate that for all energies the dose increases rapidly within the first few millimeters and then gradually achieves its maximum value at the depth of peak dose. For example, in the case of 4 MV, the percent depth dose increases from 14% to 74% in the first 2 mm, reaches 94% at a 5-mm depth and achieves its maximum value at a 10-mm depth. A practical application of this phenomenon is the case in which build-up bolus (Chapter 12) is used intentionally to maximize the dose on the

TABLE 13.2. BUILD-UP DOSE DISTRIBUTION IN POLYSTYRENE FOR A 10 × 10 cm FIELD

Depth (mm)	^{60}Co 80 cm[a]	4 MV 80 cm[a]	10 MV 100 cm[b]	25 MV 100 cm[a]
0	18.0	14.0	12.0	17.0
1	70.5	57.0	30.0	28.0
2	90.0	74.0	46.0	39.5
3	98.0	84.0	55.0	47.0
4	100.0	90.0	63.0	54.5
5	100.0	94.0	72.0	60.5
6	—	96.5	76.0	66.0
8	—	99.5	84.0	73.0
10	—	100.0	91.0	79.0
15	—	—	97.0	88.5
20	—	—	98.0	95.0
25	—	—	100.0	99.0
30	—	—	—	100.0

[a]Data from Velkley DE, Manson DS, Purdy JA, Oliver GD. Buildup region of megavoltage photon radiation sources. *Med Phys* 1975;2:14.
[b]Data from Khan FM, Moore VC, Levitt SH. Effect of various atomic number absorbers on skin dose for 10-MeV x-rays. *Radiology* 1973;109:209.

skin (e.g., covering a scar with a strip of bolus). A tissue equivalent bolus of 5- to 6-mm of thickness is usually adequate for 4 MV. Thus the thickness of bolus required to achieve 90% to 95% build-up of dose is substantially less than the depth of maximum dose.

Although the skin sparing depends on many conditions, as mentioned earlier, the effect, in general, becomes more and more pronounced as photon energy increases. For higher-energy beams, significant sparing can be achieved not only for the skin surface but also for the subcutaneous tissues.

D. Effect of Absorber-skin Distance

The electron contamination with no absorber placed in the beam is mainly caused by the secondary electron emission from the collimator (including source, flattening filter, and air). When an absorber of thickness greater than the range of secondary electrons (equilibrium thickness) is introduced in the beam, the collimator electrons are almost completely absorbed but the absorber itself becomes the principal source of electron contamination of the beam. By increasing the distance between the tray and the surface, the electron fluence incident on the skin is reduced because of divergence as well as absorption and scattering of electrons in the air. Thus skin sparing is enhanced by placing the shadow tray farther away from the skin. In the case of a ^{60}Co γ ray beam, it has been shown (27,28) that for small fields an air gap of 15 to 20 cm between the scatterer and the skin is adequate to keep the skin dose to an acceptable level (<50% of the D_{max}). This has been found to be true for higher-energy beams as well (17).

Figure 13.6 shows the effect on dose distribution in the build-up region as a Lucite shadow tray is placed in the beam at various distances from the phantom surface. Not only does the relative surface dose increase with decreasing tray-to-surface distance but the point of maximum dose buildup moves closer to the surface.

Figure 13.6 also illustrates the principle of what is known as the "beam spoiler." A low atomic number absorber, such as a Lucite shadow tray, placed at an appropriate distance from the surface, can be used to modify the build-up curve. Doppke et al. (29) have discussed the treatment of certain head and neck cancers with 10-MV x-rays using a beam spoiler to increase the dose to the superficial neck nodes.

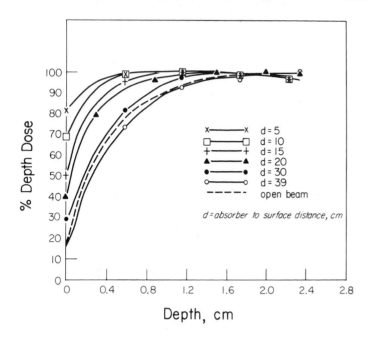

FIG. 13.6. Effect of Lucite shadow tray on dose buildup for 10-MV x-rays. Percent depth dose distribution is plotted for various tray-to-surface distances *(d)*. 10-MX x-rays, tray thickness = 1.5 g/cm², field size = 15 × 15 cm, SSD = 100 cm, and SDD = 50 cm. (From Khan FM, Moore VC, Levitt SH. Effect of various atomic number absorbers on skin dose for 10-MeV x-rays. *Radiology* 1973;109:209, with permission.)

E. Effect of Field Size

The relative skin dose depends strongly on field size. As the field dimensions are increased, the dose in the build-up region increases. This increase in dose is due to increased electron emission from the collimator and air. Figure 13.7 is a plot of relative surface dose as a function of field size for ^{60}Co, 4-MV, and 10-MV beams. These data show that skin sparing is significantly reduced for the larger field sizes.

Saylor and Quillin (24) have discussed the relative importance of field size and tray-to-skin distance for ^{60}Co γ rays. They have shown that the optimum skin sparing occurs for an *h/r* value of about 4, where *h* is the tray-to-surface distance and *r* is the radius of an

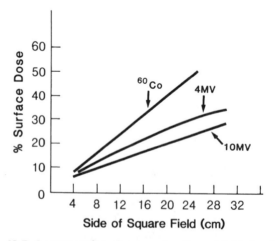

FIG. 13.7. Percent surface dose as a function of field size. ^{60}Co, Theratron 80, SSD = 80 cm, SDD = 59 cm. 4 MV, Clinac 4, SSD = 80 cm. 10 MV, LMR 13, SSD = 100 cm, SDD = 50 cm. ^{60}Co and 4-MV. (Data are from Velkley DE, Manson DJ, Purdy JA, et al. Buildup region of megavoltage photon radiation sources. *Med Phys* 1975;2:14. 10-MV data are from Khan FM, Moore VC, Levitt SH. Effect of various atomic number absorbers on skin dose for 10-MeV x-rays. *Radiology* 1973;109:209.)

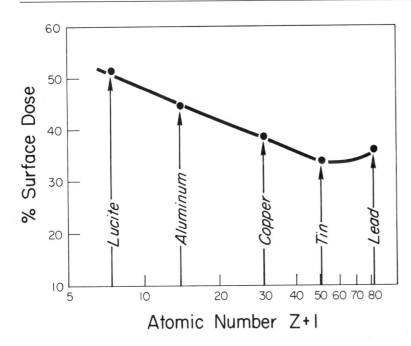

FIG. 13.8. Variation of percent surface dose with atomic number of absorber. Each absorber had a thickness of 1.5 g/cm² and was mounted underneath a Lucite shadow tray. 10-MV x-rays, field size = 15 × 15 cm and absorber-to-surface distance = 15 cm. (From Khan FM, Moore VC, Levitt SH. Effect of various atomic number absorbers on skin dose for ⁶⁰Co-MeV x-rays. *Radiology* 1973;109:209, with permission.)

equivalent circular field. This ratio can be easily achieved for the 5 × 5 cm field, because it requires a distance of 12 cm; however, for the 30 × 30 cm field, the corresponding absorber-surface distance is 67 cm, which is hardly possible for isocentric treatments.

When using large fields with a tray-to-skin distance of 15 to 20 cm, it becomes necessary to use *electron filters* to maintain the skin-sparing effect. These are discussed in the next section.

F. Electron Filters

The skin dose can be reduced by using γ ray absorbers of medium atomic number (Z in the range of 30–80). Such absorbers are commonly known as electron filters, because their introduction in the photon beam reduces the secondary electron scatter in the forward direction. Hine (30,31) studied the scattering of electrons produced by γ rays in materials of various atomic numbers. He showed that the medium atomic number absorbers give less electron scatter in the forward direction than either the low or the very high Z materials. Khan (22) and Saylor and Quillin (24) applied the results of Hine's study to the design of electron filters for the purpose of improving skin dose for ⁶⁰Co teletherapy. Later it was shown that such filters not only reduce the surface dose but also improve the build-up characteristics of large fields (32).

Figure 13.8 is a plot of relative surface dose as a function of log ($Z + 1$). These data are plotted in this manner to show agreement with the theoretical relationship discussed by Hine (30,31). As Z increases, the surface dose falls to a shallow minimum due to increased electron scattering in the absorbers. Further increases in Z result in increased surface dose due to increased production of photoelectrons and electron pairs in addition to the Compton electrons. The minimum occurs at about $Z = 50$, which is the atomic number of tin. These results qualitatively agree with those obtained for ⁶⁰Co γ rays (24,30,31).

Effectiveness of tin in reducing skin dose is demonstrated in Fig. 13.9. Greater reduction is possible by increasing filter-skin distance as discussed previously.

To preserve the light field, Saylor and Quillin (24) have suggested the use of leaded glass as an electron filter. However, breakability of leaded glass may pose a serious problem. We have used a tin sheet mounted on a pressed wood sheet that could be slipped under the Plexiglas tray at the end of the treatment set-up. In this arrangement, the tin filter must face the patient surface.

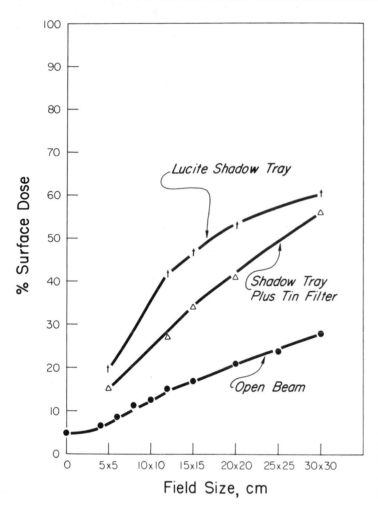

FIG. 13.9. Percent surface dose plotted as a function of field size for open beam, Lucite tray and tin filter mounted underneath the tray. 10-MV x-rays, tray-to-surface distance = 15 cm. (From Khan FM, Moore VC, Levitt SH. Effect of various atomic number absorbers on skin dose for 10-MeV x-rays. *Radiology* 1973;109:209, with permission.)

The thickness of an electron filter, in theory, should be at least equal to the maximum range of secondary electrons. For ^{60}Co, this thickness is about 0.5 g/cm^2 or 0.9 mm of tin (assuming $\rho_{tin} = 5.75$ g/cm^3). For higher energies, thicknesses less than the maximum range of electrons may be used for practical reasons.

G. Skin Sparing at Oblique Incidence

Skin dose has been shown to increase with increasing angle of incidence (33–39). Clinically, brisk reactions have been observed in patients when the beam is incident at near glancing angles. Jackson (35) has explained the increase in skin dose with increasing angle of incidence through the concept of electron range surface (ERS). The ERS is a 3-D representation of secondary electron range and distribution produced by a pencil beam of photons interacting with the medium (Fig. 13.10). Electrons generated inside the ERS volume will reach P and contribute to the dose there, whereas those generated outside, because of their inadequate range, make no contribution. The ERS for ^{60}Co γ rays is in the shape of an ellipsoid with axial dimensions of 5 × 2.4 mm (35). As illustrated in Fig. 13.10, the increase in the angle of incidence of the photon beam results in additional surface dose at P because of electron contribution from the portion of the ERS, which appears below the phantom surface (hatched curve). For tangential beam incidence, since half of the ERS is below the phantom surface, an upper estimate of the dose to the skin may be obtained by the following relationship (35,39):

$$\text{Percent skin dose} = \tfrac{1}{2}(100\% + \text{entrance dose}) \qquad (13.1)$$

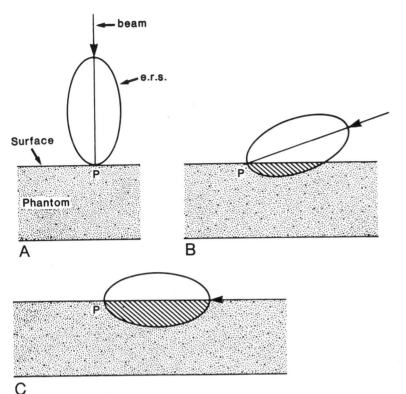

FIG. 13.10. The use of ERS to determine surface dose buildup at point *P*. **A:** Perpendicular beam incidence. **B:** Oblique beam incidence. **C:** Tangential beam incidence.

where the entrance dose represents the surface dose for normal incidence expressed as a percentage of D_{max}. The skin dose for other angles of incidence will lie between the values for the normal and the tangential incidence.

Gerbi et al. (40) did a systematic study of dose buildup for obliquely incident beams as a function of energy (6–24 MV), angle, depth, field size, and SSD. A quantity *obliquity factor* (OF) was defined as the dose at a point in phantom on central axis of a beam incident at angle $\theta°$, with respect to the perpendicular to the surface, divided by the dose at the same point and depth along central axis with the beam incident at angle 0°. The obliquity factor, therefore, represents dose enhancement due to beam obliquity for the same depth. Figure 13.11 shows that the obliquity factor at the surface increases with the increase in the angle of incidence, first gradually and then dramatically beyond 45 degrees. Thus the surface dose at large oblique angles can be significantly higher than at normal incidence. At tangential or grazing incidence, the surface dose approaches the value given by Equation 13.1.

Another important effect associated with oblique angles is that as the surface dose increases with the angle of incidence, the depth of maximum buildup decreases. The dose reaches its maximum value faster at glancing angles than at normal incidence. As a result, the dose build-up region is compressed into a more superficial region. Under these conditions, a high skin reaction becomes much more likely. Jackson (35) has discussed the possibility that if the sensitivity of the skin extends to the first or second millimeter below the surface, at glancing angles skin sparing is practically lost for the cobalt unit and greatly reduced for higher-energy beams.

13.4. SEPARATION OF ADJACENT FIELDS

Adjacent treatment fields are commonly employed in external beam radiation therapy, such as the "mantle" and "inverted-Y" fields for the treatment of Hodgkin's disease. In some cases, the adjacent fields are orthogonal, such as the craniospinal fields used in the

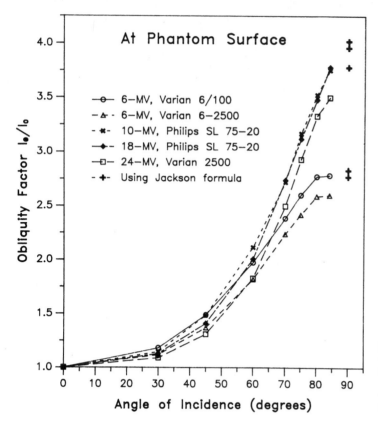

FIG. 13.11. Obliquity factor at the surface plotted as a function of beam angle for various energy beams. Jackson formula for tangential beam incidence is based on Equation 13.1. (From Gerbi BJ, Meigooni AS, Khan FM. Dose buildup for obliquely incident photon beams. *Med Phys* 1987;14:393, with permission.)

treatment of medulloblastoma. Another example is the irradiation of head and neck tumors when the lateral neck fields are placed adjacent to the anterior supraclavicular field. In each of these situations, there is a possibility of introducing very large dosage errors across the junction. Consequently, this region is at risk for tumor recurrence if it is underdosed or severe complications if it is overdosed.

The problem of adjacent fields has been extensively studied (41–53). A number of techniques have been devised to achieve dose uniformity in the field junction region. Some of the more commonly used techniques are illustrated in Fig. 13.12. Figure 13.12A has been described by Lance and Morgan (41); here fields are angled away from a common line of abutment to avoid overlap of the fields due to their geometric divergence. Figure 13.12B illustrates the methods in which the fields are separated at the skin surface to provide dose uniformity at a desired depth. The separation or gap between the fields is calculated on the basis of geometric divergence (53) or isodose curve matching (42,43). A technique using split beams (49,53) is illustrated in Fig. 13.12C. In this method, the beam is split along the plane containing the central axis by using a half-beam block or a beam-splitter, thus removing the geometric divergence of the beams at the split line. Figure 13.12D uses penumbra generators or spoilers (46,47). These lead wedges are custom designed to provide satisfactory dose distribution across the field junction.

In clinical practice, the fields are usually abutted at the surface if the tumor is superficial at the junction point. Care is however taken that the hot spot created due to the overlap of the beams at depth is clinically acceptable, considering the magnitude of the overdosage and the volume of the hot spot. In addition, the dosage received by a sensitive structure such as the spinal cord must not exceed its tolerance dose.

For the treatment of deep-seated lesions such as in the thorax, abdomen, and pelvis, the fields can be separated on the surface. It is assumed in this case that the cold spots created by the field separation are located superficially where there is no tumor.

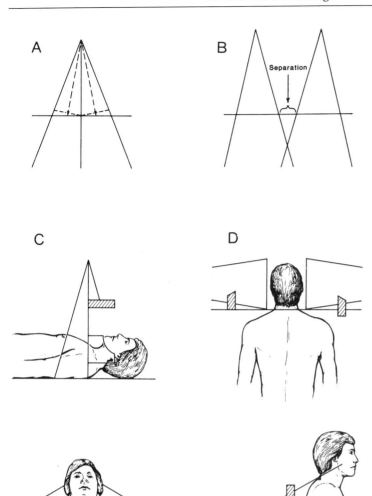

FIG. 13.12. Schematic representation of various techniques used for field matching. **A:** Angling the beams away from each other so that the two beams abut and are aligned vertically. **B:** Fields separated at the skin surface. The junction point is at depth where dose is uniform across the junction. **C:** Isocentric split beam technique for head and neck tumors. (Redrawn from Williamson TJ. A technique for matching orthogonal megavoltage fields. *Int J Radiat Oncol Biol Phys* 1979;5:111.) **D:** Craniospinal irradiation using penumbra generators. (Redrawn from Griffin TW, Schumacher D, Berry HC. A technique for cranial-spinal irradiation. *Br J Radiol* 1976;49:887.)

A. Methods of Field Separation

As stated earlier, the field separation can be accomplished geometrically or dosimetrically.

A.1. Geometric

If the geometric boundary of the field is defined by the 50% decrement line (line joining the points at depth where the dose is 50% of the central axis value at the same depth), the dose at the point of junction between the beams will add up to be 100%. The dose distribution laterally across the junction is more or less uniform, depending on the interfield scatter contribution and the penumbra characteristics of the beam.

If the two fields are incident from one side only and made to junction at a given depth (Fig. 13.13), the dose above the junction will be lower and below the junction higher than the junction dose. In the case of four fields when two fields are incident from one side and two from the parallel opposed direction (Fig. 13.14), the fields are usually made to junction at the midline depth (e.g., mantle and inverted Y fields). Such an arrangement

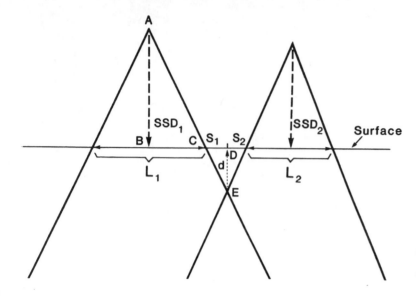

FIG. 13.13. Geometry of two adjacent beams, separated by a distance $S_1 + S_2$ on the surface and junctioning at depth d.

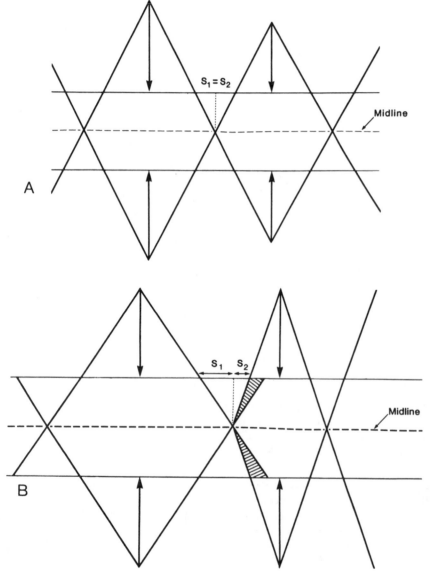

FIG. 13.14. Two pairs of parallel opposed fields. Adjacent fields are separated on the surface so that they all join at a point on the midline. **A:** Ideal geometry in which there is no three-field overlap. **B:** Arrangement in which there are two regions (shaded) of three-field overlap.

can be used to obtain almost a uniform distribution at the midline, but cold spots are created above and below the junction point.

Figure 13.13 shows the geometry of two adjacent beams that are allowed to join at a given depth d. Let L_1 and L_2 be the field lengths and SSD_1 and SSD_2 be the source-surface distances. Since triangles ABC and CDE are similar:

$$\frac{CD}{DE} = \frac{BC}{AB}$$

or

$$\frac{S_1}{d} = \frac{L_1}{2} \cdot \frac{1}{SSD_1} \tag{13.2}$$

giving

$$S_1 = \frac{1}{2} \cdot L_1 \cdot \frac{d}{SSD_1} \tag{13.3}$$

Similarly,

$$S_2 = \frac{1}{2} \cdot L_2 \cdot \frac{d}{SSD_2} \tag{13.4}$$

Thus the total separation S on the surface is given by:

$$S = S_1 + S_2 = \frac{1}{2} \cdot L_1 \cdot \frac{d}{SSD_1} + \frac{1}{2} \cdot L_2 \cdot \frac{d}{SSD_2} \tag{13.5}$$

Figure 13.14A shows an ideal geometry in which there is no overlap between a field and its adjacent opposing neighbor. The arrangement shown in Fig. 13.14B, on the other hand, creates regions of "three-field overlap" (shaded areas) where the bigger fields diverge into the opposing smaller fields. Consequently, the total dose there may exceed the central axis dose at the same depth. This will be of concern if a significant portion of the spinal cord is in the three-field overlap region.

The maximum length of three-field overlap (ΔS) occurs on the surface and is given by:

$$\Delta S = S_1 - S_2 \tag{13.6}$$

ΔS can be made equal to zero if:

$$\frac{L_1}{L_2} = \frac{SSD_1}{SSD_2} \tag{13.7}$$

Thus if the field lengths are different, the SSDs can be adjusted to eliminate the three-field overlap. Also, if the geometrically calculated gap ($S_1 + S_2$) is increased by ΔS, the three-field overlap is eliminated at the expense of a cold spot at the midline. As a compromise, one could increase the gap ($S_1 + S_2$) by an amount $\Delta S'$ just enough to eliminate the three-field overlap in a specific region such as the spinal cord. $\Delta S'$ can be calculated geometrically:

$$\Delta S' = \Delta S \cdot \frac{d' - d}{d} \tag{13.8}$$

where d' is the depth of the cord from the anterior surface and d is the midline depth.

The three-field overlap in Fig. 13.14B can also be avoided by using the same length and SSD for all the four fields and blocking the second pair (e.g., paraortic or inverted Y fields) caudally as needed. This technique is more convenient when the accelerator is equipped with asymmetric collimators that can be moved independently of each other.

Example 1

A patient is treated with parallel-opposed mantle and paraortic fields of lengths 30 and 15 cm, respectively. Calculate (a) the gap required on the surface for the beams to intersect at a midline depth of 10 cm and (b) the gap required to just eliminate the three-field overlap on the cord assumed to be at a depth of 15 cm from the anterior surface, given SSD = 100 cm for all the fields:

a. $S_1 = \frac{1}{2} \cdot L_1 \cdot \dfrac{d}{\mathrm{SSD}} = \frac{1}{2} \times 30 \times \dfrac{10}{100} = 1.5$ cm

$S_2 = \frac{1}{2} \cdot L_2 \cdot \dfrac{d}{\mathrm{SSD}} = \frac{1}{2} \times 15 \times \dfrac{10}{100} = 0.75$ cm

Total gap required $= 1.5 + 0.75 = 2.3$ cm

b. $\Delta S = S_1 - S_2 = 1.5 - 0.75 = 0.75$ cm

Length of three-field overlap on the cord:

$$\Delta S' = \Delta S \cdot \frac{d' - d}{d} = 0.75 \, \frac{15 - 10}{10} = 0.4 \text{ cm}$$

New gap required $= S_1 + S_2 + \Delta S' = 2.7$ cm

Although the previous geometric considerations provide useful criteria for field separation, one must be aware of their limitations. For example, the actual dose distribution may present a different picture than the predictions based on pure geometry of beam divergence. Patient positioning, beam alignment, field penumbra, and radiation scatter are all relevant factors that make this problem one of the most complex in radiation therapy.

Figure 13.15 shows the dose distribution for the cases discussed in Example 1. The expected three-field hot spot is seen in Fig. 13.15A when the beams intersect at the midline. This hot spot is eliminated when the gap is increased from 2.3 to 3.0 cm ($= S_1 + S_2 + \Delta S$) (Fig. 13.15B). However, the dose in the junction region has dropped considerably. Such a procedure will be justified only if the junction region is tumor free. Figure 13.15C shows the distribution when the gap is just enough to eliminate the three-field overlap at the cord, i.e., gap $= 2.7$ cm. This reduces the dose to the cord but also cools down the midjunction area by about 10%.

In practice, the choice between the options shown in Fig. 13.15 should be based on physical, clinical, and technical considerations. As usual, the guiding principles are that the tumor must receive adequate dosage and sensitive structures must not be treated beyond tolerance. If these conditions are not satisfied, other methods of field matching, discussed earlier in this chapter, may be considered.

A.2. Dosimetric

The separation of fields can be determined by optimizing the placement of fields on the contour so that the composite isodose distribution is uniform at the desired depth and the hot and cold spots are acceptable. The accuracy of this procedure depends on the accuracy of the individual field isodose curves especially in the penumbra region.

B. Orthogonal Field Junctions

Orthogonal fields denote an arrangement in which the central axes of the adjacent fields are orthogonal (i.e., perpendicular to each other). For example, orthogonal fields are used for the treatment of medulloblastoma in which the craniospinal irradiation is accomplished by lateral parallel-opposed brain fields coupled with a posterior spine field. Another common

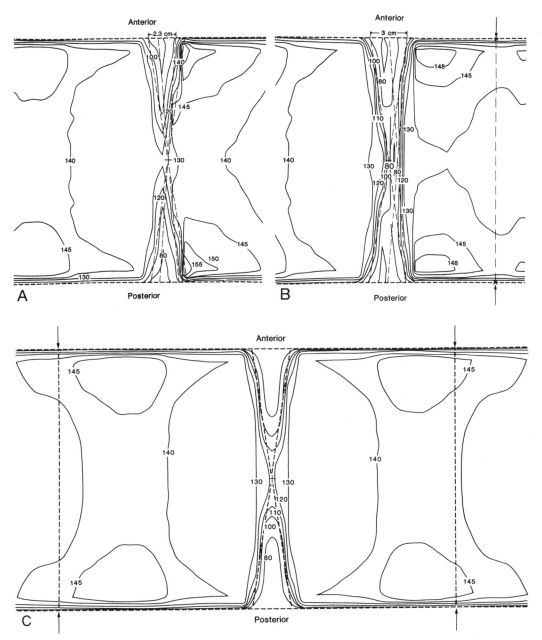

FIG. 13.15. Geometric separation of fields with all the four beams intersecting at midpoint. Adjacent field sizes: 30 × 30 cm and 15 × 15 cm; SSD = 100 cm; AP thickness = 20 cm; 4-MV x-ray beams. **A:** Field separation at surface = 2.3 cm. A three-field overlap exists in this case because the fields have different sizes but the same SSD. **B:** The adjacent field separation increased to 3 cm to eliminate three-field overlap on the surface. **C:** Field separation adjusted 2.7 cm to eliminate three-field overlap at the cord at 15 cm depth from anterior.

example is treatment of the neck by bilateral fields while an orthogonally adjacent anterior field is used to treat the supraclavicular areas.

The problem of matching orthogonal fields has been discussed by several investigators (48–52). For superficial tumors such as in the head and neck areas, it may be inadvisable to separate the adjacent fields unless the junction area is over a tumor-free region. If separation is not possible, one may use beam splitters and abut the fields along or close to their central axes (50). The matching line should be drawn each time before treatment to avoid overlap of the fields. If a sensitive structure such as the spinal cord exists in the junction region, one may additionally block an appropriate segment of the cord anteriorly or laterally, provided there is no tumor in the shielded region.

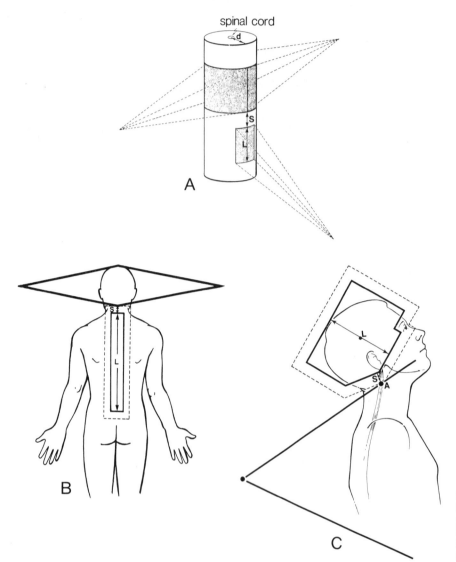

FIG. 13.16. A: A general diagram showing the separation of orthogonal fields. **B:** An example of orthogonal fields used for craniospinal irradiation. **C:** A lateral view of *B*, illustrating the geometry of orthogonal field separation.

As stated previously, field separation is possible for deep-seated tumors if there is no tumor in the superficial junction region. A geometrical method of orthogonal field separation has been described by Werner et al. (52). According to this method, one pair of opposing fields, defined by the collimating light, is allowed to diverge on the skin and the point of intersection of the field borders is marked. From this point, a distance *S* is calculated to separate the orthogonal fields. The separation *S* is given by:

$$S = \frac{1}{2} \cdot L \cdot \frac{d}{\text{SSD}} \tag{13.9}$$

where *d* is the depth at which the orthogonal fields are allowed to join. A general diagram for orthogonal field separation is illustrated in Fig. 13.16A.

B.1. Craniospinal Fields

Craniospinal irradiation involves a complex technique in which orthogonal junctions are created between the lateral brain fields and a posterior spine field. The spinal field, because of its large length, may be split into two spinal fields with a junction gap calculated according to Equation 13.5. The junction between the cranial and the spinal fields can be accomplished in several ways (48–50,52,54,55).

Technique A

Figure 13.16B presents an example showing bilateral cranial fields adjacent to a spinal field. The cranial light fields are allowed to diverge on the skin and their inferior borders meet at a point midway on the posterior neck surface. From this point, the spinal field is separated by a distance S, which is calculated from Equation 13.9 by substituting depth d of spine (from the posterior surface), length L, and SSD for the spinal field. In this diagram, the solid line represents the light field on the surface. The dashed line shows the field projected at the depth of the spinal cord. Figure 13.16C is the lateral view of Fig. 13.16B.

Technique B

The patient is positioned prone with the forehead resting on a rigid head support and the chest and abdomen resting on hard Styrofoam blocks (Fig. 13.17A). Some institutions use a half-shell plaster body cast under the patient for immobilization of head and neck relative to thorax (54,55). The spine field is simulated with the cephalad margin on the neck but without exiting through the mouth. By opening the light field, the diverging boundary of the cephalad margin of the spinal field is displayed on the lateral aspect of the neck. This boundary is marked on the patient's skin to provide a match line for the lateral cranial fields. The cranial fields are set up so that their caudad field margins are parallel with the diverging cephalad margin of the spinal field. This is accomplished by rotating the collimator of the cranial fields through an angle θ_{coll} (Fig. 13.17B).

If the cranial fields were nondivergent, the rotation of the cranial fields through θ_{coll} would be sufficient to provide the desired geometric match between the cranial and the spinal fields. However, to match the diverging cranial fields with the diverging spinal field, the couch must also be rotated through θ_{couch} in addition to the rotation of the cranial fields through θ_{coll} (Fig. 13.17C). The two angles θ_{coll} and θ_{couch}, can be calculated as:

$$\theta_{\text{coll}} = \text{arc tan}\left(\tfrac{1}{2} \cdot L_1 \cdot \frac{1}{\text{SSD}}\right) \qquad (13.10)$$

$$\theta_{\text{couch}} = \text{arc tan}\left(\tfrac{1}{2} \cdot L_2 \cdot \frac{1}{\text{SAD}}\right) \qquad (13.11)$$

where L_1 is the length of the posterior spinal field, L_2 is the length of the lateral cranial field, SSD is the source-to-surface distance for the spinal field, and SAD is the source-to-axis distance for the cranial fields, assuming the SSD technique is used for the spinal field and the SAD technique for the cranial fields. The couch is rotated toward the side the cranial field enters the head.

An alternative approach to rotating the couch is to eliminate cranial field divergence by using a half-beam block or an independent jaw to split the fields at the craniospinal junction line (Fig. 13.17D). The beam splitter is positioned at the central axis or close to it, thereby eliminating divergence of the rays at the junction line. The collimator of the cranial fields is still tilted through θ_{coll} as discussed earlier.

The technique of using independent jaw and θ_{coll} to match the craniospinal fields, has two advantages: (a) orthogonal field matching is achieved with no overlaps between the cranial and spinal fields at any depth, and (b) the independent jaw can be conveniently used to move the craniospinal junction line caudally by about a centimeter each week during the treatment course to smear out the junctional dose distribution. As long as the independent jaw splits the cranial fields within a few centimeters of the central axis, the divergence of the cranial fields into the spinal field at the matching line will be minimal.

C. Guidelines for Field Matching

1. The site of field matching should be chosen, insofar as possible, over an area that does not contain tumor or a critically sensitive organ.

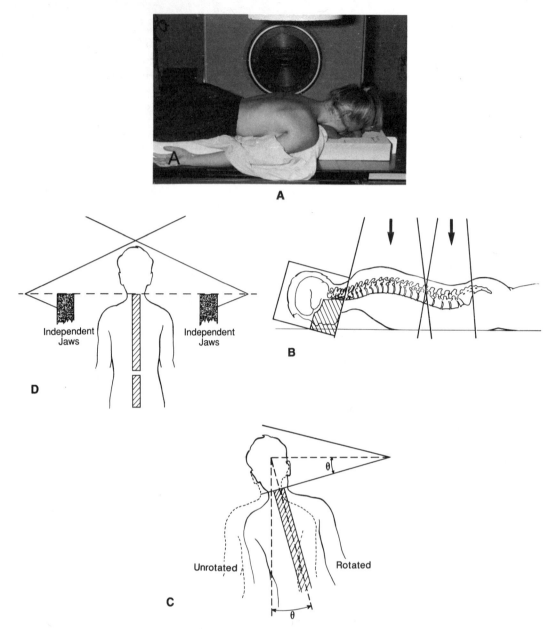

FIG. 13.17. Craniospinal irradiation technique. **A:** Patient set-up showing Styrofoam blocks and Alpha Cradle mold to provide stable position for abdomen, chest, and head. **B:** Lateral view of fields showing cranial field rotated to align with the diverging border of the spinal field. **C:** Couch rotated to provide match between the spinal field and the diverging border of the cranial field. **D:** Elimination of cranial field divergence by using an independent jaw as a beam splitter. This provides an alternative to couch rotation in C.

2. If the tumor is superficial at the junction site, the fields should not be separated because a cold spot on the tumor will risk recurrence. However, if the diverging fields abut on the skin surface, they will overlap at depth. In some cases, this may be clinically acceptable, provided the excessive dosage delivered to the underlying tissues does not exceed their tolerance. In particular, the tolerances of critical structures such as the spinal cord must not be exceeded. In the case of a superficial tumor with a critical organ located at depth, one may abut the fields at the surface but eliminate beam divergence using a beam splitter or by tilting the beams.

3. For deep-seated tumors, the fields may be separated on the skin surface so that the junction point lies at the midline. Again, care must be taken in regard to a critical structure near the junction region.

4. The line of field matching must be drawn at each treatment session on the basis of the first field treated. It is not necessary anatomically to reproduce this line every day because variation in its location will only smear the junction point, which is desirable. For the same reason some advocate moving the junction site two or three times during a treatment course.

5. A field-matching technique must be verified by actual isodose distributions before it is adopted for general clinical use. In addition, beam alignment with the light field and the accuracy of isodose curves in the penumbra region are essential prerequisites.

REFERENCES

1. Powers WE, Kinzie JJ, Demidecki AJ, et al. A new system of field shaping for external-beam radiation therapy. *Radiology* 1973;108:407.
2. Earl JD, Bagshaw MA. A rapid method for preparation of complex field shapes. *Radiology* 1967;88:1162.
3. Maruyama Y, Moore VC, Burns D, et al. Individualized lung shields constructed from lead shots embedded in plastic. *Radiology* 1969;92:634.
4. Edland RW, Hansen H. Irregular field-shaping for ^{60}Co teletherapy. *Radiology* 1969;92:1567.
5. Jones D. A method for the accurate manufacture of lead shields. *Br J Radiol* 1971;44:398.
6. Parfitt H. Manufacture of lead shields. *Br J Radiol* 1971;44:895.
7. Karzmark CJ, Huisman PA. Melting, casting and shaping of lead shielding blocks: method and toxicity aspects. *AJR* 1972;114:636.
8. Kuisk H. New method to facilitate radiotherapy planning and treatment, including a method for fast production of solid lead blocks with diverging walls for cobalt 60 beam. *AJR* 1973;117:161.
9. Khan FM, Gerbi BJ, Deibel FC. Dosimetry of asymmetric x-ray collimators. *Med Phys* 1986;13:936.
10. Brahme A. Optimal setting of multileaf collimators in stationary beam radiation therapy. *Strahlenther Onkol* 1988;164:343.
11. Boyer AL. Basic applications of a multileaf collimator. In: Mackie TR, Palta JR, eds. *Teletherapy: present and future.* College Park, MD: American Association of Physicists in Medicine, 1996.
12. Almond PR, Roosenbeek EV, Browne R, et al. Variation in the position of the central axis maximum buildup point with field size for high energy photons beams [Correspondence]. *Br J Radiol* 1970;43:911.
13. Marinello G, Dutreix A. Etude dosimétrique d'un faisceau de rayons X de 25 MV (Dosimetric study of a 25 MV x-ray beam). *J Radiol Electrol* 1973;54:951.
14. Johns HE, Rawlinson JA. Desirable characteristics of high-energy photons and electrons. In: Kramer S, Suntharalingam N, Zinniger GF, eds. *High energy photons and electrons.* New York: John Wiley & Sons, 1976:11.
15. Marbach JR, Almond PR. Scattered photons as the cause of the observed d_{max} shift with field size in high-energy photon beams. *Med Phys* 1977;4:310.
16. Padikal TN, Deye JA. Electron contamination of a high energy x-ray beam. *Phys Med Biol* 1978;23:1086.
17. Biggs PJ, Ling CC. Electrons as the cause of the observed d_{max} shift with field size in high energy photons beams. *Med Phys* 1979;6:291.
18. Velkley DE, Manson DJ, Purdy JA, et al. Buildup region of megavoltage photon radiation sources. *Med Phys* 1975;2:14.
19. Nilson B, Montelius A. Fluence perturbation in photon beams under non-equilibrium conditions. *Med Phys* 1986;13:192.
20. Rubach A, Conrad F, Bischel H. Dose build-up curves for cobalt 60 irradiations: a systematic error with pancake chamber measurements. *Phys Med Biol* 1986;31:441.
21. Gerbi BJ, Khan FM. Measurement of dose in the buildup region using fixed-separation plane-parallel ionization chambers. *Med Phys* 1990;17:17.
22. Khan FM. Use of electron filter to reduce skin dose in cobalt teletherapy. *AJR* 1971;111:180.
23. Khan FM, Moore VC, Levitt SH. Effect of various atomic number absorbers on skin dose for 10-MeV x-rays. *Radiology* 1973;109:209.
24. Saylor WL, Quillin RM. Methods for the enhancement of skin sparing in cobalt-60 teletherapy. *AJR* 1971;111:174.
25. Gray L. Relative surface doses from supervoltage radiation. *Radiology* 1973;109:437.
26. Rao PX, Pillai K, Gregg EC. Effect of shadow trays on surface dose and buildup for megavoltage radiation. *AJR* 1973;117:168.
27. Johns HE, Epp ER, Cormack DV, et al. Depth dose data and diaphragm design for the Saskatchewan 1,000 curie cobalt unit. *Br J Radiol* 1952;25:302.

28. Richardson JE, Kerman HD, Brucer M. Skin dose from cobalt 60 teletherapy unit. *Radiology* 1954;63:25.

29. Doppke K, Novack D, Wang CC. Physical considerations in the treatment of advanced carcinomas of the larynx and pyriform sinuses using 10 MV x-rays. *Int J Radiat Oncol Biol Phys* 1980;6: 1251.

30. Hine GJ. Scattering of secondary electrons produced by gamma rays in materials of various atomic numbers. *Phys Rev* 1951;82:755.

31. Hine GJ. Secondary electron emission and effective atomic numbers. *Nucleonics* 1952;10:9.

32. Leung PMK, Johns HE. Use of electron filters to improve the buildup characteristics of large fields from cobalt-60 beams. *Med Phys* 1977;4:441.

33. Burkell CC, Watson TA, Johns HE, et al. Skin effects of cobalt 60 telecurie therapy. *Br J Radiol* 1954;27:171.

34. Hughes HA. Measurements of superficial absorbed dose with 2 MV x-rays used at glancing angles. *Br J Radiol* 1959;32:255.

35. Jackson W. Surface effects of high-energy x-rays at oblique incidence. *Br J Radiol* 1971;44:109.

36. Orton CG, Seibert JB. Depth dose in skin for obliquely incident ^{60}Co radiation. *Br J Radiol* 1972;45:271.

37. Hanson WF, Grant W. Use of auxillary collimating devices in the treatment for breast cancer with ^{60}Co teletherapy units. II. Dose to the skin. *AJR* 1976;127:653.

38. Gagnon WF, Peterson MD. Comparison of skin doses to large fields using tangential beams from cobalt-60 gamma rays and 4 MV x-rays. *Radiology* 1978;127:785.

39. Gagnon WF, Horton JL. Physical factors affecting absorbed dose to the skin from cobalt-60 gamma rays and 25-MV x-rays. *Med Phys* 1979;6:285.

40. Gerbi BJ, Meigooni AS, Khan FM. Dose buildup for obliquely incident photon beams. *Med Phys* 1987;14:393.

41. Lance JS, Morgan JE. Dose distribution between adjoining therapy fields. *Radiology* 1962;79:24.

42. Glenn DW, Faw FL, Kagan RA, et al. Field separation in multiple portal radiation therapy. *AJR* 1968;102:199.

43. Faw FL, Glenn DW. Further investigations of physical aspects of multiple field radiation therapy. *AJR* 1970;108:184.

44. Page V, Gardner A, Karzmark CJ. Physical and dosimetric aspects of the radiotherapy of malignant lymphomas. II. The inverted Y technique. *Radiology* 1970;96:619.

45. Agarwal SK, Marks RD, Constable WC. Adjacent field separation for homogeneous dosage at a given depth for the 8 MV (Mevatron 8) linear accelerator. *AJR* 1972;114:623.

46. Armstrong DI, Tait JJ. The matching of adjacent fields in radiotherapy. *Radiology* 1973;108:419.

47. Hale J, Davis LW, Bloch P. Portal separation for pairs of parallel opposed portals at 2 MV and 6 MV. *AJR* 1972;114:172.

48. Griffin TW, Schumacher D, Berry HC. A technique for cranial-spinal irradiation. *Br J Radiol* 1976;49:887.

49. Williamson TJ. A technique for matching orthogonal megavoltage fields. *Int J Radiat Oncol Biol Phys* 1979;5:111.

50. Bukovitz A, Deutsch M, Slayton R. Orthogonal fields: variations in dose vs. gap size for treatment of the central nervous system. *Radiology* 1978;126:795.

51. Gillin MT, Kline RW. Field separation between lateral and anterior fields on a 6 MV linear accelerator. *Int J Radiat Oncol Biol Phys* 1980;6:233.

52. Werner BL, Khan FM, Sharma SC, et al. Border separation for adjacent orthogonal fields. *Med Dos* 1991;16:79.

53. Hopfan S, Reid A, Simpson L, et al. Clinical complications arising from overlapping of adjacent radiation fields—physical and technical considerations. *Int J Radiat Oncol Biol Phys* 1977;2:801.

54. Van Dyk J, Jenkin RDT, Leung PMK, et al. Medulloblastoma: treatment technique and radiation dosimetry. *Int J Rad Oncol Biol Phys* 1977;2:993.

55. Bentel GC, Nelson CE, Noell KT. *Treatment planning and dose calculation in radiation oncology,* 4th ed. New York: Pergamon Press, 1989:282.

ELECTRON BEAM THERAPY

High-energy electrons have been used in radiation therapy since the early 1950s. Originally, the beams were extracted mostly from betatrons although a few linear accelerators and Van de Graaff generators with relatively low electron energies were also available. In the 1970s, high-energy linear accelerators, having photon and multienergy electron beam capabilities, became increasingly available for clinical use. The surge in the commercial development of these machines was prompted largely by the clinical experience gained at a few major centers, which showed that in some commonly encountered situations "there is no alternative treatment to electron beam therapy" (1).

The most clinically useful energy range for electrons is 6 to 20 MeV. At these energies, the electron beams can be used for treating superficial tumors (less than 5 cm deep) with a characteristically sharp drop-off in dose beyond the tumor. The principal applications are (a) the treatment of skin and lip cancers, (b) chest wall irradiation for breast cancer, (c) administering boost dose to nodes, and (d) the treatment of head and neck cancers. Although many of these sites can be treated with superficial x-rays, brachytherapy, or tangential photon beams, the electron beam irradiation offers distinct advantages in terms of dose uniformity in the target volume and in minimizing dose to deeper tissues.

This chapter is intended to provide basic information on electron beam characteristics, dosimetry, and treatment planning. Most of the discussion will pertain to 6- to 20-MeV electrons, although the data at these energies can be qualitatively extrapolated to the lower or the higher energy range.

14.1. ELECTRON INTERACTIONS

As electrons travel through a medium, they interact with atoms by a variety of processes owing to Coulomb force interactions. The processes are (a) inelastic collisions with atomic electrons (ionization and excitation), (b) inelastic collisions with nuclei (bremsstrahlung), (c) elastic collisions with atomic electrons, and (d) elastic collisions with nuclei.

In inelastic collisions, some of the kinetic energy is lost as it is used in producing ionization or converted to other forms of energy such as photon energy and excitation energy. In elastic collisions, kinetic energy is not lost although it may be redistributed among the particles emerging from the collision. In low atomic number media such as water or tissues, electrons lose energy predominantly through ionizing events with atomic electrons. In higher atomic number materials, such as lead, bremsstrahlung production is more important. In the collision process with the atomic electrons, if the kinetic energy acquired by the stripped electron is large enough for it to cause further ionization, the electron is known as a secondary electron or a δ-ray. As a beam of electrons travels through a medium, the energy is continually degraded until the electrons reach thermal energies and are captured by the surrounding atoms.

A. Rate of Energy Loss

An electron traveling in a medium loses energy as a result of collisional and radiative processes. The magnitudes of the two effects for water and lead are shown in Fig. 14.1.

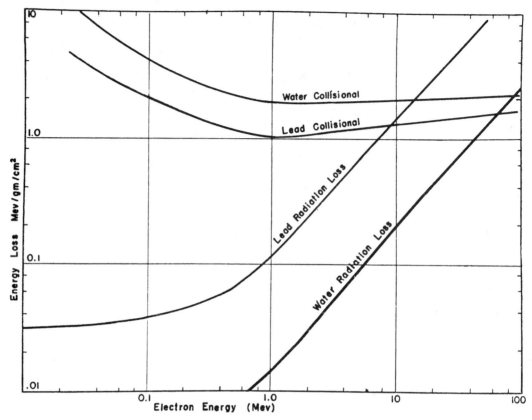

FIG. 14.1. Rate of energy loss in MeV per g/cm² as a function of electron energy for water and lead. (From Johns HE, Cunningham JR. *The physics of radiology,* 3rd ed. Springfield, IL: Charles C Thomas, 1969, with permission.)

The theoretical treatment of this subject is given elsewhere (2–5). It will suffice here to provide some important generalizations.

A.1. Collisional Losses (Ionization and Excitation)

(a) The rate of energy loss depends on the electron density of the medium. (b) The rate of energy loss per gram per centimeter squared, which is called the mass stopping power, is greater for low atomic number (Z) material than for high Z materials (compare the water curve to the lead curve in Fig. 14.1). There are two reasons for this: First, high Z materials have fewer electrons per gram than low Z materials have and, second, high Z materials have more tightly bound electrons, which are not as available for this type of interaction. (c) As seen in Fig. 14.1, the energy loss rate first decreases and then increases with increase in electron energy with a minimum occurring at about 1 MeV. Above 1 MeV, the variation with energy is very gradual. (d) The energy loss rate of electrons of energy 1 MeV and above in water is roughly 2 MeV/cm.

A.2. Radiation Losses (Bremsstrahlung)

The rate of energy loss per centimeter is approximately proportional to the electron energy and to the square of the atomic number (Z^2). Moreover, the probability of radiation loss relative to the collisional loss increases with the electron kinetic energy and with Z. That means that x-ray production is more efficient for higher energy electrons and higher atomic number absorbers.

A.3. Polarization

A high-energy electron loses more energy per gram per square centimeter in a gas than in traversing a more dense medium, because of appreciable polarization of the condensed medium (5–7). Atoms close to the electron track screen those remote from the track. This phenomenon is particularly important in dosimetry with ionization chambers when energy deposition in a medium and a gas cavity are compared. The ratio of mass stopping power of water to air varies with electron energy, and consequently, the dose conversion factor for an air ionization chamber in water (or another condensed medium) varies with depth.

A.4. Stopping Power

The total mass stopping power $(S/\rho)_{tot}$ of a material for charged particles is defined by the International Commission on Radiation Units and Measurements (ICRU) (8) as the quotient of dE by $\rho\,dl$, where dE is the total energy lost by the particle in traversing a path length dl in the material of density ρ.

$$(S/\rho)_{tot} = (S/\rho)_{col} + (S/\rho)_{rad} \tag{14.1}$$

where $(S/\rho)_{col}$ and $(S/\rho)_{rad}$ apply to collisional losses and radiation losses, respectively, discussed in previous sections A.1 and A.2.

A.5. Absorbed Dose

In calculating the energy absorbed per unit mass (absorbed dose), one needs to know the electron fluence and the "restricted" collision stopping power. Restricted collision stopping power refers to the linear energy transfer (LET) concept, that is, the rate of energy loss per unit path length in collisions in which energy is "locally" absorbed, rather than carried away by energetic secondary electrons. Thus the restricted collision mass stopping power, $(L/\rho)_{col}$, of a material for charged particles is defined (8) as the quotient of dE by $\rho\,dl$, where dE is the energy lost by a charged particle in traversing a distance dl as a result of those collisions with atomic electrons in which the energy loss is less than Δ.

$$\left(\frac{L}{\rho}\right)_{col,\Delta} = \left(\frac{dE}{\rho\,dl}\right)_{col,\Delta} \tag{14.2}$$

If Φ_E is the differentiated distribution of fluence with respect to energy $\left[\Phi_E = \dfrac{d\Phi(E)}{dE}\right]$, the absorbed dose, D, is closely approximated by:

$$D = \int_{\Delta}^{E_0} \Phi_E \cdot \left(\frac{L}{\rho}\right)_{col,\Delta} \cdot dE \tag{14.3}$$

The use of stopping powers in photon and electron dosimetry has been discussed in Chapter 8. Quantitative data on stopping powers as a function of electron energy for various elements and materials have been calculated by Berger and Seltzer (9–11) and tabulated in Table A.8 of the appendix. More extensive tables of stopping powers are given by the ICRU (12).

B. Electron Scattering

When a beam of electrons passes through a medium, the electrons suffer multiple scattering due to Coulomb force interactions between the incident electrons and, predominantly, the nuclei of the medium. As a result, the electrons acquire velocity components and displacements transverse to their original direction of motion. For most practical applications, the angular and spatial spread of a narrow, collimated beam of electrons can be approximated by a Gaussian distribution (13).

By analogy with mass stopping power, the ICRU (8) defines the mass angular scattering power of the material as the quotient $\bar{\theta}^2/\rho l$, where $\bar{\theta}^2$ is the mean square scattering angle. Following the calculations of Rossi (13), mass scattering powers for various materials and electron energies have been tabulated (14).

The scattering power varies approximately as the square of the atomic number and inversely as the square of the kinetic energy. For this reason, high Z materials are used in the construction of scattering foils. Scattering foils spread out the electron beam that emerges from the accelerator tube and are made thin to minimize x-ray contamination of the electron beam.

14.2. ENERGY SPECIFICATION AND MEASUREMENT

Although an electron beam is almost monoenergetic before striking the accelerator window, the random energy degradation that the electrons suffer as they pass through the exit window, scattering foil, monitor chambers, air, and other materials results in the beam taking on a spectrum of energies at the phantom surface. Further degradation and spread of beam energy take place with depth in the phantom (Fig. 14.2).

In clinical practice, an electron beam is usually characterized by the energy at the body surface. There are several methods that can be used to determine this energy: measurement of threshold energy for nuclear reactions; range measurements; and the measurement of Cerenkov radiation threshold (14). Of these, the range method is the most practical and convenient for clinical use.

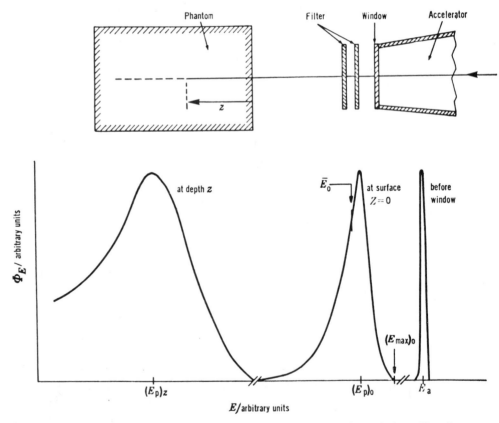

FIG. 14.2. Distribution of electron fluence in energy, Φ_E, as the beam passes through the collimation system of the accelerator and the phantom. (From ICRU. Radiation dosimetry: electrons with initial energies between 1 and 50 MeV. Report No. 21. Washington, DC: International Commission on Radiation Units and Measurements, 1972, with permission.)

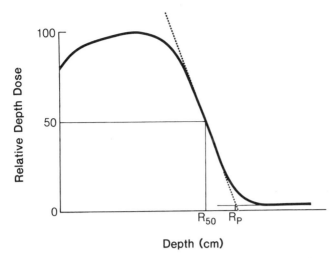

FIG. 14.3. Depth-dose curve illustrating the definition of R_p and R_{50}.

A. Most Probable Energy

The Nordic Association of Clinical Physics (15) recommends the specification of most probable energy, $(E_p)_0$ (defined by the position of the spectral peak in Fig. 14.2) at the phantom surface and the use of the following relationship:

$$(E_p)_0 = C_1 + C_2 R_p + C_3 R_p^2 \tag{14.4}$$

where R_p is the practical range in centimeters as defined in Fig. 14.3. For water, $C_1 = 0.22$ MeV, $C_2 = 1.98$ MeV cm^{-1}, and $C_3 = 0.0025$ MeV cm^{-2} (16–18). They further recommend that the field size for range measurements be no less than 12 × 12 cm for energies up to 10 MeV and no less than 20 × 20 cm for higher energies.

For the determination of range, ion chambers, diodes, or film may be used. Although the range measurements are usually made using the depth ionization curve the result is only slightly different from what would be obtained using depth dose curves (19). The practical range, R_p, is the depth of the point where the tangent to the descending linear portion of the curve (at the point of inflection) intersects the extrapolated background, as shown in Fig. 14.3.

To be in strict accordance with Equation 14.4, each point on the depth ionization curve should be corrected for beam divergence before the range is determined. The correction factor is $\left(\dfrac{f + z}{f}\right)^2$, where f is the effective source-to-surface distance (see section 14.4E for details) and z is the depth. However, this correction in R_p is clinically not significant in terms of its impact on the ionization to dose conversion factor (20).

B. Mean Energy

It has been shown (21) that the mean energy of the electron beam, $\overline{E}_0$, at the phantom surface is related to R_{50} (the depth at which the dose is 50% of the maximum dose) by the following relationship:

$$\overline{E}_0 = C_4 \cdot R_{50} \tag{14.5}$$

where $C_4 = 2.33$ MeV cm^{-1} for water. Again the divergence correction is applied to each point on the depth dose curve before determining R_{50}.

The AAPM TG-21 protocol recommended the value of C_4 as 2.33 MeV cm^{-1}. However, more recent Monte-Carlo calculations of Rogers and Bielajew (22) have shown that the value of C_4 in the energy range of clinical interest is closer to 2.4 MeV cm^{-1}.

Again, this small change in the value of C_4 as well as the divergence correction mentioned above has little impact on clinical dosimetry (20).

C. Energy at Depth

Harder (23) has shown that the most probable energy and, approximately, the mean energy of the spectrum decreases linearly with depth. This can be expressed by the relationships:

$$(E_p)_z = (E_p)_0 \left(1 - \frac{z}{R_p}\right) \tag{14.6}$$

and approximately:

$$\overline{E}_z = \overline{E}_0 \left(1 - \frac{z}{R_p}\right) \tag{14.7}$$

where z is the depth.

Equation 14.7 is important in dosimetry because for absorbed dose measurements it is necessary to know the mean electron energy at the location of the chamber.

14.3. DETERMINATION OF ABSORBED DOSE

Calorimetry is the most basic method for the determination of absorbed dose, but because of technical difficulties, the use of calorimeters is not practical in a clinical setting. Ionization chambers and Fricke dosimeters are more commonly used. Film, thermoluminescent dosimeters (TLD), and solid state diodes are used to find the ratio of the dose at one point in a phantom to the dose at another point but not usually to measure the absolute absorbed dose at a point.

Ionization chambers should be calibrated by an Accredited Dose Calibration Laboratory (ADCL) or the National Institute of Standards and Technology (NIST). However, an ADCL can usually provide calibrations only for high-energy photon beams (^{60}Co or 2-MV x-rays) but not for high-energy electron beams. The use of ionization chambers calibrated for photon beams for the measurement of absorbed dose in electron beams has been the subject of many national and international protocols (14,15,24–26). The most current recommendations are included in the protocols by Task Group 51 of the American Association of Physicists in Medicine (AAPM) (24) and the International Atomic Energy Agency (IAEA) TRS398 (25). Elements of these protocols and other related concepts were presented in Chapter 8.

A. Output Calibration

The variation of output (absorbed dose at a reference point in phantom) with field size differs considerably from one type of accelerator to another. Therefore, for every available electron energy, the output of each treatment applicator or representative field size should be measured. The output for one applicator or field size (often the 10×10 cm field), is selected as the standard to which the other output measurements are referred. Since the beam is calibrated to give 1 cGy/MU for the standard applicator at the depth of maximum dose on central axis (nominal SSD = 100 cm), the output factor for any applicator represents cGy/MU at d_{max}. This topic will be further discussed in section 14.4D.

B. Depth-dose Distribution

The depth-dose and isodose distributions can be determined by ion chambers, diodes, or films. Automatic isodose and isodensity plotters are useful in this regard and are available commercially.

B.1. Ionization Chambers

Depth ionization curves obtained with air ionization chambers can be converted into depth-dose curves by making corrections for change in stopping power ratio of water to air with depth. In addition, perturbation and displacement corrections are required for cylindrical chambers.

A general equation for obtaining percent depth dose in water (%D_W) from ion chamber measurements made in any medium or phantom is given by the following equation (20):

$$\% D_W = \left(\frac{\{M \times (\overline{L}/\rho)_{air}^{W} \times (\Phi)_{med}^{W} \times P_{repl}\}}{\{ \qquad \}_{max}} \right) \times 100 \qquad (14.8)$$

where the quantities in the numerator are determined at the effective depth of measurement and the denominator equals the value of the numerator at the depth of maximum dose.

B.2. Silicon Diodes

Silicon *p-n* junction diodes offer some advantages in terms of small size and high sensitivity (Chapter 8). However, diodes suffer from energy and temperature dependence and can be damaged by radiation. For these reasons absolute dosimetry with diodes is not recommended. Dose distributions obtained with diodes should be checked by ion chamber measurements.

Because the variation of silicon to water stopping power ratio with electron energy is quite minimal (~5% between 1 and 20 MeV), measurements made with a diode may be used directly to give depth-dose distributions. Figure 14.4 shows a comparison of depth

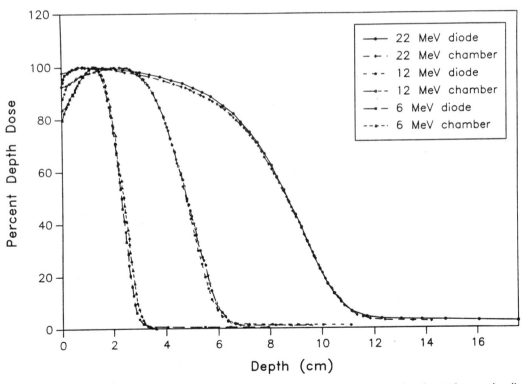

FIG. 14.4. Comparison of depth-dose curves measured with a diode and an ion chamber. Whereas the diode response was uncorrected, the chamber readings were corrected for change in $(\overline{L})_{air}^{water}$ as a function of depth, and the displacement of the effective point of measurement. (From Khan FM. Clinical electron beam dosimetry. In: Monograph No. 15. Keriakes JG, Elson HR, Born CG, eds. *Radiation oncology physics—1986.* AAPM Monograph No. 15. New York: American Institute of Physics, 1986:211, with permission.)

dose distributions obtained with an ion chamber (corrected for stopping power ratios and other effects) and a diode. The data show close agreement.

B.3. Film

Film dosimetry offers a convenient and rapid method of obtaining a complete set of isodose curves in the plane of the film. Its use for determining electron beam dose distributions is well established (27–29). It has been shown that the depth dose distributions measured by using film agree well with those by ion chambers when the latter measurements are corrected as outlined in section A (Fig. 14.5). Good agreement has also been demonstrated between film and $FeSO_4$ dosimeters used for the measurement of depth dose curves (29). The energy independence of film may be explained by the fact that the ratio of collision stopping power in emulsion and in water varies slowly with electron energy (9). Thus the optical density of the film can be taken as proportional to the dose with essentially no corrections.

Film is useful for a variety of dosimetry problems such as determining practical range, isodose curves, and beam flatness. However, film cannot be used reliably for absolute dosimetry because the optical density of a film exposed to electrons depends on many variables such as emulsion, processing conditions, magnitude of absorbed dose, and some measurement conditions, which can give rise to serious artifacts. The use of film is, therefore, restricted to relative dosimetry. Care is required to avoid air gaps adjacent to the film. In addition, the sensitometric curve (optical density as a function of absorbed dose) must be known to interpret the optical density in terms of absorbed dose. Wherever possible, a film with a linear response over the range of measured dose should be used. Errors caused by changes in the processing conditions can be minimized by developing the films at

10 MeV Electrons

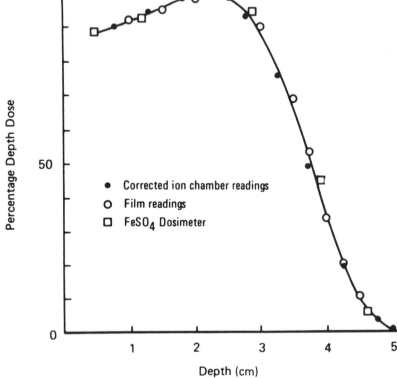

- ● Corrected ion chamber readings
- ○ Film readings
- □ $FeSO_4$ Dosimeter

FIG. 14.5. Comparison of central axis depth dose curve measured with an ion chamber, film, and $FeSO_4$ dosimeter. (From Almond PR. In: *Handbook of medical physics, Vol 1.* Boca Raton, FL: CRC Press, 1982:173, with permission.)

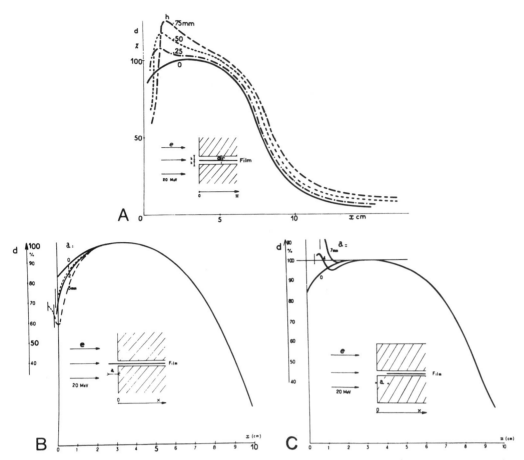

FIG. 14.6. Film artifacts created by misalignment of the film in the phantom. The effects of **(A)** air gaps between the film and the phantom, **(B)** film edge extending beyond the phantom, and **(C)** film edge recessed within the phantom. (From Dutreix J, Dutreix A. Film dosimetry of high energy electrons. *Ann NY Acad Sci* 1969;161:33, with permission.)

approximately the same time. Accuracy can also be improved by using films from the same batch.

Film can be positioned either perpendicular or parallel to the beam axis. In the latter case, precautions must be taken to align the top edge of the film with the surface of the phantom or serious artifacts and errors in the depth-dose distribution may result (28) (Fig. 14.6).

To obtain isodose curves, the film is usually placed in a plastic phantom such as polystyrene and oriented parallel to the beam axis. The film can be kept in its original paper jacket and pressed tightly between the phantom slabs. Small holes can be punched in the corners of the jacket for trapped air to escape. The film wrapping that extends beyond the phantom should be folded to one side and taped down. After processing, the film may be analyzed using a densitometer having a light aperture of about 1 mm diameter. Figure 14.7 shows an example of a film exposed to electrons and a set of isodose curves obtained by isodensity scanning. Because the effective density of transparent polystyrene is close to that of water, the resulting isodose curves can be used clinically without further correction.

Because many electron energies are often available with accelerators, an automatic film dosimetry system is a desirable thing to have in a clinical department. Automatic density plotters are commercially available, and some of them are interfaced with treatment-planning computers. Although hand processing of films gives the best results, automatic rapid processors can be used in many instances. A strict quality assurance, however, is necessary to maintain consistency in film dosimetry.

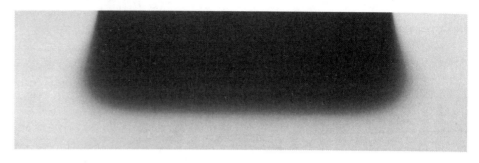

A

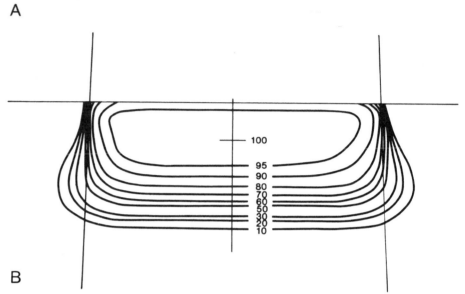

B

FIG. 14.7. Film used for obtaining isodose curves. **A:** A film exposed to 12-MeV electron beam, 14 × 8 cm cone, in a polystyrene phantom. **B:** Isodensity curves.

B.4. Phantoms

Water is the standard phantom for the dosimetry of electron beams. However, it is not always possible or practical to perform dosimetry in a water phantom. For example, plastic phantoms are more suitable when using film or plane-parallel chambers. It also is difficult to make measurements near the surface of water, because of its surface tension and the uncertainty in positioning the detector near the surface.

For a phantom to be water equivalent for electron dosimetry it must have the same linear stopping power and the same linear angular scattering power. This is approximately achieved if the phantom has the same electron density (number of electrons per cubic centimeter) and the same effective atomic number as water. Of the commonly used materials for electron dosimetry, polystyrene and electron solid water (Radiation Measurements, Inc., Middleton, WI) come closest to being water equivalent.

A depth-dose distribution measured in a nonwater phantom may be converted to that expected in a water phantom by the following relationship (20):

$$D_W\,(d_W) = D_{\mathrm{med}}(d_{\mathrm{med}})(\overline{S}/\rho)_{\mathrm{med}}^{\mathrm{water}}\,\Phi_{\mathrm{med}}^{\mathrm{water}} \tag{14.9}$$

provided the energy spectra of electrons at each position are identical. However, because of differences in stopping power and scattering power among different phantoms, it is not possible to find corresponding depths at which the energy spectra are identical. Consequently, there is no single scaling factor that can accurately transform an entire depth dose curve in a nonwater phantom to that in water. An *effective density* may be assigned to a medium to give water equivalent depth dose distribution near the therapeutic range and

TABLE 14.1. EFFECTIVE DENSITY FOR SCALING DEPTH IN NONWATER PHANTOMS TO WATER FOR ELECTRON BEAMS[a]

Material	Mass Density (g/cm³)	Effective Density Relative to Water
Water	1	1
Polystyrene (clear)	1.045	0.975
Polystyrene (high impact, white)	1.055	0.99
Acrylic	1.18	1.15
Electron solid water	1.04	1.00

[a]Recommended in AAPM. Clinical electron-beam dosimetry. AAPM Task Group No. 25. *Med Phys* 1991;18:73.

along the descending portion of the depth dose curve. The AAPM (20) has recommended that the water equivalent depth or the effective density (ρ_{eff}) may be estimated from the following relationship:

$$d_W = d_{\text{med}} \times \rho_{\text{eff}} = d_{\text{med}} \left(\frac{R_{50}^{\text{water}}}{R_{50}^{\text{med}}} \right) \qquad (14.10)$$

where R_{50} is the depth of 50% dose or detector response. Recommended values of ρ_{eff} for various phantoms are given in Table 14.1.

14.4. CHARACTERISTICS OF CLINICAL ELECTRON BEAMS

A. Central Axis Depth-dose Curves

The major attraction of the electron beam irradiation is the shape of the depth dose curve, especially in the energy range of 6 to 15 MeV. A region of more or less uniform dose followed by a rapid dropoff of dose offers a distinct clinical advantage over the conventional x-ray modalities. This advantage, however, tends to disappear with increasing energy.

It was stated earlier that high-energy electrons lose energy at the rate of about 2 MeV/cm of water or soft tissue. Beyond the maximum range of electrons, the dose is contributed only by the x-ray contamination of the beam, indicated by the tail of the depth dose curve (Fig. 14.8).

For a broad beam, the depth in centimeters at which electrons deliver a dose to the 80% to 90% isodose level, is equal to approximately one-third to one-fourth of the electron energy in MeV. Thus a 13-MeV electron beam is useful to a depth of about 3 to 4 cm, depending on the isodose level specified. As seen in Fig. 14.8, the depth dose curve falls off sharply beyond the useful depth and, therefore, the underlying tissues are spared.

The most useful treatment depth, or therapeutic range, of electrons is given by the depth of the 90% depth dose. For modern accelerators with trimmer type applicators this depth is approximately given by $E/3.2$ cm, where E is the most probable energy in MeV of the electron beam at the surface. The depth of the 80% depth dose occurs approximately at $E/2.8$ cm. The depth of D_{max} does not follow a linear relationship with energy but it covers a broad region and its value may be approximated by $0.46 E^{0.67}$ (30). Figure 14.9 shows a comparison of depth of 90% dose (R_{90}) as a function of beam energy for two different linear accelerators. These differences can be clinically significant and, therefore, underscore the requirement of using beam data that have been measured specifically for the given machine.

The choice of beam energy is much more critical for electrons than for photons. Because the dose decreases abruptly beyond the 90% dose level, the treatment depth and the required electron energy must be chosen very carefully. The guiding principle is that, when in doubt, use a higher electron energy to make sure that the target volume is well within the specified isodose curve.

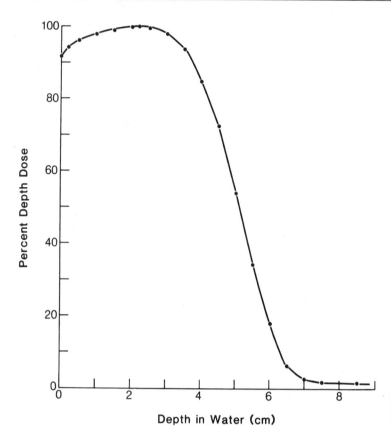

FIG. 14.8. Central axis depth dose distribution measured in water. Incident energy, $(E_p)_0 = 13$ MeV; 8 × 10 cm cone; effective source to surface distance = 68 cm.

The skin-sparing effect with the clinical electron beams is only modest or nonexistent. Unlike the photon beams, the percent surface dose for electrons increases with energy. This effect can be explained by the nature of the electron scatter. At the lower energies, the electrons are scattered more easily and through larger angles. This causes the dose to build up more rapidly and over a shorter distance. The ratio of surface dose to maximum dose is, therefore, less for the lower-energy electrons than for the higher-energy electrons. A simple illustration of this effect is seen in Fig. 14.10. For the same incident electron fluence (e^-/cm^2), the lower-energy electrons build up to a larger fluence at the depth of maximum dose than the higher-energy electrons. The increase in fluence is given by $1/\cos\theta$, where θ is the angle of scatter.

Because of differences in beam generation, beam bending, and collimation, the depth dose distribution and the surface dose can be quite different for different machines. Figure 14.11 illustrates this point by comparing central axis depth dose curves for the Sagittaire linear accelerator and the Siemen's betatron for different beam energies. In clinical practice, therefore, it is not sufficient to specify just beam energy. Isodose distributions for an individual machine, cone, and/or field size are required.

B. Isodose Curves

The scattering of electrons plays an important role in determining the shape of the isodose curves—the central axis distribution, flatness, and curvature near the field borders. Significant differences exist among the shapes of the isodose curves for different machines. These differences arise as a result of different collimation systems that the accelerators employ. The collimation system (e.g., scattering foil, monitor chambers, jaws, and cones) and the air column above the patient cause an angular dispersion of the beam as well as energy spread. Thus beams of the same energy, E_0, but passing through different collimation systems give rise to different dose distributions.

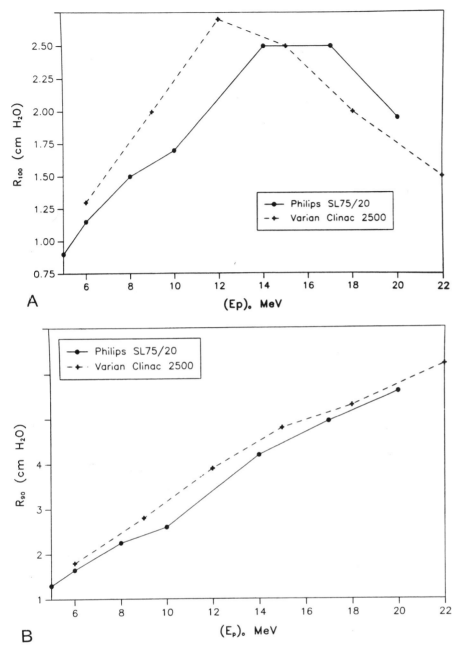

FIG. 14.9. Plots of depth dose ranges as a function of the most probable energy $(E_p)_0$ at the surface for two different linear accelerators. **A:** R_{100}, the depth of maximum dose versus $(E_p)_0$. **B:** R_{90}, the depth of 90% depth dose versus $(E_p)_0$. (From Khan FM. Clinical electron beam dosimetry. In: Keriakes JG, Elson HR, Born CG, eds. *Radiation oncology physics—1986.* AAPM Monograph No. 15. New York, American Institute of Physics, 1986:211, with permission.)

As the beam penetrates a medium, the beam expands rapidly below the surface due to scattering. However, individual spread of the isodose curves varies, depending on the isodose level, energy, field size, and collimation. Figure 14.12 shows isodose patterns for two different energy beams. Whereas for the low-energy beams all the isodose curves show some expansion, for the higher energies only the low isodose levels bulge out. The higher isodose levels tend to show lateral constriction, which becomes worse with decreasing field size.

C. Field Flatness and Symmetry

Uniformity of the electron beam is usually specified in a plane perpendicular to the beam axis and at a fixed depth. The ICRU (31) specifies beam flatness in terms of a *uniformity*

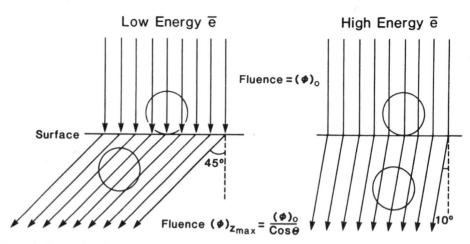

FIG. 14.10. Schematic illustration showing the increase in percent surface dose with an increase in electron energy. (From Khan FM. Clinical electron beam dosimetry. In: Keriakes JG, Elson HR, Born CG, eds. *Radiation oncology physics—1986.* AAPM Monograph No. 15. New York, American Institute of Physics, 1986:211, with permission.)

index. This is defined in a reference plane and at a reference depth as the ratio of the area where the dose exceeds 90% of its value at the central axis to the geometric beam cross-sectional area at the phantom surface. The uniformity index should exceed a given fraction (e.g., 0.80 for a 10 × 10 cm field size and at depth of maximum dose). In addition, the dose at any arbitrary point in the reference plane should not exceed 103% of the central axis value.

Figure 14.13 shows isodose curves obtained from a film exposed perpendicular to an electron beam at the depth of maximum dose. The dashed line is the boundary of the geometric beam at the surface. In this example, the homogeneity index is 0.8.

Because of the presence of lower-energy electrons in the beam, the flatness changes significantly with depth. Therefore, it has been recommended (32) that the uniformity

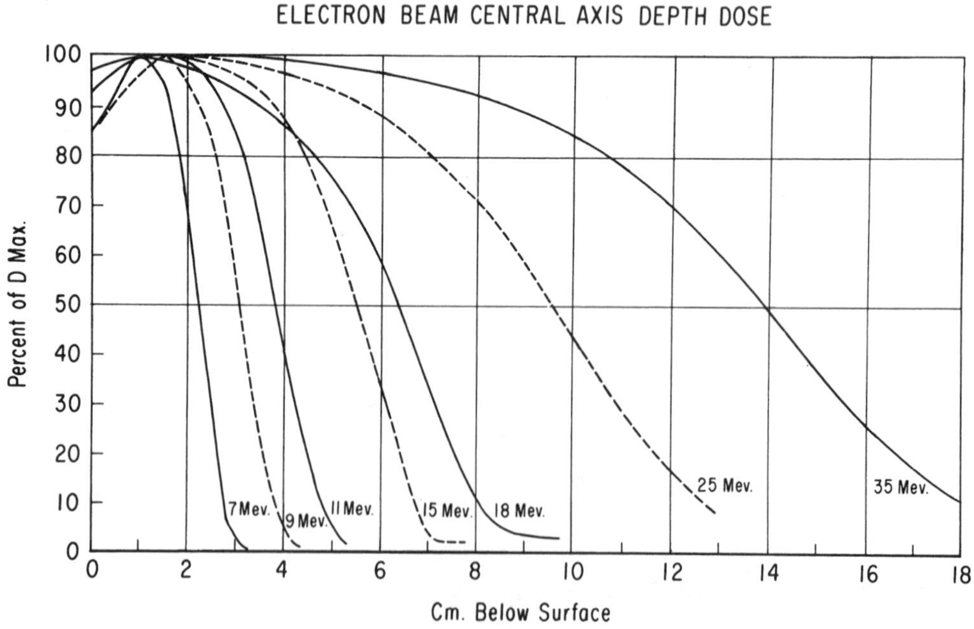

FIG. 14.11. Comparison of central axis depth-dose distributions of the Sagittaire linear accelerator *(continuous curves)* and the Siemen's betatron *(dashed curves).* (From Tapley N, ed. *Clinical applications of the electron beam.* New York: John Wiley & Sons, 1976, with permission.)

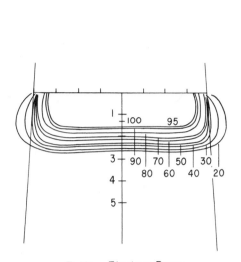

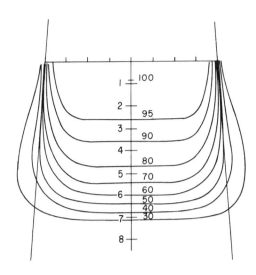

7 Mev. Electron Beam
8 cm. Circle, ∡ I, F 5, 50 cm. TSD

18 Mev. Electron Beam
8 cm. Circle, ∡ 5, F 7, 50 cm. TSD.

FIG. 14.12. Comparison of isodose curves for different energy electron beams. (From Tapley N, ed. *Clinical applications of the electron beam.* New York: John Wiley & Sons, 1976:86, with permission.)

index be defined at the depth of half the therapeutic range (e.g., one-half the depth of 85% depth dose). Furthermore, it is defined as the ratio of the areas inside the 90% and 50% isodose lines at this depth. A uniformity index of 0.70 or higher is acceptable with field sizes larger than 100 cm². The peak value in this plane should be less than 103%.

The AAPM (20) recommends that the flatness of an electron beam be specified in a reference plane perpendicular to the central axis, at the depth of the 95% isodose beyond the depth of dose maximum. The variation in dose relative to the dose at central axis should

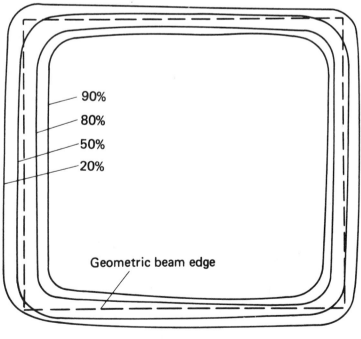

Homogeneity Index 0.8

FIG. 14.13. Isodose curves in a plane perpendicular to central axis, obtained with a film placed in a phantom at the depth of maximum dose. (From Almond PR. Radiation physics of electron beams. In: Tapley N, ed. *Clinical applications of the electron beam.* New York: John Wiley & Sons, 1976:50, with permission.)

not exceed $\pm 5\%$ (optimally to be within $\pm 3\%$) over an area confined within lines 2 cm inside the geometric edge of fields equal to or larger than 10×10 cm.

Beam symmetry compares a dose profile on one side of the central axis to that on the other. The AAPM recommends that the cross-beam profile in the reference plane should not differ more than 2% at any pair of points located symmetrically on opposite sides of the central axis.

C.1. Beam Collimation

Acceptable field flatness and symmetry are obtained with a proper design of beam scatterers and beam defining collimators. Accelerators with magnetically scanned beam do not require scattering foils. Others use one or more scattering foils, usually made up of lead, to widen the beam as well as give a uniform dose distribution across the treatment field.

The beam collimation has been significantly improved by the introduction of the dual-foil system (33). Figure 14.14 shows a typical arrangement for such a system. Whereas, the first foil widens the beam by multiple scattering, the second foil is designed to make the beam uniform in cross-section. The thickness of the second foil is differentially varied across the beam to produce a desired degree of beam widening and flattening. Analysis by Werner et al. (34) shows that the dual-foil systems compare well with the scanning beam systems in minimizing angular spread and, hence, the effect on dose distribution characteristics.

The beam-defining collimators are designed to provide a variety of field sizes and to maintain or improve the flatness of the beam. Basically, all collimators provide a primary

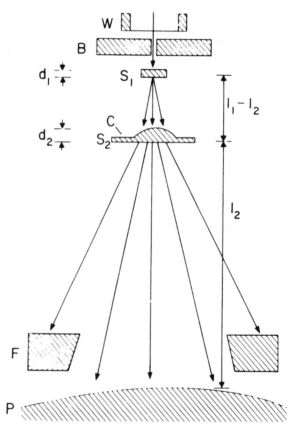

FIG. 14.14. Principle of dual-foil system for obtaining uniform electron beam field. (From Almond PR. *Handbook of medical physics, Vol I.* Boca Raton, FL: CRC Press, 1982:149, with permission.)

collimation close to the source that defines the maximum field size and a secondary collimation close to the patient to define the treatment field. The latter can be in the form of trimmer bars or a series of cones. In the electron therapy mode, the x-ray collimator jaws are usually opened to a size larger than the cone or the applicator opening. Because the x-ray jaws give rise to extensive electron scatter, they are interlocked with the individual cones to open automatically to a fixed predetermined size.

D. Field Size Dependence

The output and the central axis depth-dose distribution are field size dependent. The dose increases with field size because of the increased scatter from the collimator and the phantom. As stated previously, some electron collimators provide a fixed jaw opening, and the treatment field size is varied by various size cones, inserts, or movable trimmer bars. Such an arrangement minimizes the variation of collimator scatter, and therefore, the output variation with field size is kept reasonably small. If the collimator aperture (x-ray jaw setting) were allowed to change with the treatment field, the output would vary too widely with field size, especially for lower-energy beams. This effect is shown in Fig. 14.15, where the cone size is held fixed while the x-ray jaws are varied (35). Note that the dose rate varies by a factor of greater than 2 between small and large jaw openings at 4 MeV.

The effects of field size on output and the central axis depth dose curve due to phantom scatter alone is significant as long as the distance between the point of measurement and the edge of the field is shorter than the range of the laterally scattered electrons. When this distance is reached, there is no further increase in depth dose caused by phantom scatter. When the field is reduced below that required for lateral scatter equilibrium, the dose rate decreases rapidly. This is shown in Fig. 14.16. In these measurements, the field size at the phantom was varied without changing the photon collimator opening. For small fields, the output factor as well as depth dose can be significantly reduced compared with the broad beam distribution.

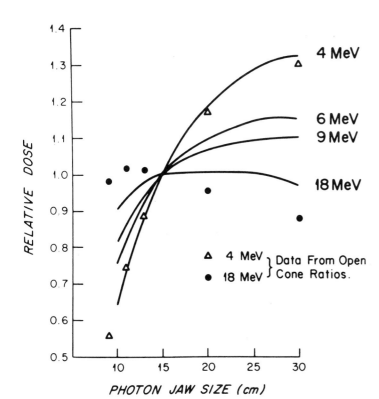

FIG. 14.15. Variation of relative dose at d_{max}, through a 10 × 10 cm cone, with change of jaw setting, relative to the recommended jaw setting. (From Biggs PJ, Boyer AL, Doppke KP. Electron dosimetry of irregular fields on the Clinac-18. *Int J Radiat Oncol Biol Phys* 1979;5:433, with permission.)

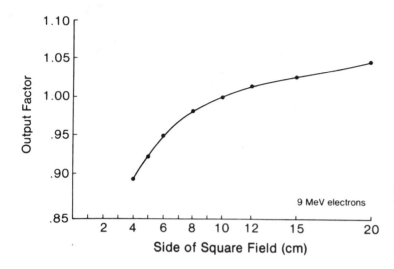

FIG. 14.16. Output factors as a function of side of square field. Primary collimator fixed, secondary collimators (trimmers) close to the phantom varied to change the field size. Data are from Therac 20 linear accelerator. (From Mills MD, Hogstrom KR, Almond PR. Prediction of electron beam output factors. *Med Phys* 1982;9:60, with permission.)

Figure 14.17 shows the change in central axis depth-dose distribution with field size. As the field size is increased, the percent depth dose initially increases but becomes constant beyond a certain field size when the lateral scatter equilibrium is reached. Furthermore the depth d_{max} shifts toward the surface for the smaller fields. Thus in clinical practice, depth-dose distribution for small fields should be measured individually in addition to the output calibration.

It has been shown (36) that the minimum field radius for the establishment of lateral scatter equilibrium at all depths on central axis is given by the following approximate

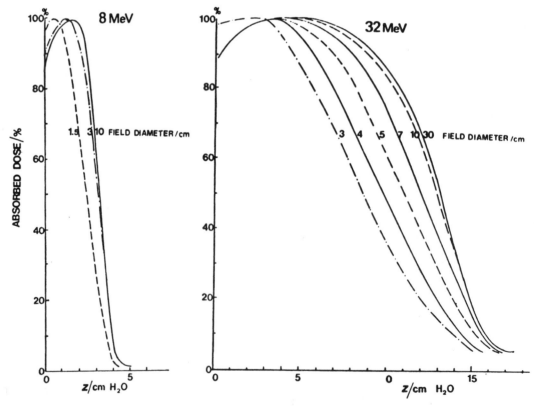

FIG. 14.17. Variation of depth-dose distribution with field size. (From ICRU. Radiation dosimetry: electron beams with energies between 1 and 50 MeV. Report No. 35. Bethesda, MD: International Commission on Radiation Units and Measurements, 1984, with permission.)

relationship:

$$R_{eq} \cong 0.88\sqrt{E_{p,o}} \qquad (14.11)$$

where R_{eq} is the field radius in cm and $E_{p,o}$ is the most probable energy in MeV. For example, the equilibrium fields for 8 MeV and 32 MeV electrons have diameters of 5cm and 10cm, respectively, which agree with the data shown in Fig. 14.17. In clinical practice, the above relationship may be used to classify fields with radius $< R_{eq}$ as small or narrow fields and radius $\geq R_{eq}$ as broad fields. As stated earlier, the depth-dose distribution for small fields is field size dependent while for broad fields it is independent of field size.

E. Field Equivalence

Exact field equivalence for electron beams cannot be established. However, it has been shown (36) that approximate equivalent circular or square fields can be determined for fields of any size, shape, and energy. The term field equivalence means that for the same incident fluence and cross-sectional beam profile, the equivalent fields have the same depth-dose distribution along the central ray. Thus field equivalence here is defined in terms of percent depth doses and not the output factors, which depend on particular jaw setting for the given applicator or other collimation conditions. According to this definition, all broad fields are equivalent because their depth-dose distribution is the same irrespective of field size. For example, 10 × 10, 10 × 15, 10 × 20, 20 × 20, etc. are all broad fields for energies up to 30 MeV (see Eq. 14.11) and hence are equivalent. Field equivalence is therefore relevant only for small fields in which the lateral scatter equilibrium does not exist and consequently, the depth-dose distribution is field size dependent.

Harder et al. (37) have shown that for a square field of cross-section (2a × 2a) the equivalent circular field has a radius R_{equiv}, given by:

$$R_{equiv} \cong 1.116a \qquad (14.12)$$

However, for a small rectangular or irregularly shaped fields, field equivalence is not as straightforward. Khan and Higgins (36) have applied Gaussian pencil beam theory to this problem and derived relationships that can be used to find approximate equivalent circular or square fields for fields of any shape. The reader is referred to their paper for further details on this subject.

F. Square Root Method

Hogstrom et al. (38) have shown that, if the change in collimator scatter with field size is not considered, the depth dose for rectangular field sizes can be extracted from square field data by the following relationships:

$$D^{X,Y} = [D^{X,X} \cdot D^{Y,Y}]^{1/2} \qquad (14.13)$$

where D is the central axis depth dose and X and Y are the field dimensions. Thus the dose for a rectangular field size can be determined from the square root of the two square field depth doses when the sides of the two square fields are equal to the two sides of the rectangular field. Referred to as the square root method, this concept has also been applied to the determination of output factors when the primary collimation is fixed and the secondary collimation close to the phantom is varied (39). It may be restated that the collimator scatter is neglected in this model. Thus the applicability of the square root method is not automatically valid for those machines in which collimator scatter varies substantially with field size.

G. Electron Source

Unlike an x-ray beam, an electron beam does not emanate from a physical source in the accelerator head. A pencil electron beam-after passing through the vacuum window

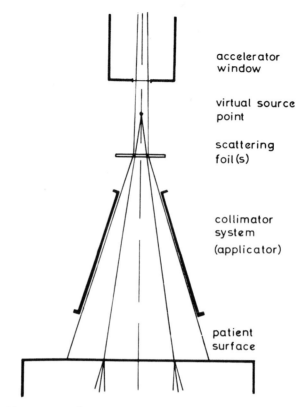

accelerator
window

virtual source
point

scattering
foil(s)

collimator
system
(applicator)

patient
surface

FIG. 14.18. Definition of virtual point source of an electron beam: the intersection point of the backprojections along the most probable directions of motion of electrons at the patient surface. (From Schroeder-Babo P. Determination of the virtual electron source of a betatron. *Acta Radiol* 1983;364[suppl]:7, with permission.)

of the accelerator, bending magnetic field, scattering foils, monitor chambers, and the intervening air column-is spread into a broad beam that *appears* to diverge from a point. This point is called the *virtual source* (40), which may be defined as an intersection point of the backprojections along the most probable directions of electron motion at the patient surface (41). This is illustrated in Fig. 14.18.

A number of methods have been suggested for the determination of virtual source position. Pohlit's (40) method consists of taking electron radiographs of a grid of copper wires at different distances from the collimator and backprojecting the images to a point, the virtual source. A multipinhole technique (41) uses double conical holes in a metal plate. Pinhole images are obtained on a film. Backprojection of the pinhole images gives the virtual source position. Meyer et al. (42) have described the method of determining field size magnification on film with distance. The virtual source point is found by the backprojection of the 50% width of the beam profiles obtained at different distances. A broad beam ($\geq 20 \times 20$ cm) is used for these measurements.

The use of virtual source-to-surface distance (SSD) does not give accurate inverse square law correction for output at extended SSDs under all clinical conditions. Measurements have shown that the virtual SSD gives correct inverse square law factor only for large field sizes (43). For small field sizes, the inverse square law correction underestimates the change in output with virtual SSD. This deviation from the inverse square law is caused by an additional decrease in output because of a loss of side-scatter equilibrium in air and in phantom that is significant for small field sizes and low electron energies. Thus the use of the virtual SSD to predict dose variation with distance requires correction factors, in addition to the inverse square law factor, as a function of field size and energy (42).

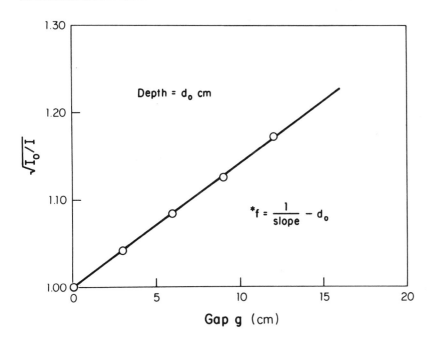

FIG. 14.19. Determination of effective SSD. (From Khan FM, Sewchand W, Levitt SH. Effect of air space on depth dose in electron beam therapy. *Radiology* 1978;126:249, with permission.)

An alternative method of correcting dose output for the air gap between the electron collimator and the patient is to determine *effective SSD,* which gives the correct inverse square law relationship for the change in output with distance. Khan et al. (44) have recommended a method that simulates as closely as possible the clinical situation. In this method, doses are measured in a phantom at the depth of maximum dose (d_m), with the phantom first in contact with the cone or at the standard SSD (zero gap) and then at various distances, up to about 20 cm from the cone end. Suppose f = effective SSD; I_0 = dose with zero gap; I_g = dose with gap g between the standard SSD point and the phantom surface. Then, if electrons obey inverse square law,

$$\frac{I_0}{I_g} = \left(\frac{f + d_m + g}{f + d_m} \right)^2 \tag{14.14}$$

or

$$\sqrt{\frac{I_0}{I_g}} = \frac{g}{f + d_m} + 1 \tag{14.15}$$

By plotting $\sqrt{\dfrac{I_0}{I_g}}$ as a function of gap g (Fig. 14.19), a straight line is obtained, the slope of which is: $\dfrac{1}{f + d_m}$. Thus, $f = \dfrac{1}{\text{slope}} - d_m$.

Although the effective SSD is obtained by making measurements at the depth d_m, its value does not change significantly with the depth of measurement (44). However, the effective SSD does change with energy and field size, especially for small field sizes and low energies. A table of effective SSDs as a function of energy and field size is necessary to meet clinical situations.

F. X-ray Contamination

The x-ray contamination dose at the end of the electron range can be determined from the tail of the depth-dose curve by reading off the dose value at the point where the tail becomes straight (Fig. 14.3). This dose in a patient is contributed by bremsstrahlung interactions of electrons with the collimation system (scattering foils, chambers, collimator jaws, etc.) and the body tissues.

TABLE 14.2. X-RAY CONTAMINATION DOSE (D_x) TO WATER, AT THE END OF THE ELECTRON RANGE AS A PERCENTAGE OF D_{max}

Energy (MeV)	D_x (%)
5	0.1
10	0.5
15	0.9
20	1.4
30	2.8
40	4.2
50	6.0

Data are for theoretical beam with no initial x-ray contamination and are extracted from Monte Carlo data of Berger MJ, Seltzer SM. Tables of energy-deposition distributions in water phantoms irradiated by point-monodirectional electron beams with energies from 1 to 60 MeV, and applications to broad beams. NBSIR 82–2451. Washington, DC: National Bureau of Standards, 1982.

Table 14.2 gives the x-ray dose for the theoretical beam, with no initial x-ray contamination. These values were extracted from the depth-dose distributions in water calculated by Berger and Seltzer (45), using a Monte Carlo program. The x-ray contamination dose from a medical accelerator depends very much on its collimation system and is usually an order of two greater than the values given in Table 14.2. In general, the x-ray contamination is least in the scanning beam type of accelerator, because the scattering foils are not used. In a modern linear accelerator, typical x-ray contamination dose to a patient ranges from approximately 0.5% to 1% in the energy range of 6 to 12 MeV; 1% to 2%, from 12 to 15 MeV; and 2% to 5%, from 15 to 20 MeV.

For regular treatment field sizes, the dose contributed by the x-ray contamination is not of much concern. However, even small amounts of x-ray contamination become critical for total body electron irradiation such as in the treatment of mycosis fungoides (section 14.8).

14.5. TREATMENT PLANNING

Most electron beam treatments are planned for a single field technique. For a relatively flat and homogeneous block of tissue, the dose distribution can be found by using the appropriate isodose chart. However, this simplicity of treatment planning is the exception rather than the rule. Surface areas are seldom flat, and in many cases, inhomogeneities, such as bone, lung, and air cavities, present dosimetric complexities.

A. Choice of Energy and Field Size

The energy of beam is dictated, in general, by the depth of the target volume, minimum target dose required, and clinically acceptable dose to a critical organ, if present in the path of the beam. In most cases, when there is no danger of overdosing a critical structure beyond the target volume, the beam energy may be set so that the target volume lies entirely within the 90% isodose curve. However, in the treatment of the breast, the energy is often chosen so that the depth dose at the chest wall-lung interface is 80% (46). The rationale for this lowering of the energy is to spare the lung, with the belief that the target volume for the chest wall irradiation is quite superficial and that a minimum of 80% (and some even advocate 70%) isodose curve is sufficient for the chest wall. Beyond the 80% depth dose, the dose falloff is characteristically rapid at these beam energies.

The choice of field size in electron beam therapy should be strictly based on the isodose coverage of the target volume. Examination of the electron isodose curves (Fig. 14.20)

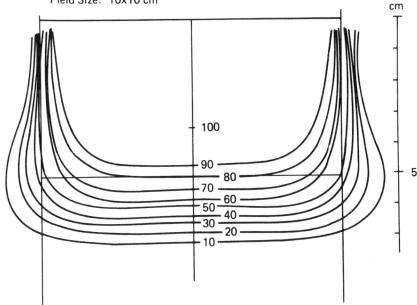

Energy: 16.0 MeV
SSD: 100 cm
Field Size: 10x10 cm

FIG. 14.20. Lateral constriction of the 80% isodose curve with depth. (From Almond PR. Radiation Physics of electron beams. In: Tapley N, ed. *Clinical applications of the electron beam.* New York: John Wiley & Sons, 1976:7, with permission.)

reveals that there is a significant tapering of the 80% isodose curve at energies above 7 MeV (46). The constriction of the useful treatment volume also depends on the field size and is worse for the smaller fields. Thus, with electrons, a larger field at the surface than one is usually accustomed to (in the case of photon beams) may be necessary to cover a target area adequately.

B. Corrections for Air Gaps and Beam Obliquity

In electron beam therapy, there is a frequent problem of treatment cone end[1] not being parallel to the skin surface. These uneven air gaps can sometimes be large as a result of the extreme curvature of the sloping surface. In these cases, it is a common practice to calculate dose distribution simply by applying inverse square law correction to the dose distribution along fan lines emanating from a virtual or effective electron source (47–49). As a result of this correction, the relative depth dose distribution for a sloping contour remains almost unchanged but the absolute value of the dose is decreased at all depths because of beam divergence. This method, however, does not take into account changes in side scatter owing to beam obliquity. This has been pointed out by Ekstrand and Dixon (50), who showed that the beam obliquity tends to (a) increase side scatter at the depth of maximum dose (d_{max}), (b) shift d_{max} toward the surface, and (c) decrease the depth of penetration (as measured by the depth of the 80% dose). These effects are evident in Fig. 14.21.

A broad electron beam can be represented by a summation of a large number of pencil or slit beams placed adjacent to each other. When the beam is incident obliquely on the patient surface, the point at the shallow depth receives greater side scatter from the adjacent pencil beams, which have traversed a greater amount of material, whereas the point at the greater depth receives less scatter. This is schematically illustrated in Fig. 14.22A. As a result of these changes in the relative orientation of the pencils, one would expect an increase in dose at shallow depths and a decrease in dose at greater depths. However, because the

---

[1] In a general sense, the cone end means a plane perpendicular to the beam axis at the nominal SSD.

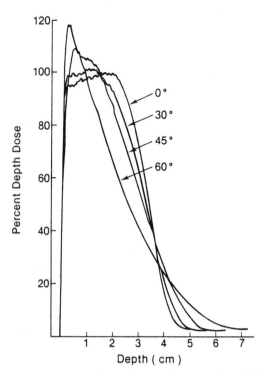

FIG. 14.21. Change in depth dose with the angle of obliquity for a 9-MeV electron beam. (From Ekstrand KE, Dixon RL. The problem of obliquely incident beams in electron beam treatment planning. *Med Phys* 1982;9:276, with permission.)

beam is divergent, the dose will also decrease at all depths as a result of the inverse square law effect, as the air gap between the cone end and the surface increases with the increase in the angle of obliquity. Thus the depth dose at a point in an obliquely incident beam is affected both by the "pencil scatter effect" and the beam divergence.

Figure 14.22B schematically represents an arrangement used frequently for the treatment of chest wall. The beam is incident vertically on a sloping surface, thus increasing the angle of obliquity as well as the air gap between the end of the cone and the surface. Let $D_0(f,d)$ be the dose at a point at depth d for a beam incident normally on a flat-surfaced phantom with an effective SSD $= f$. When the cone is placed on the chest wall, the depth dose $D(f + g,d)$ will be given by:

$$D(f + g,d) = D_0(f,d)\left(\frac{f + d}{f + g + d}\right)^2 \times OF(\theta,d) \tag{14.16}$$

where g is the air gap and $OF(\theta,d)$ is the obliquity factor for the pencil beam scatter effect discussed previously. $OF(\theta,d)$ accounts for the change in depth dose at a point if the beam angle θ changes relative to the surface without change in the distance from the point to the effective source position.

The obliquity factor becomes significant for angles of incidence approaching 45 degrees or higher. For example, a 60-degree angle of obliquity for a 9-MeV beam gives rise to $OF = 1.18$ at the d_{max}, a shift of the d_{max} to about 0.5 cm, and a shift of the 80% depth to about 1.5 cm (52). Of course, in a given clinical situation, these effects are compounded by the inverse square law effect when significantly large air gaps are caused by the sloping surface.

Khan et al. (51) have determined obliquity factors as a function of energy and depth for obliquity angles of 30 degrees, 45 degrees, and 60 degrees. These data are presented in Table 14.3. Depths are normalized to the practical range, which is approximately given by E (MeV)/2 in centimeters of water. The Z/R_p values in column 1 can be converted to

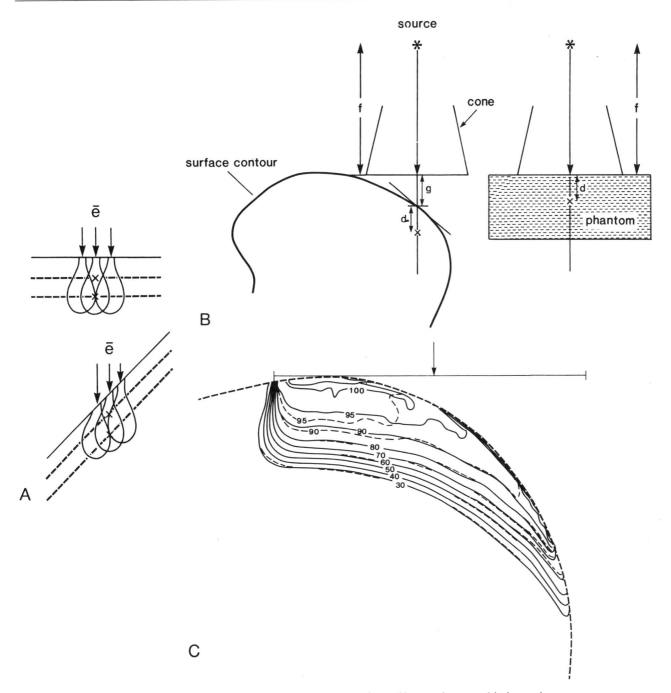

FIG. 14.22. A: A schematic illustration of how the relative orientation of pencil beams changes with the angle of obliquity. For a parallel beam, this effect would increase dose at the shallower points and decrease dose at the deeper points as the angle of obliquity is increased. (Redrawn from Ekstrand KE, Dixon RL. Obliquely incident electron beams. *Med Phys* 1982;9:276.) **B:** A diagrammatic representation of irradiation of a chest wall with sloping surface. The gap *g* and depth *d* for a point are measured along the fan line (the line joining the point to the effective source location). θ is the angle between the fan line and normal to the tangent to the sloping surface. The figure on the right represents the reference set-up, with beam incident normal, with no air gaps between the cone end and the phantom. **C:** Comparison of measured *(solid lines)* and calculated *(dashed lines)* isodose distribution for a beam incident on a polystyrene cylindrical phantom. The measured distribution represents isodensity distribution obtained with a film sandwiched in the phantom according to the procedure outlined in section 14.3B. The calculated distribution was obtained with a computer using a divergent pencil beam algorithm. Both distributions are normalized to the D_{max} in a reference set-up in which the beam is incident normally on a flat phantom with no air gaps between the cone end and the phantom. 12-MeV electrons; field size 18 × 12 cm; effective SSD = 70 cm.

TABLE 14.3. OBLIQUITY FACTORS FOR ELECTRON BEAMS[a]

Z/R_p[b]	E_0 (MeV)					
	22	**18**	**15**	**12**	**9**	**6**
(a) $\theta = 30°$						
0.0	1.00	0.98	0.98	1.00	0.94	1.01
0.1	1.00	1.00	1.00	1.00	1.00	1.08
0.2	1.00	1.00	1.01	1.02	1.05	1.11
0.3	1.01	1.00	1.02	1.03	1.05	1.06
0.4	1.01	1.01	1.02	1.00	1.00	0.96
0.5	1.00	1.00	0.98	0.96	0.92	0.86
0.6	0.95	0.94	0.92	0.90	0.86	0.79
0.7	0.92	0.90	0.87	0.86	0.86	0.83
0.8	0.93	0.85	0.82	0.90	1.00	0.96
0.9	1.09	1.00	1.20	1.11	1.44	1.00
1.0	1.42	1.54	1.50	1.50	1.30	1.00
(b) $\theta = 45°$						
0.0	1.03	1.02	1.03	1.05	0.98	1.14
0.1	1.03	1.04	1.04	1.06	1.10	1.14
0.2	1.05	1.06	1.07	1.11	1.12	1.12
0.3	1.06	1.07	1.09	1.09	1.05	1.07
0.4	1.04	1.04	1.04	1.01	0.93	0.92
0.5	1.00	0.99	0.92	0.92	0.80	0.77
0.6	0.93	0.90	0.86	0.82	0.70	0.69
0.7	0.84	0.84	0.82	0.77	0.70	0.76
0.8	0.87	0.83	0.85	0.86	0.83	1.10
0.9	1.30	1.00	1.43	1.20	1.40	1.46
1.0	2.17	2.31	2.19	2.50	2.00	2.14
(c) $\theta = 60°$						
0.0	1.06	1.06	1.10	1.14	1.14	1.30
0.1	1.10	1.12	1.17	1.20	1.23	1.21
0.2	1.12	1.14	1.15	1.16	1.17	1.08
0.3	1.07	1.07	1.07	1.02	0.98	0.90
0.4	1.00	0.96	0.93	0.86	0.79	0.70
0.5	0.87	0.84	0.79	0.74	0.67	0.56
0.6	0.75	0.74	0.69	0.63	0.58	0.51
0.7	0.70	0.68	0.67	0.62	0.57	0.56
0.8	0.75	0.71	0.67	0.74	0.77	0.87
0.9	1.21	1.00	1.29	1.14	1.60	1.40
1.0	2.31	2.46	2.75	3.0	3.2	2.45

[a]Measured on a Varian Clinac 2500 linear accelerator, by Deibel FC, Khan FM, Werner BL. Electron beam treatment planning with strip beams [abstract]. *Med Phys* 1983;10:527.
[b]Z is the depth measured along the line joining the point of measurement to the virtual electron source.

depths by multiplying with the R_p for the given energies. These obliquity factors can be used in Equation 14.15 for the calculation of dose at a point for an obliquely incident beam.

Computer algorithms have been developed (38,52–54) by which broad beam distribution is calculated by placing a set of narrow or pencil beams along the contour. The divergence correction can be taken into account by aligning central axes of the pencil beams along the fan lines and normalizing the resulting dose distribution to the dose at d_{max} for the beam incident normally on a flat-surfaced phantom. Figure 14.22C compares the calculated distribution using a pencil beam algorithm with the measured distribution obtained in a cylindrical polystyrene phantom.

Sharp surface irregularities produce localized hot and cold spots in the underlying medium due to scattering. Electrons are predominantly scattered outward by steep projections and inward by steep depressions. This can be seen in Fig. 14.23 (55). In practice, such sharp edges may be smoothed with an appropriately shaped bolus. Also, if a bolus is used to reduce beam penetration in a selected part of the field, its edges should be tapered to minimize the effect shown in Fig. 14.23.

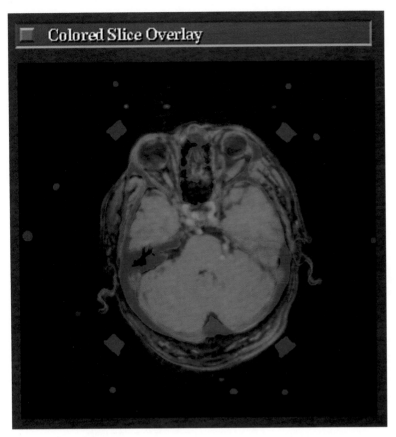

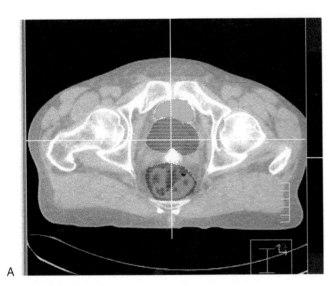

A

COLOR PLATE 19.3. Image segmentation for prostate gland treatment planning. Prostate gland, bladder, and rectum are delineated in different colors. Segmented structures are shown in transverse **(A)**, lateral **(B)**, and coronal **(C)** planes.

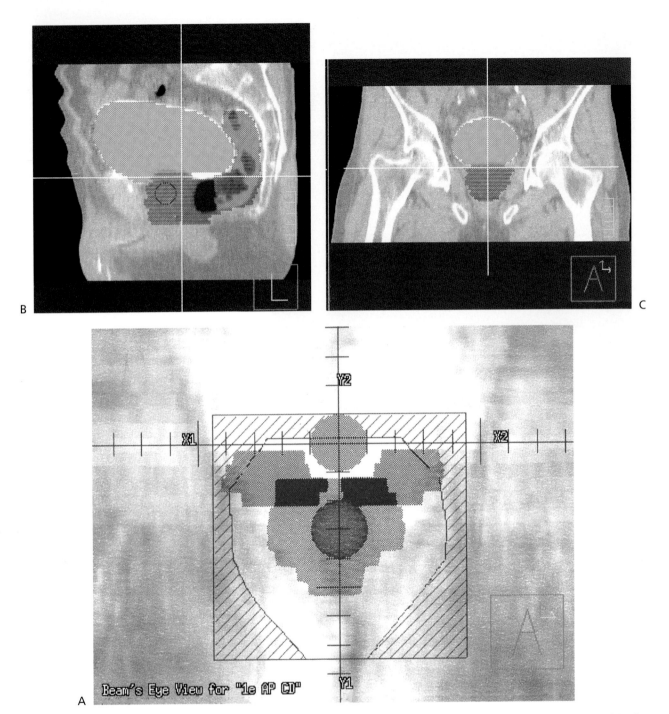

B

C

A Beam's Eye View for "1e AP CD"

COLOR PLATE 19.4. Beam's eye view of anterior-posterior **(A)** and left-right lateral **(B)** fields used in the treatment of prostate gland. Composite (initial plus boost) isodose curves for a four-field plan are displayed in transverse **(C)**, sagittal **(D)**, and coronal **(E)** planes.

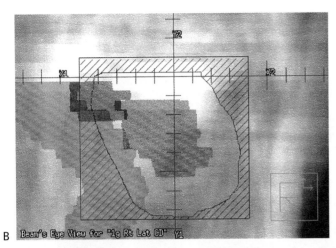

B Beam's Eye View for "1g Rt Lat CD" Y1

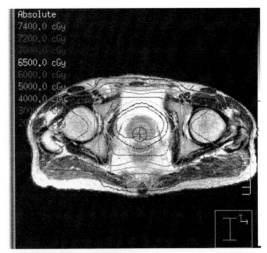

Absolute
7400.0 cGy
7200.0 cGy

6500.0 cGy

6000.0 cGy
5000.0 cGy
4000.0 cGy
3000.0
2000.0

C

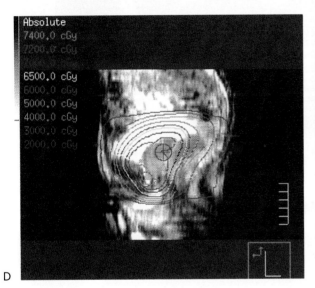

Absolute
7400.0 cGy
7200.0 cGy

6500.0 cGy

6000.0 cGy
5000.0 cGy
4000.0 cGy
3000.0 cGy
2000.0 cGy

D

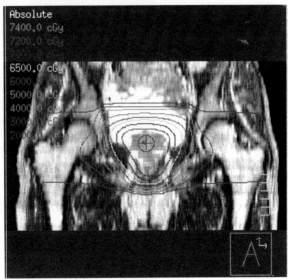

Absolute
7400.0 cGy
7200.0 cGy

6500.0 cGy

6000
5000.0 cGy
4000.0
3000.0
2000

E

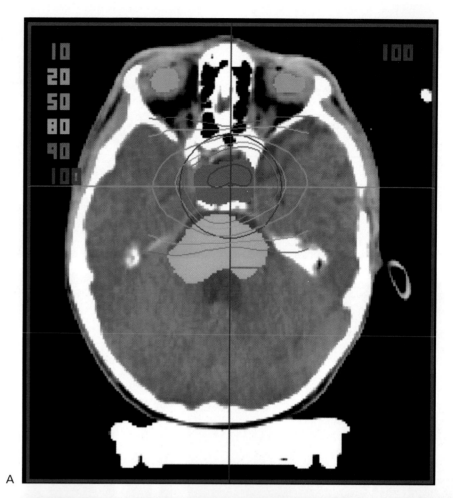

A

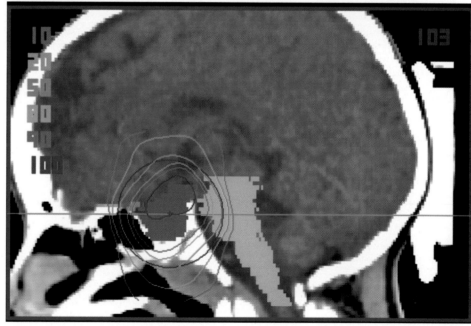

B

COLOR PLATE 19.5. A conformal stereotactic treatment plan for a pituitary tumor showing isodose curves in the transverse **(A)**, lateral **(B)**, and coronal **(C)** planes. Prescription isodose surfaces covering the target volume are displayed in frontal **(D)** and lateral **(E)** views.

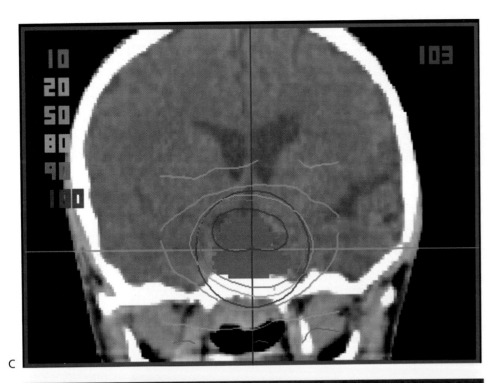

C

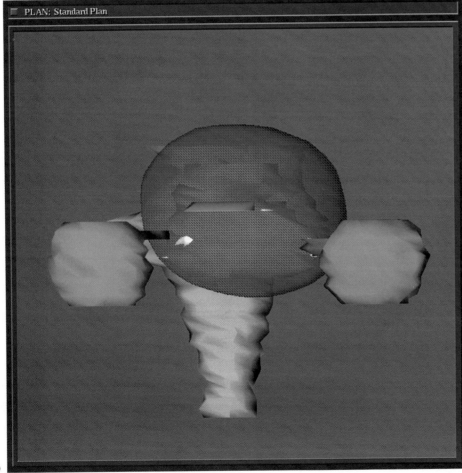

D

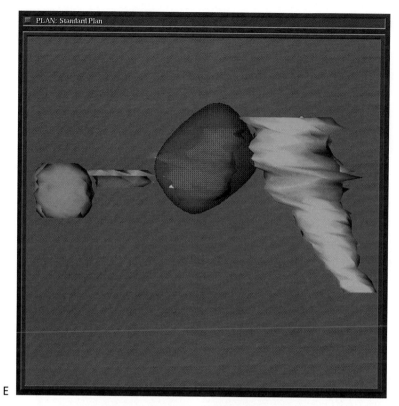

PLAN: Standard Plan

E

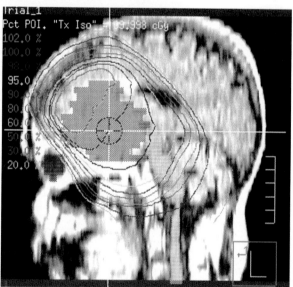

A   B

COLOR PLATE 19.6. A three-dimensional plan for the treatment of glioblastoma is displayed. Isodose curves in transverse **(A)**, lateral **(B)**, and coronal **(C)** planes are used to evaluate the plan. Cumulative DVH **(D)** is also useful in the evaluation process. Differential DVH **(E)** shown here for the tumor only, is more of an academic interest.

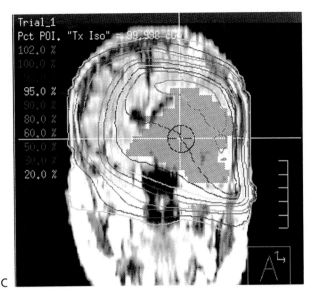

C

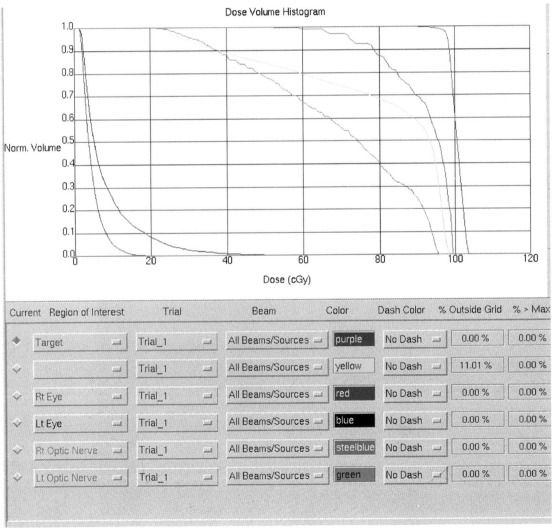

D

Dose Volume Histogram

Current	Region of Interest	Trial	Beam	Color	Dash Color	% Outside Grid	% > Max
◆	Target	Trial_1	All Beams/Sources	purple	No Dash	0.00 %	0.00 %
◇		Trial_1	All Beams/Sources	yellow	No Dash	11.01 %	0.00 %
◇	Rt Eye	Trial_1	All Beams/Sources	red	No Dash	0.00 %	0.00 %
◆	Lt Eye	Trial_1	All Beams/Sources	blue	No Dash	0.00 %	0.00 %
◇	Rt Optic Nerve	Trial_1	All Beams/Sources	steelblue	No Dash	0.00 %	0.00 %
◆	Lt Optic Nerve	Trial_1	All Beams/Sources	green	No Dash	0.00 %	0.00 %

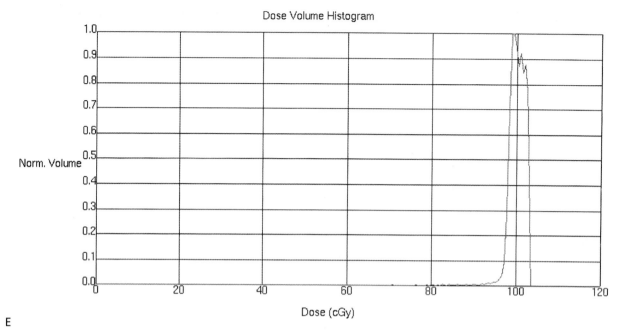

E

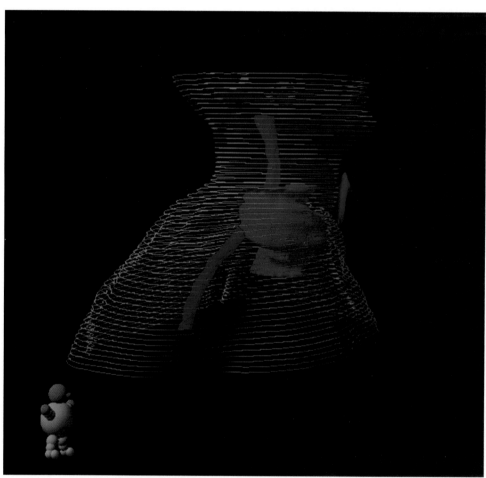

A

COLOR PLATE 20.18. A concave shape target of a thyroid tumor in close vicinity of spinal cord **(A)** and the intensity-modulated radiation therapy–generated isodose plan in a transverse slice **(B)**.

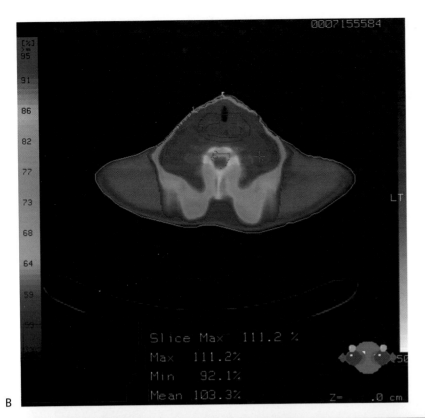

B

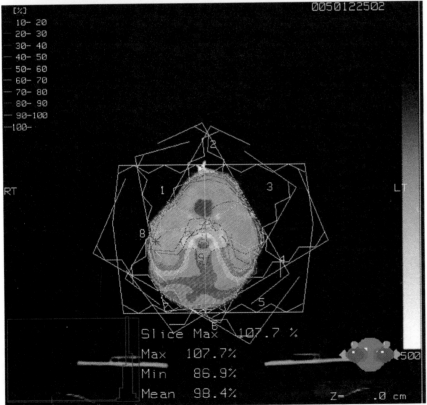

A

COLOR PLATE 20.19. Examples of IMRT-generated plans for head and neck tumors. Isodose plans **(A)** and **(B)** show transverse and sagittal dose distributions from an unknown primary in which 60 Gy were delivered to the PTV with the cord receiving no more than 42 Gy. Sample IMRT plans for optic glioma **(C)** and multiple brain metastases **(D)** were generated by CORVUS treatment planning system, a component of the NOMOS's PEACOCK system. (Courtesy of Nomos Corporation, Sewickley, PA.)

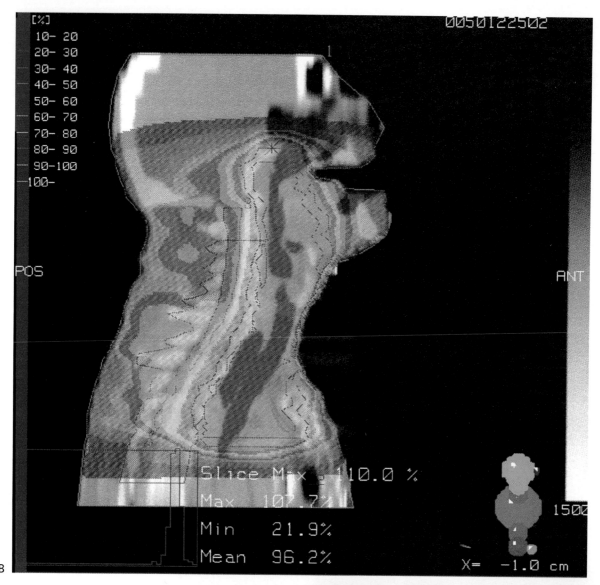

Slice Max 110.0 %
Max 107.7%
Min 21.9%
Mean 96.2%
X= -1.0 cm

B

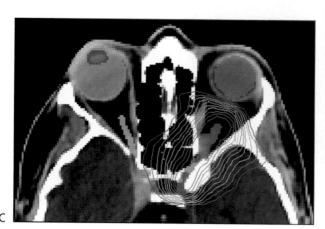

C

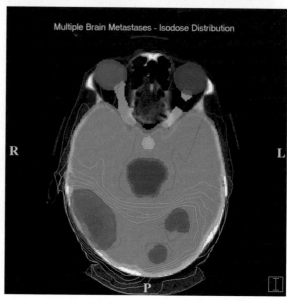

Multiple Brain Metastases - Isodose Distribution

D

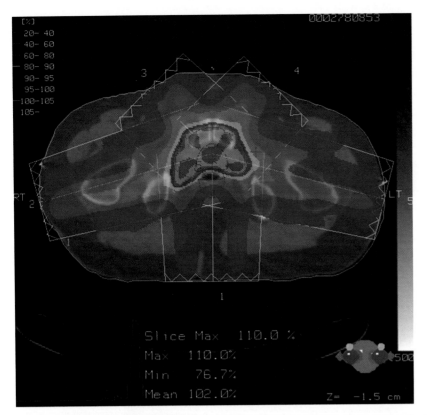

COLOR PLATE 20.20. An example of intensity-modulated radiation therapy plan for the prostate gland using five fields. Any number of intensity modulated fields may be used depending upon the degree of optimization desired in dose distribution and practical considerations of patient set-up and equipment limitations.

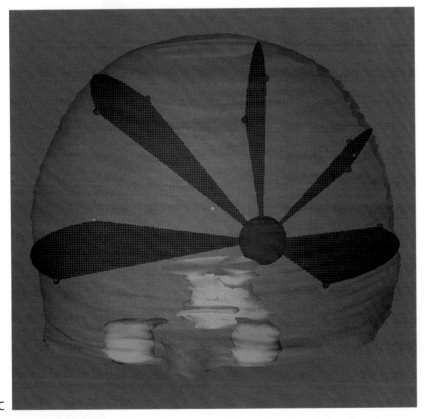

C

COLOR PLATE 21.10. An example of stereotactic radiation surgery treatment of arteriovenous malformation. **(C)** Beam arrangement using five noncoplanar arcs; isodose region (color wash) corresponding to 90% of the maximum dose is shown in anterior view **(D)** and lateral view **(E)**.

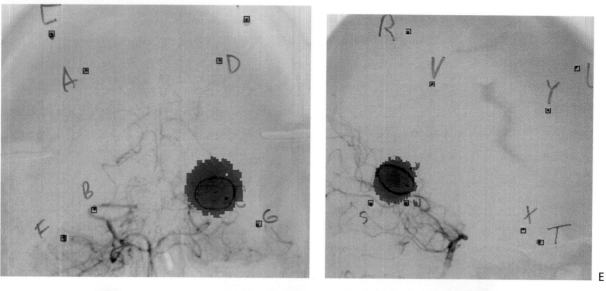

D

E

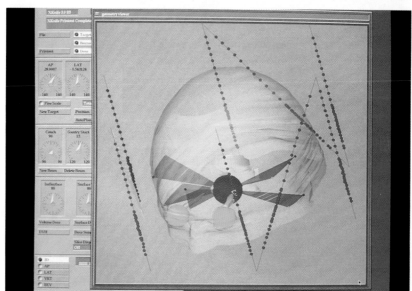

A

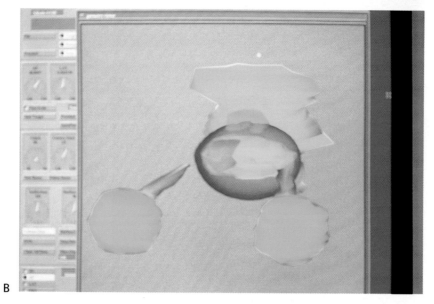

B

COLOR PLATE 21.11. Fractional stereotactic radiation therapy of pituitary adenoma. **A:** Beam arrangement with five non-coplanar arcs. **B:** Prescription surface covering the planning-treatment volume.

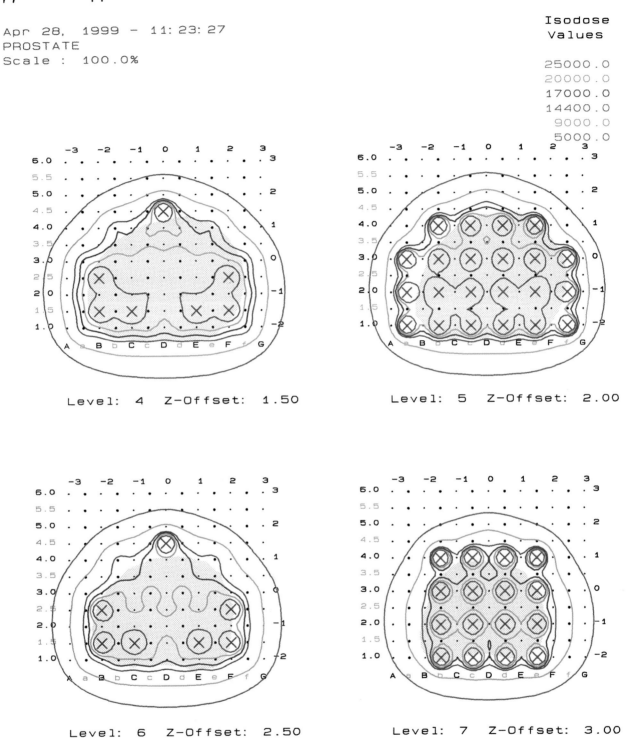

COLOR PLATE 23.1. A sample of pre-treatment plan with ^{125}I seeds showing **(A)** seeds and isodose curves in four ultrasound cross sections of prostate gland and **(B)** dose volume histogram for target (prostate gland) and normal tissue (rectum).

Dose Volume Histogram (DVH)

R   M

Apr 28, 1999 - 11:29:29
PROSTATE

-------- Target DVH   -------- Normal DVH

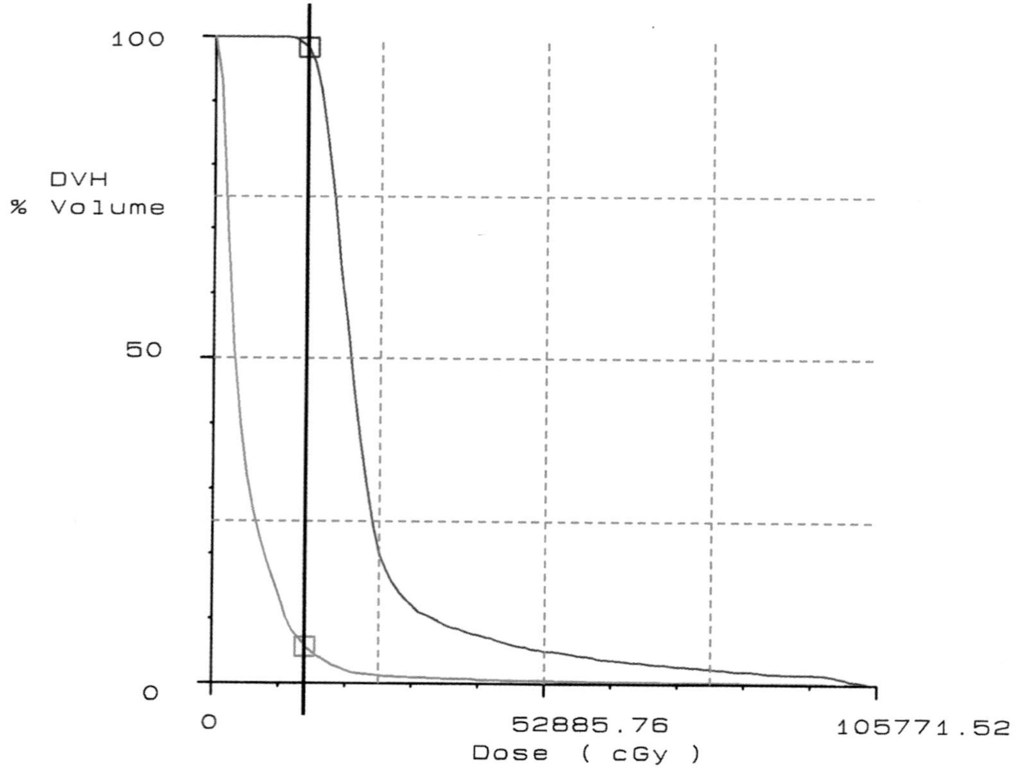

Statistical Data

Prescription   =   14400.00 cG)

Target Statistics

Volume	=	39.33 cc
□ %Volume <= Rx	=	98.31 %
Volume <= Rx	=	38.67 cc
Maximum Dose	=	105771.52 cc
Minimum Dose	=	12032.21 cc

Normal Statistics

Volume	=	287.39 cc
□ %Volume <= Rx	=	5.63 %
Volume <= Rx	=	16.19 cc
Maximum Dose	=	101112.32 cc
Minimum Dose	=	455.65 cc

DVH
% Volume

100

50

0

0   52885.76   105771.52

Dose (cGy)

B

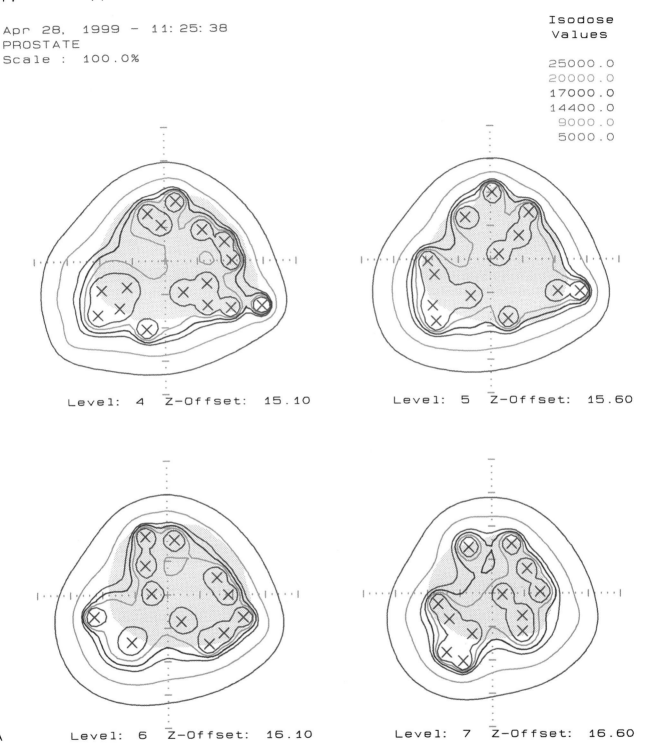

Isodose
Values

25000.0
20000.0
17000.0
14400.0
9000.0
5000.0

Level: 4   Z-Offset: 15.10

Level: 5   Z-Offset: 15.60

A   Level: 6   Z-Offset: 16.10

Level: 7   Z-Offset: 16.60

COLOR PLATE 23.2. A sample of post-treatment plan of the same patient as in Fig. 23.1 showing **(A)** seeds and isodose curves in the four ultrasound cross sections of the prostate gland and **(B)** dose volume histogram for target (prostate gland) and normal tissue (rectum).

R M

Dose Volume Histogram (DVH)

------- Target DVH   ------- Normal DVH

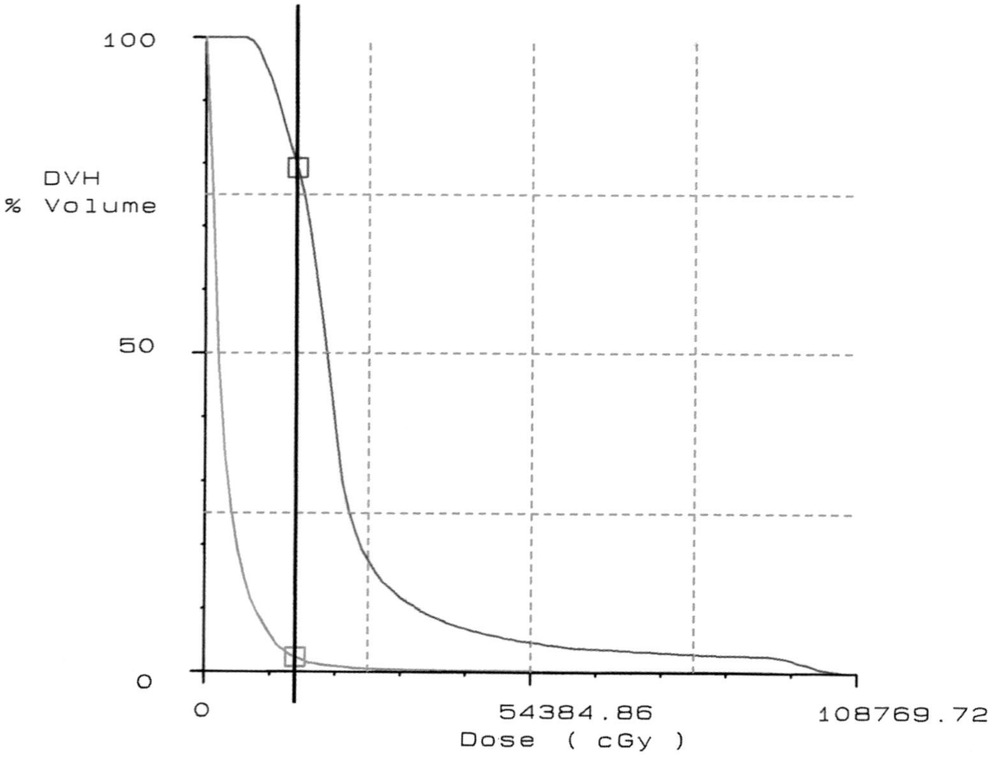

Statistical Data

Prescription = 14400.00 cG)

Target Statistics

	Volume	=	51.47	cc
□	%Volume <= Rx	=	79.25	%
	Volume <= Rx	=	40.79	cc
	Maximum Dose	=	107552.27	cc
	Minimum Dose	=	6574.52	cc

Normal Statistics

	Volume	=	447.81	cc
□	%Volume <= Rx	=	2.32	%
	Volume <= Rx	=	10.38	cc
	Maximum Dose	=	108769.72	cc
	Minimum Dose	=	272.88	cc

108769.72

54384.86

Dose (cGy)

100

DVH
% Volume

50

0   0

B

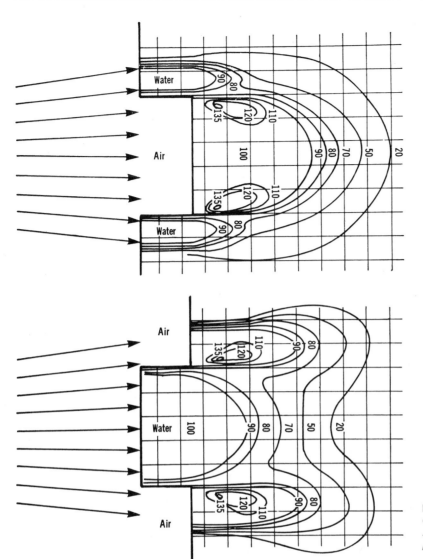

FIG. 14.23. Effect of sharp surface irregularities on electron beam isodose distributions. (From Dutreix J. Dosimetry. In: Gil y Gil, Gil Gayarre, eds. *Symposium on high-energy electrons.* Madrid: General Directorate of Health, 1970:113, with permission.)

C. Tissue Inhomogeneities

Electron beam dose distribution can be significantly altered in the presence of tissue inhomogeneities such as bone, lung, and air cavities. It is difficult to determine dose distribution within or around small inhomogeneities because of enhanced scattering effects. However, for large and uniform slabs, dose distribution beyond the inhomogeneity can be corrected by using the coefficient of equivalent thickness (CET) method (49,56–59). It is assumed that the attenuation by a given thickness z of the inhomogeneity is equivalent to the attenuation ($z \times$ CET) of water. The CET for a given material is approximately given by its electron density (electron/ml) relative to that of water. The dose at a point beyond the inhomogeneity is determined by calculating the effective depth, d_{eff}, along the ray joining the point and the virtual source of the electrons.

$$d_{eff} = d - z(1 - CET) \qquad (14.17)$$

where d is the actual depth of point P from the surface. The depth dose is read from dose distribution data for water at the effective depth. An additional correction may be applied due to the inverse square law, that is, $\left(\dfrac{f + d_{eff}}{f + d}\right)^2$, where f is the effective SSD.

C.1. Bone

The CET method is in good agreement with in vivo measurements in patients for the dose behind the mandible (60). The electron density (or CET) of a compact bone (e.g., mandible) relative to that of water is taken as 1.65. For spongy bone, such as sternum, which has a density of 1.1 g/cm^3, the electron densities are not much different from water, and therefore, CET can be assumed to be unity.

C.2. Lung

The problem of lung inhomogeneity has been studied by many investigators (56–59). Results of in vivo measurements in the lungs of dogs have shown that there is a considerable variation of CET with depth in the lung (61). This is illustrated by Fig. 14.24 for a water-cork system (simulating chest wall and lung interface). The dose near the interface is decreased due to reduced scatter from the low-density cork. Beyond a certain depth, the dose to the cork begins to increase relative to the reference curve (measured in water) as the increased penetration overtakes the reduced scatter.

Thus, in general, the CET values for lung depend on depth within the lung. Empirical equations for the CET values derived from in vivo measurements have been proposed to take this variation into account (60). An average lung CET value of 0.5 has also been suggested (56). More recent measurements (62) in anthropomorphic phantoms have shown that a CET value based on electron density gives an accuracy of approximately 10% in depth dose for typical chest wall irradiations.

The relative electron density of lung may be equated to its mass density. The studies with computed tomography (CT) have shown that the electron density of lung varies between 0.20 and 0.25 relative to that of water. Therefore, if CET is assumed equal to electron density, Equation 14.16 may be used to calculate lung correction by substituting lung density in place of CET. Figure 14.25 shows examples of uncorrected and corrected isodose distributions obtained by using pencil beams. In the case of the corrected distribution, the effective depth was calculated assuming CET equal to the lung density.

In routine treatment planning, any of the previous methods may be used as approximations. Obviously, the effective depth calculation based on electron density or some empirically derived CET is only a rough approximation, for which scattering effects are not fully taken into account.

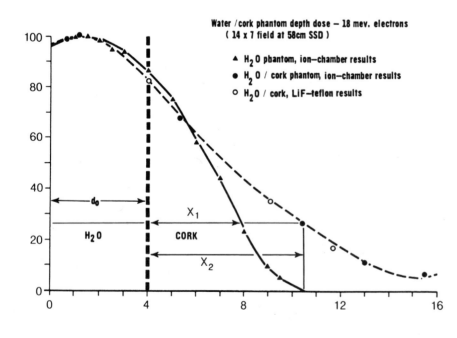

Water / cork phantom depth dose — 18 mev. electrons
(14 x 7 field at 58cm SSD)

▲ H$_2$O phantom, ion–chamber results
● H$_2$O / cork phantom, ion–chamber results
○ H$_2$O / cork, LiF–teflon results

FIG. 14.24. Depth-dose distribution in water and water-cork phantoms. CET values may be calculated from these data. CET = X_1/X_2. (Modified from Almond PR, Wright AE, Boone ML. High-energy electron dose perturbations in regions of tissue heterogeneity. *Radiology* 1967;88:1146.)

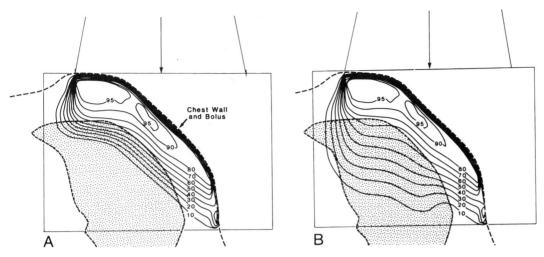

FIG. 14.25. An example of chest wall irradiation with electrons. The surface contour was irregular in shape, so bolus was used to even out chest wall thickness as well as maximize surface dose. **A:** Calculated isodose curves uncorrected for lung density. **B:** Calculated isodose curves corrected for lung density ($\rho = 0.25$ g/cm^3). 10-MeV electron beam; effective SSD = 68 cm; field size = 13 × 15 cm.

C.3. Small Inhomogeneities

Small inhomogeneities present a more complex situation because of electron scattering behind edges. Figure 14.26 schematically illustrates the effect at a single edge. For simplicity, it is assumed that the path of the electrons in medium M is along straight lines. If a material M' of a higher mass scattering power is introduced, electrons are scattered at larger angles. This causes a decrease in the electron fluence behind the slab, thus reducing the dose there. The scattered electrons, on the other hand, increase the dose in the medium M. Thus a small inhomogeneity causes cold spots and hot spots behind its edges.

Pohlit and Manegold (63) have made a systematic analysis of dose distributions behind edges of different materials. Their method can be used to get a rough estimate of the maximum values for increase and decrease of dose behind such inhomogeneities. Figure 14.27 defines angles α and β of dose perturbation. The mean angle α gives the position of the maxima of reduction and of increase of dose, and β represents the mean angle at which the effect of the inhomogeneity is practically negligible. These angles, which are related to the scattering of electrons in the medium, depend mainly on the mean electron energy $\overline{E}$ at the edge. Figure 14.28 gives these angles as a function of $\overline{E}$.

The dose distribution under the inhomogeneity but outside angle β may be calculated according to the regular CET method discussed previously. The maxima and minima of

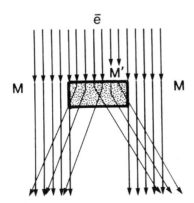

FIG. 14.26. Schematic illustration of electron scatter behind edges between materials M and M'. The scattering power of M' is greater than that of M.

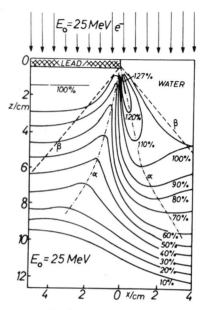

FIG. 14.27. Isodose distribution behind an edge of a thin lead slab in water. Angle α denotes the maxima of dose change and angle β of negligible change. (From Pohlit W, Manegold KH. Electron-beam dose distribution in inhomogeneous media. In: Kramer S, Suntharalingam N, Zinninger GF, eds. *High energy photons and electrons.* New York: John Wiley & Sons, 1976:243, with permission.)

dose along the boundaries of angle α may be estimated by defining a maximum change, P_{max}, in dose.

$$P_{max} = \frac{D_m - D_0}{D_0} \qquad (14.18)$$

where D_m is the dose at the highest increase or depression and D_0 is the dose in the homogeneous water phantom at that point. Figure 14.29 may be used to estimate P_{max}

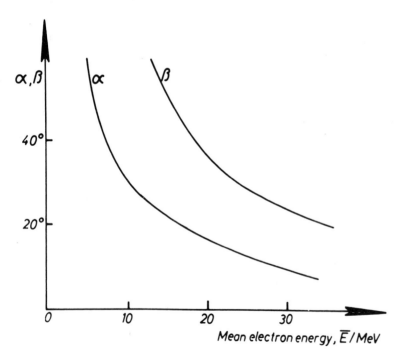

FIG. 14.28. Plot of angles α and β as a function of mean energy at the edge for inhomogeneities in water (or tissue). (From Pohlit W, Manegold KH. Electron-beam dose distribution in inhomogeneous media. In: Kramer S, Suntharalingam N, Zinninger GF, eds. *High energy photons and electrons.* New York: John Wiley & Sons, 1976:243, with permission.)

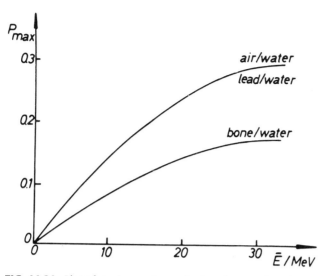

FIG. 14.29. Plot of maximum change in dose P_{max} as a function of mean electron energy at the edge of various inhomogeneities in water. (From Pohlit W, Manegold KH. Electron-beam dose distribution in inhomogeneous media. In: Kramer S, Suntharalingam N, Zinninger GF, eds. *High energy photons and electrons.* New York: John Wiley & Sons, 1976:243, with permission.)

for different energies and materials. It is important to note that the influence of an edge increases with increasing electron energy.

Scattering effects can be enhanced by adjoining scattering edges, and therefore, small inhomogeneities produce complex effects, resulting in large changes in dose caused by the overlapping of these regions.

The previous method is useful for quick-and-rough calculations. More accurate calculations require more sophisticated methods based on multiple scattering theory. Some work along these lines has been reported in the literature (34,38,54,64,65).

D. Use of Bolus and Absorbers

Bolus is often used in electron beam therapy to (a) flatten out an irregular surface, (b) reduce the penetration of the electrons in parts of the field, and (c) increase the surface dose. Ideally, the bolus material should be equivalent to tissue in stopping power and scattering power. A given bolus material should be checked by comparing depth dose distribution in the bolus with that in the water. If a scaling factor is required, it should be documented and used in treatment planning whenever the bolus is used.

A number of commercially available materials can be used as bolus, e.g., paraffin wax, polystyrene, Lucite, Superstuff, and Superflab. Usefulness of some of these materials for electron bolusing have been discussed in the literature (66,67). In my experience, Superflab[2] is excellent for bolusing. This material is transparent, flexible, and almost water equivalent.

A plate of low atomic number material such as Lucite and polystyrene is sometimes used to reduce the energy of an electron beam. Such plates are known as decelerators. The decelerator should be placed in close contact with the patient surface as with a bolus. Large air gaps between the absorber and the surface would result in scattering of electrons outside the field and reduction in dose, which may not be easily predictable unless specifically measured for those conditions. For these reasons, a flexible bolus that conforms to the surface is more desirable.

---

[2] Developed by G. R. Feaster, University of Kansas at Kansas City, and supplied by Mick Radio-Nuclear Instruments, Inc., The Bronx, New York.

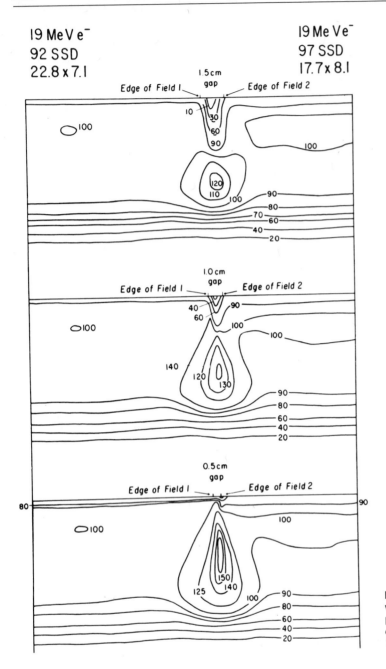

FIG. 14.30. Isodose distributions for adjacent electron fields with different gap widths. (From Almond PR. Radiation physics of electron beams. In: Tapley N, ed. *Clinical applications of the electron beam.* New York: John Wiley & Sons, 1976, with permission.)

E. Problems of Adjacent Fields

When two adjacent electron fields are overlapping or abutting, there is a danger of delivering excessively high doses in the junction region. On the other hand, separating the fields may seriously underdose parts of the tumor. Examples of combined isodose distributions for different field separations are shown in Fig. 14.30. In a clinical situation, the decision as to whether the fields should be abutted or separated should be based on the uniformity of the combined dose distribution across the target volume. Because the tumors treated with electrons are mostly superficial, the electron fields are usually abutted on the surface. The hot spots can be accepted, depending on their magnitude, extent, and location. Similar considerations apply to electron fields adjacent to x-ray fields.

When an electron field is abutted at the surface with a photon field, a hot spot develops on the side of the photon field and a cold spot develops on the side of the electron field (68). This is caused by outscattering of electrons from the electron field. Figure 14.31 shows this effect when a 9-MeV electron field is abutted with a 6-MV photon field, an

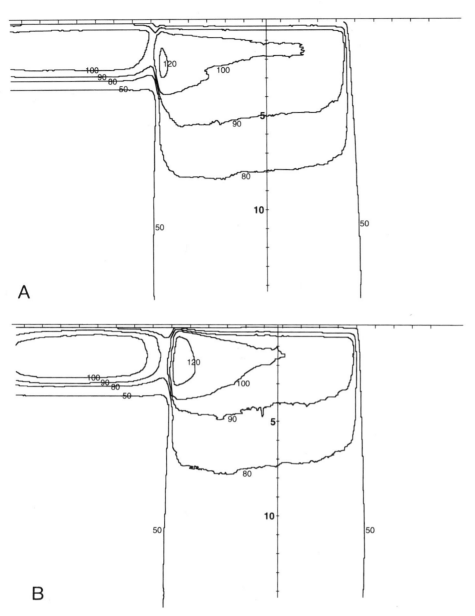

FIG. 14.31. Isodose curves in a plane perpendicular to the junction line between abutting photon and electron fields. 9-MeV Electron beam; field size = 10 × 10 cm; 6-MV photon beam; SSD = 100 cm. **A:** Electron beam at standard SSD of 100 cm. **B:** Electron beam at extended SSD of 120 cm. (From Johnson JM, Khan FM. Dosimetric effects of abutting extended SSD electron fields with photons in the treatment of head and neck cancers. *Int J Radiat Oncol Biol Phys* 1994;28:741–747, with permission.)

example typifying a clinical situation involving treatment of tumors in the neck. Whereas the photon field is used to treat the anterior neck, the electron field is used to treat the posterior neck nodes overlying the cord. Because of the limited range of the electrons, the cord can be spared, while sufficient dose can be delivered to the nodes.

An examination of the isodose distribution in Fig. 14.31 also reveals that the extent of hot and cold spots depends on the electron beam SSD. In Fig. 14.31A, the electron beam is incident at the standard SSD of 100 cm, with the distance between the applicator end and the surface being 5 cm. In Fig. 14.31B, the electron beam is incident at an extended SSD of 120 cm, exemplifying a practical situation when clearance is required between the applicator and the patient shoulder. The increased air gap between the applicator and the surface causes the electron beam profile to become less flat as a result of increased scattering of electrons by air. Consequently, the hot and cold spots spread out to cover larger areas, without significantly changing their magnitudes.

14.6. FIELD SHAPING

Extensive field shaping is sometimes required in electron beam therapy. Lead cutouts are often used to give shape to the treatment area and to protect the surrounding normal tissue or a critical organ. These cutouts are placed either directly on the skin or at the end of the treatment cone.

For lower-energy electrons (<10 MeV), less than 5 mm thickness of lead is required for adequate shielding (e.g., ≤5% transmission). Lead sheets of this thickness can be molded to conform more or less to the surface contour and, therefore, can be placed directly on the skin surface. For higher-energy electrons, however, thicker lead is required and cannot be so easily contoured. Moreover, a heavy lead mask may cause discomfort to the patient. The alternative method is to support a lead cutout at the end of the treatment cone or the field trimmers. Shields to be used in such a configuration can be designed from pure lead sheets or a low melting alloy such as Lipowitz metal (trade names: Cerrobend, Ostalloy, and Lometoy).

A. External Shielding

Several publications have reported the thickness of lead or low melting point lead alloy required for shielding in electron beam therapy (69–73). Figure 14.32 shows a set of transmission measurements through lead. The thickness for shielding can be chosen on the basis of allowable transmission (e.g., 5%). The shield thickness should be neither overly large nor so critical in measurement that a small change in thickness would cause a large change in the transmitted dose.

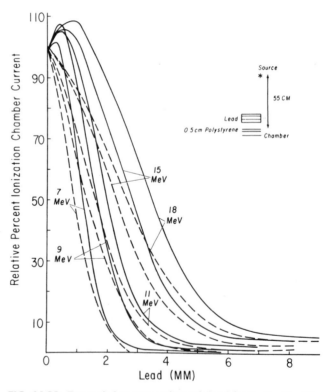

FIG. 14.32. Transmission curves through lead for 7-, 9-, 11-, 15-, and 18-MeV electrons. Measurements made with a plane-parallel chamber in a polystyrene phantom, at a depth of 0.5 cm. *Solid lines* are for 10.5 × 10.5 cm effective field size and *dashed lines* are for 6.3 × 6.3 cm effective field size. (Redrawn from Giarratano JC, Duerkes RJ, Almond PR. Lead shielding thickness for dose reduction of 7- to 28-MeV electrons. *Med Phys* 1975;2:336.)

An important consideration in electron beam shielding is to make certain that the thickness is appropriate to reduce the dose to an acceptable value. As seen in Fig. 14.32, if the lead is too thin, the transmitted dose may even be enhanced directly behind the shield. Normally, if weight or thickness is no problem, one can use a shield of thickness greater than the required minimum. But there are practical limits on the amount of lead that can be used. For example, in the case of eyeshields (74) and internal shields, it is important to use the minimum thickness of lead to obtain the desired reduction in dose.

B. Measurement of Transmission Curves

Transmission curves for a shielding material may be obtained with an ion chamber embedded in a phantom. A suitable arrangement for such measurements consists of a parallel-plate ion chamber in a polystyrene phantom. Because the maximum transmitted dose through lead occurs at a point close to the patient's surface, the measurement depth in the phantom should not exceed 5 mm (75).

The transmission curve is a plot of ionization current as a function of shield thickness. Generally, the shielding measurements made with broad beams gives an upper limit to the shielding requirements for all field sizes (69,73). However, if minimum thickness shields are needed, as for internal shielding, a transmission curve may be measured especially for the given field size and the depth of the structure to be shielded.

Although it is desirable to make measurements with the shields in the same configuration relative to the applicator and the phantom as used clinically, this is not a critical consideration. Purdy et al. (73) made measurements with the shield placed at the end of the treatment cone and at the phantom surface. They did not find significant differences in the percent transmission for the two arrangements.

Figure 14.33 shows a plot of minimum lead thickness required to stop electrons as a function of the most probable electron energy incident on lead. The transmitted dose in this case is only the result of bremsstrahlung. From these data a rule of thumb may be formulated: the minimum thickness of lead required for blocking in millimeters is given

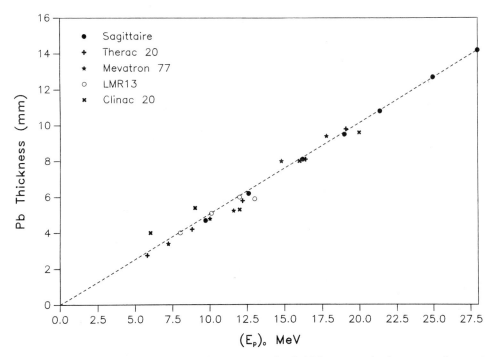

FIG. 14.33. A plot of published data for minimum lead thickness required to stop primary electrons as a function of electron energy incident on lead. (From Khan FM, et al. Clinical electron-beam dosimetry. Report of AAPM Radiation Therapy Committee Task Group No. 25. *Med Phys* 1991;18:73, with permission.)

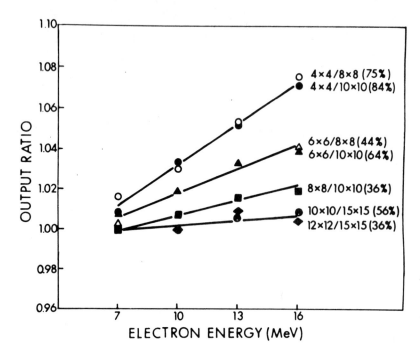

FIG. 14.34. Ratio of ionization for the open cone to the ionization for the shaped field (output ratio) as a function of beam energy. Output factor is inverse of output ratio. The field sizes for the reduced fields were defined by a lead cutout placed at the phantom surface. (From Choi MC, Purdy JA, Gerbi BJ, et al. Variation in output factor caused by secondary blocking for 7–16 MeV electron beams. *Med Phys* 1979;6:137, with permission.)

by the electron energy in MeV incident on lead divided by 2. Another millimeter of lead may be added as a safety margin. The required thickness of Cerrobend is approximately 20% greater than that of pure lead.

C. Effect of Blocking on Dose Rate

Blocking a portion of the electron beam field, in general, produces changes in the dose rate and dose distribution. The magnitude of the change depends on the extent of blocking, the thickness of lead, and the electron energy. Figure 14.34 shows increase in output ratio (or decrease in output factor) at d_{max} when a field is blocked down to a smaller size (72). If a field produced by a lead cutout is smaller than the minimum size required for maximum lateral dose buildup, the dose in the open portion is reduced (70) (Fig. 14.35).

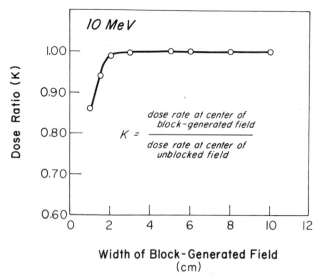

FIG. 14.35. Change of dose at D_{max} as the field size is changed using a lead cutout at the phantom surface (72).

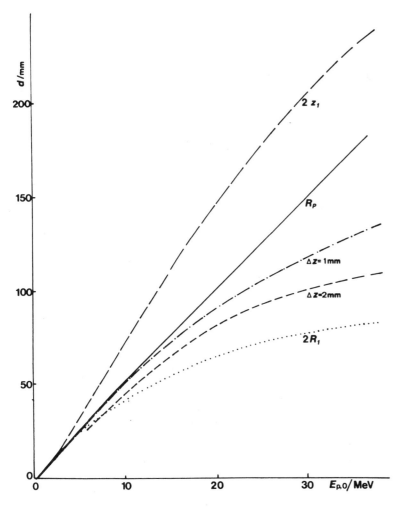

FIG. 14.36. Minimum field diameter, *d*, versus most probable energy at the surface, $E_{p,0}$, for which the depth dose distribution can be considered independent of field size. The curve labeled $2z_1$ shows maximum lateral excursion diameter of electrons. R_p is the extrapolated range. Δz is the maximum shift in the depth dose distribution for field diameter relative to broad beam. The curve $2R_1$ gives the field diameter at which the maximum dose is 1% less than its value for a broad beam. These data do not include the effects of collimator or air scatter. (From Lax I, Brahme A. On the collimation of high energy electron beams. *Acta Radiol Oncol* 1980;19:199, with permission.)

The reduction in dose also depends on the depth of measurement. Thus field shaping affects output factor as well as depth-dose distribution in a complex manner.

As the most conservative measure, a special dosimetry (e.g., output factor, depth-dose, and isodose distribution) should be measured for any irregularly shaped electron field used in the clinic. However, this is impractical because most radiation therapy fields are irregular. The ICRU (14) suggested R_p as the lower limit for field diameter, above which the field size dependence of the depth dose is negligible. That means that for a given point of interest in an irregularly shaped field, the field edges should be farther than $R_p/2$ for the lateral scatter equilibrium to be approximately achieved. For example, a 10×10 cm size field of a 12-MeV electron beam ($R_p \simeq 6$ cm) may be blocked down to 6×6 cm field without significantly affecting the depth-dose distribution.

Lax and Brahme (76) have measured field diameters above which the maximum shift of the depth-dose curve in water is less than 2 mm and the dose maximum is within 1% of its value for a broad beam. From these data (Fig. 14.36) a rough rule of thumb may be formulated: the minimum field diameter for approximate lateral scatter equilibrium (LSE) is given by E (MeV)/2.5 in centimeters of water. This rule is slightly less stringent than that of the ICRU (14) discussed above. An alternative method is to determine equilibrium radius, Req, from Equation 14.11. For an irregularly shaped field, radius in any direction must be $\geq$ Req for the establishment of LSE.

D. Internal Shielding

In some situations, such as the treatment of lip, buccal mucosa, and eyelid lesions, internal shielding is useful to protect the normal structures beyond the target volume. Lead shielding

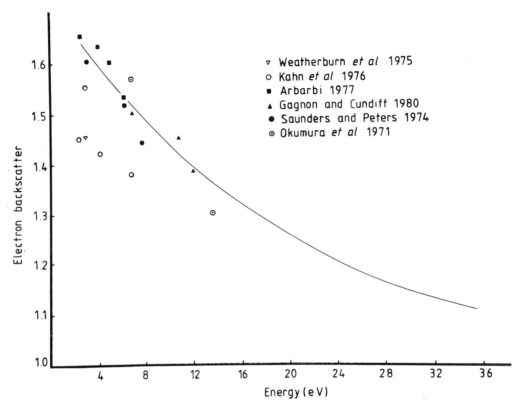

FIG. 14.37. Electron backscatter from lead as a function of mean electron energy at the interface. The *solid line* represents the best fit to the experimental data of Klevenhagen et al. (84), from which this graph is reprinted by permission.

may be used to reduce the transmitted dose to an acceptable value. However, the electron backscatter from lead enhances the dose to the tissue near the shield. This effect has been discussed by several investigators (70,77–82).

The enhancement in dose at the tissue-lead interface can be quite substantial, e.g., 30% to 70% in the range of 1 to 20 MeV, having a higher value for the lower-energy beams. Figure 14.37 shows the increase in dose (relative to homogeneous phantom) as a function of the mean energy incident at the tissue-lead interface. The scatter in the experimental data is probably due to differences in the measurement techniques and the state of angular spread of the electron beam before incidence at the interface. The curve by Klevenhagen et al. (82) represents the best fit to the experimental data for the polystyrene-lead interface and has been characterized by the following equation:

$$\text{EBF} = 1 + 0.735 \exp(-0.052\overline{E}_Z) \tag{14.19}$$

where EBF is the electron backscatter factor, defined as the quotient of the dose at the interface with the lead present to that with a homogeneous polystyrene phantom at the same point. $\overline{E}_Z$ is the average electron energy incident at the interface.

Variation of electron backscatter with atomic number Z of the scattering material has also been studied (81,82). Figure 14.38 gives the data by Klevenhagen et al. (82).

An important aspect of the electron backscatter problem is the range of the backscattered electrons. Measurements of dose in the phantom layers preceding the lead have shown (70,81,82) that for electrons in the range of 1 to 25 MeV the range of the backscattered electrons is about 1 to 2 g/cm² of polystyrene, depending on the energy of the incident electrons. The dose enhancement drops off exponentially with the distance from the interface on the entrance side of the beam. Figure 14.39 illustrates this effect for 10-MeV beam incident on a phantom with a sheet of lead placed at various depths.

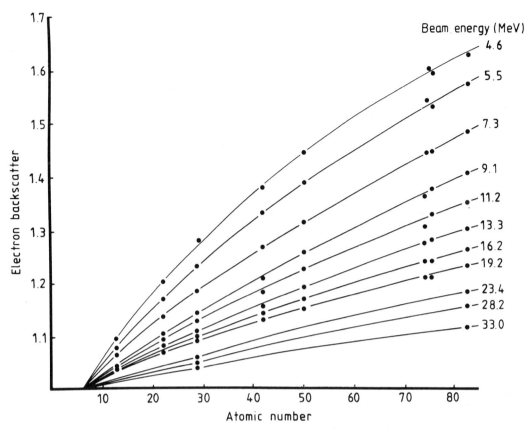

FIG. 14.38. Variation of electron backscatter with atomic number *Z* of scattering material for different electron energies at the interface. (From Klevenhagen SC, Lambert GD, Arbabi A. Backscattering in electron beam therapy for energies between 3 and 35 MeV. *Phys Med Biol* 1982;27:363, with permission.)

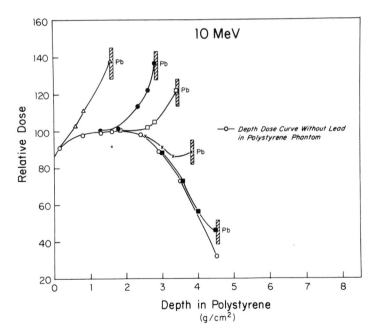

FIG. 14.39. Modification of depth dose by lead placed at various depths in a polystyrene phantom. Lead thickness = 1.7 mm. (From Khan FM, Moore VC, Levitt SH. Field shaping in electron beam therapy. *Br J Radiol* 1976;49:883, with permission.)

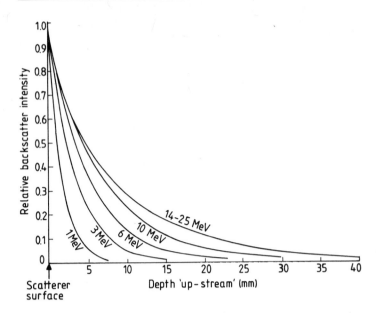

FIG. 14.40. Intensity of backscattered electrons from lead transmitted through polystyrene in the upstream direction of the primary beam. (From Lambert GD, Klevenhagen SC. Penetration of backscattered electrons in polystyrene for energies between 1–25 MeV. *Phys Med Biol* 1982;27:721, with permission.)

To dissipate the effect of electron backscatter, a suitable thickness of low atomic number absorber such as bolus may be placed between the lead shield and the preceding tissue surface. Saunders and Peters (8) recommend the use of an aluminum sheath around any lead used for internal shielding. Oral shielding has also been accomplished by special oral stents made of dental acrylic that encompasses the lead (46). Such a shield provides lead protection for the tongue and other structures as well as reduces the electron backscatter from lead reaching the buccal mucosa.

The thickness of low atomic number absorber required to absorb the backscattered electrons may be calculated using the data in Fig. 14.40. For a given energy of electrons incident on lead, the thickness of polystyrene, determined from Fig. 14.40, is converted to the absorber thickness by dividing it by its relative electron density.

Example

A buccal mucosa lesion is treated with a 9-MeV electron beam incident externally on the cheek. Assuming cheek thickness, including the lesion, to be 2 cm, calculate (a) thickness of lead required to shield oral structures beyond the cheek, (b) magnitude of electron backscatter, and (c) thickness of bolus or aluminum to absorb backscattered electrons.

For these calculations, the most probable energy and the mean energy of electrons may be assumed to be the same.

(a) Incident energy = 9 MeV; $R_p \approx 4.5$ cm. Energy at the lead-mucosa interface (at 2 cm depth) = $9 \left(1 - \dfrac{2}{4.5} \right) \approx 5$ MeV, (see Eq. 14.7) and lead thickness for shielding $\approx \dfrac{5}{2} = 2.5$ mm (Fig. 14.33).

(b) From Equation 14.18 or Fig. 14.38, electron backscatter for 5-MeV electrons incident on lead $\simeq 56\%$.

(c) From Fig. 14.40, depth upstream in polystyrene for backscattered electrons is approximately equal to 10 mm for a 10% transmission of backscatter intensity. Assuming density of polystyrene or bolus to be approximately unity and that of aluminum equal to 2.7 g/cm^3, thickness of bolus $\simeq 1$ cm and thickness of aluminum $\simeq 4$ mm.

Thus, either 1 cm of bolus or 4 mm of aluminum may be used to absorb 90% of the backscattered electrons. Considering the available space for oral shielding, one may adjust the calculated thickness of materials or the incident electron energy to provide acceptable target dose and the allowed transmitted dose through lead.

Eyeshields are designed using the same principles to protect the lens. Minimum thickness of lead is used to provide acceptable transmission value. Because a significant thickness of low Z material is required to absorb the electron backscatter, eyeshields cannot be coated with an adequate thickness of such materials without exceeding the size requirements. In such cases, it is desirable to coat the lead shield with a thin film of dental acrylic (to absorb the very low energy electrons) and calibrate the set-up for the actual enhanced dose received by the lid. Alternatively, if space allows, a 2-mm-thick aluminum sheath may be interposed between the lead shield and the eyelid to absorb the backscattered electrons.

14.7. ELECTRON ARC THERAPY

Electron beam arc technique gives excellent dose distribution for treating superficial tumors along curved surfaces. The technique was first described by Becker and Weitzel (83) in 1956. Several papers (84–91) have since appeared in the literature describing the various technical and physical aspects of electron arc therapy. For details, the reader is referred to Paliwal (92).

On the basis of isodose distribution, electron arc therapy is most suited for treating superficial volumes that follow curved surfaces such as chest wall, ribs, and entire limbs. Although all chest wall irradiations can be done with electron arcing, this technique is mostly useful in cases for which the tumor involves a large chest wall span and extends posteriorly beyond the midaxillary line. The conventional technique of using tangential photon beams in this case will irradiate too much of the underlying lung. The alternative approach of using multiple abutting electron fields is fraught with field junction problems, especially when angled beams are used. In short, it appears that for a certain class of cases, electron arc therapy has no reasonable alternative.

Not all electron accelerators are equipped with electron arc mode. However, with increasing interest in this technique, more and more linear accelerators are being made with this capability. Besides the arcing capability, certain modifications in electron collimation are necessary to make this technique feasible. For example, one needs a beam-defining aperture with adequate clearance from the patient and additional collimation close to the patient surface to sharpen the dose falloff at the arc limits (86).

Machines that cannot rotate in the electron mode may still be used to perform what is called a "pseudoarc" technique (93). In this technique, the field is defined by the x-ray jaws and the electron collimation is provided on the patient's skin surface. The beam is directed isocentrically through equally spaced large number of angles. The fields are overlapped by aligning the center of a given fixed field with the edge of its next neighboring field. Thus the pseudoarc technique is designed to achieve the results of a continuous arc by using a sufficiently large number of overlapping fields directed isocentrically.

A. Calibration of Arc Therapy Beam

Calibration of an electron arc therapy procedure requires special considerations in addition to those required for stationary beam treatments. Dose per arc can be determined in two ways: (a) integration of the stationary beam profiles and (b) direct measurement. The first method requires an isodose distribution as well as the dose rate calibration of the field (under stationary beam conditions) used for arcing. The integration procedure is illustrated in Fig. 14.41. Radii are drawn from the isocenter at a fixed angular interval $\Delta\theta$ (e.g., 10 degrees). The isodose chart is placed along each radius while the dose at point P as a fraction of the maximum dose on the central axis is recorded. Let $D_i(P)$ be this dose as the isodose chart is placed at the radius. The dose per arc at P is given by the following equation (94):

$$D_{\mathrm{arc}}(P) = \frac{\dot{D}_0 \cdot \Delta\theta}{2\pi n} \sum_{i=1}^{N} D_i(P) \cdot \mathrm{Inv}(i) \qquad (14.20)$$

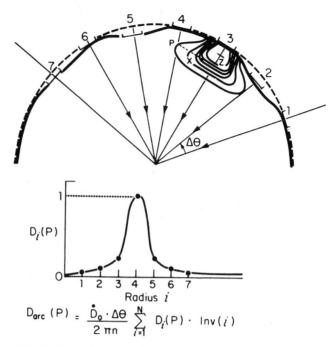

FIG. 14.41. Integration of dose per arc at a point *P. Solid line* represents an irregularly shaped patient contour and the *dotted line* is a circle approximating the contour. Isodose curves for the scanning field are placed along each radius to integrate the dose at point *P.* (From Khan FM. Calibration and treatment planning of electron beam arc therapy. In: Paliwal B, ed. *Proceedings of the symposium on electron dosimetry and arc therapy.* New York: AAPM/American Institute of Physics, 1982, with permission.)

where $\dot{D}_0$ is the dose rate per minute in the stationary field at the depth of d_{max}, n is the speed of rotation (number of revolutions per minute), and $Inv(i)$ is the inverse square law correction for an air gap between the dotted circle and the beam entry point. The term $\Delta\theta \cdot \sum_{i=1}^{N} D_i(P)$ also can be evaluated graphically as shown in Fig. 14.41.

The direct measurement of dose per arc requires a cylindrical phantom of a suitable material such as polystyrene or Lucite. A hole is drilled in the phantom to accommodate the chamber at a depth corresponding to the d_{max}. The radius of the phantom need only be approximately equal to the radius of curvature of the patient, because only a small part of the arc contributes dose to the chamber reading (94). However, the depth of isocenter must be the same as used for the treatment. The integrated reading per arc can be converted to dose per arc by using correction factors normally applicable to a stationary beam.

B. Treatment Planning

The treatment planning for electron arc therapy includes (a) choice of beam energy, (b) choice of field size, (c) choice of isocenter, (d) field shaping, and (e) isodose distribution. These are briefly considered below.

B.1. Beam Energy

The central axis dose distribution is altered due to field motion. For a small scanning field width, the depth dose curve shifts slightly and the beam appears to penetrate somewhat farther than for a stationary beam (Fig. 14.42). The surface dose is reduced and the bremsstrahlung dose at the isocenter is increased. This phenomenon is known as the "velocity effect": a deeper point is exposed to the beam longer than a shallower point, resulting in apparent enhancement of beam penetration.

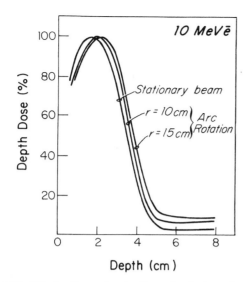

FIG. 14.42. Effect of isocenter depth on depth-dose distribution compared with a stationary beam. Cylindrical polystyrene phantoms of radii 10 and 15 cm were used. SAD = 100 cm; SSD = 64 cm; diaphragm opening = 3 × 6 cm; arc angle = 120 degrees. (From Khan FM, Fullerton GD, Lee JM, Moore VC, Levitt SH. Physical aspects of electron-beam arc therapy. *Radiology* 1977;124:497, with permission.)

B.2. Scanning Field Width

Although any field width may be used to produce acceptable isodose distribution, smaller scanning fields (e.g., width of 5 cm or less) give lower dose rate and greater x-ray contamination (86,88). However, small field widths allow almost normal incidence of the beam on the surface, thus simplifying dosimetry. Another advantage of the smaller field width is that the dose per arc is less dependent on the total arc angle. For these reasons, a geometric field width of 4 to 8 cm at the isocenter is recommended for most clinical situations.

B.3. Location of Isocenter

The isocenter should be placed at a point approximately equidistant from the surface contour for all beam angles. In addition, the depth of isocenter must be greater than the maximum range of electrons so that there is no accumulation of electron dose at the isocenter.

B.4. Field Shaping

Without electron collimation at the patient surface, the dose falloff at the treatment field borders is rather gradual. To sharpen the distribution, lead strips or cutouts should be used to define the arc limits as well as the field limits in the length direction (Fig. 14.43). Cast shielding has been found to be useful for routine electron arc therapy (91). For a greater detail of the treatment-planning process and the accessory preparation steps, the reader is referred to Leavitt et al. (95).

B.5. Isodose Distribution

This crucial information for arc therapy is not as easily available for electrons as it is for photons. Until computer programs of adequate sophistication are routinely available for electron arc therapy, this modality of treatment will probably remain inaccessible to most institutions. Of course, this problem is part of the general problem of electron beam treatment planning. However, the current surge of activity in this area as well as the CT

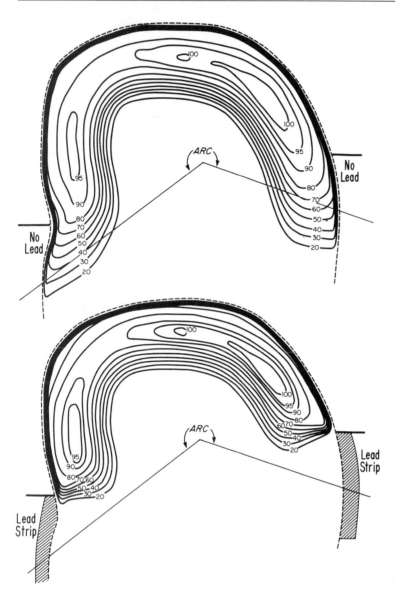

FIG. 14.43. Isodose distribution in arc rotation with and without lead strips at the ends of the arc, using a section of an Alderson Rando phantom closely simulating an actual patient cross section. Arc angle = 236 degrees; average radius of curvature = 10 cm; beam energy = 10 MeV; lead strip thickness = 6 mm; field size at the surface = 4.2 × 8.5 cm. (From Khan FM, Fullerton GD, Lee JM, Moore VC, Levitt SH. Physical aspects of electron-beam arc therapy. *Radiology* 1977;124:497, with permission.)

development provide an optimistic future for the development of sophisticated electron beam therapy techniques, including the arc.

14.8. TOTAL SKIN IRRADIATION

Electrons in the energy range of 2 to 9 MeV have been found useful for treating superficial lesions covering large areas of the body, such as mycosis fungoides and other cutaneous lymphomas. At these energies, electron beams are characterized by a rapid falloff in dose beyond a shallow depth and a minimal x-ray background (1% or less). Thus superficial skin lesions extending to about 1 cm depth can be effectively treated without exceeding bone marrow tolerance.

The treatment of mycosis fungoides with total skin irradiation was suggested at least 50 years ago (96). Since that time, various techniques have been developed and applied with success to the treatment of this disease (97–100). Basically, the methods fall into two general categories: (a) translational technique in which a horizontal patient is translated relative to a beam of electrons of sufficient width to cover the transverse dimensions of the patient and (b) large field technique in which a standing patient is treated with a combination of broad beams produced by electron scattering and large SSDs (2 to 6 m). Salient features of these techniques are discussed below.

A. Translational Technique

The translational technique has been described by a number of investigators (98,103,104). The patient lies on a motor-driven couch and is moved relative to a downward-directed beam at a suitable velocity. Alternatively, the patient may be stationary and the radiation source translated horizontally. In the latter technique, which has been described by Haybittle (103), a 24-Ci ^{90}Sr β source, in the form of a 60-cm linear array, is used. The source is contained in a shielded source housing and positioned above the couch. The maximum energy of the β particles emitted by ^{90}Sr is 2.25 MeV. However, due to the spectral distribution of β-ray energies, the effective depth of treatment in this case is only a fraction of a millimeter.

The translational technique using a 3-MeV Van de Graaff generator has been described by Wright et al. (102). A well-collimated monoenergetic electron beam is scattered just after leaving the vacuum window to improve uniformity. The beam is then collimated by an aluminum cone with a 5 mm × 45 cm defining slit. The patient is translated under this beam at a suitable speed. Williams et al. (103) have described a similar technique with a linear accelerator. No applicator is used in this technique and the x-ray collimators are fully retracted. The patient is treated anteriorly and posteriorly. The dose uniformity along the length of the patient is achieved by moving the patient through a distance sufficient that the areas treated start outside the electron beam, pass through, and finish outside the electron beam. The dose uniformity in the transverse direction is enhanced by suitably combining transversely overlapping fields.

B. Large Field Technique

Large electron fields required for total body skin irradiation can be produced by scattering electrons through wide angles and using large treatment distances. The field is made uniform over the height of the patient by vertically combining multiple fields or vertical arcing. The patient is treated in a standing position with four or six fields directed from equally spaced angles for circumferential coverage of the body surface.

B.1. Field Flatness

Low-energy electron beams are considerably widened by scattering in air. For example, a 6-MeV narrow electron beam, after passing through 4 m of air, achieves a Gaussian intensity distribution with a 50% to 50% width of approximately 1 m (104). This usually gives adequate uniformity over a patient's width. If two such fields are joined together vertically at their 50% lines, the resultant field will be uniform over a height of approximately 1 m. A proper combination of more such fields or a continuous arc can lead to a larger uniform field, sufficient to cover a patient from head to foot (Fig. 14.44).

The size and shape of an electron beam developed at a distance by air scatter can be estimated by multiple scattering theory. Holt and Perry (104) have used this approach to obtain a uniform field by combining multiple field profiles in proper proportions and angular separation (Fig. 14.44A).

In addition to air, the electron beam is scattered by a scattering foil inside or outside the collimator. However, the x-ray contamination would be increased, because unnecessarily wide beams waste electron flux to the sides.

B.2. X-ray Contamination

X-ray contamination is present in every therapy electron beam and becomes a limiting factor in total skin irradiation. Ordinarily, these x-rays are contributed by bremsstrahlung

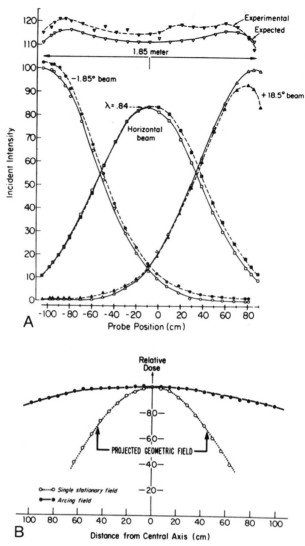

FIG. 14.44. A: Combination of three beam intensity profiles along the vertical axis to obtain a resultant beam profile. The central beam is directed horizontally, whereas the others are directed at 18.5 degrees from the horizontal. λ is a weighting factor used in an equation developed by Holt and Perry. (From Holt JG, Perry DJ. Some physical considerations in whole skin electron beam therapy. *Med Phys* 1982;9:769, with permission.) **B:** Vertical beam profile at the treatment plane for a stationary single field and an arcing field. (From Sewchand W, Khan FM, Williamson J. Total-body superficial electron-beam therapy using a multiple-field pendulum-arc technique. *Radiology* 1979;130:493, with permission.)

interactions produced in the exit window of the accelerator, scattering foil, ion chambers, beam-defining collimators, air, and the patient. The bremsstrahlung level can be minimized if the electron beam is scattered by air alone before incidence on the patient. This would necessitate some modifications in the accelerator, such as removing the scattering foil and other scatterers in the collimation system. Various safety interlocks would be required to make this separation feasible for routine clinical use. Such a system was developed at Memorial Hospital, New York, on a Varian Clinac-6 (105).

In the Stanford technique, described by Karzmark et al. (97,106,107), the electron beam, after emerging from the accelerator window, is scattered by a mirror (0.028-inch Al), an aluminum scatterer located externally at the front of the collimator (0.037-inch

Al), and about 3 m of air before incidence on the patient. The x-ray contamination incident on the patient is reduced by angling the beam 10 degrees to 15 degrees above and below the horizontal. Because the x-rays produced in the scatterers at the collimators are preferentially directed along the central axes, they largely miss the patient. In addition, this set-up provides a large electron field with sufficient dose uniformity in the vertical dimensions of the patient.

B.3. Field Arrangement

In the Stanford technique, the patient is treated with six fields (anterior, posterior, and four obliques) positioned 60 degrees apart around the circumference of the patient. Each field is made up of two component beams, pointing at a suitable angle with respect to the horizontal. The patient treatment positions and the full six-field treatment cycle are illustrated in Fig. 14.45.

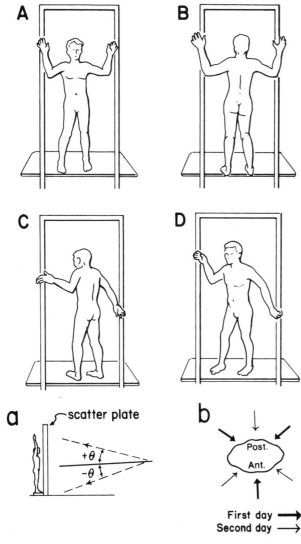

FIG. 14.45. Patient positions for the six-field Stanford technique. Patient is treated by two beams at each position, one beam directed 15 degrees below horizontal and the other 15 degrees above horizontal. (From Page V, Gardner A, Karzmark CJ. Patient dosimetry in the treatment of large superficial lesions. *Radiology* 1970;94:635, with permission.)

The Memorial technique (105) also uses dual fields to obtain field flatness in the vertical direction. The patient is treated from four directions, the anterior, the posterior, and each of the laterals. Holt and Perry (104) reexamined this technique and found that at least six fields are required to achieve adequate uniformity. They recommend eight fields, treating with four fields 1 day, and rotated four the next.

A multiple field arc technique used at the University of Minnesota has been described by Sewchand et al. (108). In this technique, the beam describes an up-and-down arc as the gantry of the linear accelerator rotates in an oscillatory manner analogous to a pendulum. Six fields are used for each cycle of treatment, as in the Stanford technique. The advantage of this technique is that the dose distribution in the vertical plane can be made reproducibly uniform over the height of any patient standing at a distance of about 4 m. However, if the electron beam is scattered by a scattering foil at the position of the collimators, this technique contributes higher x-ray contamination to the patient than does the stationary dual field technique. This problem may be minimized by removing scattering foils and allowing the electron beam to be scattered by air alone, as in the Memorial technique.

B.4. Dose Distribution

The depth-dose distribution in a single large field incident on a patient will depend on the angle of incidence of the beam relative to the surface contour. For an oblique beam, the depth-dose curve and its d_{max} shift toward the surface. When multiple large fields are directed at the patient from different angles, the composite distribution shows a net shift with apparent decrease in beam penetration. This shift of the relative depth doses closer to the surface has been explained by Bjarngard et al. (109) as being due to greater path lengths taken by the obliquely incident electrons in reaching a point.

Although a dose uniformity of $\pm 10\%$ can be achieved over most of the body surface using the six-field technique, areas adjacent to surface irregularities vary substantially due to local scattering. Areas such as inner thighs and axillae, which are obstructed by adjacent body structures, require supplementary irradiation.

The total bremsstrahlung dose in the midline of the patient for the multiple field technique is approximately twice the level of a single field. This factor of two has been experimentally observed by a number of investigators (104,108,110).

C. Modified Stanford Technique

The Stanford technique of six dual fields described earlier requires modifications of the accelerator such as removing the scattering foil and installing a scatterer at the front end of the collimator. These changes would require safety interlocks to prevent operation of the accelerator in this configuration for conventional electron beam treatments. Most institutions, including the University of Minnesota, have adopted the Stanford technique in principle without making alterations in the accelerator hardware. Because the regular scattering foils and various interlocks are left in place, no special precautions are required in preparing the machine for total skin irradiation.

In some accelerators (e.g., Varian Clinac C series) a high dose rate mode is installed to allow an output of more than 2,000 monitor units per minute. This significantly speeds up the treatments. Because conventional electron cones are not used, the electron field is collimated by a special wide-aperture insert attached at the end of the collimator. It is preset via interlock to a wider jaw setting and a specific electron energy, selected for high dose rate mode of operation. Some institutions use an acrylic scatter plate ($\simeq 1$ cm in thickness) in front of the patient to provide additional scatter to the electron beam (Fig. 14.45).

To shorten the treatment time, the patient is treated with three dual fields per day, for example, day 1: one dual field from the anterior, two dual oblique fields from the posterior; day 2: one dual field posterior and two dual fields anterior oblique. A complete cycle of six dual fields is thus completed in 2 days (Fig. 14.45). A source-to-patient distance of about 4 m is sufficient for this technique.

C.1. Dual Field Angle

A low-energy electron beam is considerably widened in size by scattering in air. For example, a 9-MeV electron beam, after transversing 4 m of air and an acrylic scatter plate, attains a Gaussian dose profile measuring a 90% to 90% isodose width of about 60 cm, which is usually sufficient to cover a patient's width. Along the height of the patient, two fields, one directed toward the head and the other toward the feet, are angled such that in the composite dose distribution a ± 10% dose uniformity can be obtained over a length of about 200 cm.

A method of determining dual field angle by film dosimetry has been described by Khan (111). A series of dosimetry films in their jackets are mounted on a vertical board, larger than the height of a typical patient, and are positioned at the treatment distance. The scatter plate is placed in front of the films as in actual treatment. The films are exposed to a single electron field directed at 10 degree to 15 degree angle with respect to the horizontal axis. The films are scanned for the optical density profile in the vertical direction. The profile is then placed side by side with its mirror image and separated by a distance such that the combined profile shows not more than ± 10% variation within about 200 cm (Fig. 14.46A). The separation between the two profiles gives the desired angle between the dual fields. A confirmatory composite profile is then measured by exposing the films to the dual fields with the interfield angle determined above (Fig. 14.46B). Figure 14.47 shows a transverse beam profile for the dual field arrangement.

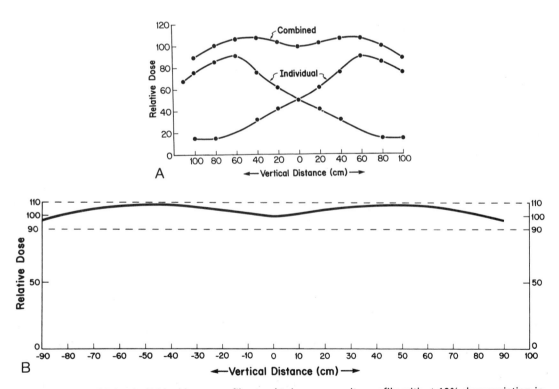

FIG. 14.46. Combining individual beam profiles to obtain a composite profile with ± 10% dose variation in the vertical direction. **A:** Data for 9 MeV; SSD = 410 cm; scatter plate to phantom distance = 20 cm; individual profile beam angle = 12 degrees relative to horizontal axis. A dual field angle $\theta = \pm 11$ degrees is obtained by combining the profiles as shown. **B:** Confirmatory beam profile for the dual field using $\theta = \pm 11$ degrees. (From Khan FM. Total skin electron therapy: technique and dosimetry. In: Purdy JA, ed. *Advances in radiation oncology physics.* AAPM Monograph No. 19. New York, American Institute of Physics, 1990:466, with permission.)

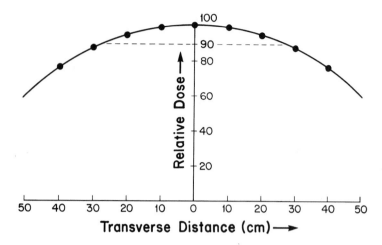

FIG. 14.47. Transverse dose profile showing width of the profile within ±90% dose relative to central axis. (From Khan FM. Total skin electron therapy: technique and dosimetry. In: Purdy JA, ed. *Advances in radiation oncology physics.* AAPM Monograph No. 19. New York, American Institute of Physics, 1990:466, with permission.)

C.2. Calibration

A thin window (≤ 0.05 g/cm^2) plane-parallel chamber is a suitable instrument for measuring depth dose distribution for the low-energy beams used for this technique. Because plane-parallel chambers are presently not calibrated by the calibration laboratories, they may be calibrated by intercomparison with a calibrated Farmer-type chamber, using a high-energy (≥ 10 MeV) electron beam (20).

The AAPM (112) recommends that the total skin irradiation dose be measured at the calibration point located at the surface of the phantom and the horizontal axis. This dose for a single dual field is called the *calibration point dose, D_P.*

A plane-parallel chamber, embedded in a polystyrene phantom, is positioned to first measure the depth dose distribution along the horizontal axis for the single dual field (the depth dose distribution can also be measured by a film sandwiched in a polystyrene phantom and placed parallel to the horizontal axis). The surface dose measurement is made at a depth of 0.2 mm (20). Suppose M is the ionization charge measured, the calibration point dose to polystyrene, $(D_P)_{\text{Poly}}$, is given by:

$$(D_P)_{\text{Poly}} = M \cdot C_{T,P} \cdot N_{\text{gas}} \cdot \left(\frac{\overline{L}}{\rho}\right)^{\text{Poly}}_{\text{air}} \cdot P_{\text{ion}} \cdot P_{\text{repl}} \tag{14.21}$$

The symbols are defined in Chapter 8. The calibration point dose to water, $(D_P)_W$, can then be determined as:

$$(D_P)_W = (D_P)_{\text{Poly}} \cdot (\overline{S}/\rho)^W_{\text{Poly}} \cdot \Phi^W_{\text{Poly}} \tag{14.22}$$

The electron fluence factor Φ^W_{Poly} is approximately unity, because the calibration measurement is made close to the surface. P_{repl} can also be equated to unity for the plane-parallel chambers. The parameters $\overline{L}/\rho$ and $\overline{S}/\rho$ are determined for the mean energy of electrons at the depth of measurement, which is given by Equation 14.7.

The *treatment skin dose,* $(\overline{D}_S)_{\text{Poly}}$ is defined by the AAPM (112) as the mean of the surface dose along the circumference of a cylindrical polystyrene phantom 30 cm in diameter and 30 cm high that has been irradiated under the total skin irradiation conditions with all six dual fields. If $(D_P)_{\text{Poly}}$ is the calibration point dose for the single dual field, then

$$(\overline{D}_S)_{\text{Poly}} = (D_P)_{\text{Poly}} \cdot B \tag{14.23}$$

where B is a factor relating the treatment skin dose with the calibration point dose, both measured at the surface of a cylindrical polystyrene phantom. Typically, B ranges between 2.5 and 3 for the Stanford type technique.

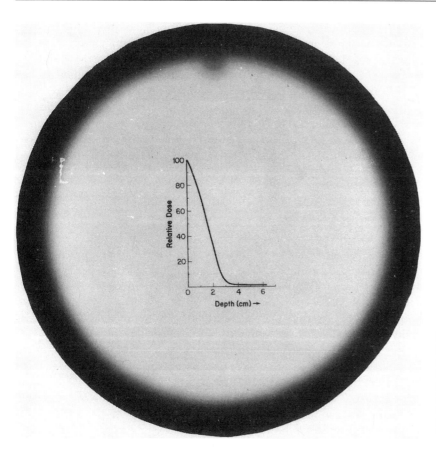

FIG. 14.48. Composite depth-dose distribution for six dual fields obtained with a dosimetry film sandwiched in a cylindrical polystyrene phantom exposed under treatment conditions. Irradiation conditions are given in Fig. 14.46. (From Khan FM. Total skin electron therapy: technique and dosimetry. In: Purdy JA, ed. *Advances in radiation oncology physics.* AAPM Monograph No. 19. New York: American Institute of Physics, 1990:466.)

The treatment skin dose for a water phantom, $(\overline{D}_S)_W$, can be calculated from Equations 14.21 and 14.22:

$$(\overline{D}_S)_W = (D_P)_W \cdot B \qquad (14.24)$$

The factor B can also be determined by taping a film strip in its light-tight paper to the surface of the cylindrical polystyrene phantom, specified above, and exposing it to a single dual field. Another filmstrip taped around the phantom is exposed to six dual fields. By relating optical densities to doses in the two cases, factor B can be determined from Equation 14.22.

The composite depth-dose distribution for the six dual fields may be determined by sandwiching a dosimetry film (in its paper jacket) in the cylindrical polystyrene phantom and cutting the excess film so that the edges conform to the circular surface of the phantom. A black tape is wrapped around the phantom over the film edges to make the film light-tight. The phantom, with the film parallel to the horizontal axis, is exposed to the six dual fields, duplicating actual treatment conditions. After appropriate processing, the film is scanned for optical density distribution, which is related to dose distribution by a reference sensitometric curve. Figure 14.48 gives the results of such a measurement.

C.3. In Vivo Dosimetry

Although an overall surface dose uniformity of $\pm 10\%$ can be achieved at the treatment distance, in a plane perpendicular to the horizontal axis and within an area equivalent to a patient's dimensions, there are localized regions of extreme nonuniformity of dose on the patient's skin. Excessive dose (e.g., 120%–130%) can occur in areas with sharp body projections, curved surfaces, or regions of multiple field overlaps. Low-dose regions occur when the skin is shielded by other parts of the body or overlying body folds. From in vivo measurements, areas receiving a significantly less dose can be identified for local boost. If eyelids need to be treated, internal eyeshields can be used, but the dose to the inside of the lids should be assessed, taking into account the electron backscatter from lead.

Thermoluminescent dosimeters (TLD) are most often used for in vivo dosimetry. For these measurements, the TLD must be thin (<0.5 mm) to minimize the effect of dose gradient across the dosimeters. TLD chips are commercially available that meet these specifications. These chips can be sealed in thin polyethylene sheets to avoid contamination. The reference chips may be calibrated in a polystyrene phantom using an electron beam of approximately the same mean energy incident on the TLDs as in the in vivo measurement conditions. The desired mean energy may be obtained by selecting an appropriate incident beam energy and depth (Eq. 14.7).

14.9. TREATMENT-PLANNING ALGORITHMS

Early methods of electron beam dose computation were based on empirical functions that used ray line geometrics, assuming broad beam dose distribution. Inhomogeneity corrections were incorporated using transmission data measured with large slabs of heterogeneities. These methods have been reviewed by Sternick (113).

Major limitations of the empirical methods based on broad beams and slab geometries are their inability to predict effects on dose distribution of small fields, sudden changes in surface contour, small inhomogeneities, and oblique beam incidence. An improvement over the empirical methods came about with the development of algorithms based on the age-diffusion equation by Kawachi (114) and others in the 1970s. These methods have been reviewed by Andreo (115). Although these algorithms are able to use semiempirically derived pencil beams that can be placed along the surface contour to predict effects of small fields and surface irregularity, their accuracy to calculate inhomogeneity correction is limited. They use effective path lengths between the virtual source and the point of calculation but the effects of anatomy and small tissue heterogeneities in three dimensions are not fully accounted for.

Major advancement in electron beam treatment planning occurred in the early 1980s (38,54,65,116). Methods were developed that were based on Gaussian pencil beam distributions calculated with the application of Fermi-Eyges multiple scattering theory (117). For a detailed review of these algorithms the reader is referred to Brahme (118) and Hogstrom, Starkschall, and Shiu (119).

Pencil beam algorithms based on multiple scattering theory are the algorithms of choice for electron beam treatment planning. A brief discussion is presented to familiarize the users of these algorithms with the basic theory involved.

A. Pencil Beam Based on Multiple Scattering Theory

Assuming small-angle multiple scattering approximation, an elementary pencil beam penetrating a scattering medium is very nearly Gaussian in its lateral spread at all depths. Large-angle scattering events could cause deviations from a pure Gaussian distribution, but their overall effect on dose distributions is considered to be small. The spatial dose distribution for a Gaussian pencil beam can be represented thus:

$$d_p(r, z) = d_p(o, z)e^{-r^2/\sigma_r^2(z)} \tag{14.25}$$

where $d_p(r, z)$ is the dose contributed by the pencil beam at a point at a radial distance r from its central axis and depth z, $d_p(o, z)$ is the axial dose and $\sigma_r^2(z)$ is the mean square radial displacement of electrons as a result of multiple Coulomb scattering. It can be shown that $\sigma_r^2 = 2\sigma_x^2 = 2\sigma_y^2$ where σ_x^2 and σ_y^2 are the mean square lateral displacements projected on the X, Y, and Y, Z planes. The exponential function in Equation (14.25) represents the off-axis ratio for the pencil beam, normalized to unity at $r = 0$.

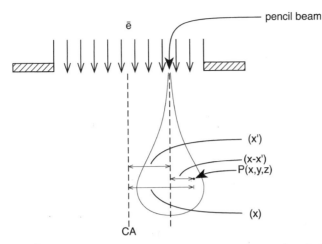

FIG. 14.49. A pencil beam coordinate system. (From Khan FM. Dose distribution algorithms for electron beams. In: Khan FM, Potish RA, eds. *Treatment planning in radiation oncology.* Baltimore: Williams & Wilkins, 1998:113–122, with permission.)

Another useful form of Equation (14.25) is:

$$d_p(r, z) = D_\infty(o, z) \frac{e^{-r^2/\sigma_r^2(z)}}{\pi \sigma_r^2(z)} \tag{14.26}$$

where $D_\infty(o, z)$ is the dose at depth z in an infinitely broad field with the same incident fluence at the surface as the pencil beam. The Gaussian distribution function in Equation 14.26 is normalized so that the area integral of this function over a transverse plane at depth z is unity.

In Cartesian coordinates Equation (14.26) can be written as:

$$d_p(x, y, z) = D_\infty(o, o, z) \frac{e^{-\frac{(x-x')^2 + (y-y')^2}{2\sigma^2(x', y', z)}}}{2\pi \sigma^2(x', y', z)} \tag{14.27}$$

where $d_p(x, y, z)$ is the dose contributed to point (x, y, z) by a pencil beam whose central axis passes through (x', y', z) (Fig 14.49).

The total dose distribution in a field of any size and shape can be calculated by summing all the pencil beams:

$$D(x, y, z) = \iint d_p(x - x', y - y', z)dx' dy' \tag{14.28}$$

The integration of a Gaussian function within finite limits cannot be performed analytically. To evaluate this function necessitates the use of error function (erf). Thus convolution calculus shows that for an electron beam of a rectangular cross section (2a × 2b), the spatial dose distribution is given by:

$$D(x, y, z) = D_\infty(o, o, z) \cdot \frac{1}{4} \left(\text{erf} \frac{a + x}{\sigma_r(z)} + \text{erf} \frac{a - x}{\sigma_r(z)} \right) \left(\text{erf} \frac{b + y}{\sigma_r(z)} + \text{erf} \frac{b - y}{\sigma_r(z)} \right) \tag{14.29}$$

where the error function is defined thus:

$$\text{erf}(x) = \frac{2}{\sqrt{\pi}} \int_o^x e^{-t^2} dt \tag{14.30}$$

The error function is normalized so that $\text{erf}(\infty) = 1$ (it is known that the integral $\int_0^\infty e^{-t^2} dt = \frac{\sqrt{\pi}}{2}$). Error function values for $0 < x < \infty$ can be obtained from tables published in mathematics handbooks (120). The quantity $D_\infty(o, o, z)$ is usually determined

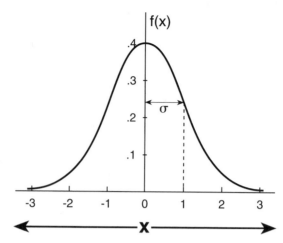

FIG. 14.50. A plot of normal distribution function given by Equation 14.29 for $\sigma = 1$. The function is normalized to unity for limits $\infty \times \infty$. (From Khan FM. Dose distribution algorithms for electron beams. In: Khan FM, Potish RA, eds. *Treatment planning in radiation oncology.* Baltimore: Williams & Wilkins, 1998:113–122, with permission.)

from the measured central axis depth-dose data of a broad electron field (e.g., 20 × 20 cm).

A.1. Lateral Spread Parameter, σ

Gaussian function is characterized by its lateral spread parameter, σ, which is similar to the standard deviation parameter of the familiar normal frequency distribution function:

$$f(x) = \frac{1}{\sqrt{2\pi}\sigma} e^{-\frac{x^2}{2\sigma^2}} \tag{14.31}$$

The previous function is plotted in Fig. 14.50 for $\sigma = 1$. The function is normalized so that its integral between the limits $-\infty < x < +\infty$ is unity.

The dose distribution in a pencil electron beam incident on a uniform phantom looks like a teardrop or onion (Fig. 14.51). The lateral spread (or σ) increases with depth until

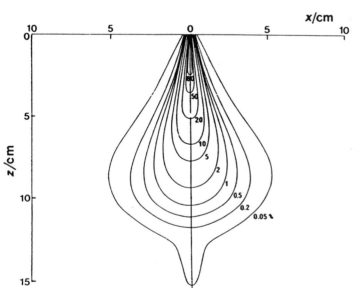

FIG. 14.51. Pencil beam dose distribution measured with a narrow beam of 22 MeV energy incident on a water phantom. (From ICRU Report 35. *Radiation dosimetry: electron beams with energies between 1 and 50 MeV.* Bethesda, MD: International Commission on Radiation Units and Measurements 1984:36, with permission.)

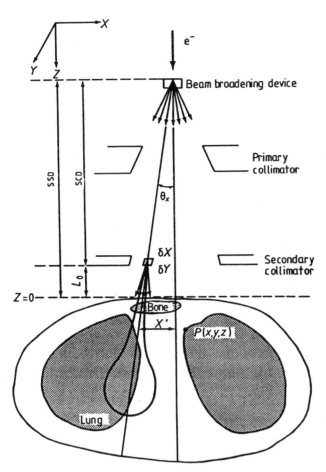

FIG. 14.52. Schematic representation of the Hogstrom algorithm for electron beam treatment planning. (From Hogstrom KR, Mills MD, Almond PR. Electron beam dose calculation. *Phys Med Biol* 1981;26:445, with permission.)

a maximum spread is achieved. Beyond this depth there is a precipitous loss of electrons as their larger lateral excursion causes them to run out of energy.

Eyges (117) predicted σ theoretically by extending the small-angle multiple scattering theory of Fermi to slab geometry of any composition. Considering $\sigma_x(z)$ in the x-z plane,

$$\sigma_x^2(z) = \frac{1}{2} \int \left(\frac{\theta^2}{\rho l}(z') \right) \rho(z')(z - z')^2 \, dz' \qquad (14.32)$$

where $\theta^2/\rho l$ is the mass angular scattering power and ρ is the density of the slab phantom.

There are limitations to the previous Eyges equation. As pointed out by Werner et al. (54), σ, given by Equation 14.32, increases with depth indefinitely which is contrary to what is observed experimentally in a narrow beam dose distribution. Also, Equation 14.32 is based on small-angle multiple Coulomb scattering, hence ignores the probability of large-angle scatter. This results in an underestimate of σ. Correction factors have been proposed to overcome these problems (54,121,122).

Practical implementation of the above algorithm was carried out by Hogstrom et al. in 1981 (38) and was subsequently adopted by several commercial treatment-planning systems. Figure 14.52 shows a schematic representation of the Hogstrom algorithm. The pencil beam σ is calculated using the Fermi-Eyges equation (Eq. 14.32). By correlating electron linear collision stopping power and linear angular scattering power relative to that of water with CT numbers, effective depth and σ are calculated for inhomogeneous media. Thus the method allows pixel-by-pixel calculation of heterogeneity correction.

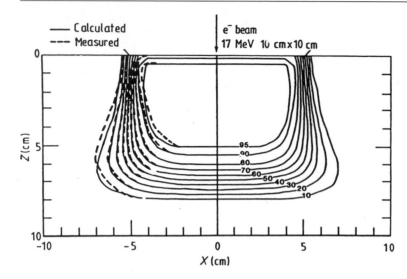

FIG. 14.53. Comparison of calculated and measured isodose distribution. (From Hogstrom KR, Mills MD, Almond PR. Electron beam dose calculation. *Phys Med Biol* 1981;26:445, with permission.)

Figure 14.53 shows a comparison of calculated and measured isodose curves as an example. Starkschall et al. (123) have extended the Hogstrom algorithm to three dimensions. An irregularly shaped field is divided into strip beams and each strip is divided into segments so that σ of the pencil beams and effective depths are calculated in three dimensions. Integration of the pencils is carried out over all strips and segments.

REFERENCES

1. Fletcher GH. Introduction. In: Tapley N, ed. *Clinical applications of the electron beam.* New York: John Wiley & Sons, 1976:1.
2. Evans RD. *The atomic nucleus.* New York: McGraw-Hill, 1955.
3. Johns HE, Laughlin JS. Interaction of radiation with matter. In: Hine G, Brownell G, eds. *Radiation dosimetry.* New York: Academic Press, 1956:49.
4. National Council on Radiation Protection and Measurements (NCRP). Stopping powers for use with cavity ionization chambers. Report No. 27. Handbook 79. Washington, DC: National Bureau of Standards, 1961.
5. Sternheimer RM. The density effect for the ionization loss in various materials. *Phys Rev* 1952; 88:851.
6. Fermi E. The ionization loss of energy in gases and condensed materials. *Phys Rev* 1940;57:485.
7. Laughlin JS, Beattie JW. Ranges of high energy electrons in water. *Phys Rev* 1951;83:692.
8. ICRU. Radiation quantities and units. Report No. 33. Washington, DC: International Commission on Radiation Units and Measurements, 1980.
9. Berger MJ, Seltzer SM. Tables of energy losses and ranges of electrons and positrons. NASA SP-3012. Washington, DC: National Aeronautics and Space Administration, 1964.
10. Berger MJ, Seltzer SM. Additional stopping power and range tables for protons, mesons, and electrons. NASA SP-3036. Washington, DC: National Aeronautics and Space Administration, 1966.
11. Berger MJ, Seltzer SM. *Stopping powers and ranges of electrons and positrons,* 2nd ed. Washington, DC: U.S. Department of Commerce, National Bureau of Standards, 1983.
12. ICRU. Stopping powers for electrons and positrons. Report No. 37. Bethesda, MD: International Commission on Radiation Units and Measurements, 1984.
13. Rossi BB. *High energy particles.* Englewood Cliffs, NJ: Prentice-Hall, 1956.
14. ICRU. Radiation dosimetry: electrons with initial energies between 1 and 50 MeV. Report No. 21. Washington, DC: International Commission on Radiation Units and Measurements, 1972.
15. Nordic Association of Clinical Physics (NACP). Procedures in external radiation therapy dosimetry with electron and photon beams with maximum energies between 1 and 50 MeV. *Acta Radiol* 1980;19:55.
16. Markus B. Beitrage zur Entwicklung der Dosimetrie schneller. *Elektronen Strahlentherapie* 1964; 123:350, 508 and 1964;124:33.
17. Nusse M. Factors affecting the energy-range relation of fast electrons in aluminum. *Phys Med Biol* 1969;14:315.
18. Harder D, Schulz HJ. Some new physical data for electron beam dosimetry. In: Proceedings of the European Congress of Radiology. Amsterdam: Excerpta Medica, 1971.

19. Svensson H, Hettinger G. Dosimetric measurements at the nordic medical accelerators. I. Characteristics of the radiation beam. *Acta Radiol* 1971;10:369.
20. Khan FM, Doppke K, Hogstrom KR, et al. Clinical electron-beam dosimetry. Report of AAPM Radiation Therapy Committee Task Group No. 25. *Med Phys* 1991;18:73.
21. Brahme A, Svensson H. Specification of electron beam quality from the central-axis depth absorbed-dose distribution. *Med Phys* 1976;3:95.
22. Rogers DWO, Bielajew AF. Differences in electron depth-dose curves calculated with EGS and ETRAN and improved energy-range relationships. *Med Phys* 1986;13:687.
23. Harder D. Energiespectren Schneller Elecktronen in Verschiedenen Tiefen. In: Montreux, Zuppinger A, Poretti G, eds. *Symposium on high-energy electrons.* Berlin: Springer-Verlag, 1965:260.
24. AAPM. Task Group 51. Protocol for clinical reference dosimetry of high-energy photon and electron beams. *Med Phys* 1999;26:1847–1870.
25. IAEA. Technical Reports Series No. 398. Absorbed dose determination in external beam radiotherapy. Vienna: International Atomic Energy Agency, 2000.
26. American Association of Physicists in Medicine (AAPM). A protocol for the determination of absorbed dose from high energy photons and electrons. RTC Task Group No. 21. *Med Phys* 1983;10:741.
27. Loevinger R, Karzmark CJ, Weissbluth M. Radiation dosimetry with high energy electrons. *Radiology* 1961;77:906.
28. Dutreix J, Dutreix A. Film dosimetry of high energy electrons. *Ann NY Acad Sci* 1969;161:33.
29. Hettinger G, Svensson H. Photographic film for determination of isodose from betatron electron radiation. *Acta Radiol* 1967;5:74.
30. Khan FM, Higgins PD. Calculation of depth dose and dose per monitor unit for irregularly shaped electron fields: an addendum. *Phys Med Biol* 1999;44:N77–N80.
31. ICRU. Radiation dosimetry: electron beams with energies between 1 and 50 MeV. Report No. 35. Bethesda, MD: International Commission on Radiation Units and Measurements, 1984.
32. Almond PR. Characteristics of current medical electron accelerator beams. In: Chu F, ed. *Proceedings of the symposium on electron beam therapy.* New York: Memorial Sloan-Kettering Cancer Center, 1979:43.
33. Mandour MA, Harder D. Systematic optimization of the double-scatterer system for electron beam field flattening. *Strahlentherapie* 1978;154:328.
34. Werner BL, Khan FM, Deibel FC. Model for calculating depth dose distributions for broad electron beam. *Med Phys* 1983;10:582.
35. Biggs PJ, Boyer AL, Doppke KP. Electron dosimetry of irregular fields on the Clinac-18. *Int J Radiat Oncol Biol Phys* 1979;5:433.
36. Khan FM, Higgins PD. Field equivalence for clinical electron beams. *Phys Med Biol* 2001;46:N9–N14.
37. Harder D, Schröder-Babo P, Abou Mandour M. Private communication, 1982.
38. Hogstrom KR, Mills MD, Almond PR. Electron beam dose calculations. *Phys Med Biol* 1981;26:445.
39. Mills MD, Hogstrom KR, Almond PR. Prediction of electron beam output factors. *Med Phys* 1982;9:60.
40. Pohlit W. Dosimetrie Zur Betatrontherapie. Stuttgart: Verlag, 1965.
41. Shroder-Babo P. Determination of the virtual electron source of a betatron. *Acta Radiol* 1983;364[suppl]:7.
42. Meyer JA, Palta JR, Hogstrom KR. Determination of relatively new electron dosimetry measurement techniques on Mevatron 80. *Med Phys* 1984;11:670.
43. Jamshidi A, Kuchnir FT, Reft SC. Determination of the source position for the electron beam from a high-energy linear accelerator. *Med Phys* 1986;13:942.
44. Khan FM, Sewchand W, Levitt SH. Effect of air space on depth dose in electron beam therapy. *Radiology* 1978;126:249.
45. Berger MJ, Seltzer SM. Tables of energy-deposition distributions in water phantoms irradiated by point-monodirectional electron beams with energies from 1 to 60 MeV, and applications to broad beams. NBSIR 82–2451. Washington, DC: National Bureau of Standards, 1982.
46. Tapley N, ed. *Clinical applications of the electron beam.* New York: John Wiley & Sons, 1976.
47. Okumura Y. Correction of dose distribution for air space in high energy electron therapy. *Radiology* 1972;103:183.
48. Khan FM, Lee JMF. Computer algorithm for electron beam treatment planning. *Med Phys* 1979;6:142.
49. Holt JG, Mohan R, Caley R, et al. Memorial electron beam AET treatment planning system. In: Orton CG, Bagne F, eds. *Practical aspects of electron beam treatment planning.* New York: American Institute of Physics, 1978.
50. Ekstrand KE, Dixon RL. Obliquely incident electron beams. *Med Phys* 1982;9:276.
51. Khan FM, Deibel FC, Soleimani-Meigooni A. Obliquity correction for electron beams. *Med Phys* 1985;12:749.
52. McKenzie AL. Air-gap correction in electron treatment planning. *Phys Med Biol* 1979;24:628.

53. Deibel FC, Khan FM, Werner BL. Electron beam treatment planning with strip beams [abst.]. *Med Phys* 1983;10:527.
54. Werner BL, Khan FM, Deibel FC. Model for calculating electron beam scattering in treatment planning. *Med Phys* 1982;9:180.
55. Dutreix J. Dosimetry. In: Gil y Gil, Gil Gayarre, eds. *Symposium on high-energy electrons.* Madrid: General Directorate of Health, 1970:113.
56. Laughlin JS. High energy electron treatment planning for inhomogeneities. *Br J Radiol* 1965;38:143.
57. Laughlin JS, Lundy A, Phillips R, et al. Electron-beam treatment planning in inhomogeneous tissue. *Radiology* 1965;85:524.
58. Almond PR, Wright AE, Boone ML. High-energy electron dose perturbations in regions of tissue heterogeneity. *Radiology* 1967;88:1146.
59. Dahler A, Baker AS, Laughlin JS. Comprehensive electron-beam treatment planning. *Ann NY Acad Sci* 1969;161:189.
60. Almond PR. Radiation physics of electron beams. In: Tapley N, ed. *Clinical applications of the electron beam.* New York: John Wiley & Sons, 1976:7.
61. Boone MLM, Almond PR, Wright AE. High energy electron dose perturbation in regions of tissue heterogeneity. *Ann NY Acad Sci* 1969;161:214.
62. Prasad SC, Bedwinek JM, Gerber RL. Lung dose in electron beam therapy of chest wall. *Acta Radiol* 1983;22:91.
63. Pohlit W, Manegold KH. Electron-beam dose distribution in inhomogeneous media. In: Kramer S, Suntharalingam N, Zinninger GF, eds. *High energy photons and electrons.* New York: John Wiley & Sons, 1976:243.
64. Goitein M. A technique for calculating the influence of thin inhomogeneities on charged particle beams. *Med Phys* 1978;5:258.
65. Perry DJ, Holt JG. A model for calculating the effects of small inhomogeneities on electron beam dose distributions. *Med Phys* 1980;7:207.
66. Bagne F, Tulloh ME. Low energy electrons. In: Orton CG, Bagne F, eds. *Practical aspects of electron beam treatment planning.* AAPM Publication. New York: American Institute of Physics, 1978:80.
67. Sharma SC, Deibel FC, Khan FM. Tissue equivalence of bolus materials for electron beams. *Radiology* 1983;146:854.
68. Johnson JM, Khan FM. Dosimetric effects of abutting extended SSD electron fields with photons in the treatment of head and neck cancers. *Int J Radiat Oncol Biol Phys* 1994;28:741–747.
69. Giarratano JC, Duerkes RJ, Almond PR. Lead shielding thickness for dose reduction of 7- to 28-MeV electrons. *Med Phys* 1975;2:336.
70. Khan FM, Moore VC, Levitt SH. Field shaping in electron beam therapy. *Br J Radiol* 1976;49:883.
71. Goede MR, Gooden DS, Ellis RG, et al. A versatile electron collimation system to be used with electron cones supplied with Varian's Clinac 18. *Int J Radiat Oncol Biol Phys* 1977;2:791.
72. Choi MC, Purdy JA, Gerbi BJ, et al. Variation in output factor caused by secondary blocking for 7–16 MeV electron beams. *Med Phys* 1979;6:137.
73. Purdy JA, Choi MC, Feldman A. Lipowitz metal shielding thickness for dose reduction of 6–20 MeV electrons. *Med Phys* 1980;7:251.
74. Asbell SO, Sill J, Lightfoot DA, et al. Individualized eye shields for use in electron beam therapy as well as low-energy photon irradiation. *Int J Radiat Oncol Biol Phys* 1980;6:519.
75. Khan FM, Werner BL, Deibel FC. Lead shielding for electrons. *Med Phys* 1981;8:712.
76. Lax I, Brahme A. On the collimation of high energy electron beams. *Acta Radiol Oncol* 1980;19:199.
77. Okumura Y, Mori T, Kitagawa T. Modification of dose distribution in high energy electron beam treatment. *Radiology* 1971;99:683.
78. Weatherburn H, McMillan KTP, Stedford B, et al. Physical measurements and clinical observations on the backscatter of 10 MeV electrons from lead shielding (correspondence). *Br J Radiol* 1975;48:229.
79. Saunders JE, Peters VG. Backscattering from metals in superficial therapy with high energy electrons. *Br J Radiol* 1974;47:467.
80. Nusslin F. Electron back-scattering from lead in a Perspex phantom (correspondence). *Br J Radiol* 1974;48:467.
81. Gagnon WF, Cundiff JH. Dose enhancement from backscattered radiation at tissue-metal interfaces irradiated with high energy electrons. *Br J Radiol* 1980;53:466.
82. Klevenhagen SC, Lambert GD, Arbabi A. Backscattering in electron beam therapy for energies between 3 and 35 MeV. *Phys Med Biol* 1982;27:363.
83. Becker J, Weitzel G. Neue Formen der Bewegungstrahlung beim 15 MeV-Betatron der Siemens-Reinger-Werke. *Strahlentherapie* 1956;101:180.
84. Benedetti GR, Dobry H, Traumann L. Computer programme for determination of isodose curves for electron energies from 5–42 MeV. *Electromedica (Siemens)* 1971;39:57.

85. Rassow J. On the telecentric small-angle pendulum therapy with high electron energies. *Electromedica (Siemens)* 1972;40:1.

86. Khan FM, Fullerton GD, Lee JM, et al. Physical aspects of electron-beam arc therapy. *Radiology* 1977;124:497.

87. Ruegsegger DR, Lerude SD, Lyle D. Electron beam arc therapy using a high energy betatron. *Radiology* 1979;133:483.

88. Kase KR, Bjarngard BE. Bremsstrahlung dose to patients in rotational electron therapy. *Radiology* 1979;133:531.

89. Leavitt DD. A technique for optimization of dose distributions in electron rotational therapy [abst.]. *Med Phys* 1978;5:347.

90. Blackburn BE. A practical system for electron arc therapy. In: Paliwal B, ed. *Proceedings of the symposium on electron dosimetry and arc therapy.* New York: AAPM/American Institute of Physics, 1982:295.

91. Thomadsen B. Tertiary collimation of moving electron beams. In: Paliwal B, ed. *Proceedings of the symposium on electron dosimetry and arc therapy.* New York: AAPM/American Institute of Physics, 1982:315.

92. Paliwal B, ed. Proceedings of the symposium on electron dosimetry and arc therapy. New York: AAPM/American Institute of Physics, 1982.

93. Boyer AL, Fullerton GD, Mira MD, et al. An electron beam pseudoarc technique. In: Paliwal B, ed. *Proceedings of the symposium on electron dosimetry and arc therapy.* New York: AAPM/American Institute of Physics 1982:267.

94. Khan FM. Calibration and treatment planning of electron beam arc therapy. In: Paliwal B, ed. *Proceedings of the symposium on electron dosimetry and arc therapy.* New York: AAPM/American Institute of Physics, 1982:249.

95. Leavitt DD, Peacock LM, Gibbs FA, et al. Electron arc therapy: physical measurements and treatment planning techniques. *Int J Radiat Oncol Biol Phys* 1985;11:987.

96. Trump JG, Wright KA, Evans WW, et al. High energy electrons for the treatment of extensive superficial malignant lesions. *AJR* 1953;69:623.

97. Karzmark CJ, Loevinger R, Steel RE. A technique for large-field, superficial electron therapy. *Radiology* 1960;74:633.

98. Szur L, Silvester JA, Bewley DK. Treatment of the whole body surface with electrons. *Lancet* 1962;1:1373.

99. Fuks Z, Bagshaw MA. Total-skin electron treatment of mycosis fungoides. *Radiology* 1971;100:145.

100. Heller EH. The management of cutaneous manifestations of lymphoma by means of electron beam. *Australas J Dermatol* 1972;13:11.

101. Haybittle JL. A 24 curie strontium 90 unit for whole-body superficial irradiation with beta rays. *Br J Radiol* 1964;37:297.

102. Wright KA, Granke RC, Trump JG. Physical aspects of megavoltage electron therapy. *Radiology* 1956;67:533.

103. Williams PC, Hunter RD, Jackson SM. Whole body electron therapy in mycosis fungoides—successful translational technique achieved by modification of an established linear accelerator. *Br J Radiol* 1979;52:302.

104. Holt JG, Perry DJ. Some physical considerations in whole skin electron beam therapy. *Med Phys* 1982;9:769.

105. Edelstein GR, Clark T, Holt JG. Dosimetry for total-body electron-beam therapy in the treatment of mycosis fungoides. *Radiology* 1973;108:691.

106. Karzmark CJ. Large-field superficial electron therapy with linear accelerators. *Br J Radiol* 1964;37:302.

107. Karzmark CJ. Physical aspects of whole-body superficial therapy with electrons. *Frontiers Radiat Ther Oncol* 1968;2:36.

108. Sewchand W, Khan FM, Williamson J. Total-body superficial electron-beam therapy using a multiple-field pendulum-arc technique. *Radiology* 1979;130:493.

109. Bjarngard BE, Chen GTY, Piontek RN, et al. Analysis of dose distributions in whole body superficial electron therapy. *Int J Radiat Oncol Biol Phys* 1977;2:319.

110. Tetenes PJ, Goodwin PN. Comparative study of superficial whole-body radiotherapeutic techniques using a 4-MeV nonangulated electron beam. *Radiology* 1977;122:219.

111. Khan FM. Total skin electron therapy: technique and dosimetry. In: Purdy JA, ed. *Advances in radiation oncology physics.* AAPM Monograph No. 19. New York: American Institute of Physics, 1990:466.

112. AAPM. Total skin electron therapy technique and dosimetry. Report No. 23. New York: American Institute of Physics, 1988.

113. Sternick E. Algorithms for computerized treatment planning. In: Orton CG, Bagne F, eds. *Practical aspects of electron beam treatment planning.* New York: American Institute of Physics, 1978:52.

114. Kawachi K. Calculation of electron dose distribution for radiotherapy treatment planning. *Phys Med Biol* 1975;20:571.

115. Andreo P. Broad beam approaches to dose computation and their limitations. In: Nahum AE, ed. *The computation of dose distributions in electron beam radiotherapy.* Kungalv, Sweden: mimiab/goatab, 1985:128.

116. Jette D. The application of multiple scattering theory to therapeutic electron dosimetry. *Med Phys* 1983;10:141.

117. Egyes L. Multiple scattering with energy loss. *Phys Rev* 1948;74:1534.

118. Brahme A. Brief review of current algorithms for electron beam dose planning. In: Nahum AE, ed. *The computation of dose distributions in electron beam radiotherapy.* Kungalv, Sweden: miniab/gotab, 1985:271.

119. Hogstrom KR, Starkschall G, Shiu AS. Dose calculation algorithms for electron beams. In: Purdy JA, ed. *Advances in radiation oncology physics.* American Institute of Phyiscs Monograph 19. New York: American Institute of Physics, 1992:900.

120. Beyer WH. *Standard mathematical tables,* 25th ed. Boca Raton: CRC Press, 1978:524.

121. Lax I, Brahme A. Collimation of high energy electron beams. *Acta Radiol Oncol* 1980:19;199.

122. Lax I, Brahme A, Andreo P. Electron beam dose planning using Gaussian beams. In: Brahme A, ed. *Computed electron beam dose planning.* Acta Radiol 1983;364[suppl]:49.

123. Starkschall G, Shie AS, Buynowski SW, et al. Effect of dimensionality of heterogeneity corrections on the implementation of a three-dimensional electron pencil-beam algorithm. *Phys Med Biol* 1991;36:207.

BRACHYTHERAPY

Brachytherapy is a method of treatment in which sealed radioactive sources are used to deliver radiation at a short distance by interstitial, intracavitary, or surface application. With this mode of therapy, a high radiation dose can be delivered locally to the tumor with rapid dose fall-off in the surrounding normal tissue. In the past, brachytherapy was carried out mostly with radium or radon sources. Currently, use of artificially produced radionuclides such as ^{137}Cs, ^{192}Ir, ^{198}Au, ^{125}I, and ^{103}Pd is rapidly increasing.

New technical developments have stimulated increased interest in brachytherapy: the introduction of artificial isotopes, afterloading devices to reduce personnel exposure, and automatic devices with remote control to deliver controlled radiation exposure from high-activity sources. Although electrons are often used as an alternative to interstitial implants, brachytherapy continues to remain an important mode of therapy, either alone or combined with external beam.

15.1. RADIOACTIVE SOURCES

From the time of its discovery in 1898, radium has been the most commonly used isotope in brachytherapy. However, artificial radioisotopes offer special advantages in some situations because of their γ ray energy, source flexibility, source size, and half-life. Table 15.1 lists the most commonly used sources for brachytherapy with their relevant physical properties.

A. Radium

A.1. Decay

Radium is the sixth member of the uranium series, which starts with $^{238}_{92}$U and ends with stable $^{206}_{82}$Pb (Fig. 2.3). Radium disintegrates with a half-life of about 1,600 years to form radon.

$$^{226}_{88}\text{Ra} \xrightarrow[\sim 1,600 \text{ years}]{} {}^{222}_{86}\text{Rn} + {}^{4}_{2}\text{He}$$

The product nucleus radon is a heavy inert gas that in turn disintegrates into its daughter products as shown in Fig. 2.3. As a result of the decay process from radium to stable lead, at least 49 γ rays are produced with energies ranging from 0.184 to 2.45 MeV. The average energy of the γ rays from radium in equilibrium with its daughter products and filtered by 0.5 mm of platinum is 0.83 MeV (1). A filtration of at least 0.5 mm platinum provided by the source case is sufficient to absorb all the α particles and most of the β particles emitted by radium and its daughter products. Only γ rays are used for therapy.

Because the half-life for radioactive decay is much greater for ^{226}Ra than for any of its daughter products, radium, when placed in a sealed container, achieves a secular equilibrium with its daughters (Fig. 2.5). The time required to establish equilibrium is approximately 1 month from the time of encapsulation.

TABLE 15.1. PHYSICAL CHARACTERISTICS OF RADIONUCLIDES USED IN BRACHYTHERAPY

Radionuclide	Half-Life	Photon Energy (MeV)	Half-Value Layer (mm lead)	Exposure Rate Constant (Rcm²/mCi-h)
²²⁶Ra	1,600 yr	0.047–2.45 (0.83 avg)	12.0	8.25^{ab} (Rcm²/mg-h)
²²²Rn	3.83 days	0.047–2.45 (0.83 avg)	12.0	10.15^{ac}
⁶⁰Co	5.26 yr	1.17, 1.33	11.0	13.07^c
¹³⁷Cs	30.0 yr	0.662	5.5	3.26^c
¹⁹²Ir	73.8 days	0.136–1.06 (0.38 avg)	2.5	4.69^c
¹⁹⁸Au	2.7 days	0.412	2.5	2.38^c
¹²⁵I	59.4 days	0.028 avg	0.025	1.46^c
¹⁰³Pd	17.0 days	0.021 avg	0.008	1.48^c

[a]In equilibrium with daughter products.
[b]Filtered by 0.5 mm Pt.
[c]Unfiltered.

A.2. Source Construction

The radium is supplied mostly in the form of radium sulfate or radium chloride which is mixed with an inert filler and loaded into cells about 1 cm long and 1 mm in diameter. These cells are made of 0.1- to 0.2-mm-thick gold foil and are sealed to prevent leakage of radon gas. The sealed cells are then loaded into the platinum sheath, which in turn is sealed. Radium sources are manufactured as needles or tubes in a variety of lengths and activities (Fig. 15.1).

A.3. Source Specification

Radium sources are specified by: (a) active length, the distance between the ends of the radioactive material; (b) physical length, the distance between the actual ends of the source; (c) activity or strength of source, milligrams of radium content; and (d) filtration, transverse thickness of the capsule wall, usually expressed in terms of millimeters of platinum.

Linear activity of a source can be determined by dividing the activity by the active length. Figure 15.1 illustrates three types of radium needles used for implants: needles of uniform linear activity, needles with higher activity at one end (Indian club), and needles with high activity at both ends (dumbbell). Uniform linear activity needles may be "full intensity" (0.66 mg/cm) or "half intensity" (0.33 mg/cm). Needles also are constructed with linear activities of 0.5 and 0.25 mg/cm. Tubes for intracavitary and mold therapy are usually furnished in multiples of 5 mg of radium filtered by 1 mm platinum.

RADIUM NEEDLES

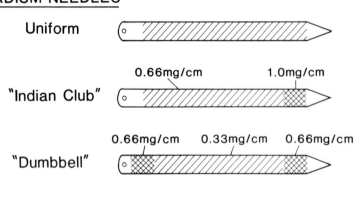

FIG. 15.1. Types of radium sources used in interstitial and intracavitary therapy.

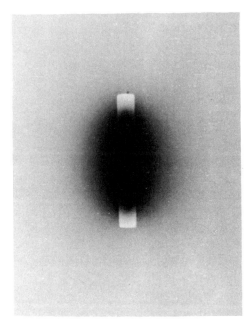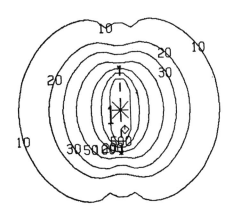

FIG. 15.2. An autoradiograph of a cesium-137 tube. Isodose curves are shown for the same source in the diagram on the *right*.

To test the uniformity of activity distribution, an autoradiograph is obtained by placing the source on an unexposed x-ray film for a time long enough to obtain reasonable darkening of the film. The source may be radiographed at the same time to show physical dimensions of the source superimposed on the autoradiograph. Figure 15.2 shows an autoradiograph obtained in this manner. The exposed film may be scanned with a densitometer to obtain optical density distribution. Uniformity of activity distribution can thus be assessed from such a distribution.

A.4. Exposure Rate Constant[1]

The activity of a radioactive nuclide emitting photons is related to the exposure rate by the exposure rate constant, Γ_δ (see section 8.8 for derivation). In brachytherapy, this constant is usually expressed as numerically equal to the exposure rate in R/h at a point 1 cm from a 1 mCi *point* source. In the case of radium, the source strength is specified in terms of milligrams of radium instead of mCi.

The International Commission on Radiation Units and Measurements (ICRU) (4) has recommended that Γ_δ for radium filtered by 0.5 mm platinum be taken as

---

[1] ICRU (2) defines the exposure rate constant as:

$$\Gamma_\delta = \frac{l^2}{A}\left(\frac{dx}{dt}\right)_\delta$$

where $(dx/dt)_\delta$ is the exposure rate due to photons of energy greater than δ, at a distance l from a point source of activity A. Special units of Γ_δ are Rm^2 h^{-1}Ci^{-1} or any convenient multiple of these.

This quantity replaces, but is not identical to, the specific γ ray constant. The latter applied to γ rays only and did not include the exposure rate of emitted x-rays such as characteristic x-rays and internal bremsstrahlung.

A further change has been made by the ICRU (3). A new quantity, called *air kerma rate constant*, has been recommended to replace the exposure rate constant. This quantity is still named Γ_δ, but is now defined as:

$$\Gamma_\delta = \frac{l^2}{A}\left(\frac{dk_{air}}{dt}\right)_\delta$$

where k_{air} is the air kerma. The SI unit for this quantity is m^{2}Jkg^{-1}h^{-1}Ci^{-1}. When the special names, gray (Gy) and becquerel (Bq) are used, the unit becomes m^{2}Gy Bq^{-1} sec^{-1}.

TABLE 15.2. EXPOSURE RATE CONSTANT FOR RADIUM POINT SOURCE FILTERED BY VARIOUS THICKNESSES OF PLATINUM

Filtration (mm Pt)	Γ_δ (Rcm^{2}h^{-1}mg^{-1})
0	9.09
0.5	8.25
0.6	8.14
0.7	8.01
0.8	7.90
0.9	7.81
1.0	7.71
1.5	7.25
2.0	6.84

From Shalek RJ, Stovall M. Dosimetry in implant therapy. In: Attix FH, Roesch WC, eds. *Radiation dosimetry.* Vol. 3. New York: Academic Press, 1969:chap 31, with permission.

8.25 Rcm^{2}h^{-1} mg^{-1}. Table 15.2 gives Γ_δ factors for radium with other filtrations. These values are based on relative transmission measurements versus platinum thickness (5) and normalized to $\Gamma_\delta = 8.25$ for 0.5 mm platinum.

A.5. Radon Hazard

Leakage of radon gas from a radium source represents a significant hazard if the source is broken. The sources are, however, doubly encapsulated to prevent such an occurrence. Spontaneous rupture of a sealed radium source due to pressure build-up of helium gas (from α particle disintegrations) is considered unlikely. Van Roosenbeek et al. (6) have calculated that sources encapsulated in platinum may remain safely sealed for more than 400 years.

B. Cesium-137

Cesium-137 is a γ ray-emitting radioisotope that is used as a radium substitute in both interstitial and intracavitary brachytherapy. It is supplied in the form of insoluble powders or ceramic microspheres, labeled with ^{137}Cs, and doubly encapsulated in stainless-steel needles and tubes. The advantages of ^{137}Cs over radium are that it requires less shielding (compare half-value layers in Table 15.1) and is less hazardous in the microsphere form. With a long half-life of about 30 years, these sources can be used clinically for about 7 years without replacement, although the treatment times have to be adjusted to allow for radioactive decay (2% per year).

^{137}Cs emits γ rays of energy 0.662 MeV. The decay scheme shows that ^{137}Cs transforms to ^{137}Ba by the process of β^- decay but 93.5% of the disintegrations are followed by γ rays from the ^{137}Ba metastable state. The β particles and low-energy characteristic x-rays are absorbed by the stainless-steel material, so that the clinical source is a pure γ emitter.

It should be emphasized that Γ_δ is defined in terms of an ideal point source. Any practical source will have a finite size and would necessitate corrections for photon attenuation and scattering.

The γ rays from cesium have nearly the same penetrating power as radium γ rays in tissue. Meisberger et al. (7) have compared the measured and calculated depth-dose values along the transverse axes of the sources and showed that the exposure in water to exposure in air ratio is the same for radium and cesium for depths up to 10 cm. Significant differences, however, exist between radium and cesium doses at points along oblique angles (near the longitudinal axis) due to the filtration effect (8,9). Not only is the attenuation of γ rays in steel and platinum quite different but also cesium emits monoenergetic γ rays while radium emits γ rays of wide energy range.

The exposure rate constant Γ_δ for unfiltered ^{137}Cs is 3.26 Rcm^2 mCi^{-1} h^{-1} (10). Comparing this with the Γ_δ of 8.25 Rcm^2 mg^{-1} h^{-1} for radium filtered by 0.5 mm Pt, the conversion factor is 8.25/3.26 = 2.53 mCi of ^{137}Cs/mg of ^{226}Ra. However, along the transverse axes of clinical sources (cesium with 0.5 mm steel and radium with 0.5 mm Pt filtration), the mean conversion factor has been calculated to be 2.55 for cesium needles and 2.59 for cesium tubes (9).

C. Cobalt-60

^{60}Co has been used for brachytherapy but is rarely used now. The main advantages of ^{60}Co is its high specific activity, which allows fabrication of small sources required for some special applicators. However, it is more expensive than ^{137}Cs and has a short half-life (5.26 years), necessitating more frequent replacement and a complex inventory system.

Cobalt brachytherapy sources are usually fabricated in the form of a wire that is encapsulated in a sheath of platinum iridium or stainless steel. The sources can be used to replace ^{226}Ra in intracavitary applications. Curie-sized cobalt sources have also been used in a unit called the Cathetron (11–13). This is a remote-loading device and provides high dose rates for intracavitary therapy, e.g., 250–300 cGy/min at point "A" (see section 15.7B for definition of point A).

D. Iridium-192

Iridium-192 (alloy of 30% Ir and 70% Pt) sources are fabricated in the form of thin flexible wires which can be cut to desired lengths. Nylon ribbons containing iridium seeds 3 mm long and 0.5 mm in diameter, spaced with their centers 1 cm apart, are also commonly used. Both the wires and the seed ribbons are quite suitable for the afterloading technique (14,15) (see section 15.6B).

^{192}Ir has a complicated γ ray spectrum with an average energy of 0.38 MeV. Because of the lower energy, these sources require less shielding for personnel protection (compare half-value layers in Table 15.1). ^{192}Ir has the disadvantage of a short half-life (73.8 days). However, the half-life is long compared to the average treatment time so that the sources can be used in nonpermanent implants similar to radium and cesium. The activity varies by only a few percent during an average implant duration.

Many values have been cited in the literature for Γ_δ for ^{192}Ir. The differences in the calculated values arise because different spectroscopic data were used by each investigator. This problem has been discussed in detail by Glasgow and Dillman (16). Basing their calculations on the most recent nuclear spectroscopy data for ^{192}Ir, they recommend a value of 4.69 Rcm^2 h^{-1} mCi^{-1}.

E. Gold-198

Seeds or "grains" consisting of a radioactive isotope of gold, ^{198}Au, are used for interstitial implants. They are used in the same way as radon seeds have been used for permanent implants. ^{198}Au has a half-life of 2.7 days and emits a monoenergetic γ ray of energy 0.412 MeV. β rays of maximum energy 0.96 MeV are also emitted but are absorbed by the 0.1-mm-thick platinum wall surrounding the seed. A gold seed is typically 2.5 mm long with an outer diameter of 0.8 mm.

Because of its lower γ ray energy, personnel protection problems with gold are easier to manage than those of radon. Moreover, radon seeds continue to exhibit low-level γ activity for many years due to bremsstrahlung, arising from high-energy β particles emitted by its long-lived daughter products. It is suspected that this chronic irradiation may be carcinogenic (17). For these reasons, gold seeds replaced radon seeds for many years, until ^{125}I seeds gained more widespread acceptance.

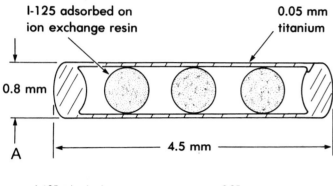

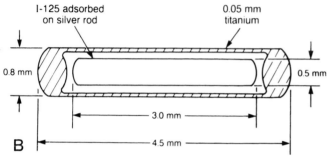

FIG. 15.3. Schematic diagram of ^{125}I seeds. **A:** Model 6702. **B:** Model 6711. (From Medical Products Division, 3M Co., New Brighton, MN, with permission.)

F. Iodine-125

[125]I has gained a wide use for permanent implants in radiation therapy (18,19). The advantages of this isotope over radon and [198]Au are its long half-life (59.4 days), which is convenient for storage, and its low photon energy, which requires less shielding. However, the dosimetry of ^{125}I is much more complex than the conventional interstitial sources.

Three ^{125}I seed models, designated 6701, 6702 and 6711, have been manufactured,[2] which are identical in size and encapsulation but differ in the active source design. The earlier model 6701 is now obsolete. Figure 15.3 shows the design of the currently used seeds. The encapsulation consists of a 0.05-mm-thick titanium tube welded at both ends to form a cylindrical capsule of dimensions 4.5×0.8 mm. The model 6702 seed contains ion-exchange resin beads, which are impregnated with ^{125}I in the form of the iodide ion. The model 6711 seed contains a silver wire with the active material, silver iodide (AgI), adsorbed on its surface.

In the new seed design, namely model 6711, the silver wire is readily visible on radiographs and shows seed position as well as orientation. The model 6702 seed is radiographically less visible although the titanium end welds can be seen when surrounded by reduced thickness of tissue.

[125]I decays exclusively by electron capture to an excited state of [125]Te, which spontaneously decays to the ground state with the emission of a 35.5-keV γ photon. Characteristic x-rays in the range of 27 to 35 keV also are produced due to the electron capture and internal conversion processes. Titanium encapsulation serves to absorb liberated electrons and x-rays with energies less than 5 keV. The model 6711 seed emits two additional photons at 22.1 keV and 25.2 keV energies. These are fluorescent (characteristic) x-rays produced by the interaction of ^{125}I photons with the silver wire (20).

Because of the presence of titanium end welds, the dose distribution around iodine seeds is highly anisotropic (Fig. 15.4). This can pose problems of creating cold spots near the source ends. The users of ^{125}I implants either ignore this problem or try to minimize the extent of cold spots by creating random seed distributions. Although the basic problem

---

[2] Medical Products Division/3M, New Brighton, Minnesota.

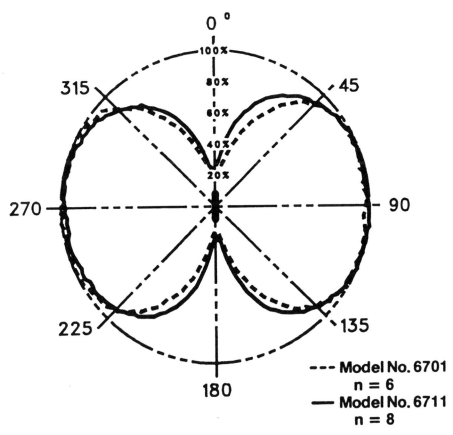

FIG. 15.4. Angular photon fluence distribution from ^{125}I seeds. The relative photon fluence in any direction is proportional to the radial distance from the seed to the plotted curve. *n* is the number of seeds used to obtain average results. (From Ling CC, Yorke ED, Spiro IS, et al. Physical dosimetry of ^{125}I seeds of a new design for interstitial implant. *Int J Radiat Oncol Biol Phys* 1983;9:1747, with permission.)

still remains, most treatment-planning systems do not take into account anisotropy around individual sources.

Significant differences exist in the published values of exposure rate constant for ^{125}I. Schulz et al. (21) have reported a calculated value of 1.464 Rcm^2 mCi^{-1} h^{-1} for an unfiltered point source. As will be discussed, the use of the exposure rate constant for unfiltered point sources to calculate dose distribution around actual sources of complex design such as ^{125}I has serious accuracy limitations.

G. Palladium-103

^{103}Pd seeds have recently become available for use in brachytherapy. Their clinical applications are similar to those of ^{125}I. Having a shorter half-life (17 days) than that of ^{125}I (59.4 days), ^{103}Pd may provide a biologic advantage in permanent implants because the dose is delivered at a much faster rate (22).

The palladium-103 seed model 200^3 consists of a laser-welded titanium tube containing two graphite pallets plated with ^{103}Pd (Fig. 15.5). A lead marker between the pallets provides radiographic identification.

^{103}Pd decays by electron capture with the emission of characteristic x-rays in the range of 20 to 23 keV (average energy 20.9 keV) and Auger electrons. The photon fluence distribution around the source is anisotropic due to the self-absorption by the source

---

^{3} Manufactured by Theragenics Corp., Norcross, Georgia.

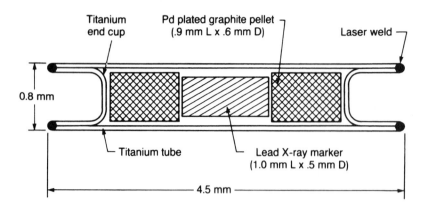

Titanium end cup

Pd plated graphite pellet (.9 mm L x .6 mm D)

Laser weld

0.8 mm

Titanium tube

Lead X-ray marker (1.0 mm L x .5 mm D)

4.5 mm

FIG. 15.5. Schematic diagram of ^{103}Pd seed (model 200). (From Theragenics Corp., Norcross, GA, with permission.)

pallets, the welds, and the lead x-ray marker (Fig. 15.6). The dosimetry data for ^{103}Pd is sparse. The reader is referred to Meigooni et al. (23) and Chiu-Tsao and Anderson (24) for dose-distribution data.

15.2. CALIBRATION OF BRACHYTHERAPY SOURCES

A. Specification of Source Strength

The strength of a brachytherapy source may be specified in several ways.

A.1. Activity

The source strength for any radionuclide may be specified in terms of millicuries (mCi). The exposure rate at any particular point is proportional to the product of activity and its exposure rate constant. Errors, however, may be introduced in this method from the fact that corrections must be applied for the source and wall filtration and that the exposure rate constant may not be known accurately. It should be recalled that the accuracy of the

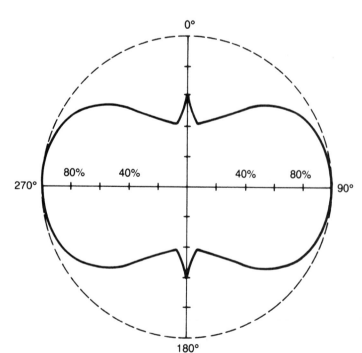

FIG. 15.6. Photon fluence distribution in air for ^{103}Pd seed. (From Meli JA, Anderson LL, Weaver KA. Dose distribution. In: Interstitial Collaborative Working Group, ed. *Interstitial brachytherapy.* New York: Raven, 1990:21, with permission.)

exposure rate constant depends critically on the accurate knowledge of the spectroscopic data and the relevant absorption coefficients.

A.2. Exposure Rate at a Specified Distance

The National Council on Radiation Protection and Measurements (NCRP) (25) recommends that the strength of any γ emitter should be specified directly in terms of exposure rate in air at a specified distance such as 1 m. This specification can be carried out simply by measuring exposure rate in free air at a distance sufficiently large that the given source can be treated as a point. A long distance measurement geometry minimizes the dependence of the calibration upon the construction of the source and the detector because both can be treated as points. In addition, the effect of oblique transmission of photons through the source capsule becomes negligible.

Loevinger (26) has recommended calibration of brachytherapy sources in terms of absorbed dose in water, close to the source. However, such calibrations are not routinely available. So, until these are available, the exposure rate calibration, far from the source, remains the most appropriate method.

A.3. Equivalent Mass of Radium

There are historical reasons that make it convenient to specify brachytherapy sources in terms of the equivalent mass of radium. Because some users, especially the physicians who are accustomed to radium sources, continue to use mg-Ra eq, it has been suggested (25) that the exposure rate could be expressed in terms of "effective" equivalent mass of radium. This conversion is simply made by dividing the exposure rate at 1 m by the exposure rate constant of radium (point source filtered by 0.5 mm Pt) at 1 m. It should, however, be emphasized that the best way to calibrate and specify brachytherapy sources is still in terms of exposure rate or air kerma rate at a distance of 1 m. The effective mg-Ra eq should be used only to provide output comparison with radium sources.

Example

An iridium-192 source has been calibrated and its strength is specified as 0.495 mR/h at 1 m. What is the strength of this source in terms of effective mg-Ra eq?

Exposure rate constant of radium filtered by 0.5 mm Pt $= 8.25$ R·cm^2/h·mg $= 0.825$ mR·m^2/h·mg

$$\text{Effective mg-Ra eq} = \frac{0.495}{0.825} = 0.600 \text{ mg}$$

Note that such a conversion of units must explicitly specify the radium source in terms of a point source and its filtration.

A.4. Apparent Activity

If the source is calibrated in terms of exposure rate at 1 m, its strength may be specified as *apparent activity*. It is defined as the activity of a *bare point* source of the same nuclide that produces the same exposure rate at 1 m as the source to be specified. The apparent activity of a brachytherapy source is determined by dividing the measured exposure rate at 1 m with the exposure rate constant of the unfiltered source at 1 m.

It is a common practice with the vendors of brachytherapy sources to specify source strength as apparent activity, although the original calibration is done in terms of exposure rate. In order for the user to calculate exposure rate from the apparent activity, the exposure rate constant to be used must be the same as the one used by the vendor. Thus the exposure rate constant is used as a dummy constant in this conversion, that is, a purely arbitary value would do, provided its product with the apparent activity yields the same exposure rate as determined by the original calibration.

A.5. Air Kerma Strength

Although exposure rate at a specified distance is the method of choice in designating source strength, the quantity exposure is in the process of being phased out. Most of the standards laboratories have already replaced exposure by the quantity air kerma. In keeping with these trends the AAPM recommended the quantity *air kerma strength* for the specification of brachytherapy sources.

The air kerma strength is defined (27) as the product of air kerma rate in "free space" and the square of the distance of the calibration point from the source center along the perpendicular bisector, that is,

$$S_K = \dot{K}_l \cdot l^2 \tag{15.1}$$

where S_K is the air kerma strength and $\dot{K}_l$ is the air kerma rate at a specified distance l (usually 1 m). Recommended units for air kerma strength are $\mu Gy m^2 h^{-1}$.

Because no single system is being currently followed universally, it is instructive to derive relationships between the different quantities being used for source strength specification.

From Equations 8.6 and 8.13 (see Chapter 8) kerma is related to exposure by:

$$K = X\left(\frac{\overline{W}}{e}\right)\frac{\overline{\mu}_{tr}/\rho}{\overline{\mu}_{en}/\rho} \tag{15.2}$$

where K is kerma, X is exposure, $\overline{W}/e$ is the average energy absorbed per unit charge of ionization in air, $\overline{\mu}_{tr}/\rho$ and $\overline{\mu}_{en}/\rho$ are, respectively, the average values of the mass transfer coefficient and the mass energy absorption coefficient of air for the photons. Also,

$$\overline{\mu}_{en}/\rho = \overline{\mu}_{tr}/\rho(1 - g) \tag{15.3}$$

where g is the fraction of the energy lost to bremsstrahlung. However, in the energy range of brachytherapy photons and for the air medium $\overline{\mu}_{en}/\rho \simeq \overline{\mu}_{tr}/\rho$. Therefore,

$$K = X\left(\frac{\overline{W}}{e}\right) \tag{15.4}$$

From Equations 15.1 and 15.4,

$$S_K = \dot{X}_l\left(\frac{\overline{W}}{e}\right)l^2 \tag{15.5}$$

Thus the exposure calibration of a brachytherapy source can be readily converted to air kerma strength by the use of Equation 15.5. If exposure rate is measured in R/h at $l =$ 1 m,

$$S_K = \dot{X}(R/h)(0.876 \text{ cGy/R})(1 m)^2$$

where 0.876 cGy/R is the value of $\overline{W}/e$ for dry air (see section 8.3) or:

$$S_K = \dot{X}(R/h)(8.76 \times 10^3 \text{ m}^2 \mu Gy/R) \tag{15.6}$$

Milligram Radium Equivalent

By definition, 1 mg-Ra eq gives 8.25×10^{-4} R/h at 1 m; therefore, in terms of air kerma strength (from Eq. 15.6),

1 mg-Ra eq = $(8.25 \times 10^{-4} \text{ R/h})(8.76 \times 10^3 \text{ m}^2 \mu Gy/R)$

$$= 7.227 \mu Gy \text{ m}^2 h^{-1} \tag{15.7}$$

or

$$1\,\mu Gy\,m^2\,h^{-1} = 0.138\ mg\text{-Ra eq} \qquad (15.8)$$

Apparent Activity

By definition, 1 unit of apparent activity, App, gives exposure rate at 1 m equal to the exposure rate constant of the specified source at 1 m. Using the exposure rate constants given in Table 15.1 and Equation 15.6, $1\,\mu Gy\,m^2\,h^{-1} = 0.348$ mCi for ^{137}Cs; 0.243 mCi for ^{192}Ir; 0.486 mCi for ^{198}Au; 0.787 for ^{125}I; and 0.773 for ^{103}Pd. These apparent activities per unit air kerma strength may be used to convert source strengths calibrated in air kerma strengths to apparent activities in millicuries.

Example

An ^{192}Ir seed calibrated by an accredited dose calibration laboratory (ADCL) has air kerma strength of 5.00 $\mu Gy\,m^2\,h^{-1}$. What is the strength of the source (*a*) in units of mg-Ra eq and (*b*) in units of mCi (apparent activity)?

Using the conversion factors derived above,

$$\begin{aligned}
(a)\ \text{equivalent mass of radium} &= 5.00 \times 0.138 \\
&= 0.69\ mg\text{-Ra eq} \\
(b)\ \text{apparent activity} &= 5.00 \times 0.243 \\
&= 1.22\ mCi
\end{aligned}$$

B. Exposure Rate Calibration

The National Institute of Standards and Technology (NIST) has established exposure rate calibration standards for some of the brachytherapy sources, e.g., ^{226}Ra, ^{60}Co, ^{137}Cs, and ^{192}Ir. The NIST method consists of calibrating a working standard of each type using open-air geometry and a series of spherical graphite cavity chambers (28,29). A given source is then calibrated by intercomparison with the working standard using a 2.5-liter spherical aluminum ionization chamber, positioned at a distance of about 1 m. A similar procedure is used for calibrating a radium source except that the working standards of radium have been calibrated in terms of actual mass of radium.

Because of their lower exposure rate and shorter half-life, ^{192}Ir is calibrated in a slightly different manner (29). A composite source containing about 50 seeds is calibrated in terms of exposure rate at 1 m in open-air scatter-free geometry, as in the case of ^{137}Cs sources, using spherical graphite chambers. Each seed is then measured individually in a well-type ionization chamber to calibrate the chamber. This well-type ionization chamber now serves as the working standard for calibrating ^{192}Ir seeds.

^{125}I seeds are calibrated at the NIST in terms of exposure rate in free space at 1 m using a free-air ionization chamber (30). For routine calibrations a well-type ionization chamber is used whose calibration is maintained by a free-air chamber as the primary standard.

Calibration of clinical sources should be directly traceable to NIST or one of the AAPM-ADCLs. This means that the sources should be calibrated by direct comparison with a NIST- or ADCL-calibrated source of the same kind, i.e., the same radionuclide with the same encapsulation, size, and shape. If a well-type ionization chamber is used, it should bear a calibration factor determined with a NIST- or ADCL-calibrated source of the same kind.

B.1. Open-air Measurements

Figure 15.7 is a schematic representation of an open-air measurement geometry for the calibration of brachytherapy sources. The arrangement consists of a large source to ion

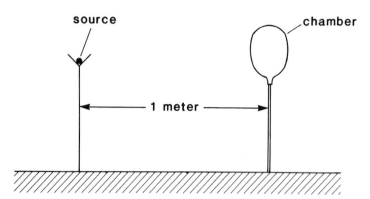

FIG. 15.7. Schematic drawing of open air geometry for exposure rate calibration of brachytherapy sources.

chamber distance relative to source and detector dimensions. The apparatus is set up as far away as possible from potential scattering surfaces. Because the output from brachytherapy sources is low at large distances, the chamber volume should be large, for example, 100 ml or larger. A signal-to-noise ratio greater than 100:1 should be achievable.

Because of the difficulty in obtaining "good geometry" conditions, the open-air method is a time-consuming measurement. It is not suitable for routine calibration checks required in a busy department. A well-type ionization chamber is more suited to routine measurements.

B.2. Well-type Ion Chambers

Routine calibration of brachytherapy sources is usually carried out with a "re-entrant"-type ion chamber in which the walls of the chamber surround the source, approximating a 4π measurement geometry. Examples of such chambers are those designed by the British National Physics Laboratory (31), a re-entrant chamber designed by Radiological Physics Center (32), a spherical aluminum chamber designed by NIST (33), and commercially available dose calibrators (34–36).

Figure 15.8 is a schematic drawing of a dose calibrator, Capintec Model CRC-10. This unit consists of an aluminum wall ion chamber filled with argon gas under high pressure. The collection potential applied to the chamber is about 150 V. A source holder is devised to reproduce the source geometry in relation to the surrounding chamber walls.

The dose calibrator is traditionally used for assay of radiopharmaceuticals in which the instrument response is interpreted as activity in units of millicuries. These activity calibrations of various isotopes are based on relative chamber response measured by intercomparison with the respective standards calibrated by NIST directly in terms of activity (37). However, these standards are usually in the form of an aqueous suspension of the isotope sealed in a glass ampule. These vendor calibrations of the instrument are, therefore, not valid for brachytherapy sources because of differences in construction between brachytherapy and standard sources. Even the practice of using a radium standard for calibrating different sources is prone to significant errors due to energy dependence of the instrument (35,36,38). In addition, the response of well chambers is known to depend on the source position in the well and on the length of the source (32). Correction factors must be determined for these effects for a given instrument and the type of sources to be calibrated.

The energy dependence of the chamber arises from absorption and scattering of photons and secondary electrons in the chamber walls and the gas. Besides this intrinsic energy dependence, oblique filtration through the source encapsulation affects the chamber response both by photon absorption and by producing changes in the energy spectrum. This effect of source construction on the chamber response has been studied in detail by Williamson et al. (34,39) for commonly used brachytherapy sources. These authors conclude: "In these apparatuses, all one can count on is a linear response with respect to

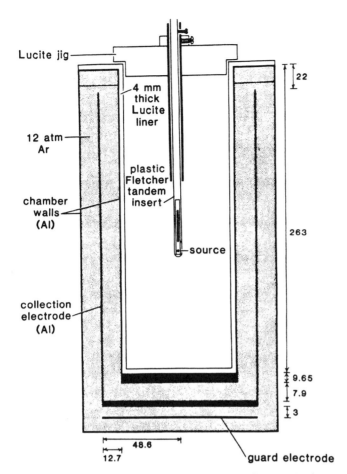

FIG. 15.8. Schematic drawing of a dose calibrator, Capintec Model CRC-10. (From Williamson JF, Khan FM, Sharma SC, et al. Methods for routine calibration of brachytherapy sources. *Radiology* 1982;142:511, with permission.)

exposure rate given fixed energy, filtration, and source position. For each isotope, an exposure calibrated standard is needed" (34). These studies support the recommendations that the brachytherapy sources should be calibrated in terms of exposure rate using exposure calibrated standards of the same kind (25,26).

15.3. CALCULATION OF DOSE DISTRIBUTIONS

A. Exposure Rate

Exposure rate distribution around a linear brachytherapy source can be calculated using the Sievert integral, introduced by Sievert (40) in 1921. The method (1,41) consists of dividing the line source into small elementary sources and applying inverse square law and filtration corrections to each. Consider a source of active length L and filtration t (Fig. 15.9). The exposure rate dI at a point $P(x, y)$ contributed by the source element of length dx is given by:

$$dI(x, y) = \frac{A}{L} \cdot \Gamma \cdot dx \cdot \frac{1}{r^2} \cdot e^{-\mu' \cdot t \cdot \sec \theta} \qquad (15.9)$$

where A and Γ are the activity and exposure rate constant of the unfiltered source and μ' is the effective attenuation coefficient for the filter. Other variables are defined by Fig. 15.9.

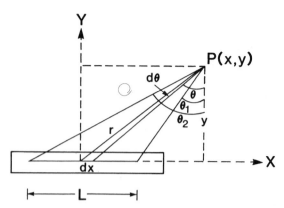

FIG. 15.9. Diagram illustrating geometrical relationships used in calculation of exposure at point *P,* from a linear source.

Making use of the following relationships:

$$r = y \sec \theta$$
$$x = y \tan \theta$$
$$dx = y \sec^2 \theta \, d\theta$$

and integrating Equation 15.9, we obtain the exposure rate *I(x, y)* for the whole source.

$$I(x, y) = \frac{A\Gamma}{Ly} \int_{\theta_1}^{\theta_2} e^{-\mu' \cdot t \cdot \sec \theta} \, d\theta \tag{15.10}$$

The above Sievert integral can be evaluated by numerical methods (1).

If the source intensity is specified in terms of exposure rate $\dot{X}_s$ at a specified distance *s* far from the source, i.e., $s \gg L$, then the Sievert integral can be written as:

$$I(x, y) = \frac{\dot{X}_s \cdot s^2}{Ly} \cdot e^{\mu' t} \int_{\theta_1}^{\theta_2} e^{-\mu' \cdot t \cdot \sec \theta} \, d\theta \tag{15.11}$$

Alternatively, if the source strength is specified in terms of equivalent mass of radium, m_{eq}, such that $\dot{X}_s = m_{eq} \cdot \Gamma_{Ra} \cdot s^{-2}$, then:

$$I(x, y) = \frac{m_{eq} \cdot \Gamma_{Ra}}{Ly} \cdot e^{\mu' t} \int_{\theta_1}^{\theta_2} e^{-\mu' \cdot t \cdot \sec \theta} \, d\theta \tag{15.12}$$

If the source strength is specified in air kerma strength, then:

$$I(x, y) = \frac{S_K}{Ly \left(\frac{\overline{W}}{e} \right)} \cdot e^{\mu' t} \int_{\theta_1}^{\theta_2} e^{-\mu' \cdot t \cdot \sec \theta} \, d\theta \tag{15.13}$$

Several additional corrections are applied to compute the exposure rate accurately using the Sievert integral. A correction for self-absorption in the source material, although small for clinical sources, has been used by Shalek and Stovall (1). Wall thickness, *t,* should be corrected for the internal radius of the source, because some photons traverse a thickness of filter greater than the radial thickness of the wall (42,43). Depending on the type of source and filtration, the energy spectrum may be significantly altered by the filter. Not only is an "effective attenuation coefficient" needed but this coefficient varies with filter thickness (43,44). This problem becomes more severe when the effects of oblique filtration are considered (45).

In the case of ^{226}Ra encapsulated in platinum, measured values of μ' (43,44) may be used (Fig. 15.10). However, if such data are not available for a given source-filter

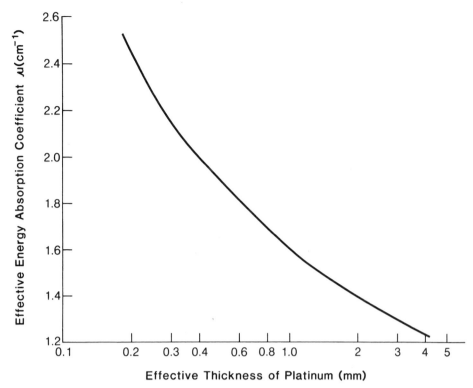

FIG. 15.10. Effective energy absorption coefficients of radium gamma rays in platinum. (Data are from Whyte GN. Attenuation of radium gamma radiation in cylindrical geometry. *Br J Radiol* 1955;28:635; and Keyser GM. Absorption correction for radium standardization. *Can J Phys* 1951;29:301.)

combination, calculated values have to be used. Williamson et al. (45) give the following expression for μ' as a function of filter thickness d:

$$\mu'(d) = -\left(\frac{1}{d}\right) \ln \left[\frac{\sum_i p_i E_i (\mu_{en}/\rho)^{air}_i \, e^{-\mu^i_{en} \cdot d}}{\sum_i p_i E_i (\mu_{en}/\rho)^{air}_i} \right] \tag{15.14}$$

where p_i denotes the number of photons with energy E_i emitted per disintegration, and $(\mu_{en}/\rho)^{air}_i$ is the mass energy absorption coefficient in air for photon of energy E_i.

Because the Sievert integral uses the energy absorption coefficient, the underlying assumption is that the emitted energy fluence is exponentially attenuated by the filter thickness traversed by the photons. This is an approximation that has been shown to work well for ^{226}Ra and ^{192}Ir seeds in the region bounded by the active source ends (1,45). However, Monte Carlo simulations (45) have shown that beyond the end of the active source region, the Sievert approach introduces significant errors and practically breaks down in the extreme oblique directions.

A.1. Effect of Inverse Square Law

Figure 15.11 compares the radial exposure rate distribution of a line source of radium with that of a point source of radium, both filtered by 1 mm Pt. Whereas the curve for the point source represents an inverse square law function, the linear source curve was obtained using the Sievert integral. The exposure rate constant for ^{226}Ra with 1 mm Pt filter was assumed to be 7.71 Rcm^2 mg^{-1} h^{-1}. It is evident from Fig. 15.11 that for the linear source, the exposure rate is less than that predicted by the inverse square law, especially at points close to the source. This is as expected because the photons reaching these points from the source extremities travel larger distances and suffer oblique filtration which is greater than the radial wall thickness. As the distance is increased, however, these effects of the

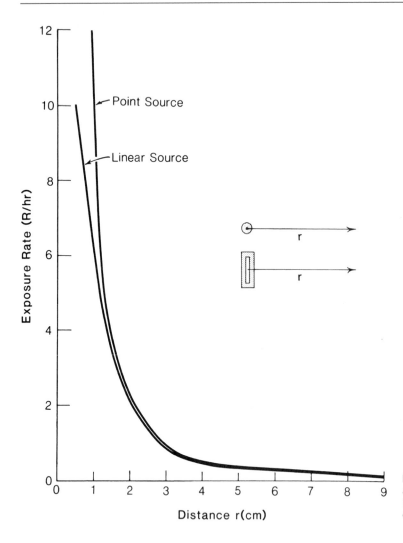

FIG. 15.11. Plot of exposure rate from 1-mg ^{226}Ra source as a function of radial distance. Point source with 1.0 mm Pt filtration. Linear source with 1.0 mm Pt filtration, 1.5 cm active length.

linear source approach those of the point source and, therefore, its exposure rate curve approaches inverse square law.

B. Absorbed Dose in Tissue

The Sievert integral gives the exposure rate distribution in air and considers only the inverse square law and filtration effects. When a source is implanted in the tissue, one needs to consider, in addition, attenuation as well as scattering in the surrounding tissue. The exposure rate calculated at a point in tissue can then be converted into absorbed dose rate by using the appropriate roentgen-to-rad factor (see Chapter 8).

Several investigators have experimentally determined the ratio of exposure in water to exposure in air as a function of distance for a number of isotopes. Because of the large discrepancies between various sets of experimental data, Meisberger et al. (46) formulated a third order polynomial to fit the average of their theoretical and all available experimental data (46–52). This polynomial is commonly used for routine calculation of absorbed dose in tissue in various computer programs.

More recently, Webb and Fox (53) calculated the dose distribution around point γ ray emitters in water by the Monte Carlo method. Their results agree very well with Meisberger's average or "selected" curve.

The radial dependence of dose in a water medium, with the inverse square law removed can also be represented by $D_r = B_r e^{-\mu r}$ where μ denotes the linear attenuation coefficient and B_r is a build-up factor at distance r from the source. This expression is similar to the

TABLE 15.3. CONSTANTS k_a AND k_b DETERMINED BY USE OF MONTE CARLO DATA

Isotope	μ (cm²/g)	k_a	k_b
^{60}Co	0.0632	0.896	1.063
^{226}Ra	0.0811	1.17	1.19
^{137}Cs	0.0858	1.14	1.20
^{198}Au	0.105	1.48	1.32
^{192}Ir	0.113	1.59	1.36

Data from Kornelsen RO, Young MEJ. Brachytherapy build-up factors. *Br J Radiol* 1981;54:136.

ratio of exposure in water to exposure in air. Evans (54) has suggested that B_r may be represented by:

$$B_r = 1 + k_a(\mu r)^{kb} \qquad (15.15)$$

where k_a and k_b are constants. Kornelsen and Young (55) have fitted the Monte Carlo data of Webb and Fox (53) to determine the constants k_a and k_b. These are given in Table 15.3. Figure 15.12 shows the curves calculated by these authors.[4]

Figure 15.12 shows that at short distances, the attenuation of the primary photons is very much compensated for by the contribution of scattered photons with the result that the exposure in water is almost equal to the exposure in air at the same point. However, tissue attenuation overtakes scattering at larger distances. For radium sources, the net reduction is about 1% per cm of intervening tissue up to 5 cm.

It is instructive to study the dose falloff with distance in tissue. Figure 15.13 is a plot of percent dose as a function of distance in water for point sources of ^{60}Co, ^{226}Ra, ^{137}Cs, ^{198}Au, ^{192}Ir, and ^{125}I. These plots also are compared with the inverse square law function $(1/r^2)$. These data show that over a distance of about 5 cm the percent dose rates for ^{226}Ra, ^{60}Co, and ^{137}Cs are about equal and show a slight decrease below inverse square law due to tissue attenuation. The curves for ^{192}Ir and ^{198}Au, on the other hand, are practically indistinguishable from the inverse square law curve up to about 5 cm. The dose distribution for ^{125}I progressively deviates from the inverse square law as a result of increased tissue attenuation for this isotope. However, up to about 1 cm, all the curves are indistinguishable due to the severity of the inverse square law effect at such short distances.

Absorbed dose rate tables for linear radium sources have been published by Shalek and Stovall (1) which take into account attenuation and scattering in tissue. Similar data also are available for ^{137}Cs and ^{125}I (9,56). Such tables are useful for manual calculations as well as for checking the accuracy of computer calculations.

C. Modular Dose Calculation Model: TG-43

The traditional method of calculating dose in a medium (sections 15.3A and 15.3B) using Sievert integral requires the determination of μ', the effective attenuation coefficient for the filter as a function of thickness and the tissue attenuation factors. Both of these parameters are difficult to measure or calculate, especially for sources of complex design such as ^{125}I and ^{103}Pd. It is, therefore, advantageous to calculate dose rates from quantities measured solely in the medium. The data for a particular source can be compiled in a tabular form as a function of position. A modular approach has been proposed by the AAPM Task Group 43 in which the effects of several physical factors on dose rate distribution are considered separately (57). The dose rate, $\dot{D}(r,\theta)$ at point P with polar coordinates (r,θ) in a medium

---

[4] The authors appear to have normalized the dose values to unity at $r = 1$ cm. Spot checks of Fig. 15.12 revealed that the tissue attenuation correction factor is given by D_r/D_1, where D_1 is the dose at 1 cm.

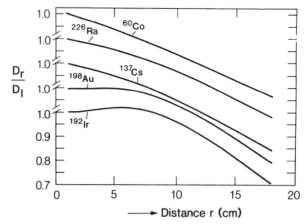

FIG. 15.12. Attenuation correction factor in water as a function of distance for a point source. Curves are calculated by Equation 15.15 and fitted to Monte Carlo data. See text for details.

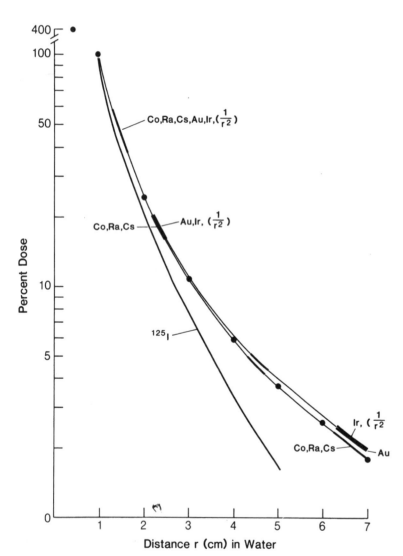

FIG. 15.13. Percent dose variation with distance in water for point sources of ^{60}Co, ^{226}Ra, ^{137}Cs, ^{198}Au, ^{192}Ir, and ^{125}I. Function ($1/r^2$) represents inverse square falloff. (^{125}I data are from Krishnaswamy V. Dose distribution around an ^{125}I seed source in tissue. *Radiology* 1976;126:489.) The other isotope data were calculated from Fig. 15.12 in addition to the inverse square law.

TABLE 15.4. RECOMMENDED DOSE RATE CONSTANTS IN WATER

Seed	cGy hr^{-1} U^{-1}	cGy mCi^{-1} hr^{-1}
^{125}I model 6702	0.919	1.16
^{125}I model 6711	0.847	1.07
^{192}Ir	1.11	4.55

The units for U are μGy m^2 h^{-1} or cGy cm^2 h^{-1}.
From Meli JA, Anderson LL, Weaver KA. Dose distribution. In:
Interstitial Collaborative Working Group, ed. *Interstitial brachytherapy.* New York: Raven, 1990:21, with permission.

(e.g., water) from the center of a source of air kerma strength S_K can be expressed as:

$$\dot{D}(r, \theta) = \Lambda S_K \frac{G(r, \theta)}{G(1, \pi/2)} F(r, \theta) g(r) \tag{15.16}$$

where Λ is the dose rate constant, defined as the dose rate per unit air kerma strength (U) at 1 cm along the transverse axis of the seed and has units of cGy h^{-1} U^{-1}, i.e.,

$$\Lambda = \dot{D}(1, \pi/2)/S_K \tag{15.17}$$

The dose rate constant, Λ, depends on the type of source, its construction, and its encapsulation. The values recommended for ^{125}I seeds (models 6702 and 6711) and ^{192}Ir seed are listed in Table 15.4.

$G(r, \theta)$ is the geometry factor (cm^{-2}) that accounts for the geometric falloff of the photon fluence with distance from the source and depends on the distribution of radioactive material. For a point source, $G(r, \theta) = 1/r^2$ and for uniformly distributed line source, $G(r, \theta) = (\theta_2 - \theta_1)/Ly$.[5]

$F(r, \theta)$ is the anisotropy factor normalized at $\theta = \pi/2$ (transverse axis), with the geometric factor factored out, that is,

$$F(r, \theta) = \frac{\dot{D}(r, \theta) G(r, \pi/2)}{\dot{D}(r, \pi/2) G(r, \theta)} \tag{15.18}$$

The anisotropy factor accounts for the angular dependence of photon absorption and scatter in the encapsulation and the medium.

The radial dose function, $g(r)$, accounts for radial dependence of photon absorption and scatter in the medium along the transverse axis and is given by:

$$g(r) = \frac{\dot{D}(r, \pi/2) G(1, \pi/2)}{\dot{D}(1, \pi/2) G(r, \pi/2)} \tag{15.19}$$

Again the geometric factor is factored out from the dose rates in defining $g(r)$.

Table 15.5 is an example of the geometry factor calculated for a 3-mm-long line source. Table 15.6 provides anisotropy and radial dose function data measured for ^{125}I seeds, models 6702 and 6711.

Because anisotropy is not as serious a problem for ^{192}Ir seeds as it is for ^{125}I seeds, iridium seeds may be treated as point sources in a dose calculation formalism. For a point source, Equation 15.16 reduces to:

$$\dot{D}(r) = \Lambda S_K \frac{g(r)}{r^2} \phi_{an} \tag{15.20}$$

where ϕ_{an} is the average anisotropy factor. It is defined as the ratio of 4π averaged dose rate at a given radial distance divided by the dose rate at the same distance along the transverse

---

[5] These results can be ascertained by substituting $\mu' = 0$ in Equation 15.10 and separating out the geometric factor.

TABLE 15.5. EXAMPLE OF THE GEOMETRY FACTOR, $G(r, \theta)$, FOR A 3.0-MM LINE SOURCE

θ (deg)	$r = 0.5$ cm	$r = 1.0$ cm
0	4.396	1.023
10	4.377	1.022
20	4.323	1.019
30	4.246	1.015
90	3.885	0.993

From Meli JA, Anderson LL, Weaver KA. Dose distribution. In: Interstitial Collaborative Working Group, ed. *Interstitial brachytherapy.* New York: Raven, 1990:21, with permission.

axis. ϕ_{an} for ^{192}Ir seeds may be equated to unity. The data for $g(r)$ for ^{192}Ir seeds are given in Table 15.7.

D. Isodose Curves

The above methods can be used to calculate absorbed dose to a matrix of points around a source. The isodose curves are then constructed by interpolation between points, connecting those points receiving the same dose. Because of the complex and time-consuming calculations required to generate isodose curves, the job is ideally suited for computers. Presently, almost all commercial treatment planning computers offer brachytherapy software that can perform sophisticated treatment planning involving three-dimensional distribution of multiple sources.

Experimental determination of isodose curves is sometimes necessary to check new calculation algorithms. Film and thermoluminescent dosimetry (TLD) (see chapter 8) require the least apparatus for such measurements. Film offers a high resolution but has a serious limitation of energy dependence, that is, increased sensitivity to low-energy photons

TABLE 15.6. THE ANISOTROPY FACTOR, $F(r, \theta)$, AND RADIAL DOSE FUNCTION, $g(r)$, FOR ^{125}I MODELS 6702 AND 6711

Model	r(cm)[a]	Anisotropy Factor					Radial Dose Function
		0°	10°	20°	30°	90°	
6702	0.5	0.448	0.544	0.701	0.815	1.0	1.04
	1.0	0.501	0.598	0.758	0.866	1.0	1.00
	2.0	0.537	0.628	0.781	0.874	1.0	0.851
	3.0	0.572	0.656	0.798	0.873	1.0	0.670
	4.0	0.605	0.683	0.814	0.872	1.0	0.510
	5.0	0.634	0.707	0.826	0.871	1.0	0.389
	6.0	0.651	0.719	0.828	0.870	1.0	0.302
	8.0						0.178
	10.0						0.131
6711	0.5	0.376	0.448	0.627	0.783	1.00	1.04
	1.0	0.369	0.464	0.658	0.799	1.00	1.00
	2.0	0.419	0.503	0.683	0.791	1.00	0.832
	3.0	0.474	0.551	0.715	0.800	1.00	0.632
	4.0	0.493	0.579	0.736	0.813	1.00	0.463
	5.0	0.478	0.583	0.743	0.823	1.00	0.344
	6.0						0.264
	8.0						0.145
	10.0						0.0820

[a]For $r < 0.5$ cm $g(r) = 1.00 \pm 0.1$.
From Meli JA, Anderson LL, Weaver KA. Dose distribution. In: Interstitial Collaborative Working Group, ed. *Interstitial brachytherapy.* New York: Raven, 1990:21, with permission.

TABLE 15.7. THE RADIAL DOSE FUNCTION, *g*(*r*), FOR
¹⁹²IR

r(cm)	*g*(*r*)
0.5	0.994
1.0	1.00
2.0	1.01
3.0	1.02
4.0	1.01
5.0	0.996
6.0	0.972
8.0	0.912
10.0	0.887

From Meli JA, Anderson LL, Weaver KA. Dose distribution. In:
Interstitial Collaborative Working Group, ed. *Interstitial*
brachytherapy. New York: Raven, 1990:21, with permission.

present in the nuclides' γ ray spectrum and the scattered radiation. TLD shows energy dependence (58) also but to a lesser degree than the film.

Automatic isodose plotters (59,60) also have been used to measure isodose curves. One of the γ ray detectors used in these instruments is a small scintillation detector. The scintillation counter is connected to an automatic isodose recording device. The output of the scintillation counter is independently calibrated by comparison with a calibrated source of the same kind. A silicon diode detector connected to a radiation field scanner also has been used for relative close distribution measurements (20). Small size and almost complete energy independence make it quite suitable for these measurements.

Figure 15.14 shows an example of isodose curves around a radium needle. Examination of the curves indicates that close to the source they are more or less elliptical. At large distances, the isodose curves become circles, because the source behaves as a point source. The dip in the curves close to the source axis is due to the effect of oblique filtration.

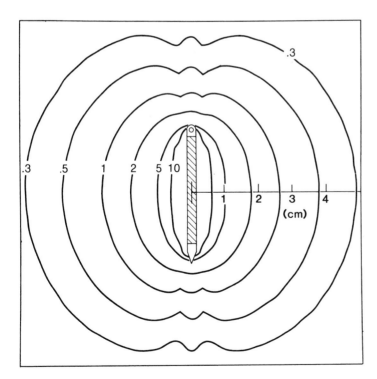

FIG. 15.14. Isodose curves in terms of rad/h around a 1-mg radium source. Active length = 3.0 cm; filtration = 0.5 mm Pt.

15.4. SYSTEMS OF IMPLANT DOSIMETRY

The objectives of treatment planning are (*a*) to determine the distribution and type of radiation sources to provide optimum dose distribution and (*b*) to provide a complete dose distribution in the irradiated volume. Numerous systems of dosimetric planning have been devised over the past 50 years. Of these the Paterson-Parker system (61) and the Quimby system (62) have received the most widespread use. These and other systems were designed during the times when computers were not available for routine treatment planning. Extensive tables and elaborate rules of source distribution were devised to facilitate the process of manual treatment planning. Then a more significant development occurred: the use of digital computers to calculate isodose distributions for individual patients (63–65). This gave the radiation therapist freedom to deviate from the established systems. Although, the old systems with their rules and tables are still being used, the computer treatment planning is fast replacing the traditional systems. Some of these methods will be reviewed here to illustrate the basic problems and concepts of brachytherapy planning.

A. The Paterson-Parker System

The Paterson-Parker or Manchester system (61) was developed to deliver uniform dose (within ± 10%) to a plane or volume. The system specified rules of source distribution to achieve the dose uniformity and provided dosage tables for these idealized implants. These tables are reproduced in the appendix.

A.1. Planar Implant

In the case of planar implants the uniformity of dose is achieved in parallel planes at 0.5 cm from the implanted plane and within the area bounded by the projection of the peripheral needles on that plane. The "stated" dose, determined from the Paterson-Parker tables, is 10% higher than the minimum dose. The maximum dose should not exceed 10% above the stated dose to satisfy the uniformity criterion. The dose is, however, much more nonuniform within the plane of implant. For example, the dose at the surface of the needles is about five times the stated dose.

The distribution rules for the planar implants are:

1. The ratio between the amount of radium in the periphery and the amount of radium over the area itself depends on the size of the implant, for example:

Area	*Fraction Used in Periphery*
Less than 25 cm^2	$2/3$
25–100 cm^2	$1/2$
Over 100 cm^2	$1/3$

2. The spacing of the needles should not be more than 1 cm from each other or from the crossing ends.
3. If the ends of the implant are uncrossed (Fig. 15.15B or C), the effective area of dose uniformity is reduced.[6] The area is, therefore, reduced by 10% for each uncrossed end for table reading purposes.
4. In the case of multiple implant planes, the radium should be arranged as in rules 1–3, and the planes should be parallel to each other.

---

[6] If it is not possible to cross an end, one can increase the size of the implant by using longer needles so that the effective area of dose uniformity adequately covers the tumor. Again, 10% is deducted from the implant area for each uncrossed end for table reading purposes.

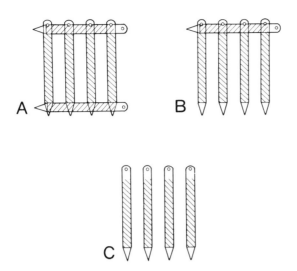

FIG. 15.15. Examples of three planar implants. **A:** Both ends crossed. **B:** One end uncrossed. **C:** Both ends uncrossed.

A.2. Volume Implants

Some tumors are better implanted using three-dimensional shapes such as cylinders, spheres, or cuboids.

1. The total amount of radium is divided into eight parts and distributed as follows for the various shapes. The cylinder is composed of belt, four parts; core, two parts; and each end, one part (Fig. 15.16). The sphere is made up of shell, six parts, and core, two parts. The cuboid consists of each side, one part; each end, one part; and core, two parts.

2. The needles should be spaced as uniformly as possible, not more than 1 cm apart. There should be at least eight needles in the belt and four in the core.

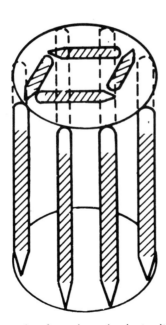

FIG. 15.16. Example of a volume implant with one end uncrossed. The implant has eight needles in the belt, four in the core (not shown), and four at one end. Whereas the needles in the belt and core are 1 mg each, the crossing needles at the end are 0.5 mg each, thus satisfying the Paterson-Parker rule of radium distribution.

3. If the ends of the volume implant are uncrossed, 7.5% is deducted from the volume for uncrossed end for table reading purposes.

For a volume implant, the prescribed dose is stated 10% higher than the minimum dose within the implanted volume.

A.3. Paterson-Parker Tables

The Paterson-Parker tables (61) are designed to give milligram hours/1,000 roentgens (mg-h/1,000 R) for implants of various sizes, both for planar and volume implants (see Tables A.12.1 and A.12.2 in the appendix). To convert Paterson-Parker roentgens to cGy in tissue, one needs to make the following corrections: (*a*) Exposure rate constant (Γ): the tables assume $\Gamma = 8.4$ Rcm^2/mg-h instead of the current value of 8.25 Rcm^2/mg-h. (*b*) A roentgen:cGy factor of 0.957 should be used to convert exposure into dose in muscle. (*c*) Oblique filtration: Paterson-Parker tables do not take into account increased attenuation by oblique filtration by the platinum capsule, giving rise to a 2% to 4% error for typical implants. (*d*) Paterson-Parker tables are based on exposure in air. Corrections are needed for tissue attenuation and scattering (section 15.3B).

Stovall and Shalek (66) have demonstrated that for typical planar and volume implants a combined factor of 0.90 selects an isodose curve approximately equivalent to the Paterson-Parker dosage. Thus the mg-h/1,000 R in the original Paterson-Parker tables should be considered equivalent to mg-h/900 cGy.

A.4. Determination of Implant Area or Volume

Dosage tables for interstitial implants require the knowledge of area or volume of implant. If the needles are close to the surface, one can determine the size of the implant directly. If not, it has to be determined radiographically.

Orthogonal Radiographs

Three-dimensional localization of individual sources can be obtained by orthogonal (perpendicular) radiographs, such as anteroposterior (AP) and lateral (Lat) views. It is important that the central axes of the anteroposterior and lateral x-ray beams meet at a point, approximately in the middle of the implant. This can be easily achieved by an isocentric radiographic unit, such as a treatment simulator. For the above isocentric geometry, the film magnification factor is given by SFD/SAD, where SFD is source-to-film distance and SAD is source-to-axis distance. Alternatively, a circular object, such as a metallic ring, may be taped to the patient at the level of the implant. The ratio of the largest outside diameter of the ring image to the actual outside diameter of the ring gives the magnification factor.

To determine the width or length of an implant, one needs to determine the distance between two points, three dimensionally. Figure 15.17 illustrates the principle of deriving this information from orthogonal radiographs. Let $A(x_1, y_1, z_1)$ and $B(x_2, y_2, z_2)$ be the two points in question. Then by the application of the Pythagorean theorem, it can be shown that:

$$AB = (x_2 - x_1)^2 + (y_2 - y_1)^2 + (z_2 - z_1)^2 \tag{15.21}$$

Equation 15.21 can also be written as:

$$AB = \sqrt{a^2 + c^2} \tag{15.22}$$

where a is the length of the image of AB on one of the radiographs and c is the projection of the image of AB to the baseline in the other radiograph (the baseline is a line perpendicular to the intersection of the radiographs, usually parallel to the edges of the films). Figure 15.17 assumes a magnification factor of unity. However, in actual practice, a and c will have to be corrected for film magnification.

a) Lateral Radiograph

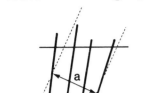

b) Anteriorposterior Radiograph

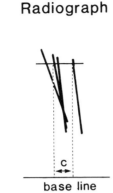

base line

FIG. 15.17. Orthogonal radiographs of an implant. Baseline is parallel to the edge of the film.

Thus, by determining the width of the implant image on one film and its width projected to the baseline on the other, one can calculate the actual width of the implant. The length of the implant can also be determined the same way but is usually given by the known active length of the needles.

Example

Figure 15.17 shows the anteroposterior and lateral radiographs of a planar implant that was planned according to the Paterson-Parker system. Assume a magnification factor of 1.4 for both films. Determine the time to deliver 6500 cGy at 0.5 cm from the plane of implant.

Given width of the implant image on the lateral radiograph $= a = 3.8$ cm
Projection of AP image on baseline $= c = 0.9$ cm
Peripheral needles $= 3 \times 2$ mg
Central needles $= 2 \times 1$ mg
All needles have active length of 3 cm and 0.5 mm Pt filtration.
Treatment distance $= 0.5$ cm from the plane of implant

$$\text{Width of implant} = \sqrt{\left(\frac{3.8}{1.4}\right)^2 + \left(\frac{0.9}{1.4}\right)^2} = 2.79 \text{ cm}$$

Length of implant $= 3$ cm
Area of implant $= 2.79 \times 3 = 8.4$ cm^2

Because one end is uncrossed, the area for table reading purposes $= 8.4 - 10\%$ $(8.4) = 7.6$ cm^2. From Paterson-Parker table (Table A.12.1 in the appendix), the mg-h/1,000 R or mg-h/900 cGy required $= 200$.

$$\text{mg-h required to deliver 6,500 cGy} = 200 \times \frac{6,500}{900} = 1,444$$

$$\text{time required} = \frac{1,444 \text{ mg-h}}{8 \text{ mg}} = 181 \text{ h}$$

$$\text{dose rate} = \frac{6,500}{181} = 36 \text{ cGy/h}$$

B. The Quimby System

The Quimby system (62) of interstitial implantation is characterized by a uniform distribution of sources of equal linear activity. Consequently, this arrangement of sources results in a nonuniform dose distribution, higher in the central region of treatment. For planar implants, the Quimby table gives the milligram-hours required to produce 1,000 R in the center of the treatment planes, up to 3 cm distance from the plane of implant. The stated dose is thus the maximum dose in the plane of treatment. For volume implants, the stated dose is the minimum dose within the implanted volume.

The original Quimby tables, like the Manchester tables, are based on an exposure rate constant of 8.4 Rcm^2/mg-h instead of the currently accepted value of 8.25 Rcm^2/mg-h. Also, other corrections, namely the roentgen:cGy factor, oblique filtration, and tissue attenuation, have to be applied as in the case of the Paterson-Parker tables.

Shalek and Stovall compared the Quimby and the Paterson-Parker systems for selected idealized cases and found that fundamental differences exist between the two systems. They caution against the use of these systems interchangeably. "It is imperative that a radiation therapist use one radium system to the exclusion of the other" (1).

C. The Memorial System

The Memorial system, as described by Laughlin et al. (64) in 1963, is an extension of the Quimby system and is characterized by complete dose distributions around lattices of point sources of uniform strength spaced 1 cm apart. Based on computer-generated dose distributions, tables were constructed that gave milligram-hours to deliver 1,000 rads at designated points, for example, "minimum peripheral" and "reference maximum dose" points in the plane 0.5 cm from the source plane for the planar implants. For volume implants, similar data points within the implanted volume as well as "central line peripheral dose" points were chosen. These tables use proper exposure rate constant and include the effects of oblique filtration and tissue attenuation.

Another method, known as the "dimension averaging" technique also has been used at Memorial Hospital for permanent implants (67,68). The method is based on the rationale that radiation tolerance of tissue depends on the size of the implant and the smaller volumes could be intentionally given larger doses. According to this method, the total activity required for an implant is directly proportional to the average of the three dimensions of the implant region.

Mathematically,

$$A = K \cdot \overline{d} \qquad (15.23)$$

where A is the activity in mCi and d is the averaged dimension, that is, $\overline{d} = (a + b + c)/3$, where a, b, and c are the three mutually perpendicular dimensions. The constant K of proportionality is based on clinical experience: $K = 10$ for ^{222}Rn and $K = 5$ for ^{125}I.

In addition to the total activity required for an implant, one needs to know the number of seeds and the spacing between seeds. Anderson (68) has described a nomogram for ^{125}I seed spacing that takes into account the elongation factor for the implant shape, for example, spheroid or cylinder.

D. The Paris System

The Paris system (69) of dosimetry is intended primarily for removable implants of long line sources, such as ^{192}Ir wires. The system prescribes wider spacing for longer sources or larger treatment volumes. As summarized in Table 15.8, the sources are of uniform linear activity and are implanted in parallel lines. The details of the system are described by Pierquin et al. (70).

In the Paris system the dose specification is based on an isodose surface, called the *reference isodose.* However, in practice, the value of the reference isodose is fixed at 85% of the "basal dose," which is defined as the average of the minimum dose between sources. It has been shown that the reference isodose for a Paris implant surrounds the implant within a few millimeters, and its value is approximately equal to 85% of the basal dose (71). Figure 15.18 illustrates how the basal dose is calculated in different patterns of implants using the Paris system.

TABLE 15.8. RULES OF INTERSTITIAL IMPLANT SYSTEMS

Characteristic	Paterson-Parker	Quimby	Paris	Computer[a]
Linear strength	Variable (full intensity, 0.66 mg Ra/cm; half intensity, 0.33 mg Ra/cm)	Constant (full intensity, 1 mg Ra/cm; half intensity, 0.5 mg Ra/cm)	Constant (0.6–1.8 mg Ra eq/cm)	Constant (0.2–0.4 mg Ra eq/cm)
Source distribution	Planar implants: Area <25 cm², 2/3 Ra in periphery; area 25 to 100 cm², 1/2 Ra in periphery. Area >100 cm², 1/3 Ra in periphery	Uniform	Uniform	Uniform
	Volume implants Cylinder: belt, four parts; core, two parts; each end, one part. Sphere: shell, six parts; core, two parts. Cube: each side, one part; core, two parts.	Uniform distribution of sources throughout the volume	Line sources arranged in parallel planes	Line sources arranged in parallel planes or cylindric volumes
Line source spacing	Constant approximately 1 cm apart from each other or from crossing ends	Same as Paterson-Parker	Constant, but selected according to implant dimensions-larger spacing used in large volumes; 8 mm minimum to 15 mm maximum separation	Constant, 1–1.5 cm, depending on size of implant (larger spacing for larger size implants)
Crossing needles	Crossing needles required to enhance dose at implant ends	Same as Paterson-Parker	Crossing needles not used; active length 30% to 40% longer than target length	Crossing needles not required; active length of sources 30% to 40% longer than target length

[a]The computer system used at the University of Minnesota Hospital.
From Khan FM. Brachytherapy: rules of implantation and dose specification. In: Levitt SH, Khan FM, Potish RA, eds. *Technological basis of radiation therapy*. Philadelphia: Lea & Febiger, 1992:113, with permission.

E. Computer System

An implant system that has evolved through the use of computers but bears no formal name is used in many institutions in the United States. I will call it the *computer system*. The implantation rules are very simple: the sources of uniform strength are implanted, spaced uniformly (e.g., 1.0 to 1.5 cm, with larger spacing for larger size implants), and cover the entire target volume.

It is realized that the implantation of uniform activity sources gives rise to an implant that is "hotter" in the middle than in the periphery, as is the case with the Quimby and the Paris systems. However, this dose inhomogeneity is accepted with the belief that the central part of the target would need higher doses to sterilize than the periphery.

In the computer system, the target volume is designed with sufficient safety margins so that the peripheral sources can be placed at the target boundary with adequate coverage of the tumor. The dose is specified by the isodose surface that just surrounds the target or the implant. An important criterion is followed: It is better to implant a larger volume than to select a lower value isodose curve to increase the coverage. If the target volume is designed with adequate safety margins, the peripheral sources should then be implanted on the outer surface of the target volume. Also, the active length of the line sources should be suitably longer (≃40% longer) than the length of the target volume because of uncrossed ends.

Figure 15.19A shows isodose distribution in the central cross-sectional plane for a computer system volume implant (two parallel planes). The prescription isodose curve just surrounds the peripheral sources. Figure 15.19B shows the isodose pattern in the longitudinal plane through the middle of implant to assess adequate coverage by the

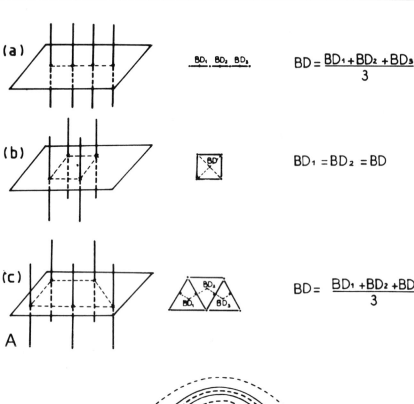

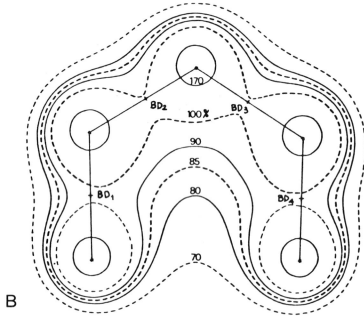

FIG. 15.18. Determination of basal dose (BD) in implants using the Paris system. **A:** Line sources implanted in patterns of (a) single plane, (b) squares, and (c) triangles. **B:** Isodose curves in central plane of a volume implant using the Paris system. The isodose values are normalized to the average basal dose, which is given by 1/4 ($BD_1 + BD_2 + BD_3 + BD_4$). (From Dutreix A, Marinello G. In: Pierquin B, Wilson JF, Chassagne D, eds. *Modern brachytherapy.* New York: Masson, 1987, with permission.)

prescription isodose curve in this plane. In fact, target volume coverage can be viewed in any plane or three-dimensionally, provided volumetric data for the target are available.

15.5. COMPUTER DOSIMETRY

The older dosimetry systems are based on idealized implants conforming to certain distribution rules. In actual practice, however, such ideal distributions are seldom realized. With a computer, it is possible to preplan not only implants but a complete isodose distribution, corresponding to the final source distribution. The rapid turnaround time with the modern computer systems allows the therapist to modify the implant, if necessary, on the basis of 3-D dose distribution.

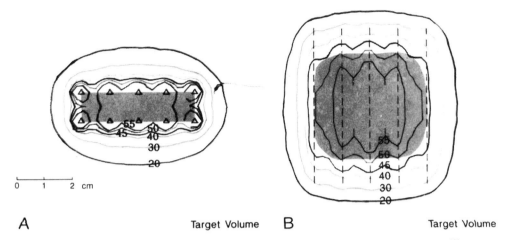

FIG. 15.19. Isodose curves for a volume implant using two parallel planes containing five ^{192}Ir line sources per plane. **A:** Central cross-sectional plane. **B:** Longitudinal plane through middle of implant. Prescription dose is specified on the 45 cGy/h isodose curve, which just encloses the implant in the central cross-sectional plane. (From Khan FM. Brachytherapy: rules of implantation and dose specification. In: Levitt SH, Khan FM, Potish RA, eds. *Technological basis of radiation therapy.* Philadelphia: Lea & Febiger, 1992:113, with permission.)

Computer calculation of a brachytherapy dose distribution consists of repeated calculation of dose at a point for each of the implant sources. The total dose at a given point is determined by summing the individual source contributions. Point dose rates are computed for each of a grid of points arranged in a cubic lattice so that isodose curves may be generated in any arbitrary plane. The isodose patterns can also be magnified and superimposed on an implant radiograph for viewing the distribution in relation to the patient's anatomy.

A. Localization of Sources

Dose calculation algorithms require spatial coordinates for each radioactive source. Three-dimensional reconstruction of the source geometry is usually accomplished by using a set of two radiographs, exposed with either orthogonal or "stereo-shift" geometry. Most programs allow input of the film coordinates using a digitizer.

A.1. Orthogonal Imaging Method

As discussed in section 15.4A.4, the orthogonal radiographs are taken at right angles, with the central axes of the x-ray beams meeting approximately in the middle of the implant. Usually, AP film and lateral film, exposed isocentrically, provide such a geometry. The coordinate system is conventionally established with the x axis from the right to the left of the patient, the y axis from inferior to superior, and the z axis from posterior to anterior. The anteroposterior film represents a magnified view of the implant image projected onto the x–y plane while the lateral film presents the image projected onto the z–y plane. The origin of the coordinate system is chosen to be a point identified to be the same on both films such as one end of a source. The sources can be identified by comparing the y coordinates of the ends on both films. For example, a source end having the smallest y coordinate on one film will have the smallest y coordinate on the other film also, because the y axis is common to both films. After all the sources have been identified, the tip and end of each linear source image are sampled with a digitizer, sampling each end sequentially from one film to the other. The source coordinates on each film are corrected for magnification and stored in the computer as x, y, and z coordinates of each source end. The program also determines errors in source localization by comparing the y coordinates (which should be the same) of a source end on both films and comparing the calculated physical length with the actual physical length of the source. If (x_1, y_1, z_1) and (x_2, y_2, z_2) are the coordinates

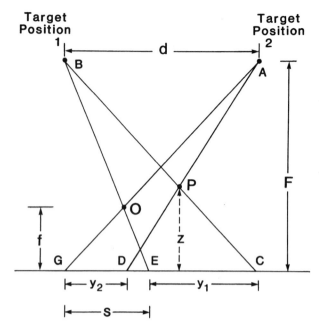

FIG. 15.20. Diagram illustrating stereo-shift method of source localization. (Drawing is modified from Anderson LL. Dosimetry of interstitial radiation therapy. In: Hilaris BS, ed. *Handbook of interstitial brachytherapy.* Acton, MA: Publishing Sciences Group, 1975:87.)

of the two ends of the source, then the length L of the source is given by:

$$L = \sqrt{(x_2 - x_1)^2 + (y_2 - y_1)^2 + (z_2 - z_1)^2} \qquad (15.24)$$

A.2. Stereo-shift Method

The stereo-shift method of source localization consists of taking two radiographs of the same view but the patient or the x-ray tube is shifted a certain distance (e.g., 20 cm) between the two exposures. The principle of the method is illustrated in Fig. 15.20. Suppose both films are anteroposterior, parallel to the $x–y$ plane of the patient as the tube is shifted in the y direction between films. A tabletop fiducial marker is used to serve as origin at O. Because the x, y coordinates of a point source or a source end can be obtained from either of the films, the z coordinates can be derived as follows. Let:

   $P =$ point to be localized three dimensionally
   $y_1 =$ distance between images of P and O on the first film
   $y_2 =$ distance between images of P and O on the second film
   $s =$ film shift in the origin O due to tube shift
   $d =$ tube shift distance
   $F =$ target-to-film distance
   $f =$ table-to-film distance

From similar triangles APB and CPD

$$\frac{d}{y_1 + s - y_2} = \frac{F - z}{z} \qquad (15.25)$$

Also, from similar triangles AOB and EOG

$$\frac{d}{s} = \frac{F - f}{f} \qquad (15.26)$$

From Equations 15.25 and 15.26, we get

$$z = F\frac{(F-f)(y_2-y_1)-d\cdot f}{(F-f)(y_2-y_1)-d\cdot F} \qquad (15.27)$$

The accuracy of the orthogonal film method is generally better than that of the stereo-shift method (72). For example, small errors in the measurement of y coordinates produces a large error in the z values. However, the stereo-shift method is more suitable for cases in which sources cannot be easily identified by orthogonal films such as a large number of seeds or some sources being masked by overlying bone.

B. Dose Computation

Earlier computer programs were used mostly to obtain linear source tables, build-up factors, and scatter factors. Later, programs became available (63–65) to calculate isodose distributions for individual patients. Currently, almost all treatment-planning software packages provide brachytherapy dosimetry. Most of these programs use either the Sievert integral directly or precalculated dose tables for different types of sources. Some, but not all, use tissue attenuation corrections, discussed in section 15.3B.

For radium and other long-lived isotopes, the dose rates, presented in the form of isodose curves, can be directly used to calculate implant duration. In the case of temporary implants of relatively short-lived isotopes such as ^{192}Ir, the computer calculates cumulated dose, using decay correction for the implant duration. An approximate time for the implant duration can first be determined from dose rate $\dot{D}_0$ without decay correction and the total dose to be delivered. The cumulated dose D_c is then given by:

$$D_c = \dot{D}_0\cdot T_{av}(1 - e^{-t/T_{av}}) \qquad (15.28)$$

where T_{av} is the average life and t is the implant duration.

For permanent implants such as ^{125}I or ^{198}Au, cumulated dose (to complete decay) is given by:

$$D_c = \dot{D}_0\cdot T_{av} = 1.44\cdot \dot{D}_0\cdot T_{1/2} \qquad (15.29)$$

15.6. IMPLANTATION TECHNIQUES

Brachytherapy sources are applied in three ways: external applicators or molds, interstitial implantation, and intracavitary therapy. A choice of one technique or the other is dictated primarily by the size and location of the tumor. For example, surface molds are used to treat small superficial areas, such as the ear or the lip; interstitial therapy is indicated when the tumor is well-localized and can be implanted directly according to accepted rules of distribution; intracavitary therapy is used when applicators containing radioactive sources can be introduced into body cavities. In all these cases, owing to the short treatment distance, the geometry of source distribution is critical.

A. Surface Molds

Plastic molds are prepared (73) to conform to the surface to be treated and the sources are securely positioned on the outer surface of the mold. The distance between the plane of the sources to the skin surface is chosen to give a treatment distance of usually 0.5 to 1.0 cm. The dosimetry and source distribution rules are the same for external molds as for interstitial sources (61).

B. Interstitial Therapy

In interstitial therapy, the radioactive sources are fabricated in the form of needles, wires, or seeds, which can be inserted directly into the tissue. There are basically two types of interstitial implants: temporary and permanent. In a temporary implant, the sources are removed after the desired dose has been delivered (e.g., radium needles, iridium wires, or iridium seeds). In a permanent implant, the sources are left permanently in the implanted tissues (e.g., ^{198}Au and ^{125}I seeds). In general, a temporary implant provides better control of source distribution and dosimetry than a permanent implant. However, the permanent implant is a one-time procedure and is a preferred method for some tumors such as those in the abdominal and thoracic cavities.

A major improvement in temporary implant technique occurred with the introduction of "afterloading" techniques (74,75) in which the sources are loaded into tubes previously implanted in the tissues. This procedure eliminates exposure in the operating room, x-ray room, and the areas through which the patient is transported. "Dummy" sources are used for radiographic localization and dosimetry. The radioactive sources are loaded after the patient is returned to his or her room and the implant has been evaluated.

Figure 15.21 illustrates the basic principles of the afterloading technique described by Henschke et al. (74). Stainless steel needles (e.g., 17 gauge) are first implanted in and around the tumor. The nylon tubes are threaded through the needles, and the needles are then withdrawn, leaving the nylon tubes in place. The nylon tubes are secured in position by buttons on the skin surface. The tube ends are then usually cut off a few centimeters beyond the buttons.

Many variations of the above procedure have been published in the literature. Further details can be obtained from Hilaris (76).

The simplest device for permanent implants is a single-seed inserter consisting of a stainless-steel needle. Each seed is individually loaded into the tip of this needle and, after insertion into the tissue, the seed is pushed out by a stylet. This technique, however, is unsatisfactory for the implantation of deep-seated tumors and volume implants requiring many seeds.

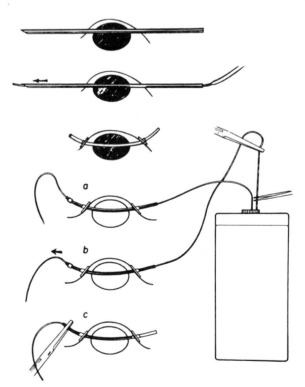

FIG. 15.21. Illustration of an afterloading technique for ^{192}Ir seeds. (From Hilaris BS, ed. *Handbook of interstitial brachytherapy.* Acton, MA: Publishing Sciences Group, 1975:87, with permission.)

An afterloading technique has also been adopted for the permanent implants (77). The first step in this technique consists of inserting unloaded 17-gauge stainless-steel needles into the tumor. The needles are spaced 1 to 2 cm apart, depending on the size of the tumor. The needles are then afterloaded with radioactive seeds, using a special implantation instrument that allows insertion of several seeds at different depths, determined by a gauge as the needle is withdrawn.

Seed-introducing guns (76,78) have been devised that allow preloading of radioactive seeds into a magazine from which they are pushed into the needle, and then into the tissue. These instruments are convenient to use and can provide greater precision than possible with single seed inserters. Modern techniques of seed implants are discussed in Chapter 23.

C. Intracavitary Therapy

C.1. Uterine Cervix

Intracavitary therapy is mostly used for cancers of the uterine cervix, uterine body, and vagina. A variety of applicators have been designed to hold the sources in a fixed configuration. A cervix applicator basically consists of a central tube, called the tandem, and lateral capsules or "ovoids." The ovoids are separated from each other by spacers.

Since the first application of radium in the treatment of cancer of the uterus in 1908, several techniques have evolved, most of which are modifications of the Stockholm technique (79) and the Paris technique (80). The Manchester system, which evolved from the Paris technique, uses a rubber uterine tandem to hold one to three radium tubes and rubber ovoids, separated by a rubber spacer, to each hold a radium tube. The radiation is delivered in at least two applications. In the Fletcher-Suit applicator (75,81) (Fig. 15.22) the tandem and the ovoids (or the colpostats) are made of stainless steel and then secured to hollow handles to permit afterloading of the sources. Tables have been devised with various combinations of external beam therapy and intracavitary radium using standard loadings (82).

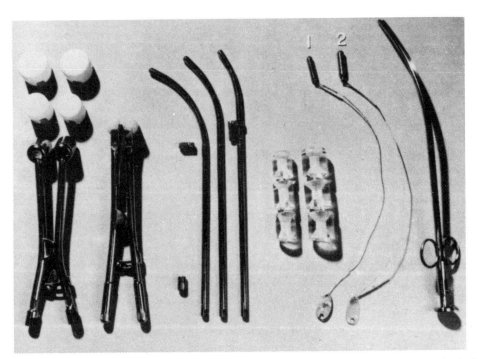

FIG. 15.22. A Fletcher-Suite applicator set. (From Fletcher GH. *Textbook of radiotherapy,* 2nd ed. Philadelphia: Lea & Febiger, 1973:620, with permission.)

C.2. Uterine Corpus

Cancer of the uterine body can be treated with radium or cesium sources using Heyman capsules (83). These capsules are available in different sizes, each containing 5 to 10 mg-Ra eq source. The Heyman technique consists of packing the uterine cavity with multiple sources. Tables have been published that specify dose to the inside surface of the uterine cavity in terms of milligram-hours (83). These dosages have been established on the basis of various measurements, and therefore, individual patient calculations are usually not required.

15.7. DOSE SPECIFICATION: CANCER OF THE CERVIX

Pierquin et al. (70) have reviewed various systems of dose specification for the cervix treatment. Whereas no single system has been devised that can meet all the criteria of dose specification, three systems are described that are most commonly used in many forms and combinations.

A. Milligram-Hours

One of the oldest system of dose specification for the brachytherapy treatment of cervix is the milligram-hours, that is, the product of total source strength and the implant duration. The rationale for this system is based on extensive clinical data that have been accumulated using particular applicators and guidelines for source loading and implant duration for various stages of the disease. The most notable example of this system is the *Fletcher guidelines,* which were developed on the basis of M. D. Anderson experience (84).

It is obvious that the dose specification by milligram-hours alone is not adequate. It lacks the information on source arrangement, position of tandem relative to the ovoids, packing of the applicators, tumor size, and patient anatomy. By computer dosimetry, it is easy to show that a dose specification system based on milligram-hours alone is fraught with large uncertainties in the dose distribution from patient to patient. Although the milligram-hours is an important treatment parameter, it cannot be made the sole basis of dose-response curve.

B. The Manchester System

The Manchester system is one of the oldest and the most extensively used systems in the world. It is characterized by doses to four points: point *A,* point *B,* a bladder point, and a rectum point. The duration of the implant is based on the dose rate calculated at point *A,* although the dose at the other points is taken into consideration in evaluating a treatment plan. With the availability of the treatment planning computers, most users of the Manchester system examine the isodose distributions in the frontal and sagittal planes in addition to obtaining dose at the four designated points. Point *A* still remains the point of dose prescription.

Point *A* was originally defined as 2 cm superior to the lateral vaginal fornix and 2 cm lateral to the cervical canal (Fig. 15.23) (85). Later, it was redefined to be 2 cm superior to the external cervical os (or cervical end of the tandem), and 2 cm lateral to the cervical canal (86). Point *B* is defined 3 cm lateral to point *A.*

Ideally, a point *A* represents the location where the uterine vessels cross the ureter. It is believed that the tolerance of these structures is the main limiting factor in the irradiation of the uterine cervix. The anatomic significance of point *A,* however, has been questioned by several investigators (70,84,87). The critics point out the following limitations of point *A: (a)* it relates to the position of the sources and not to a specific anatomic structure; (*b*) dose to point *A* is very sensitive to the position of the ovoid sources relative to the tandem sources, which should not be the determining factor in deciding on implant duration; and

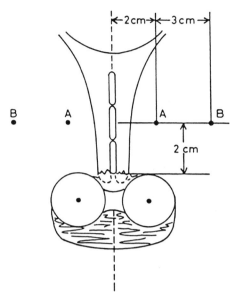

FIG. 15.23. Original definition of points *A* and *B,* according to the Manchester system. (From Meredith WJ. *Radium dosage: the Manchester system.* Edinburgh: Livingstone, 1967, with permission.)

(*c*) depending on the size of the cervix, point *A* may lie inside the tumor or outside the tumor (Fig. 15.24). Thus, dose prescription at point *A* could risk underdosage of large cervical cancers or overdosage of small ones.

B.1. Dose to Bladder and Rectum

The colpostats in the Fletcher-Suit applicator are partially shielded at the top and the bottom to provide some protection to bladder and rectum. However, dosimetrically it is difficult to demonstrate the extent of protection actually provided by these shields.

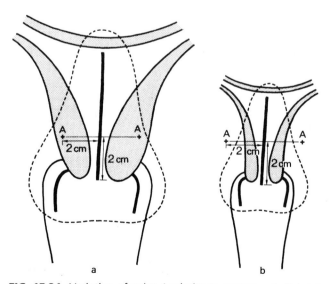

FIG. 15.24. Variation of point *A* relative to anatomy. **A:** Point *A* inside large cervix, resulting in underdosage. **B:** Point *A* outside small cervix, resulting in overdosage. (From Pierquin B, Wilson JF, Chassagne D, eds. *Modern brachytherapy.* New York: Masson, 1987, with permission.)

The dose to bladder and rectum depends on the distribution of sources in a given application. If this dose is assessed to be too high either by measurement or calculation, one has the option of altering the geometry of the sources. Although various instruments, including intracavitary ionization chambers, are available for such measurements, the calculation method has been found to be more reliable in this case. The localization of bladder and rectum can be performed using radiographs taken with contrast media in the bladder and rectum. The maximum dose to bladder and rectum should be, as far as possible, less than the dose to point *A* (e.g., 80% or less of the dose to point *A*).

C. The International Commission on Radiation Units and Measurements System

The ICRU has recommended a system of dose specification that relates the dose distribution to the target volume, instead of the dose to a specific point (88). The dose is prescribed as the value of an isodose surface that just surrounds the target volume.

Figure 15.25 illustrates the concept of target volume when only intracavitary treatment is given and when intracavitary and external beam therapy are combined. For the intracavitary treatment, the target volume includes the cervix region and the corpus.

Table 15.9 summarizes the ICRU system of dose specifications, which includes recording of various treatment parameters. These parameters are discussed.

Description of the Technique. Minimum information should include the applicator type, source type and loading and orthogonal radiographs of the application.

Total Reference Air Kerma. By this parameter is meant the total air kerma strength of sources times the implant duration. This is similar to the total milligram-hours of radium or total mg-Ra eq-h except that the sources are calibrated in units of air kerma strength, that is, μGy m^2 h^{-1}.

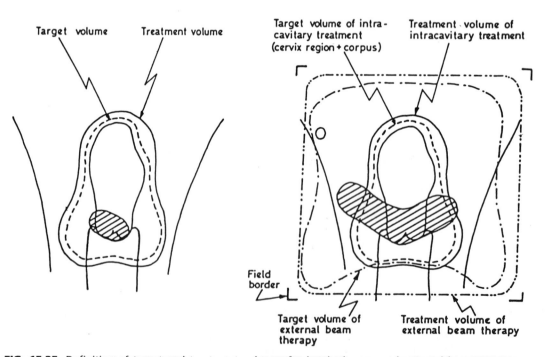

A. ONLY INTRACAVITARY TREATMENT

B. COMBINED INTRACAVITARY AND EXTERNAL BEAM THERAPY

FIG. 15.25. Definition of target and treatment volumes for brachytherapy and external beam treatment. (From ICRU. Dose and volume specification for reporting intracavitary therapy in gynecology. ICRU Report No. 38. Bethesda, MD: International Commission on Radiation Units and Measurements, 1985, with permission.)

TABLE 15.9. DATA NEEDED FOR REPORTING INTRA-CAVITARY THERAPY IN GYNECOLOGY (ICRU)

Description of the technique
Total reference air kerma
Description of the reference volume
   Dose level if not 60 Gy
   Dimensions of reference volume (height, width, thickness)
Absorbed dose at reference points
   Bladder reference point
   Rectal reference point
   Lymphatic trapezoid
   Pelvic wall reference point
Time-dose pattern

From ICRU. Dose and volume specification for reporting intracavitary therapy in gynecology. ICRU report no. 38. Bethesda, MD: International Commission on Radiation Units and Measurements, 1985.

Reference Volume. The reference volume is the volume of the isodose surface that just surrounds the target volume. The value of this isodose surface, based on the Paris experience (70), is set at 60 Gy.

The prescription isodose value of 60 Gy includes the dose contribution from the external beam. The reference volume for the intracavitary part of the treatment should be identified and its dimensions recorded. Figure 15.26 shows how the height (d_h), width

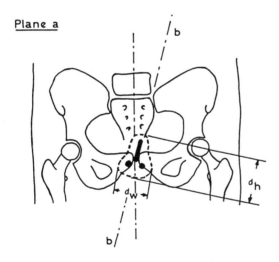

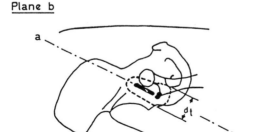

FIG. 15.26. Determination of the reference isodose surface dimensions. d_w, width; d_h, height; d_t, thickness. (From ICRU. Dose and volume specification for reporting intracavitary therapy in gynecology. ICRU Report No. 38. Bethesda, MD: International Commission on Radiation Units and Measurements, 1985, with permission.)

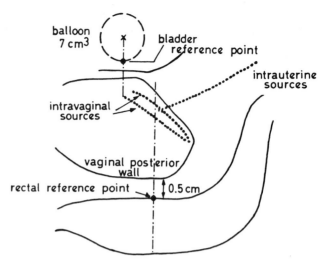

FIG. 15.27. Localization of bladder and rectum points. (From ICRU. Dose and volume specification for reporting intracavitary therapy in gynecology. ICRU Report No. 38. Bethesda, MD: International Commission on Radiation Units and Measurements, 1985, with permission.)

(d_w), and thickness (d_t) of the pear-shaped reference volume can be measured from the oblique frontal and oblique sagittal planes. The reference volume is approximated by ($d_h \times d_w \times d_t$) cm^3.

C.1. Absorbed Dose at Reference Points

Bladder Point. The bladder point is localized by using a Foley catheter, with the balloon filled with a contrast material. On the frontal radiograph, the bladder point is marked at the center of the balloon; on the lateral radiograph, the bladder point is obtained on a line drawn anteroposteriorly through the center of the balloon, at the posterior surface (Fig. 15.27).

Rectal Point. The rectal point is identified on the frontal radiograph at the midpoint of the ovoid sources (or at the lower end of the intrauterine source). On the lateral radiograph, the rectal point is located on a line drawn from the middle of the ovoid sources, 5 mm behind the posterior vaginal wall (Fig. 15.27). The posterior vaginal wall may be visualized by using radiopaque gauze for the vaginal packing.

Lymphatic Trapezoid of Fletcher. These points correspond to the paraaortic and iliac nodes and are shown in Fig. 15.28.

Pelvic Wall Points. On the anteroposterior radiograph, the pelvic wall points are located at the intersection of a horizontal tangent to superior aspect of the acetabulum and a vertical line touching the medial aspect of the acetabulum. On the lateral view, these points are marked as the highest middistance points of the right and left acetabulums (Fig. 15.29).

Time Dose Pattern. The duration and time sequence of the implant relative to the external beam treatment should be recorded.

D. Commentary

Several papers have discussed the pros and cons of various dose specification systems for the intracavitary treatment of cervix cancer (70,88–90). At present, universal agreement does not exist as to the superiority of any one system. The problem is perhaps with the nature of brachytherapy—a highly empirical discipline, no more sophisticated than gourmet cooking. However, as in cooking, there is a little bit of everything: art, science, technique, and taste. Although dose specification systems should be endorsed by appropriate committees,

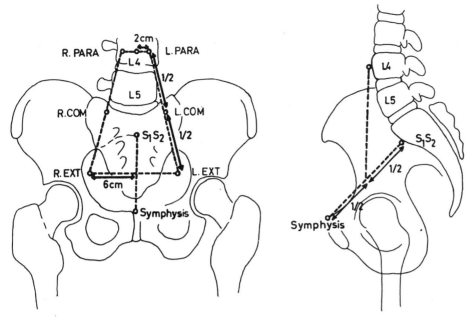

FIG. 15.28. Determination of reference points corresponding to the lymphatic trapezoid of Fletcher. (From ICRU. Dose and volume specification for reporting intracavitary therapy in gynecology. ICRU Report No. 38. Bethesda, MD: International Commission on Radiation Units and Measurements, 1985, with permission.)

I would like to take the author's privilege and express my opinion on the subject of dose specification for cervix treatment.

1. Established technique guidelines should be followed to take advantage of the vast amount of clinical data that have been accumulated with excellent results.
2. By using semirigid applicator such as Fletcher-Suit and the recommended source loadings one ensures consistency of technique. However, the dose distribution patterns will vary from patient to patient, depending on the packing and the source geometry achieved.
3. The most significant parameters that determine the clinical outcome, in terms of tumor control and complications, are the mg Ra eq-h or the total reference air kerma, source loading, and the type of applicator used.
4. Dose to the ICRU recommended reference points provide useful information in regard to the tolerance and adequacy of treatment.
5. For each application, the isodose distribution should be viewed at least in the frontal and sagittal planes (containing the initial straight part of the tandem). The target (cervix regions and corpus) should be visualized on the isodose patterns to determine the isodose surface value that just surrounds the target volume. This should be called the minimum target dose.
6. The implant duration should be based on the minimum target dose rate.

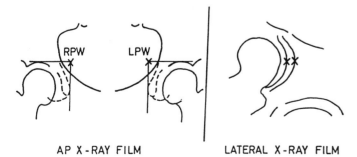

FIG. 15.29. Definition of pelvic wall points. *Left,* Anteroposterior view. *Right,* Lateral view. (From ICRU. Dose and volume specification for reporting intracavitary therapy in gynecology. ICRU Report No. 38. Bethesda, MD: International Commission on Radiation Units and Measurements, 1985, with permission.)

It is realized that the weakness of the whole system lies in the inability to visualize the target volume. Unless the target volume can be accurately determined and superimposed on the isodose pattern, one cannot determine the minimum target dose.

In summary, the ICRU system of dose specification is probably the best that can be achieved at this time. Its greatest weakness, however, is in the determination of reference volume. Further progress needs to be made in the determination and delineation of target volume so that the cervix dose can be specified by the minimum target dose.

15.8. REMOTE AFTERLOADING UNITS

Most brachytherapy is now practiced with devices that allow loading of radioactive sources after the source containers (applicators or catheters) are put in place in the patient and have been checked out radiographically for proper positioning using radiopaque markers or source dummies. Traditionally, the afterloading techniques require manual handling of radioactive material during source preparation and loading of the sources into the previously inserted applicators. Although these procedures, when carried out properly, pose no greater risk to patients and personnel than the nationally or internationally accepted standards, they are not state of the art in minimizing radiation hazards. Remotely controlled afterloading devices are now available that eliminate the direct handling of the radioactive sources. In addition, the sources can be instantly loaded and unloaded, making it possible to provide patient care with the sources retracted into their shielded position.

Remote afterloaders are available for either low-dose rate (LDR) or high-dose rate (HDR) brachytherapy and for interstitial or intracavitary treatments. With the LDR units, it is possible to use the same type of applicators (e.g., Fletcher-Suit) and dose rates as used in conventional brachytherapy. The room shielding requirements are the same except that instead of using mobile shields for staff protection, sources are automatically retracted whenever required for patient care and reinserted after each interruption.

The HDR remote afterloader treatments are performed in a fully shielded room with safety requirements comparable with those required for a cobalt teletherapy unit. For example, the walls are shielded, the room is equipped with door interlocks that retract the source when the door is opened or when the emergency button is pushed, radiation monitors are installed with visible and audible alarms, the patient is monitored via remote closed-circuit television camera and intercommunication devices, and the emergency procedures are posted at the control station. In practice, HDR equipment is often housed in existing cobalt or accelerator rooms.

^{192}Ir is the most commonly used radioisotope in remote afterloaders, although ^{137}Cs or ^{60}Co sources also are used in some units. The sources are contained in a storage safe when not in use. Several channels for source transport and a mechanism to move the source(s) from the storage safe into the applicator(s) in the patient are provided. The most common method of source transfer is the steel drive cable to which the source is welded. The cable is moved by a stepping motor. In one system (Selectron), source trains with source pallets and inactive spacers are moved by microprocessor controlled pneumatic devices.

HDR remote afterloading implants are achieved by moving a single high-strength (e.g., 10 Ci) ^{192}Ir source, welded to the end of a flexible cable, through one or many available channels. The source can be precisely positioned at any point in the implanted catheters or applicators. By programming *dwell position* and *dwell time* of the source, desired isodose distributions can be obtained. These high-dose rate units can be used for interstitial, interluminal, or intracavitary implant (see Chapter 22 for details).

A single-source system (micro-Selectron-PDR) also has been adopted to provide equivalent LDR brachytherapy, using pulsed brachytherapy principle (91). In this unit a single ^{192}Ir source of activity in the range of 0.5 to 1.0 Ci is used. The dose is delivered in several pulses of programmable duration and frequency.

Some of the commercially available remote afterloading systems include the Curietron, the micro-Selectron, the Gamma Med, and the Buchler unit. Many of these systems come in different models with specialized functions. For a review of these systems see Glasgow (92).

A. Advantages

1. The major advantage of the remote afterloaders is the elimination or reduction of exposure to medical personnel.
2. Well-designed systems can provide the capability of optimizing dose distributions beyond what is possible with manual afterloading.
3. Treatment techniques can be made more consistent and reproducible.
4. In LDR remote afterloading, sources can be retracted into shielded position to allow better patient care under normal as well as emergency conditions.
5. HDR remote afterloading permits treatment on an outpatient basis, using multiple fraction regimens.
6. HDR remote afterloading is suited for treating large patient populations that would otherwise require prolonged hospitalization if treated by LDR brachytherapy.

B. Disadvantages

1. Remote afterloading devices are expensive and require a substantial capital expenditure ($200,000–$300,000) for equipment acquisition.
2. In the case of HDR, additional costs must be considered for room shielding (if not located in an existing shielded facility) and installing ancillary imaging equipment.
3. Locating HDR in an existing radiation therapy room compounds the problem of patient scheduling unless the room is dedicated to HDR brachytherapy.
4. No significant improvements are expected in clinical outcome over state-of-the-art conventional LDR brachytherapy, although the issue is still controversial and needs further investigation.
5. Quality assurance requirements for remote afterloading devices are significantly greater because of the greater complexity of the equipment and frequent source changes.

C. High-dose Rate versus Low-dose Rate

Whereas remote afterloading is undoubtedly a superior technique when it comes to radiation protection and reproducibility of treatment, the question of how HDR compares with LDR in clinical outcome is a highly controversial issue. If HDR is or can be made equivalent to LDR, this would be a victory for HDR, because of its other advantages such as its ability to treat large patient populations, convenience of treating on an outpatient basis, etc. However, the question is not close to being settled, because the outcome data in terms of survival rates and early and late tissue complication rates for the HDR technique to date are not sufficient to draw definitive conclusions. The reader is referred to selected papers to understand these issues (93–97).

REFERENCES

1. Shalek RJ, Stovall M. Dosimetry in implant therapy. In: Attix FH, Roesch WC, eds. *Radiation dosimetry, Vol 3.* New York: Academic Press, 1969.
2. ICRU. Radiation quantities and units. Report No. 19. Washington, DC: International Commission on Radiation Units and Measurements, 1971.
3. ICRU. Radiation quantities and units. Report No. 33. Washington, DC: International Commission on Radiation Units and Measurements, 1980.
4. ICRU. Radioactivity. Report No. 10C. Washington, DC: International Commission on Radiation Units and Measurements, 1963.
5. Whyte GN. Attenuation of radium gamma radiation in cylindrical geometry. *Br J Radiol* 1955; 28:635.
6. Van Roosenbeek E, Shalek RJ, Moore EB. Safe encapsulation period for sealed medical radium sources. *AJR* 1968;102:697.
7. Meisberger LL, Keller RJ, Shalek RJ. The effective attenuation in water of gamma rays of gold 198, iridium 192, cesium 137, radium 226, and cobalt 60. *Radiology* 1968;90:953.
8. Horsler AFC, Jones JC, Stacey AJ. Cesium 137 sources for use in intracavitary and interstitial radiotherapy. *Br J Radiol* 1964;37:385.

9. Krishnaswamy V. Dose distribution about ^{137}Cs sources in tissue. *Radiology* 1972;105:181.

10. Attix FH. Computed values of specific gamma ray constant for ^{137}Cs and ^{60}Co. *Phys Med Biol* 1968;13:119.

11. O'Connell D, Joslin CA, Howard N, et al. The treatment of uterine carcinoma using the cathetron. *Br J Radiol* 1967;40:882.

12. Joslin CAF, Smith CW. The use of high activity ^{60}Co sources for intracavitary and surface mould therapy. *Proc R Soc Med* 1970;63:1029.

13. Snelling MD, Lambert HE, Yarnold JR. The treatment of carcinoma of the cervix and endometrium at the Middlesex Hospital. *Clin Radiol* 1979;30:253.

14. Henschke UK, Hilaris BS, Mahan GD. Afterloading in interstitial and intracavitary radiation therapy. *AJR* 1963;90:386.

15. Pierquin B, Chassagne D, Baillet F, et al. L'endocurietherapie des Cancers de la Langue Mobile et due Plancher buccal par l'iridium-192. *Rev Med* 1971;31:1947.

16. Glasgow GP, Dillman LT. Specific γ-ray constant and exposure rate constant of ^{192}Ir. *Med Phys* 1979;6:49.

17. Boggs RF, Williams KD, Schmidt GD. Radiological health aspects of spent radon seeds. *Radiat Health Data Rep* 1969;10:185.

18. Hilaris BS, ed. *Handbook of interstitial brachytherapy.* Acton, MA: Publishing Science Group, 1975.

19. Kim JH, Hilaris BS. Iodine 125 source in interstitial tumor therapy. *AJR* 1975;123:163.

20. Ling CC, Yorke ED, Spiro IJ, et al. Physical dosimetry of ^{125}I seeds of a new design for interstitial implant. *Int J Radiat Oncol Biol Phys* 1983;9:1747.

21. Schulz RJ, Chandra P, Nath R. Determination of the exposure rate constant for ^{125}I using a scintillation detector. *Med Phys* 1980;7:355.

22. Orton CG. Time-dose-factors (TDFs) in brachytherapy. *Br J Radiol* 1974;47:603.

23. Meigooni AS, Sabnis S, Nath R. Dosimetry of Pd-103 brachytherapy sources for permanent implants—endocuriether/hyperthermia. *Oncology* 1990;6:107.

24. Chiu-Tsao ST, Anderson LL. Thermoluminescent dosimetry of ^{103}Pd seeds (model 200) in solid water phantom. *Med Phys* 1990;18:449.

25. National Council on Radiation Protection and Measurements (NCRP). Specification of gamma-ray brachytherapy sources. NCRP Report No. 41. Washington, DC: U.S. Government Printing Office, 1974.

26. Loevinger R. The role of standards laboratory in brachytherapy. In: Shearer DR, ed. Recent advances in brachytherapy physics (AAPM Med. Phys. Monograph No. 7). New York: American Institute of Physics, 1981.

27. American Association of Physicists in Medicine. Specification of brachytherapy source strength. AAPM Report No. 21. New York: American Institute of Physics, 1987.

28. Loftus TP. Standardization of cesium-137 gamma-ray sources in terms of exposure units (roentgens). *J Res Natl Bur Stand (US)* 1970;74A:1–6.

29. Loftus TP. Standardization of iridium-192 gamma-ray sources in terms of exposure. *J Res Natl Bur Stand (US)* 1980;85:19–25.

30. Loftus TP. Exposure standardization of ^{125}I seeds used for brachytherapy. *J Res Bur Stand* 1984; 89:295.

31. Dale JWG, Perry WE, Pulfer RF. A beta-gamma ionization chamber for substandards of radioactivity. I and II. *Int J Radiat Isotopes* 1961;10:65.

32. Berkley LW, Hanson WF, Shalek RJ. Discussion of the characteristics and results of measurements with a portable well ionization chamber for calibration of brachytherapy sources. In: Shearer DR, ed. *Recent advances in brachytherapy physics.* New York: American Institute of Physics, 1981.

33. Loftus TP. Standardization of iridium-192 gamma ray sources in terms of exposure. *J Res Natl Bur Stand (US)* 1979;80:19.

34. Williamson JF, Khan FM, Sharma SC, et al. Methods for routine calibration of brachytherapy sources. *Radiology* 1982;142:511.

35. Kubiatowciz DO. Calibration of cesium-137 brachytherapy sources. In: Shearer DR, ed. *Recent advances in brachytherapy physics.* New York: American Institute of Physics, 1981.

36. Cobb PD, Chen TS, Kase KR. Calibration of brachytherapy iridium-192 sources. *Int J Radiat Oncol Biol Phys* 1981;7:259.

37. Suzuki A, Suzuki MN, Weis AM. Analysis of a radioisotope calibration. *J Nucl Med Technol* 1976; 4:193.

38. Boyer AL, Cobb PD, Kase KR, et al. In: Shearer DR, ed. *Recent advances in brachytherapy physics.* New York: American Institute of Physics, 1981.

39. Williamson JF, Morin RL, Khan FM. Dose calibrator response to brachytherapy sources: a Monte Carlo and analytic evaluation. *Med Phys* 1983;10:135.

40. Sievert RM. Die Intensitätsverteilung der Primären γ-Strahlung in der Nähe medizinischer Radiumpräparate. *Acta Radiol* 1921;1:89.

41. Young MEJ, Batho HF. Dose tables for linear radium sources calculated by an electronic computer. *Br J Radiol* 1964;37:38.

42. Evans RD, Evans RO. Studies of self absorption in gamma-ray sources. *Rev Mod Phys* 1948;20:305.

43. Keyser GM. Absorption correction for radium standardization. *Can J Phys* 1951;29:301.

44. Whyte GN. Attenuation of radium gamma radiation in cylindrical geometry. *Br J Radiol* 1955;28:635.

45. Williamson JF, Morin RL, Khan FM. Monte Carlo evaluation of the Sievert integral for brachytherapy dosimetry. *Phys Med Biol* 1983;28:1021.

46. Meisberger LL, Keller R, Shalek RJ. The effective attenuation in water of the gamma rays of gold-198, iridium-192, cesium-137, radium-226, and cobalt-60. *Radiology* 1968;90:953.

47. Van Dilla MA, Hine GJ. Gamma-ray diffusion experiments in water. *Nucleonics* 1952;10:54.

48. Ter-Pogossian M, Ittner WB III, Aly SM. Comparison of air and tissue doses for radium gamma rays. *Nucleonics* 1952;10:50.

49. Wooton P, Shalek RJ, Fletcher GH. Investigation of the effective absorption of radium and cobalt gamma radiation in water and its clinical significance. *AJR* 1954;71:683.

50. Reuss A, Brunner F. Phantommessungen mit den Mikroionisationskammern des Bomke-Dosimeters an Radium and Kobalt 6. *Stahlentherapie* 1957;103:279.

51. Kenney GN, Kartha KIP, Cameron JR. Measurement of the absorption and build-up factor for radium, cobalt 60 and cesium 137. *Phys Med Biol* 1966;11:145.

52. Meredith WJ, Greene D, Kawashima K. The attenuation and scattering in a phantom of gamma rays from some radionuclides used in mould and interstitial gamma-ray therapy. *Br J Radiol* 1966;39:280.

53. Webb S, Fox RA. The dose in water surrounding point isotropic gamma-ray emitters. *Br J Radiol* 1979;52:482.

54. Evans RD. *The atomic nucleus.* New York: McGraw-Hill, 1955:732.

55. Kornelsen RO, Young MEJ. Brachytherapy build-up factors. *Br J Radiol* 1981;54:136.

56. Krishnaswamy V. Dose distribution around an ^{125}I seed source in tissue. *Radiology* 1976;126:489.

57. Nath R, Anderson LL, Luxton G, et al. Dosimetry of interstitial brachytherapy sources: recommendations of the AAPM Radiation Therapy Committee Task Group no. 43. *Med Phys* 1995;22:209–234.

58. Camerson JR, Suntharalingam N, Kenney GN. *Thermoluminescence dosimetry.* Madison: University of Wisconsin Press, 1968.

59. Hine GJ, Friedman M. Isodose measurements of linear radium sources in air and water by means of an automatic isodose recorder. *AJR* 1950;64:989.

60. Cole A, Moore EB, Shalek RJ. A simplified automatic isodose recorder. *Nucleonics* 1953;11:46.

61. Merredith WJ, ed. *Radium dosage: the Manchester system.* Edinburgh: Livingstone, Ltd, 1967.

62. Glasser O, Quimby EH, Taylor LS, et al. *Physical foundations of radiology,* 3rd ed. New York: Harper & Row, 1961.

63. Stovall M, Shalek RJ. A study of the explicit distribution of radiation in interstitial implantation. I. A method of calculation with an automatic digital computer. *Radiology* 1962;78:950.

64. Laughlin JS, Siler WM, Holodny EI, et al. A dose description system for interstitial radiation therapy. *AJR* 1963;89:470.

65. Powers WE, Bogardus CR, White W, et al. Computer estimation of dosage of interstitial and intracavitary implants. *Radiology* 1965;85:135.

66. Stovall M, Shalek RJ. The M.D. Anderson method for the computation of isodose curves around interstitial and intracavitary radiation sources. III. Roentgenograms for input data and the relation of isodose calculations to the Paterson Parker system. *AJR* 1968;102:677.

67. Henschke UK, Cevc P. Dimension averaging-a simple method for dosimetry of interstitial implants. *Radiat Biol Ther* 1968;9:287.

68. Anderson LL. Dosimetry of interstitial radiation therapy. In: Hilaris BS, ed. *Handbook of interstitial brachytherapy.* Acton, MA: Publishing Sciences Group, 1975:87.

69. Pierquin B, Dutreix A, Paine C. The Paris system in interstitial radiation therapy. *Acta Radiol Oncol* 1978;17:33.

70. Pierquin B, Wilson JF, Chassagne D, eds. *Modern brachytherapy.* New York: Masson, 1987.

71. Dutreix A. Can we compare systems for interstitial therapy? *Radiother Oncol* 1988;13:127.

72. Sharma SC, Williamson JF, Cytacki E. Dosimetric analysis of stereo and orthogonal reconstruction of interstitial implants. *Int J Radiat Oncol Biol Phys* 1982;8:1803.

73. Paterson R. *The treatment of malignant disease by radiotherapy.* Baltimore: Williams & Wilkins, 1963.

74. Henschke UK, Hilaris BS, Mahan GD. Afterloading in interstitial and intracavitary radiation therapy. *AJR* 1963;90:386.

75. Suit HD, Moore EB, Fletcher GH, et al. Modifications of Fletcher ovoid system for afterloading using standard-size radium tubes (milligram and microgram). *Radiology* 1963;81:126.

76. Hilaris BS, ed. *Handbook of interstitial brachytherapy.* Acton, MA: Publishing Science Group, 1975.

77. Henschke UK. Interstitial implantation with radioisotopes. In: Hahn PF, ed. *Therapeutic use of artificial radioisotopes.* New York: John Wiley & Sons, 1956:375.

78. Jones CH, Taylor KW, Stedeford JBH. Modification to the Royal Marsden Hospital gold grain implantation gun. *Br J Radiol* 1965;38:672.

79. Heyman J. The technique in the treatment of cancer uteri at radium-hemmet. *Acta Radiol* 1929;10:49.

80. Regaud C. Radium therapy of cancer at the radium institute of Paris. *AJR* 1929;21:1.

81. Fletcher GH, Shalek RJ, Cole A. Cervical radium applicators with screening in the direction of bladder and rectum. *Radiology* 1953;60:77.

82. Fletcher GH. *Textbook of radiotherapy*, 2nd ed. Philadelphia: Lea & Febiger, 1973:620.

83. Heyman J, Reuterwall O, Benner S. The radium-hemmet experience with radiotherapy in cancer of the corpus of the uterus. *Acta Radiol* 1941;22:11.

84. Fletcher GH. Squamous cell carcinoma of the uterine cervix. In: Fletcher GH, ed. *Textbook of radiotherapy*, 3rd ed. Philadelphia: Lea & Febiger, 1980:720.

85. Tod MC, Meredith WJ. A dosage system for use in the treatment of cancer of the uterine cervix. *Br J Radiol* 1938;11:809.

86. Tod M, Meredith WJ. Treatment of cancer of the cervix uteri-a revised "Manchester method." *Br J Radiol* 1953;26:252.

87. Schwaz G. An evaluation of the Manchester system of treatment of carcinoma of the cervix. *AJR* 1969;105:579.

88. ICRU. Dose and volume specification for reporting intracavitary therapy in gynecology. ICRU Report No. 38. Bethesda, MD: International Commission on Radiation Units and Measurements, 1985.

89. Potish RA. Cervix cancer. In: Levitt SH, Khan FM, Potish RA, eds. *Technological basis of radiation therapy*. Philadelphia: Lea & Febiger, 1992:289.

90. Khan FM. Brachytherapy: rules of implantation and dose specification. In: Levitt SH, Khan FM, Potish RA, eds. *Technological basis of radiation therapy*. Philadelphia: Lea & Febiger, 1992:113.

91. Hall EJ, Brenner DJ. Conditions for the equivalence of continuous to pulsed low dose rate brachytherapy. *Int J Radiat Oncol Biol Phys* 1991;20:181.

92. Glasgow GP. High dose rate afterloaders: dosimetry and quality assurance. In: Purdy JA, ed. *Advances in radiation oncology physics*. AAPM Monograph No. 19. New York: American Institute of Physics, 1990:770.

93. Speiser B. Advances of high dose rate remote afterloading: physics or biology. *Int J Radiat Oncol Biol Phys* 1991;20:1133.

94. Orton C, Seyedsadr M, Somnay A. Comparison of high and low dose rate remote afterloading for cervix cancer and the importance of fractionation. *Int J Radiat Oncol Biol Phys* 1991;21:1425.

95. Hall E, Brenner D. The dose-rate effect revisited: radiobiological considerations of importance in radiotherapy. *Int J Radiat Oncol Biol Phys* 1991;21:1403.

96. Stitt J, Fowler J, Thomadsen B, et al. High dose rate intracavitary brachytherapy for carcinoma of the cervix: the Madison system: I-clinical and biological considerations. *Int J Radiat Oncol Biol Phys* 1992;24:335.

97. Eifel PJ. High-dose-rate brachytherapy for carcinoma of the cervix: high tech or high risk? *Int J Radiat Oncol Biol Phys* 1992;24:383.

RADIATION PROTECTION

Radiation exposure limits or standards were introduced as early as the start of the twentieth century when the potential hazards of radiation were realized. One of the first standard setting bodies was the International Commission on Radiological Protection (ICRP), which continues its function through its series of publications. These reports form the basis for many national protection guidelines. In the United States, the National Council on Radiation Protection and Measurements (NCRP) has functioned as a primary standard-setting body through its separate publications. One of the agencies with regulatory powers in this country is the Nuclear Regulatory Commission (NRC), which has control over the use of all reactor-produced materials (e.g., ^{60}Co and ^{192}Ir). The naturally occurring radioactive materials (e.g., radium and radon) and x-ray machines are regulated by individual states.

16.1. DOSE EQUIVALENT

Because the biologic effects of radiation depend not only on dose but also on the type of radiation, the dosimetric quantity relevant to radiation protection is the dose equivalent (H). It is defined as:

$$H = D \cdot Q \qquad (16.1)$$

where D is the absorbed dose and Q is the quality factor for the radiation.[1]

The SI unit for both dose and dose equivalent is joules per kilogram, but the special name for the SI unit of dose equivalent is sievert (Sv).

$$1 \text{ Sv} = 1 \text{ J/kg}$$

If dose is expressed in units of rad, the special unit for dose equivalent is called the rem.

$$H(\text{rem}) = D(\text{rad}) \cdot Q$$

Because Q is a factor and has no units,

$$1 \text{ rem} = 10^{-2} \text{ J/kg}$$

The use of quality factor in radiation protection is analogous to the use of relative biological effectiveness (RBE) in radiation biology. However, the quality factor is a somewhat arbitrarily chosen conservative value based on a range of RBEs related to the linear energy transfer (LET) of the radiation. Thus the Q factor encompasses RBEs in a very broad sense, independent of the organ or tissue or of the biologic endpoint under consideration.

Although the dose equivalent for particular situations can be calculated (1), it is convenient for quick-and-rough calculations to have a table of practical quality factors available. Table 16.1 gives these approximate factors for a variety of radiations used in radiation therapy.

---

[1] The distribution factor (N) once used in this equation has been deleted.

TABLE 16.1. RECOMMENDED QUALITY FACTORS

Radiation	Quality Factor
X-rays, γ rays, and electrons	1
Thermal neutrons	5
Neutrons, heavy particles	20

Data are from NCRP. *Recommendations on limits for exposure to ionizing radiation.* Report no. 91. Bethesda, MD: National Council on Radiation Protection and Measurements, 1987, with permission.

16.2. EFFECTIVE DOSE EQUIVALENT

Whole body exposures are rarely uniform. For a given exposure received, internally or externally, dose equivalents for various tissues may differ markedly. Also, tissues vary in sensitivity to radiation-induced effects. To take into account these nonuniform irradiation situations the concept of *effective dose equivalent* has been adopted by the ICRP and the NCRP.

The effective dose equivalent (H_E), is defined as "the sum of the weighted dose equivalents for irradiated tissues or organs" (2). Mathematically,

$$H_E = \sum W_T H_T \tag{16.2}$$

where W_T is the weighting factor of tissue T and H_T is the mean dose equivalent received by tissue T.

The weighting factors represent the proportionate risk (stochastic) of tissue when the body is irradiated uniformly. They are derived from *risk coefficients* (i.e., risk per unit dose equivalent). Table 16.2 gives the weighting factors and the corresponding risk coefficients for various types of tissues and organs.

A. Risk Estimates

The risk estimates given in Table 16.2 include an assumption of full expression of the cancer risk and an assumption of a population distribution over all ages and both sexes. The genetic component includes severe genetic effects for the first two generations. In the total risk coefficient, the somatic risk is 125×10^{-4} Sv^{-1} (125×10^{-6} rem^{-1}), which for radiation protection purposes is rounded off to 1×10^{-2} Sv^{-1} (1×10^{-4} rem^{-1}). The genetic component of the risk is 40×10^{-4} Sv^{-1} (0.4×10^{-4} rem^{-1}).

TABLE 16.2. RECOMMENDED VALUES OF THE WEIGHTING FACTORS W_T, FOR CALCULATING EFFECTIVE DOSE EQUIVALENT AND THE RISK COEFFICIENTS FROM WHICH THEY WERE DERIVED

Tissue (T)	Risk Coefficient	W_T
Gonads	40×10^{-4} Sv^{-1} (40×10^{-6} rem^{-1})	0.25
Breast	25×10^{-4} Sv^{-1} (25×10^{-6} rem^{-1})	0.15
Red bone marrow	20×10^{-4} Sv^{-1} (20×10^{-6} rem^{-1})	0.12
Lung	20×10^{-4} Sv^{-1} (20×10^{-6} rem^{-1})	0.12
Thyroid	5×10^{-4} Sv^{-1} (5×10^{-6} rem^{-1})	0.03
Bone surface	5×10^{-4} Sv^{-1} (5×10^{-6} rem^{-1})	0.03
Remainder	50×10^{-4} Sv^{-1} (50×10^{-6} rem^{-1})	0.30
Total	165×10^{-4} Sv^{-1} (165×10^{-6} rem^{-1})	1.00

From NCRP. *Recommendations on limits for exposure to ionizing radiation.* Report no. 91. Bethesda, MD: National Council on Radiation Protection and Measurements, 1987, with permission.
Values are from ICRP. *Recommendations of the International Commission on Radiological Protection.* Report no. 26. New York: Pergamon Press, 1977.

TABLE 16.3. ESTIMATED TOTAL EFFECTIVE DOSE EQUIVALENT RATE FOR A MEMBER OF THE POPULATION IN THE UNITED STATES AND CANADA[a] FROM VARIOUS SOURCES OF NATURAL BACKGROUND RADIATION

Source	Total Effective Dose Equivalent Rate (mSv/y)[b]					
	Lung	Gonads	Bone Surfaces	Bone Marrow	Other Tissues	Total
W_T	0.12	0.25	0.03	0.12	0.48	1.0
Cosmic	0.03	0.07	0.008	0.03	0.13	0.27
Cosmogenic	0.001	0.002	—	0.004	0.003	0.01
Terrestrial	0.03	0.07	0.008	0.03	0.14	0.28
Inhaled	2.0	—	—	—	—	2.0
In the body	0.04	0.09	0.03	0.06	0.17	0.40
Rounded totals	2.1	0.23	0.05	0.12	0.44	3.0

[a]The effective dose equivalent rates for Canada are approximately 20% lower for the terrestrial and inhaled components.
[b]1mSv = 100 mrem.
From NCRP. Exposure of the population in the United States and Canada from natural background radiation. Report no. 94. Bethesda, MD: National Council on Radiation Protection and Measurements, 1987, with permission.

16.3. BACKGROUND RADIATION

Radiation is a part of the natural environment. This background radiation is contributed principally by three sources: terrestrial radiation, cosmic radiation, and radiation from radioactive elements in our bodies. Table 16.3 gives average values of background radiation to which various parts of the body are exposed annually. The total effective dose equivalent for a member of the population in the United States from various sources of natural background radiation is approximately 3.0 mSv/year (300 mrem/year).

The terrestrial radiation varies over the earth because of differences in the amount of naturally occurring elements in the earth's surface. In addition, building materials may incorporate naturally occurring radioactive materials. Many buildings may have elevated levels of radon emitted by naturally occurring uranium-238 in the soil. It has been estimated (3) that the average annual dose equivalent to bronchial epithelium from radon decay products is approximately 24 mSv (2.4 rem).

Cosmic radiation levels change with elevation. For example, air travel exposes individuals to increased radiation exposure. It has been estimated that at 30,000 feet the dose equivalent is approximately 0.5 mrem/hour (4).

The internal irradiation arises mainly from ^{40}K in our body, which emits β and γ rays and decays with a half-life of 1.3×10^9 years.

In addition to the background radiation, the population is exposed to radiation from various medical procedures—the planned exposure of patients, as distinct from occupational exposures received by health personnel. It was estimated by the U.S. Public Health Service that the average annual genetically significant dose equivalent[2] in 1970 was approximately 20 mrem/year from radiologic procedures.

Under ordinary circumstances, exposures from natural background radiation and medical procedures are not included in the occupational exposure controls for the individual cases.

16.4. LOW-LEVEL RADIATION EFFECTS

A vast literature exists on the biologic effects of radiation. Discussions pertinent to radiation protection can be found in reports of the United Nations Scientific Committee on the Effects of Atomic Radiation (6).

---

[2] The genetically significant dose equivalent is the per capita dose equivalent when the long-term genetic effects of radiation are averaged over the whole population. This dose is expected to produce the same total genetic injury to the population as do the actual doses received by the various individuals (5).

Whereas large doses of radiation produce identifiable effects within a relatively short period, the effects are difficult to ascertain at low doses (e.g., less than 10 cGy). The difficulty is due mainly to the extremely low frequency with which these effects might occur. The statistical problems are enormous in identifying small effects in the constant presence of spontaneously occurring effects. However, certain effects have been demonstrated in humans and other mammals at doses lower than those required to produce acute radiation syndrome but greatly in excess of dose limits recommended by the standards setting bodies. Thus exposures to low-level radiation may produce (a) genetic effects, such as radiation-induced gene mutations, chromosome breaks, and anomalies; (b) neoplastic diseases, such as increased incidence of leukemia, thyroid tumors, and skin lesions; (c) effect on growth and development, such as adverse effects on fetus and young children; (d) effect on life span, such as diminishing of life span or premature aging; and (e) cataracts or opacification of the eye lens.

The harmful effects of radiation may be classified into two general categories: *stochastic* effects and *nonstochastic* effects. The NCRP (2) defines these effects as follows.

A stochastic effect is one in which "the probability of occurrence increases with increasing absorbed dose but the severity in affected individuals does not depend on the magnitude of the absorbed dose." In other words, a stochastic effect is an all or none phenomenon, such as the development of a cancer or genetic effect. Although the probability of such effects occurring increases with dose, their severity does not.

A nonstochastic effect is one "which increases in severity with increasing absorbed dose in affected individuals, owing to damage to increasing number of cells and tissues." Examples of nonstochastic effects are radiation-induced degenerative changes such as organ atrophy, fibrosis, lens opacification, blood changes, and decrease in sperm count.

Whereas no threshold dose can be predicted for stochastic effects, it is possible to set threshold limits on nonstochastic effects that are significant or seriously health impairing. However, for the purpose of radiation protection, a cautious assumption is made that "the dose-risk relationship is strictly proportional (linear) without threshold, throughout the range of dose equivalent and dose equivalent rates of importance in routine radiation protection."

Many analysts believe that these two assumptions may overestimate the biologic effects at low dose levels. Some have proposed a linear quadratic dose-response curve that assigns relatively reduced effects to low doses. However, in the absence of more reliable data it seems prudent to adopt a conservative model, the nonthreshold linear response, for predicting low dose effects. For further discussion of dose-response models, the reader is referred to references 7 to 10.

16.5. EFFECTIVE DOSE EQUIVALENT LIMITS

NCRP (2) recommendations on exposure limits of radiation workers are based on the following criteria: (a) at low radiation levels the nonstochastic effects are essentially avoided; (b) the predicted risk for stochastic effects should not be greater than the average risk of accidental death among workers in "safe" industries; and (c) ALARA principle should be followed, for which the risks are kept *as low as reasonably achievable*, taking into account social and economic factors.

It is important to compare radiation risks with the risks in other industries when setting radiation protection standards. Table 16.4 gives data on annual fatality rates from accidents in different occupations. On the basis of these data, "safe" industries are defined as "those having an associated annual fatality accident rate of 1 or less per 10,000 workers, that is, an average annual risk of 10^{-4} (2). The available data for the radiation industries show average fatal accident rate of less than 0.3×10^{-4} (11). From this perspective, the radiation industries compare favorably with the "safe" industries. For radiation protection purposes, the total risk coefficient is assumed to be 1×10^{-2} Sv^{-1} (1×10^{-4} rem^{-1}).

TABLE 16.4. ANNUAL FATALITY RATES FROM ACCIDENTS IN DIFFERENT OCCUPATIONS[a]

Occupation	Number of Workers $\times 10^3$	Annual Fatal Accident Rate (per 10,000 Workers)
Trade	24,000	0.5
Manufacturing	19,900	0.6
Service	28,900	0.7
Government	15,900	0.9
Transportation and utilities	5,500	2.7
Construction	5,700	3.9
Agriculture	3,400	4.6
Mining, quarrying	1,000	6.0
All industries (U.S.)	104,300	1.1

[a]Certain occupations have higher annual fatal accident rates than those given here.
Reprinted from NCRP. Recommendations on limits for exposure to ionizing radiation. Report no. 91. Bethesda, MD: National Council on Radiation Protection and Measurements, 1987, with permission. Data are from NSC. *Accident facts 1984.* Chicago: National Safety Council, 1985.

A. Occupational and Public Dose Limits

Table 16.5 gives occupational and public dose equivalent limits as recommended by the NCRP (2). These limits do not include exposure received from medical procedures or the natural background. Radiation workers are limited to an annual effective dose equivalent of 50 mSv (5 rem) and the general public is not to exceed one tenth of this value (0.5 rem) for infrequent exposure and 1 mSv (0.1 rem) for continuous or frequent exposure. Higher

TABLE 16.5. SUMMARY OF RECOMMENDATIONS

A. Occupational exposures (annual)		
1. Effective dose equivalent limit (stochastic effects)	50 mSv	(5 rem)
2. Dose equivalent limits for tissues and organs (nonstochastic effects)		
a. Lens of eye	150 mSv	(15 rem)
b. All others (e.g., red bone marrow, breast, lung, gonads, skin, and extremities)	500 mSv	(50 rem)
3. Guidance: cumulative exposure	10 mSv × age	(1 rem × age in yr)
B. Planned special occupational exposure, effective dose equivalent limit	see section 15[a]	
C. Guidance for emergency occupational exposure	See section 16[a]	
D. Public exposures (annual)		
1. Effective dose equivalent limit, continuous or frequent exposure	1 mSv	(0.1 rem)
2. Effective dose equivalent limit, infrequent exposure	5 mSv	(0.5 rem)
3. Remedial action recommended when:		
a. Effective dose equivalent	>5 mSv	(>0.5 rem)
b. Exposure to radon and its decay products	>0.007 Jhm^{-3}	(>2 WLM)
4. Dose equivalent limits for lens of eye, skin, and extremities	50 mSv	(5 rem)
E. Education and training exposures (annual)		
1. Effective dose equivalent	1 mSv	(0.1 rem)
2. Dose equivalent limit for lens of eye, skin, and extremities	50 mSv	(5 rem)
F. Embryo-fetus exposures		
1. Total dose equivalent limit	5 mSv	(0.5 rem)
2. Dose equivalent limit in a month	0.5 mSv	(0.05 rem)
G. Negligible individual risk level (annual) effective dose equivalent per source or practice	0.01 mSv	(0.001 rem)

[a]In NCRP Report no. 91.
From NCRP. Recommendations on limits for exposure to ionizing radiation. Report no. 91. Bethesda, MD: National Council on Radiation Protection and Measurements, 1987, with permission.

limits are set for some organs and areas of the body that involve nonstochastic effects and are less sensitive to radiation than others. For example, the annual occupational dose equivalent limit to the lens of the eye is 150 mSv (15 rem) and to other organs is 500 mSv (50 rem).

The NCRP has discontinued its previous recommendation of the age-proration formula for the cumulative limit, that is, (age − 18) × 5 rem. The new guidance is that the numerical value of the individual worker's lifetime effective dose equivalent in tens of mSv (rem) does not exceed the value of his or her age in years.

Students under the age of 18 who may be exposed to radiation as a result of their educational or training activities should not receive more than 1 mSv (0.1 rem) per year.

B. Dose Limits for Pregnant Women

The pregnant woman who is a radiation worker can be considered as an occupationally exposed individual, but the fetus cannot. The total dose equivalent limit to an embryo-fetus is 5 mSv (0.5 rem), with the added recommendation that exposure to the fetus should not exceed 0.5 mSv (0.05 rem) in any one month.

Premenopausal women must be informed of the potential risk of exposure to the fetus and methods available to minimize the exposure. If there is a possibility of the fetus receiving more than 5 mSv (0.5 rem) during the gestation period, the employee should discuss her options with her employer. Once a pregnancy is made known, the dose equivalent limit of 0.5 mSv (0.05 rem) in any one month should be the guiding principle. Even if there is practically no possibility of this limit being exceeded, it is prudent to assign pregnant workers to duties that involve potential exposure much lower than the recommended limit. For example, some institutions have developed a policy of not assigning pregnant technologists to work with cobalt-60 teletherapy units (because of constant radiation leakage from the source housing) or to handle brachytherapy sources. Such measures come under the ALARA principle, that is, the principle of limiting the dose of exposed persons (in this case the fetus) to levels as low as is reasonably achievable, taking into account economic and social factors.

C. Negligible Individual Risk Level

A negligible individual risk level (NIRL) is defined by the NCRP (2) as "a level of average annual excess risk of fatal health effects attributable to irradiation, below which further effort to reduce radiation exposure to the individual is unwarranted." The NCRP also states that "the NIRL is regarded as *trivial* compared to the risk of fatality associated with ordinary, normal societal activities and can, therefore, *be dismissed from consideration.*"

The concept of NIRL is applied to radiation protection because of the need for having a reasonably negligible risk level that can be considered as a threshold below which efforts to reduce the risk further would not be warranted or, in the words of the NCRP, "would be deliberately and specifically curtailed."

To avoid misinterpretation of the relationships between the NIRL, ALARA, and maximum permissible levels, the NCRP points out that the NIRL should not be thought of as an acceptable risk level, a level of significance, or a limit. Nor should it be the goal of ALARA, although it does provide a lower limit for application of the ALARA process. The ALARA principle encourages efforts to keep radiation exposure as low as reasonably achievable, considering the economic and social factors.

The annual NIRL has been set at a risk of 10^{-7}, corresponding to a dose equivalent of 0.01 mSv (0.001 rem). This corresponds to a lifetime (70 years) risk of 0.7×10^{-5}.

Example

Calculate the risk for (a) radiation workers, (b) members of the general public, and (c) NIRL, corresponding to respective annual effective dose equivalent limits (Table 16.5). Assume risk coefficient of 10^{-2} Sv^{-1} (10^{-4} rem^{-1}).

a. Annual effective dose equivalent limit for:

radiation workers = 50 mSv (5 rem)
Annual risk $= 5 \text{ rem} \times (10^{-4} \text{ rem}^{-1})$
        $= 5 \times 10^{-4}$

b. Annual effective dose equivalent limit for members of:

general public = 1 mSv (0.1 rem)
Annual risk $= 0.1 \text{ rem} \times (10^{-4} \text{ rem}^{-1})$
       $= 10^{-5}$

c. Annual effective dose equivalent limit for NIRL:

     $= 0.01 \text{ mSv} (0.001 \text{ rem})$
Annual risk $= 0.001 \text{ rem} \times (10^{-4} \text{ rem}^{-1})$
     $= 10^{-7}$

16.6. STRUCTURAL SHIELDING DESIGN

Radiation protection guidelines for the design of structural shielding for radiation installations are discussed in the NCRP Reports 49 and 51 (12,13). These reports contain the necessary technical information as well as recommendations for planning new facilities and remodeling existing facilities. The reader is referred to these reports for comprehensive details on this subject. This section will discuss only some of the basic factors that are considered in the calculation of barrier thicknesses.

Protective barriers are designed to ensure that the dose equivalent received by any individual does not exceed the applicable maximum permissible value. The areas surrounding the room are designated as *controlled* or *noncontrolled,* depending on whether or not the exposure of persons in the area is under the supervision of a radiation protection supervisor. For protection calculations, the dose equivalent limit is assumed to be 0.1 rem/week for the controlled areas and 0.01 rem/week for the noncontrolled areas. These values approximately correspond to the annual limits of 5 rem/year and 0.5 rem/year, respectively.

Protection is required against three types of radiation: the primary radiation; the scattered radiation; and the leakage radiation through the source housing. A barrier sufficient to attenuate the useful beam to the required degree is called the *primary barrier.* The required barrier against stray radiation (leakage and scatter) is called the *secondary barrier.* The following factors enter into the calculation of barrier thicknesses.

1. *Workload (W).* For x-ray equipment operating below 500 kVp, the workload is usually expressed in milliampere minutes per week, which can be computed by multiplying the maximum mA with approximate minutes/week of beam "on" time. For megavoltage machines, the workload is usually stated in terms of weekly dose delivered at 1 m from the source. This can be estimated by multiplying the number of patients treated per week with the dose delivered per patient at 1 m. *W* is expressed in rad/week at 1 m.
2. *Use Factor (U).* Fraction of the operating time during which the radiation under consideration is directed toward a particular barrier. Although the use factors vary depending on the techniques used in a given facility, typical values are given in Table 16.6.
3. *Occupancy Factor (T).* Fraction of the operating time during which the area of interest is occupied by the individual. If more realistic occupancy factors are not available, values given in Table 16.7 may be used.
4. *Distance (d).* Distance in meters from the radiation source to the area to be protected. Inverse square law is assumed for both the primary and stray radiation.

TABLE 16.6. TYPICAL USE FACTOR FOR PRIMARY PROTECTIVE BARRIERS

Location	Use Factor
Floor	1
Walls	$\frac{1}{4}$
Ceiling	$\frac{1}{4}$–$\frac{1}{2}$, depending on equipment and techniques

A. Primary Radiation Barrier

Suppose the maximum permissible dose equivalent for the area to be protected is P (e.g., 0.1 rad/week for controlled and 0.01 rad/week for noncontrolled area).[3] If B is the transmission factor for the barrier to reduce the primary beam dose to P in the area of interest, then:

$$P = \frac{WUT}{d^2} \cdot B \tag{16.3}$$

Therefore, the required transmission factor B is given by:

$$B = \frac{P \cdot d^2}{WUT} \tag{16.4}$$

By consulting broad beam attenuation curves (Figs. 16.1 and 16.2) for the given energy beam, one can determine the barrier thickness required. More data on beam attenuation are available from the NCRP (13).

The choice of barrier material, for example, concrete, lead, or steel, depends on structural and spatial considerations. Because concrete is relatively cheap, the walls and roof barriers are usually constructed out of concrete. Lead or steel can be used where space is at a premium. For megavoltage x and γ radiation, equivalent thickness of various materials can be calculated by comparing tenth value layers (TVL) for the given beam energy. If such information is not available specifically for a given material, relative densities can be used in most cases. Densities and TVLs for different materials and beam energies are available from the NCRP (13).

B. Secondary Barrier for Scattered Radiation

Radiation is scattered from the patient in all directions. The amount of scattered radiation depends on the beam intensity incident on the scatterer, the quality of radiation, the area of the beam at the scatterer, and the scattering angle. The ratio of scattered dose to the incident dose may be denoted by α. Table 16.8 gives values of α for various angles and beam qualities. For megavoltage beams, α is usually assumed to be 0.1% for 90 degrees scatter.

The scattered radiation, in general, has lower energy compared with the incident energy. However, the softening of the beam as a result of Compton scatter depends on the incident energy and the direction of scatter. For orthovoltage radiation, the quality of scattered radiation is usually assumed to be the same as that of the incident beam. For megavoltage beams, on the other hand, the maximum energy of the 90-degree scattered photons is 500 keV. Therefore, the transmission of this scattered radiation through a barrier is estimated to be approximately the same as that for a 500-kVp useful beam. At smaller scattering angles, however, the scattered beam has greater penetrating power (14). In addition, a greater fraction of the incident beam is scattered at smaller angles.

Suppose a transmission factor of B_s is required to reduce the scattered dose to an acceptable level P in the area of interest; then:

$$P = \frac{\alpha \cdot WT}{d^2 \cdot d'^2} \cdot \frac{F}{400} \cdot B_s \tag{16.5}$$

---

[3] For x and γ radiations, one can assume 1 rad = 1 rem.

TABLE 16.7. TYPICAL OCCUPANCY FACTORS

Full occupancy ($T = 1$)
  Work areas, offices, nurses' stations
Partial occupancy ($T = \frac{1}{4}$)
  Corridors, restrooms, elevators with operators
Occasional occupancy ($T = \frac{1}{8}-\frac{1}{16}$)
  Waiting rooms, restrooms, stairways, unattended elevators,
    outside areas used only for pedestrians or vehicular traffic

where α is the fractional scatter at 1 m from the scatterer, for beam area of 400 cm^2 incident at the scatterer, d is the distance from source to the scatterer, d' is the distance from the scatterer to the area of interest, and F is the area of the beam incident at the scatterer. The use factor for the secondary barrier is considered unity.

Thus the barrier transmission B_s is given by:

$$B_s = \frac{P}{\alpha WT} \cdot \frac{400}{F} \cdot d^2 \cdot d'^2 \tag{16.6}$$

The required thickness of concrete or lead can be determined for appropriate transmission curves given by the NCRP (13) or Figs. 16.1 and 16.2.

C. Secondary Barrier for Leakage Radiation

The leakage requirements of therapeutic source assemblies have been revised and are currently described in the NCRP Report 102 (15). This report supersedes the previous NCRP Report 33. The new recommendations are summarized below:

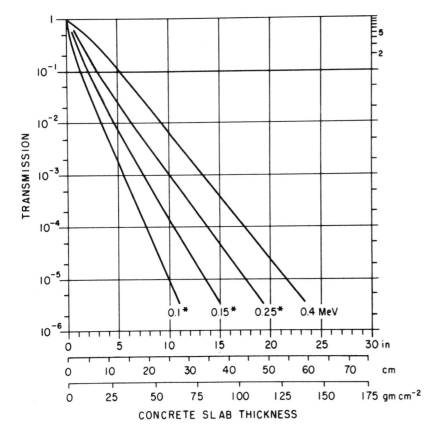

FIG. 16.1. Transmission through concrete (density 2.35 g cm^{-3}) of x-rays produced by 0.1- to 0.4-MeV electrons, under broad-beam conditions. Electron energies designated by an asterisk were accelerated by voltages with pulsed wave form; unmarked electron energies were accelerated by a constant potential generator. Curves represent transmission in dose-equivalent index ratio. (Reprinted with permission from NCRP. Radiation protection design guidelines for 0.1–100 MeV particle accelerator facilities. Report No. 51. Washington, DC: National Council on Radiation Protection and Measurements, 1977.)

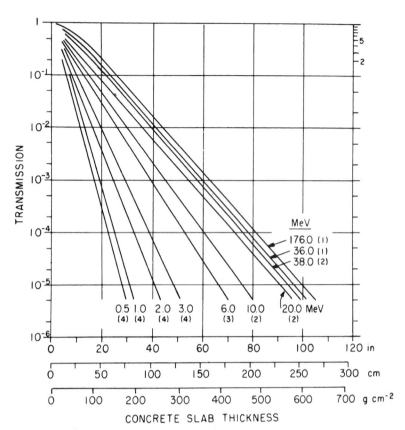

FIG. 16.2. Transmission of thick-target x-rays through ordinary concrete (density 2.35 g cm^{-3}), under broadbeam conditions. Energy designations on each curve (0.5 to 176 MeV) refer to the monoenergetic electron energy incident on the thick x-ray production target. *Curves* represent transmission to dose equivalent index ratio. (Reprinted with permission from NCRP. Radiation protection design guidelines for 0.1–100 MeV particle accelerator facilities. Report No. 51. Washington, DC: National Council on Radiation Protection and Measurements, 1977.)

1. *5 to 50 kVp.* The leakage exposure rate[4] shall not exceed 0.1 R in any 1 hour at any point 5 cm from the source assembly.

2. *Greater than 50 kVp and less than 500 kVp.* The leakage exposure rate at a distance of 1 m from the source shall not exceed 1 R in any 1 hour. In addition, these assemblies shall limit exposure rate to 30 R/h at 5 cm from the surface of the assembly.

3. *Greater than 500 kVp.* The absorbed dose rate due to leakage radiation (excluding neutrons) at any point outside the maximum field size, but within a circular plane of radius 2 m that is perpendicular to and centered on the central axis at the normal treatment distance, shall not exceed 0.2% of the useful beam dose rate at the treatment distance. Except for the area defined above, the leakage dose rate from the source assembly at any point at a distance of 1 m from the electron path between the source and the target shall not exceed 0.5% of the useful beam dose rate at the treatment distance. The neutron contribution to the dose within the useful beam shall be kept well below 1% of the x-ray dose. Outside the useful beam, the neutron dose should be reduced to as low as practicable.

4. *Cobalt teletherapy.* Leakage dose rate from this source housing with the beam in the "off" position shall not exceed 2 mrad/hour on the average and 10 mrad/hour maximum in any direction, at a distance of 1 m from the source. With the beam in the "on" position, the leakage dose rate from the source housing shall not exceed 0.1% of the useful beam dose rate, both measured at a distance of 1 m from the source. In addition, for sources that give rise to a useful beam dose rate of less than 1,000 rad/hour at 1 m, the leakage from the source housing shall not exceed 1 rad/h at 1 m from the source.

---

[4] The NCRP Report 102 (14) uses the quantity kerma rate instead of exposure rate to conform with the SI units. As an approximation the quantities exposure, air kerma, and dose are assumed here to have the same numerical value. For exact relationship, refer to Chapter 8.

TABLE 16.8. RATIO, α, OF SCATTERED TO INCIDENT EXPOSURE[a]

Scattering Angle (From Central Ray)	γ Rays	X-Rays	
	^{60}Co	4 MV	6 MV
15			9×10^{-3}
30	6.0×10^{-3}		7×10^{-3}
45	3.6×10^{-3}	2.7×10^{-3}	1.8×10^{-3}
60	2.3×10^{-3}		1.1×10^{-3}
90	0.9×10^{-3}		0.6×10^{-3}
135	0.6×10^{-3}		0.4×10^{-3}

[a]Scattered radiation measured at 1 m from phantom when field area is 400 cm^2 at the phantom surface; incident exposure measured at center of field but without phantom.
From NCRP. Medical x-ray and gamma-ray protection for energies up to 10 MeV. Structural shielding design and evaluation. Report no. 34. Washington, DC: National Council on Radiation Protection and Measurements, 1970, with permission.
Data also are available in NCRP. Radiation protection design and guidelines for 0.1–100 MeV particle accelerator facilities. Report no. 51. Washington, DC: National Council on Radiation Protection and Measurements, 1977.

Because leakage radiation is present whenever the machine is operated, the use factor for leakage is unity. Suppose the required secondary barrier for leakage radiation has a transmission factor of B_L to reduce the leakage dose to the maximum permissible level P (rem/week).

For therapy units below 500 kVp:

$$P = \frac{WT}{d^2 \cdot 60\,I} \cdot B_L \qquad (16.7)$$

where I is the maximum tube current. The number 60 is used to convert leakage limit of 1 R/hour to 1/60 R/minute, because the workload W is expressed in terms of mA-minute/week.

For a megavoltage therapy unit,

$$P = \frac{0.001\,WT}{d^2} \cdot B_L \qquad (16.8)$$

The factor 0.001 is the 0.1% leakage limit through the source housing.[5]

Thus the transmission factor B_L for the leakage barrier is given by:

$$B_L = \frac{P \cdot d^2 \cdot 60\,I}{WT} \quad \text{[Therapy below 500 kVp]} \qquad (16.9)$$

and

$$B_L = \frac{P \cdot d^2}{0.001\,WT} \text{[Therapy above 500 kVp]} \qquad (16.10)$$

The quality of leakage radiation is approximately the same as that of the primary beam. Therefore, the transmission curve for the primary beam should be used to determine the leakage barrier thickness (Figs. 16.1, 16.2).

For megavoltage therapy installations, the leakage barrier usually far exceeds that required for the scattered radiation, because the leakage radiation is more penetrating than the scattered radiation. For the lower-energy x-ray beams, however, the difference between the barrier thickness for the leakage and for the scattered radiation is relatively less.

A barrier designed for primary radiation provides adequate protection against leakage and scattered radiation. If a barrier is designed for stray radiation only, the thickness is computed for leakage and scattered radiations separately. If the thicknesses of the two

[5]Any leakage limit may be used in Equation 16.8. However, most megavoltage units do not exceed the limit of 0.1% for source housing.

barriers differ by at least three HVLs, the thicker of the two will be adequate. If the difference is less than three HVLs, one HVL should be added to the larger one to obtain the required secondary barrier.

D. Door Shielding

Unless a maze entranceway is provided, the door must provide shielding equivalent to the wall surrounding the door. For megavoltage installations, a door that provides direct access to the treatment room will have to be extremely heavy. It will require a motor drive as well as a means of manual operation in case of emergency. A maze arrangement, on the other hand, drastically reduces the shielding requirements for the door. The function of the maze is to prevent direct incidence of radiation at the door. With a proper maze design, the door is exposed mainly to the multiply scattered radiation of significantly reduced intensity and energy. For example, in Fig. 16.3, radiation is scattered at least twice before incidence on the door. Each Compton scatter at 90 degrees or greater will reduce the energy to 500 keV or less. The intensity will also be greatly reduced at each large angle scatter. The door shielding in this case can be calculated by tracing the path of the scattered radiation from the patient to the door and repeatedly applying Equation 16.6. For megavoltage units, the attenuation curves for the 500-kVp x-rays may be used to determine the door shielding from multiply scattered x-rays. In most cases, the required shielding turns out to be less than 6 mm of lead.

E. Protection against Neutrons

High-energy x-ray beams (e.g., >10 MV) are contaminated with neutrons. These are produced by high-energy photons and electrons incident on the various materials of target, flattening filter, collimators, and other shielding components. The cross-sections for (e,n) reactions are smaller by a factor of about 10 than those for (γ,n) reactions. Because of this, the neutron production during electron beam therapy mode is quite small compared with that during the x-ray mode.

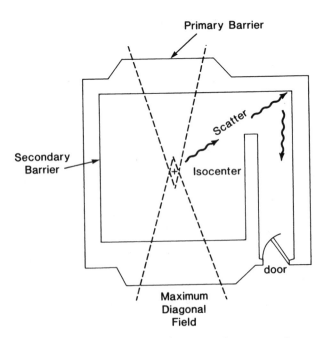

FIG. 16.3. Schematic diagram of a megavoltage x-ray therapy installation (drawing not to scale). Radiation scatter from patient can reach the door, as shown.

The neutron contamination increases rapidly as the energy of the beam is increased from 10 to 20 MV, and then remains approximately constant above this. Measurements have shown (16–18) that in the 16 to 25 MV x-ray therapy mode the neutron dose equivalent along central axis is approximately 0.5% of the x-ray dose and falls off to about 0.1% outside the field. Sohrabi and Morgan (17) have listed a wide range of neutron contamination values that have been reported in the literature for some medical accelerators.

The energy spectrum (19) of emitted neutrons within the x-ray beam is similar to the uranium fission spectrum, showing a broad maximum in the range of 1 MeV. The neutron energy is considerably degraded after multiple scattering from walls, roof, and floor, and consequently, the proportion of the fast neutron (>0.1 MeV) reaching the inside of the maze is usually small.

Concrete barriers designed for x-ray shielding are sufficient for protection against neutrons. However, the door must be protected against neutrons that diffuse into the maze and reach the door. Reflections from the walls cause a reduction in the neutron fluence and, depending on the accelerator configuration, a decrease in neutron fluence of two orders of magnitude (10^{-2}) from machine location to the inside of the maze can be expected (20). The shielding required for the door can be further reduced by the maze design. In general, a longer maze (>5 m) is desirable in reducing the neutron fluence at the door. Finally, a few inches of a hydrogenous material such as polyethylene can be added to the door to thermalize the neutrons and reduce the neutron dose further. A steel or lead sheet may be added to the door to protect against scattered x-rays, as discussed previously.

When thermal neutrons are absorbed by the nuclei of atoms within the shielding door, energetic γ radiations (called the neutron-capture γ rays) are produced. These radiations have a spectrum of energies ranging up to 8 MeV, but most have energies in the region of 1 MeV. Unless the neutron fluence at the door is high such as in the case of a short maze, the intensity of capture γ rays generated within the shielding door is usually low. Because the capture γ rays have high energy, thick sheets of lead are required to provide effective attenuation. Thus it is more desirable to reduce the neutron fluence incident at the door such as by designing a longer maze than to have a high neutron fluence at the door and add prohibitive amounts of lead shielding to the door to attenuate the capture γ rays.

Computation of shielding requirements for a high-energy installation requires many considerations that cannot be discussed in adequate detail in this text. The reader is referred to the literature for further guidance (13,19,21,22).

16.7. PROTECTION AGAINST RADIATION FROM BRACHYTHERAPY SOURCES

This subject has been dealt with in detail in NCRP Report 40 (23). In this section, only a brief review will be given of some practical guidelines that have been developed for safe handling and use of brachytherapy sources.

A. Storage

Lead-lined safes with lead-filled drawers are commercially available for storing brachytherapy sources. In choosing a particular safe, consideration should be given to the adequacy of shielding, distribution of sources, and time required for personnel to remove sources from, and return sources to, the safe.

The storage area for radium should be ventilated by a direct filtered exhaust to the outdoors, because of the possibility of radon leaks. A similar arrangement is recommended for encapsulated powdered sources or sources containing microspheres. This precaution is taken so that if a source ruptures, the radionuclide is not drawn into the general ventilation system of the building.

The storage rooms are usually provided with a sink of cleaning source applicators. The sink should be provided with a filter or trap to prevent loss of source.

B. Source Preparation

A source preparation bench should be provided close to the safe. The preparation and dismantling of source applicators should be carried out behind a suitable barrier to shield the operator adequately. Many facilities are equipped with a protective "L-block," usually constructed of lead. A lead glass viewing window provides some protection by providing shielding as well as a suitable distance between the face of the operator and the sources.

Brachytherapy sources must never be touched with the hands. Suitably long forceps should be used to provide as much distance as practical between sources and the operator.

Besides various kinds of protective shielding available for brachytherapy applications, the operator must be aware of the effectiveness of time and distance in radiation protection. Exposures of individuals can be greatly reduced if, as far as practical, the time spent in the vicinity of the sources is minimized and the distance from the sources is maximized.

Certain brachytherapy techniques have the advantages of giving reduced exposure to personnel. For example, afterloading techniques involve no exposure to operating room personnel or x-ray technologists. Some exposure is received during the loading and removal of sources, but even these exposures can be reduced by using mobile protective shields. The use of low-energy sources in place of radium or radon is another example of how personnel exposure can be minimized.

C. Source Transportation

The sources can be transported in lead containers or leaded carts. The thickness of lead required will depend on the type of source and the amount of radioactive material to be transported. A table of required thickness for various conditions is given by the NCRP (23).

D. Leak Testing

Various methods of leak testing of a sealed source are available (23). A radium source can be checked for radon leaks by placing it in a small test tube with some activated carbon or a ball of cotton. After 24 hours, the carbon or the cotton ball can be counted in a scintillation-well counter. It is sometimes convenient to leak test the entire stock of radium by pumping the air from the safe and passing it through on an activated charcoal filter. The filter is counted for α activity. If a leak is detected, then individual sources will have to be tested to isolate the defective source.

Periodic leak testing of radium is usually specified by state regulations. A source is considered to be leaking if a presence of 0.005 μCi or more of removable contamination is measured. The leaking source should be returned to a suitable agency that is authorized for the disposal of radioactive materials.

16.8. RADIATION PROTECTION SURVEYS

After the installation of radiation equipment, a qualified expert must carry out a radiation protection survey of the installation. The survey includes checking equipment specifications and interlocks related to radiation safety and evaluation of potential radiation exposure to individuals in the surrounding environment.

A. Radiation Monitoring Instruments

The choice of a particular radiation detector or dosimeter depends on the type of measurement required. In radiation protection surveys, low levels of radiation are measured and, therefore, the instrument must be sensitive enough to measure such low levels. The detectors most often used for x-ray measurements are the ionization chambers, Geiger

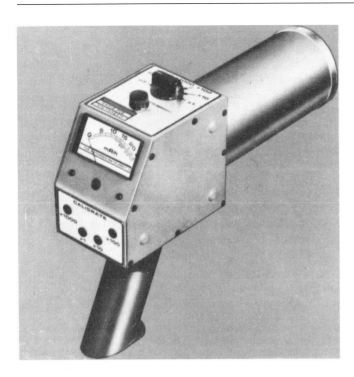

FIG. 16.4. A Cutie Pie survey meter. (Courtesy of the Victoreen Instrument Division, Cleveland, OH.)

counters, thermoluminescent dosimeters (TLD), and photographic film. The TLD and film dosimetry have been discussed in Chapter 8. In this section, the Geiger counter and an ionization chamber suitable for low-level radiation measurements will be briefly described.

A.1. Ionization Chamber

An ionization chamber used for low-level x-ray measurements (of the order of milliroentgens per hour) has a large volume (~600 ml) to obtain high sensitivity (Fig. 16.4). A direct-current voltage is applied between the outer shell and the central electrode to collect ionization charge produced by radiation in the internal air volume when the chamber is exposed to radiation. This causes an ion current to flow in the external circuit. These currents are extremely small, however, and special electrometer circuitry, including a current amplifier, is required to measure them. The output current is directly proportional to the exposure rate.

An ion chamber survey meter is usually calibrated for exposure in a γ ray beam from a cesium or a radium brachytherapy source using an open-air measurement geometry (see section 15.2B.1). For accurate usage at middle and high energies, the energy response curve for the chamber should be used to correct the exposure. Additional corrections for scale linearity, air temperature, and pressure and angular dependence may also be necessary.

A.2. Geiger-Müller Counters

The Geiger-Müller counter (G-M tube) consists essentially of a cylindrical cathode with a fine wire stretched along the axis of the cylinder. The tube is filled with a special mixture of gases at a pressure of about 100 mm Hg. The voltage applied to the electrodes is much higher than the saturation voltage applied to an ionization chamber. Potential is so high that the particles from the original ionization become energetic enough to produce further secondary ionization giving rise to "gas amplification." If the voltage is high enough that an "avalanche" of charge is generated by the original ionizing event, independent of its size, the detector is called a Geiger-Müller counter.

The G-M tube is much more sensitive than the ionization chamber. For example, the Geiger counter can detect individual photons or individual particles that could never be observed in a ionization chamber. However, this detector is not a dose-measuring device. Although a Geiger counter is useful for preliminary surveys to detect the presence of radiation, ionization chambers are recommended for quantitative measurement. Because of their inherently slow recovery time ($\sim$50 to 300 μs), they can never record more than 1 count/machine pulse. Thus a G-M counter could significantly underestimate radiation levels when used to count radiation around pulsed machines such as accelerators.

A.3. Neutron Detectors

Neutrons can be detected with the aid of their various interactions. In a hydrogenous material, neutrons produce hydrogen recoils or protons that can be detected by ionization measurements, proportional counters, scintillation counters, cloud chambers, or photographic emulsions. Neutrons can also be detected by their induced nuclear reactions. Certain materials, called activation detectors, become radioactive when exposed to neutrons. The detector, after exposure to the neutron field, is counted for β or γ ray activity.

Neutron measurements in or near the primary x-ray beam can be made with passive detectors such as activation detectors, without being adversely affected by pulsed radiation. An activation detector can be used either as a bare threshold detector or inside a moderator such as polyethylene. An example of bare threshold detector is phosphorus (in the form of phosphorus pentoxide) that has been successfully used by several investigators to measure neutrons in as well as outside the primary beam (18,24). A phosphorus detector can monitor both fast and slow or thermal neutrons, using $^{31}P(n,p)^{31}Si$ and $^{31}P(n,\gamma)^{32}P$ reactions. The activation products ^{31}Si and ^{32}P are essentially pure β emitters and are counted using a calibrated liquid scintillation spectrometer. The problem of photon interference (activation of the detector by photons) is minimal with this detector.

Moderated activation systems suffer from photoneutron production in the moderator itself. Therefore, these detectors are primarily useful outside the primary beam. Examples of the moderated activation detectors are activation remmeters and moderated foil detectors. A gold foil placed in a polyethylene cylinder (24 cm long and 22 cm in diameter) has been used by Rogers and Van Dyk (25) for measurements outside the primary photon beam. McCall et al. (26) have developed a system in which a gold foil is surrounded by a polyethylene cylinder covered by a layer of cadmium and boron to absorb thermal neutrons. The activity induced in the gold foil is measured by using a calibrated Ge(Li) detector system.

Outside the treatment room, it is a common practice to use two detectors that respond predominantly to one or the other radiation. For example, a conventional air-filled ionization chamber with nonhydrogenous walls (carbon) predominantly measures photons, and its response to neutrons can be negligible because the n:γ ratio outside the shield is usually small and the neutrons are low energy. An ion chamber with hydrogenous walls, on the other hand, can detect both neutrons and x-rays. An ion chamber that can be filled with either argon or propane to obtain a predominantly photon or photon plus neutron response, respectively, has also been used to estimate photon and neutron exposure rates outside the shield of a medical accelerator (27). Also, proportional counters, with filling gases such as BF_3, are often used inside moderators to detect thermalized neutrons with good discrimination against signals produced by photons. Such a gas proportional counter, used either in the counting mode or current measurement, may be regarded as an ionization chamber with internal gas multiplication. The voltage is high enough so that ionization by collision occurs and, as a result, the current due to primary ionization is increased manyfold. The basis of the detection system is the reaction $^{10}B(n,\alpha)^7Li$, whereby the α particles can be counted or the ionization current caused by them is measured. A moderated BF_3 counter will also count proton recoil particles produced by neutrons in the hydrogenous material.

Figure 16.5 shows one of the commercially available neutron survey meters, the Eberline Neutron Rem Counter. The instrument consists of a BF_3 proportional counter surrounded by a 9-inch cadmium-loaded polyethylene sphere to moderate the neutrons. The counter operates typically at 1,600 to 2,000 V and can be used for measuring neutrons

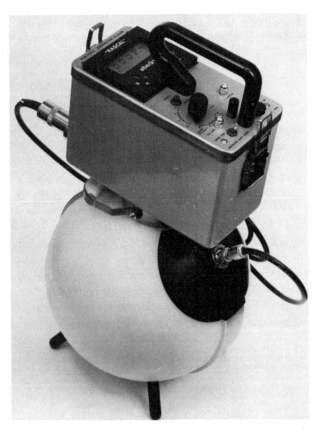

FIG. 16.5. A portable neutron rem counter, "Rascal." (Courtesy of Eberline, Santa Fe, NM.)

from thermal to approximately 10-MeV energy. The response is displayed in terms of count rate, mR/hour, and millirem/hour. The survey meter is calibrated using an NIST-calibrated Pu-Be neutron source.

B. Equipment Survey

Some of the design specifications (15) related to patient and personnel safety can be determined by visual inspection. Various operational and beam-limiting interlocks are checked out as part of the field testing of the machine. The leakage radiation through the source housing may be measured as follows:

(a) The collimator opening is blocked with at least 10 half-value layers of lead.
(b) Sheets of prepacked film may be wrapped around the source housing to locate areas of high radiation leakage.
(c) Using an ionization chamber of appropriate volume or sensitivity (e.g., survey meter), the dose rate is determined at a distance of 1 m from the source, as a function of the primary beam dose rate at 1 m. These measurements should be made in selected directions in which leakage is expected to be maximum.
(d) In the case of ^{60}Co teletherapy, the leakage radiation through the source housing with the beam "on" position is determined in the same manner as above. In the beam "off" condition, however, measurements are made in 14 different directions to determine the average and maximum leakage dose rate (15). A calibrated ionization chamber such as a Cutie Pie is a suitable instrument for these measurements.

The leakage limits through the source assemblies for various energy radiation generators were discussed in section 16.6C. If a unit is equipped with a beam interceptor to reduce structural shielding requirements, the radiation transmitted through the interceptor must not exceed 0.1% of the useful beam. It should also reduce by the same factor the radiation scattered by the patient through an angle of up to 30 degrees from the central ray.

C. Area Survey

Areas outside the treatment room that are accessible to any individual should be designed as controlled or noncontrolled, depending on whether the exposure of persons in the area is monitored or not. Exposure levels in these areas should be measured with the beam oriented in various possible directions. The transmitted radiation through the primary barrier should be measured with the beam of maximum size directly incident at the barrier. Measurements outside the secondary barriers should be made with a phantom at the treatment position. Other operational conditions such as total body irradiation may present special treatment conditions that should be considered in the area survey.

The results of the survey should be evaluated by taking into account the actual operating conditions, including workload, use factor, occupancy factor, and attenuation and scattering of the useful beam by the patient. The environmental safety will be considered acceptable if no person is likely to receive more than the applicable dose equivalent limit.

The survey data based on instantaneous dose rate measurements should be supplemented with cumulative radiation measurements and personnel monitoring over appropriate time periods.

If, as a result of a radiation survey, supplementary shielding is added to the protective barriers, a survey should be made to evaluate the adequacy of the shielding after the modification.

16.9. PERSONNEL MONITORING

Personnel monitoring must be used in controlled areas for occupationally exposed individuals. Cumulative radiation monitoring is mostly performed with film badges, although TLD badges are also used in some case. Because the badge is mostly used to monitor whole body exposure, it should be worn on the chest or abdomen. Special badges may also be used to measure exposure to specific parts of the body (e.g., hands) if higher exposures are expected during particular procedures.

Although film monitoring is a simple and convenient method of personnel monitoring, it has certain drawbacks. The energy dependence poses a major problem especially when an individual is exposed to both soft- and high-energy radiation. However, some information is obtained concerning beam quality by placing filters of different materials and thickness to partly cover the film. By comparing the film darkening under the filter with that of the part without filter gives some indication of the penetration ability of the radiation.

Radiation monitoring during a particular procedure may also be performed with pocket dosimeters. These instruments are useful where exposure needs to be monitored more frequently than possible with the regular film badge service.

16.10. NUCLEAR REGULATORY COMMISSION REGULATIONS

The United States NRC (USNRC) controls the use of all reactor-produced materials (byproduct materials) in this country. The use of naturally occurring radioactive materials (e.g., radium) and x-ray machines is regulated by individual states. Also, the USNRC has an agreement with a number of states, called the *agreement states,* that allows these states to enforce the NRC regulations.

The NRC regulations that govern the medical use of byproduct materials are contained in the Code of Federal Regulations 10 CFR Part 35 (28). These regulations, for the most part, are based on the recommendations of various advisory groups such as the NCRP, the

ICRP, and the AAPM. However, some regulations are enacted in response to problems that are brought to the attention of the NRC. All new regulations go through the usual public and congressional hearing process as is customary for the enactment of any federal regulation.

Technical details and legal ramifications of the NRC regulations are beyond the scope of this book. These regulations may change from time to time. For a complete text of these regulations, the reader is referred to the most up-to-date NRC document. In this section, a summary will be presented of current regulations that pertain to teletherapy and brachytherapy use of radioisotopes.

A. License

License is required from the NRC (or the agreement state) for possession or use of byproduct materials. A license is issued after a detailed review of the applicant's education and training, administrative requirements, technical requirements, management program, etc. Any subsequent changes in the conditions stipulated in the license require approval by the NRC in the form of license amendments.

B. Administrative Requirements

B.1. ALARA Program

A written radiation program is required that includes the ALARA principles (see section 16.5). The program must be communicated to the workers and be reviewed periodically to ensure that a reasonable effort is being made to keep individual and collective occupational doses ALARA.

B.2. Radiation Safety Officer

A radiation safety officer (RSO) must be appointed who will have the responsibility of implementing the radiation protection program. The licensee, through the RSO, must ensure that the program is conducted in accordance with the approved procedures and regulatory requirements.

B.3. Radiation Safety Committee

Each medical institution licensee shall establish a radiation safety committee to oversee the use of byproduct material. The committee must include the radiation safety officer, authorized user, nurse, and a representative of management who is neither the RSO nor an authorized user. The charge of the committee is outlined in the 10 CFR Part 35 document (28). The committee must meet at least quarterly.

B.4. Quality Management Program

The licensee must maintain a written quality management program. This program must include the following objectives:

1. A *written directive* is prepared before administration. The directive must specify the dosage and the quantities of the radioactive material to be administered.
2. Patient identity is verified by more than one method before administration.
3. The final plans of treatment and related calculations are in accordance with the written directive.
4. Each administration is in accordance with the written directive.
5. Any unintended deviation from the written directive is identified and evaluated in terms of a *recordable event* or a *misadministration*.

Recordable Event. A recordable event means the administration of (a) a radiopharmaceutical dosage that differs from the prescribed dosage by more than 10%, (b) a weekly calculated administered teletherapy dose that is greater than the weekly prescribed dose by 15%, and (c) a calculated brachytherapy-administered dose that differs from the prescribed dose by more than 10% of the prescribed dose.

Misadministration. Misadministration means the administration of (a) radiation therapy to the wrong patient; (b) radiopharmaceutical dosage that differs from the prescribed dose by more than 20% of the prescribed dose; (c) a calculated γ stereotactic radiation surgery dose that differs from the prescribed dose by more than 10%; (d) a teletherapy dose when the treatment consists of three or fewer fractions and the calculated total administered dose differs from the total prescribed dose by more than 10% of the total prescribed dose, when the calculated weekly administered dose is 30% greater than the weekly prescribed dose, or when the total administered dose differs from the total prescribed dose by more than 20% of the total prescribed dose; and/or (e) brachytherapy involving a sealed source that is leaking, when for a temporary implant one or more sealed sources are not removed after completion of the procedure, or when the calculated administered dose differs from the prescribed dose by more than 20% of the prescribed dose.

6. In case of misadministration the licensee must (a) notify the NRC Operations Center by telephone no later than the next calendar day after discovery of the misadministration; (b) submit a written report to the appropriate NRC regional office within 15 days of the discovery of the misadministration; and (c) notify the referring physician and the patient no later than 24 hours of the misadministration, unless the referring physician takes the responsibility of informing the patient or based on medical judgment, telling the patient would be harmful. If the patient was notified, a written report should be sent to the patient within 15 days of the discovery of the misadministration.

7. The licensee shall develop procedures for conducting a review of the quality management program at intervals no greater than 12 months. This review must include (a) an audit of a representative sample of patient administration, (b) all recordable events, and (c) all misadministrations.

C. Technical Requirements

1. The licensee authorized to use radiopharmaceuticals must possess a dose calibrator to measure activity administered to each patient. The calibrator must be checked for constancy of response, accuracy of calibration, linearity, and source geometry dependence. The records of these checks must be retained for 3 years.

2. The licensee must possess calibrated *survey instruments.* Calibration of the survey meter must be done annually and following repair. This calibration must include (a) all scales with readings up to 1,000 mrem/h, (b) two separate readings on each scale, (c) conspicuous indication on the instrument of the apparent exposure rate from a dedicated check source, and (d) a description of the calibration procedure. Records of each survey instrument calibration must be retained for 3 years.

3. A licensee in possession of *sealed* sources or *brachytherapy sources* must follow the radiation safety instructions supplied by the manufacturer and maintain the instructions for the duration of source use in a legible form convenient to the users: (a) The licensee must leak test the source before its first use unless the licensee has a leak test certificate from the supplier. Subsequent leak tests must be performed at intervals not to exceed 6 months. If the leakage test reveals the presence of 0.005 μCi or more of removable contamination, the source must be withdrawn from use and appropriately stored; (b) The licensee must conduct a quarterly physical inventory of all sources in possession, and (c) measure ambient dose rates quarterly in all areas where such sources are stored and retain records of these surveys for 3 years.

4. A licensee may not *release a patient* administered a radiopharmaceutical from confinement for medical care until either the measured dose rate at a distance of 1 m from the

patient is less than 5 mrem/h or the activity remaining in the patent is less than 30 μCi. In the case of a permanent brachytherapy implant, the patient must not be released until the measured dose at a distance of 1 m from the patient is less than 5 mrem/h. A patient with a temporary implant must not be released until all sources have been removed and the patient surveyed with a radiation detector to confirm that all sources have been removed. A record of patient surveys have to be retained by the licensee for 3 years.

5. Promptly after removing sources from the patient, the licensee (a) shall return the sources to the storage and (b) count the number to ensure that all sources taken from the storage have been returned. Immediately after implanting sources in a patient, the licensee shall make a radiation survey of the patient and the area of use to confirm that no sources have been misplaced. The records of the above activities shall be retained by the licensee for 3 years.

6. A licensee shall provide radiation safety instructions to all personnel caring for the patient undergoing implant therapy. These instruction records shall be retained for 3 years.

7. A licensee shall not house a patient receiving implant therapy in the same room with another patient who is not receiving radiation therapy. Exceptions must be justified by other relevant provisions of the NRC. The patient's door shall be posted with a "Radioactive Materials" sign. Visits by individuals under age 18 shall be authorized only on a patient-by-patient basis with the approval of the authorized user and the RSO. The radiation safety officer must be notified immediately if the patient dies or has a medical emergency.

D. Teletherapy

The following regulations govern the use of teletherapy units for medical use that contain a sealed source of cobalt-60 or cesium-137.

1. *Maintenance and repair.* Only a person specifically licensed by the commission (or an agreement state) to perform teletherapy unit maintenance and repair shall (a) install, relocate, or remove a teletherapy sealed source or a teletherapy unit containing a sealed source and (b) maintain, adjust, or repair the source drawer or other mechanism that could expose the source, reduce the shielding around the source, or result in increased radiation levels.

2. *License amendments.* Amendments are required in case of (a) any change in treatment room shielding, (b) any change in the unit location within the room, (c) relocation of the teletherapy unit, (d) use of the unit in a manner that would increase the radiation levels outside the treatment room, and (e) an individual not listed on the license being allowed to perform the duties of the teletherapy physicist.

3. *Safety instructions.* A licensee shall (a) post safety instructions at the teletherapy unit console informing the operator of procedures to follow before turning the beam on and emergency procedure in case of source movement failure and (b) provide education and training to all individuals who operate a teletherapy unit. The records shall be kept for 3 years.

4. *Safety precautions.* A licensee shall (a) control access to the teletherapy room by a door; (b) install door interlocks to prevent the beam from turning on when the door is open, to turn the beam off when the door is opened, and prevent the beam from turning back on after a door interlock interruption without closing the door and resetting beam "on/off" control at the console; (c) install a permanent radiation monitor capable of continuously monitoring beam status; and (d) equip teletherapy room to permit continuous observation of the patient from the teletherapy unit console during irradiation.

5. *Dosimetry equipment.* A licensee shall have a calibrated dosimetry system that must have been calibrated by the NIST or by a calibration laboratory accredited by the American Association of Physicists in Medicine (AAPM). The calibration of the dosimeter must

have been performed within the previous 2 years and after any repair. The 2-year interval for calibration may be extended to 4 years if chamber intercomparisons are carried out according to the NRC specifications; see 10 CFR Part 35.630 (28). The licensee shall retain a record of each chamber calibration and intercomparison for the duration of the license.

6. *Full calibration.* A licensee shall perform full calibration measurements on the teletherapy unit (a) before the first medical use of the unit; (b) if spot check measurements indicate that the output differs more than 5% from the output obtained at the last full calibration, corrected for radioactive decay; (c) following replacement of source or relocation of the unit; (d) following repair of the unit; and (e) at intervals not exceeding 1 year. Full calibration measurements must include (a) output for the range of field sizes and distances used clinically, (b) light field versus radiation field coincidence, (c) radiation field uniformity and its dependence on beam orientation, (d) timer constancy and linearity, (e) on/off error (shutter correction), and (f) accuracy of distance measuring and localization devices. Full calibration measurements must be made using protocols published by the AAPM, either the one described in reference 29 or 30. Full calibration measurements must be performed by the licensee's teletherapy physicist. A licensee shall retain a record of each calibration for the duration of the teletherapy unit source.

7. *Periodic spot checks.* A licensee shall perform output spot checks once in each calendar month. These checks must include (a) timer constancy and linearity, (b) on/off error, (c) light field versus radiation field coincidence, (d) accuracy of all distance measuring and localization devices, and (e) the output for one typical set of operating conditions and its comparison with the value obtained at last full calibration, corrected for radioactive decay. In addition to the above checks, the licensee shall perform safety checks once in each calendar month of (a) door interlock, (b) interlocks for restrictions on beam orientation (if installed), (c) beam condition indicator lights on the console, and (d) patient viewing system. In case of malfunction of a safety mechanism, the licensee shall lock the control console in the off position and not use the unit until necessary repairs have been made.

8. *Radiation surveys.* Before medical use, after each installation of a teletherapy source, and after making any change for which an amendment is required, the licensee shall perform a radiation survey of the facility. The survey must verify that (a) the leakage from the source head with the beam in the off position does not exceed 2 mrem/hour on the average and 10 mrem/hour maximum, both measured at a distance of 1 m from the source and (b) dose rates outside the room in the restricted and unrestricted areas do not exceed the limits specified by the NRC in 10 CFR Parts 20.101–20.105 (28). The maximum permissible whole-body exposure for individuals in the restricted area is 1.25 rem per calendar quarter. In the unrestricted area, radiation levels must not exceed 2 mrem in any 1 hour, 100 mrem in any 1 week, and 0.5 rem in any 1 year.

9. *Five-year inspection.* A licensee shall have the teletherapy unit fully inspected and serviced during teletherapy source replacement or at intervals not to exceed 5 years, whichever comes first. This inspection and servicing may only be performed by persons specifically licensed to do so by the commission or an agreement state.

E. Training and Experience Requirements

Training and experience requirements for the licensee, radiation safety officer, and teletherapy physicist are listed under 10 CFR Parts 35.900 to 35.972 (28).

REFERENCES

1. Relative Biological Effectiveness Committee of the ICRP and ICRU. Report of the RBE Committee to the International Commission on Radiological Protection and on Radiological Units and Measurements. *Health Phys* 1963;9:357.

2. NCRP. Recommendations on limits for exposure to ionizing radiation. Report No. 91. Bethesda, MD: National Council on Radiation Protection and Measurements, 1987.

3. NCRP. Ionizing radiation exposure of the population of the United States. Report No. 93. Bethesda, MD: National Council on Radiation Protection and Measurements, 1987.

4. Friedell HI. Radiation protection—concepts and trade-offs. In: Perception of risk, proceedings of the National Council on Radiation Protection and Measurements. Washington, DC, 1980.

5. NCRP. Basic radiation protection criteria. Report No. 39. Washington, DC: National Council on Radiation Protection and Measurements, 1971.

6. United States Scientific Committee on the Effects of Atomic Radiation. Report of the United Nations Scientific Committee on the Effects of Atomic Radiation. General Assembly, Official Records: 13th Session Suppl. No. 17 (A/3838) (1958); 17th Session, Suppl. No. 16 (A/5216) (1962); 21st Session, Suppl. No. 14 (A/6314) (1966); 24th Session, Suppl. No. 13 (A/7613) (1969). New York: United Nations.

7. Elkind MM. The initial part of the survival curve: implication for low-dose-rate radiation responses. *Radiat Res* 1977;71:1.

8. Withers HR. Response of tissues to multiple small dose fractions. *Radiat Res* 1977;71:24.

9. Brown MM. The shape of the dose-response curve for radiation carcinogenesis: extrapolation to low doses. *Radiat Res* 1977;71:34.

10. Upton AC. Radiological effects of low doses: implications for radiological protection. *Radiat Res* 1977;71:51.

11. Department of Energy. *U.S. Department of Energy injury and property damage summary.* Springfield, VA: National Technical Information Service, 1984.

12. NCRP. Structural shielding design and evaluation for medical use of x rays and gamma rays of energies up to 10 MeV. Report No. 49. Washington, DC: National Council on Radiation Protection and Measurements, 1976.

13. NCRP. Radiation protection design guidelines for 0.1–100 MeV particle accelerator facilities. Report No. 51. Washington, DC: National Council on Radiation Protection and Measurements, 1977.

14. Karzmark CJ, Capone T. Measurements of 6 MV x-rays. II. Characteristics of secondary radiation. *Br J Radiol* 1968;41:224.

15. NCRP. Medical x-ray, electron beam and gamma-ray protection for energies up to 50 MeV. Report No. 102. Bethesda, MD: National Council on Radiation Protection and Measurements, 1989.

16. Axton E, Bardell A. Neutron production from electron accelerators used for medical purposes. *Phys Med Biol* 1972;17:293.

17. Sohrabi M, Morgan KZ. Neutron dosimetry in high energy x-ray beams of medical accelerators. *Phys Med Biol* 1979;24:756.

18. Price KW, Nath R, Holeman GR. Fast and thermal neutron profiles for a 25-MV x-ray beam. *Med Phys* 1978;5:285.

19. NCRP. Shielding for high-energy electron accelerator installations. Report No. 31. Washington, DC: National Committee on Radiation Protection and Measurements, 1964.

20. Deye JA, Young FC. Neutron production from a 10 MV medical linac. *Phys Med Biol* 1977;22:90.

21. ICRP. Protection against electromagnetic radiation above 3 MeV and electrons, neutrons, and protons. Report No. 4. New York: Pergamon Press, 1964.

22. Kersey R. Estimation of neutron and gamma radiation doses in the entrance mazes of SL 75–20 linear accelerator treatment rooms. *Medicamundi* 1979;24:151.

23. NCRP. Protection against radiation from brachytherapy sources. Report No. 40. Washington, DC: National Council on Radiation Protection and Measurements, 1972.

24. Bading JR, Zeitz L, Laughlin JS. Phosphorus activation neutron dosimetry and its application to an 18-MV radiotherapy accelerator. *Med Phys* 1982;9:835.

25. Rogers DWO, Van Dyk G. Use of a neutron remmeter to measure leakage neutrons from medical electron accelerators. *Med Phys* 1981;8:163.

26. McCall RC, Jenkins TM, Shore RA. Transport of accelerator produced neutrons in a concrete room. *IEEE Trans Nucl Sci* 1979;NS-26:1593.

27. Schulz RJ. Argon/propane ionization—chamber dosimetry for mixed x-ray/neutron fields. *Med Phys* 1978;5:525.

28. Nuclear Regulatory Commission. Code of federal regulations, 10 CFR Part 0–50. Washington, DC: U.S. Government Printing Office, 1993.

29. AAPM. Protocol for the dosimetry of x- and gamma-ray beams with maximum energies between 0.6 and 50 MeV. *Phys Med Biol* 1971;16:379.

30. AAPM. A protocol for the determination of absorbed dose from high energy photon and electron beams. *Med Phys* 1983;10:741.

QUALITY ASSURANCE

The term *quality assurance* (QA) describes a program that is designed to control and maintain the standard of quality set for that program. For radiation oncology, a quality assurance program is essentially a set of policies and procedures to maintain the quality of patient care. The general criteria or standards of quality are usually set collectively by the profession. It is expected that a QA program designed specifically for an institution will meet those standards.

Model QA programs in radiation oncology have been proposed by professional organizations such as the American College of Radiology (ACR) (1), the American Association of Physicists in Medicine (AAPM) (2,8), and the American College of Medical Physics (ACMP) (3). These programs incorporate many of the standards and criteria developed by the National Council on Radiation Protection and Measurements (NCRP), the International Commission on Radiation Units and Measurements (ICRU), the International Commission on Radiological Protection (ICRP), and the International Electrotechnical Commission (IEC). In addition, mandatory programs with QA components have been instituted by the Nuclear Regulatory Commission (NRC) and the individual states. The Joint Commission for Accreditation of Health Care Organizations (JCAHO) has also set minimum standards of QA that are required of hospitals seeking accreditation.

Despite the many standard-setting bodies and the regulatory agencies, the standards of radiation oncology practice are quite varied across the United States. A patterns of care study (4), using Hodgkin's disease, prostate cancer, and cervix cancer as examples, showed correlations between patient outcome and facility equipment, structure, technical support, and physician characteristics. These data underscore the importance of quality assurance in providing patients the best chance for cure.

The major reason for the lack of commitment to QA by many institutions is financial. An adequate QA program requires increased staffing and up-to-date equipment, both of which can be expensive. According to the analysis by Peters (5), the total cost of the QA program in radiation therapy amounts to approximately 3% of the annual billing for combined technical and professional charges. Because QA programs are voluntary (with the exception of the NRC or the state-mandated component), the only incentive to establishing these programs is a desire to practice good radiation therapy or avoid malpractice suits. However, the latter has not been a sufficient deterrent to effect change.

17.1. GOALS

The Inter-Society Council for Radiation Oncology specifies the goals of a QA program in what is called the "Blue Book" (6):

> The purpose of a Quality Assurance Program is the objective, systematic monitoring of the quality and appropriateness of patient care. Such a program is essential for all activities in

Radiation Oncology. The Quality Assurance Program should be related to structure, process and outcome, all of which can be measured. Structure includes the staff, equipment and facility. Process covers the pre- and post-treatment evaluations and the actual treatment application. Outcome is documented by the frequency of accomplishing stated objectives, usually tumor control, and by the frequency and seriousness of treatment-induced sequelae.

That "such a program is essentially for all activities in radiation oncology" emphasizes the need for a comprehensive QA program that includes administrative, clinical, physical, and technical aspects of radiation oncology. Operationally no single personnel has the expertise to cover all these areas. Therefore, teamwork is essential among administrators, radiation oncologists, nurses, medical physicists, and therapy technologists. For a QA program to be effective, all the staff involved with the radiation oncology service must be well-coordinated and committed to QA.

The American College of Radiology has recommended that a quality assurance committee (QAC) be formed with appropriate personnel (e.g., radiation oncologist, physicist, dosimetrist, therapist, nurse, and administrator) to represent the various aspects of radiation oncology (7). This committee will meet on a regular basis to review the QA program and oversee its implementation. If there were a hospital-wide QA program, the radiation oncology QAC would coordinate its activities with the hospital QAC.

The multidisciplinary nature of a radiation oncology QA program precludes a comprehensive coverage of the subject in this book. Only the physical aspects of radiation oncology QA will be presented here. For further details, the reader is referred to reports generated by the various organizations (1–3,8).

17.2. PHYSICS STAFFING

The physics component of quality assurance in radiation oncology is one of the major responsibilities of the radiation physicist. Adequate physics staffing, in proportion to patient load and equipment, is required to carry out these responsibilities properly. The Blue Book recommends at least one physicist per center for up to 400 patients treated annually (Table 17.1). Additional physicists are recommended in the ratio of one per 400 patients treated annually. These recommendations are for clinical service only. Additional personnel will be required for research, teaching, or administrative functions.

Many of the clinical physics tasks that have been traditionally performed by physicists can be delegated to dosimetrists or physics assistants. For example, dosimetrists can assist in routine QA checks, computer treatment planning, and monitor unit calculations and brachytherapy source preparations. A physicist in this case has a role in establishing the procedures, directing the activities, and reviewing the results.

In treatment planning, Fig. 17.1 illustrates how physics support is usually organized in this country. Arrangement *A* in which the physician practically works alone or does not seek consultation from the physics team is obviously not appropriate and is contrary to the concept of multidisciplinary approach to radiation oncology. Arrangement *B* is not satisfactory either but is prevalent in many institutions. There may be several reasons why an essential member of the team, the physicist, is excluded in this case from the clinical process. Economics is one reason, as physicists are usually higher salaried than the dosimetrists. Other reasons may include having physicists who lack clinical training or a well-defined role in the clinic. Nonetheless, Arrangement *C* is probably the best approach, as it involves teamwork among personnel whose responsibilities are matched with their credentials.

The Blue Book recommendation on dosimetrist staffing is one per 300 patients treated annually. In some institutions, dosimetrists perform physics work only, whereas in others they also do simulations. The relative proportion of a dosimetrist's effort to various tasks is dictated by the individual needs of the department, the scope of the physics activities, and the extent of other physics and technical support available.

TABLE 17.1. MINIMUM[a] PERSONNEL REQUIREMENTS FOR CLINICAL RADIA-TION THERAPY

Category	Staffing
Radiation oncologist-in-chief	One per program
Staff radiation oncologist	One additional for each 200–250 patients treated annually; no more than 25–30 patients under treatment by a single physician
Radiation physicist	One per center for up to 400 patients annually; additional in ratio of one per 400 patients treated annually
Treatment-planning staff	
Dosimetrist or physics assistant	One per 300 patients treated annually
Physics technologist (mold room)	One per 600 patients treated annually
Radiation therapy technologist	
Supervisor	One per center
Staff (treatment)	Two per megavoltage unit up to 25 patients treated daily per unit; four per megavoltage unit up to 50 patients treated daily per unit
Staff (simulation)	Two for every 500 patients simulated annually
Staff (brachytherapy)	As needed
Treatment aid	As needed, usually one per 300–400 patients treated annually
Nurse[b]	One per center for up to 300 patients treated annually and an additional one per 300 patients treated annually
Social worker	As needed to provide service
Dietitian	As needed to provide service
Physical therapist	As needed to provide service
Maintenance engineer/electronics technician	One per 2 megavoltage units or 1 megavoltage unit and a simulator if equipment serviced inhouse

[a]Additional personnel will be required for research, education, and administration. For example, if 800 patients are treated annually with three accelerators, one ^{60}Co teletherapy unit, a superficial x-ray machine, one treatment planning computer, the clinical allotment for physicists would be two to three. A training program with eight residents, two technology students and a graduate student would require another 1 to 1.5 FTEs. Administration of this group would require 0.5 FTE. If the faculty had 20% time for research, a total of five to six physicists would be required.
[b]For direct patient care. Other activities supported by LVNs and nurses aides.
From ISCRO. Radiation oncology in integrated cancer management. Reston, VA: American College of Radiology, 1991, with permission.

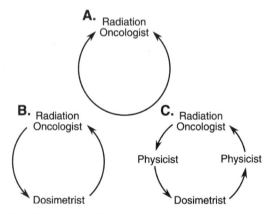

FIG. 17.1. Patterns of interaction among treatment planning personnel. **A:** Radiation oncologist works alone. **B:** Radiation oncologist and dosimetrists generate a treatment plan. **C:** Teamwork between radiation oncologist, physicist and dosimetrist.

A. Training

Besides the adequacy of physics staffing in terms of number of personnel in relation to the patient load or equipment, education and training of these personnel are of critical importance. The greatest weakness in this regard has been the physicist's training. Most physicists are hired with less-than-adequate clinical training. Structured clinical training programs have been traditionally nonexistent. Certification boards for physicists exist, but the entry requirements for the examination still do not mandate residency-type clinical training as is required of the physicians. As a result, there is an unchecked influx of inadequately trained physicists into the field.

The physicist's training problems are being addressed at the national level (9–11). Physics residency programs are now being instituted, although at a much slower pace than needed. It is hoped that eventually clinical medical physicists will go through nationally accredited residency programs before taking the board examinations or assuming independent clinical responsibilities.

Just as formalized clinical training is important for physicians and physicists, it is also important for dosimetrists. Efforts are being made by the American Association of Medical Dosimetrists to formalize the training of dosimetrists by establishing training curricula, accreditation, and professional certification.

B. Qualifications

Qualifications of a clinical medical physicist have been debated in the past, but recently a consensus has developed among the various national organizations. A radiation oncology physicist is considered qualified if he or she has an M.S. or Ph.D. degree in physics, medical physics, or a closely related field and a certification in radiation oncology physics by the American Board of Radiology, the American Board of Medical Physics, or another appropriate certifying body.

A qualified medical dosimetrist has a minimum of high school diploma and a certification by the American Association of Medical Dosimetrists. Most certified dosimetrists also are certified radiation therapy technologists.

C. Roles and Responsibilities

The roles and responsibilities of the physics team have been discussed in the literature (11–13) and are summarized in Table 17.2. As emphasized previously, the physicist must direct the physics team and assume full responsibility of the physics data and procedures applied to the patients, irrespective of whether these activities are carried out by the physicist, dosimetrist, or other personnel. This unambiguous responsibility of physics procedures by

TABLE 17.2. ROLES AND RESPONSIBILITIES OF PHYSICISTS

Equipment (Teletherapy, Brachytherapy, Simulator)	Treatment Planning (Teletherapy and Brachytherapy)	Dosimetry	Radiation Protection	Academic/ Administrative
Selection, specifications	Management/QA of treatment-planning computer	Dose calculation formalism	Regulatory	Teaching
Acceptance testing	Beam data management	Special treatment techniques	Radiation survey	Research
Commissioning, beam data measurement	Simulation consultation	Special dosimetry	Personnel monitoring	Developmental
Calibration	Patient data for treatment planning	*In vivo* dosimetry	Facility design	Administrative
Quality assurance	Technique optimization; isodose planning; plan analysis/evaluation; treatment aids; beam modifiers			

From Khan FM. Residency training for medical physicists. *Int J Radiat Oncol Biol Phys* 1992;24:853, with permission.

the physicist is based on the same rationale as the physician's control of medical prescription. Nonconformity to this principle can pose a serious risk to the patient.

The radiation oncologist undoubtedly has the overall responsibility for the conduct of the entire treatment process. Because of that role, it is his or her responsibility to ensure that an adequate and competent physics team is in place and that the roles of different personnel on the team are appropriately defined. It has been recognized that inadequacy of physics support translates into substandard or less than optimal patient care (4,6).

Calibration of radiation generators or sources is the exclusive responsibility of the medical physicist. No other personnel has the expertise to perform this most critical function. Because of the absolute necessity of the calibration procedure before the machine can be released for patient treatment, all institutions manage to acquire physics support at least sufficient to provide periodic calibration of the radiation equipment. However, these periodic calibrations, outside of a well-structured quality assurance program, are inadequate and cannot ensure continued safety of machine operation on a daily basis (14).

Next to calibration and quality assurance of radiation equipment is the physicist's role in treatment planning. Although the treatment planning process involves sophisticated physics concepts in designing and optimizing patient treatments, most institutions do not involve physicists sufficiently in this process. As discussed previously (Fig. 17.1), some physicians tend to work alone or with dosimetrists to design treatment plans. It should be realized that the absence of physicist from the treatment-planning scene takes away an important element of quality control, namely, the optimization and scientific authentication of the treatment plan.

The physicist's direct involvement in the treatment-planning process is possible only if the consultation is sought by the radiation oncologist. If the latter is not accustomed, by training or experience, to such interactions, the physicist is not brought into the treatment-planning loop. Consequently, an important member of the treatment-planning team is bypassed.

At some institutions, the physicist's role in treatment planning has been made indispensable. For example, at the University of Minnesota the physicist's consultation is made as important as other consultations, such as those sought from the medical oncologist, the surgeon, or the radiologist. To prevent bypassing the physics consultation, each patient is assigned a physicist who is available at the time of simulation to assist the radiation oncologist in formulating the best possible treatment plan. Subsequent physics work is the designated physicist's responsibility, although he or she may be assisted by the dosimetrist or other technical personnel. The final treatment plan is approved by the radiation oncologist after discussing the plan with the physicist. Also, the physicist is present at the time of first treatment and subsequent treatments, if needed, to ensure proper implementation of the plan.

Not all the clinical physics procedures need to be performed by physicists. Many of the technical tasks can be delegated to dosimetrists so that physicists can devote time to essential developmental activities. Every radiation oncology department needs to develop new programs as well as revise the old ones to keep current with advancements in the field. Responsibility often rests with the physicist to implement these advances while maintaining the quality of care. Examples from the past three decades include development of linear accelerator technology, computer imaging, 3-D treatment planning, conformal and dynamic therapy, and remote afterloading brachytherapy. Whereas these technologies were not developed exclusively by physicists, they had an important role in their design and clinical application. Along with these major advancements came the innovations in treatment techniques, for example, mantle fields, total body irradiation, electron beam therapy, intensity-modulated radiation therapy, stereotactic radiosurgery, low-energy source brachytherapy, and high dose rate brachytherapy. These refinements form an integral part of the physicist's responsibilities and are often not separated from his or her routine clinical duties. It is, therefore, important to recognize the need of providing sufficient technical support to the physicist for a proper fulfillment of his or her role.

17.3. EQUIPMENT

High-quality patient care cannot be achieved or maintained without appropriate equipment. Tumors occur in many forms, shapes, and locations. Unless radiation can be effectively delivered to the tumor site with minimal side effects, the whole treatment process becomes no more than a costly exercise—costly in terms of economics as well as human life. For any institution to embark on a radiation therapy program, foremost attention must be paid to its capability of providing optimal care to all the patients who will be referred to it. Thus the available equipment must be suitable to treat effectively the many different kinds of cancers that are presented in the clinic.

A. External Beam Units

The type or quality of radiation beam is dictated by the type and location of cancer to be treated. Most head and neck cancers can be treated with low-energy megavoltage units: cobalt-60 or linear accelerators in the energy range of 4 to 6 MV. That does not mean that a facility equipped with only one of these units is capable of providing quality care to all patients with head and neck cancers. On the contrary, institutions whose sole treatment equipment is one of these units are not in a position to undertake complex and sophisticated treatment techniques required for most head and neck cancers. Depending on the kind and stage of the disease, an optimal treatment plan may call for other types of beams such as a combination of low- and high-energy photon beams or an electron beam. A facility equipped with a single-energy beam tends to follow suboptimal treatment plans or obsolete treatment techniques when the best available radiation therapy equipment is a cobalt unit.

Because of the wide variety of cancers normally seen in a radiation therapy clinic, it is necessary to have at least two qualities of photon beams: a low-energy (cobalt-60 or 4 to 6 MV x-rays) and a high-energy (10 MV or higher) beam. In addition, electron beams of several different energies between 6 and 20 MeV must be available because approximately 30% of patients require an electron beam for boost or an entire course of treatment.

A dual-energy linear accelerator can provide all the beams necessary for modern radiation therapy. These machines are usually equipped with one low- and one high-energy photon beam and a number of electron energies up to 18 or 20 MeV. That provides sufficient capability to treat any cancer that needs external beam.

Additional machines are required if the patient load exceeds about 30 patients per day. Although it is possible to treat more than 30 patients per machine per day, higher patient loads necessitate hurried treatments and consequently allow less attention to detail. It is important for a radiotherapy facility to be equipped not only with appropriate type and quality of beams but also with a sufficient number of machines to handle the patient load.

B. Brachytherapy Sources

Certain cancers need brachytherapy, usually in combination with external beam. Cancer of the uterine cervix and some other gynecologic malignancies are best treated with these techniques. Unless the center has the policy not to treat patients for whom the brachytherapy is the treatment of choice, brachytherapy equipment must be available to provide quality care to patients who need this form of therapy.

For intracavitary application, radium and cesium are equally effective as far as the therapeutic effects are concerned. Cesium has replaced radium mainly on the basis of radiation protection considerations pertaining to storing and handling of these sources. For interstitial implants, iridium-192 is the best available source although iodine-125 offers some advantages for particular techniques, for example, permanent implants or temporary brain implants with high-intensity sources.

Availability of brachytherapy sources and equipment adds to the comprehensiveness of a center to provide radiation therapy. Again, if this capability is not available, a patient's treatment may be compromised if the institution does not have a suitable alternative or rationalizes the use of external beam alone not on the basis of merit but on the nonavailability of brachytherapy service.

Afterloading procedures are the standard of practice in brachytherapy. The therapeutic quality of the procedure is little affected by whether the afterloading is done by the bedside or remotely. An institution can provide quality brachytherapy by using conventional afterloading applicators. The need for the remote afterloaders (the LDR or the HDR) is based primarily on considerations such as minimizing radiation exposure to personnel or handling large patient loads. Again, if it can be established that the remote afterloading will improve patient care (e.g., by allowing better nursing care or optimizing source placement), a case can be made to acquire such equipment. High-tech equipment such as the remote afterloaders can be very expensive and can drive up the cost of patient care. Therefore, the additional cost must be justified on the basis of cost versus patient benefit analysis.

C. Simulator

The simulator is an essential tool for planning and designing radiation therapy treatments. Because of the poor imaging quality of the treatment beam and the logistic difficulty of obtaining time on the treatment machine, a simulator is the appropriate equipment to image the treatment fields and optimize their placement before actual treatment. Because the simulator offers the same beam geometry as the treatment machine, simulator films are used to outline the field shape and dimensions for custom designing field blocks. The simulator room is the place where different techniques can be modeled and solutions to technical problems devised.

An essential requirement for simulation is the geometric accuracy that must be maintained at the same level as that of the treatment machine. If the simulated field cannot be accurately reproduced under the treatment machine, the whole simulation process becomes a useless exercise. Inaccurate simulation can result in erroneous treatment.

Besides the mechanical and radiation field accuracy of a simulator, its imaging quality cannot be overemphasized. Unless anatomic structures can be made visible with reasonable clarity, fields cannot be accurately outlined, negating the very purpose of simulation.

Fluoroscopic capability of a simulator is a desirable option because it allows iterative field adjustments and viewing before a final radiograph is obtained. Nonavailability of fluoroscopic option results in an increased number of film retakes and, in the long run, is not cost-effective. Moreover, too many repeats could deter from optimization of the simulation process.

New developments in simulation are taking place in the area of computed tomography (CT) simulation. A large number of CT scans taken through the region of the body to be simulated can be processed to produce a digital reconstructed radiography (DRR) in any plane. The DRR corrected for beam divergence is like the simulator radiograph, except that it is created from individual CT slices. If targets and critical structures are outlined on each CT slice, a DRR can be created to provide any simulator view with the target and the critical structures highlighted in different shades of color. The DRR view is used to optimize the design and placement of treatment fields before a simulation film is taken for verification.

17.4. DOSIMETRIC ACCURACY

Available evidence for effectively treating certain types of cancers points to the need for an accuracy of approximately $\pm 5\%$ in dose delivery (15,16). This is indeed a very stringent requirement, considering the uncertainties in equipment calibration, treatment planning, and patient set-up. Further reduction in the dose accuracy limit will be not only very difficult but probably of marginal value.

Calculation of overall uncertainty in a radiation therapy procedure is a complex problem, because some errors are random while others can be systematic. Loevinger and Loftus

TABLE 17.3. UNCERTAINTY[a] IN THE CALIBRATION OF AN ION CHAMBER

Step	Uncertainty (Percent)
Physical constants	1.1
Standard beam, NIST	0.5
Secondary standard, NIST	0.4
Field instrument, ADCL	1.0
Cumulative	1.6

ADCL, Accredited Dose Calibration Laboratory; NIST, National Institute of Standards and Technology.
[a]95% confidence interval.
From ICRU. Determination of absorbed dose in a patient irradiated by beams of x or gamma rays in radiotherapy procedures. Report no. 24. Washington DC: International Commission on Radiation Units and Measures, 1976, with permission.

(15) have proposed a model in which the random and systematic errors are statistically treated the same way. Individual uncertainties are represented by standard deviations that are then added in quadrature to determine the cumulative uncertainty. The combined standard deviation may be multiplied by two to obtain an uncertainty with a 95% confidence interval.

Table 17.3 gives an estimate of uncertainty in the calibration of a treatment beam with a field ion chamber (e.g., 0.6 cm^3 Farmer-type chamber). The analysis shows that an ion chamber suitable for calibrating radiation therapy beams and provided with a ^{60}Co exposure calibration factor from an accredited dosimetry calibration laboratory (ADCL) has a cumulative uncertainty of approximately 1.5% (two standard deviations). Calibration of beams with this chamber will introduce additional uncertainties such as in the measurement procedure and in the parameters of the dosimetry protocol. The overall uncertainty of the treatment beam calibration using current protocols is estimated to be about 2.5% under optimal conditions (15).

Table 17.4 gives uncertainties in the various steps involved in delivering a certain dose to a patient at a reference point such as at the isocenter. The estimate of the uncertainties in these steps is approximate and arrived at by considering the various procedures as they may be typically carried out. These uncertainties could be further refined and broadened to include uncertainties in the dose distribution within the target volume and the surrounding structures (2).

A QA program must address not only the issues of random and systematic errors inherent in the procedures but also the possibilities of human error such as in reading an instrument, selecting a treatment parameter, making arithmetic computations, or interpreting a treatment plan. Although human errors cannot be eliminated altogether, the

TABLE 17.4. OVERALL UNCERTAINTY[a] IN DOSE DELIVERED AT A POINT IN A PATIENT

Step	Uncertainty (Percent)
Ion chamber calibration	1.6
Calibration procedure	2.0
Dose calculation parameters and methods	3.0
Effective depth	2.0
SSD	2.0
Wedges	2.0
Blocking trays	2.0
Cumulative	5.6

SSD, source-to-surface distance.
[a]95% confidence interval.

probability of their occurrence can be minimized by a well-designed QA program. An undue relaxation of a QA program or the lack of it can be construed as professional negligence.

17.5. EQUIPMENT SPECIFICATIONS

Acquisition of a major piece of equipment involves many steps: justification of need, market evaluation of different makes and models, checks of vendors' business relations and service record, calling up users for their opinions, writing bid specifications, making final evaluation, and doing price negotiations. Even if the institution does not require closed bids, it is important to prepare detailed specifications and obtain a formal written response from the vendor before deciding on the purchase.

Most vendors list their equipment specifications in company brochures that are available on request. These specifications should be carefully compared with other vendors' specifications. Formal bid specifications can then be written for the product that most closely meets the institution's needs. For an impartial bid process, the specifications should be as generic as possible, so that all major vendors have a fair chance of responding to the bids. Specifications that the institution considers essential must be identified so that vendors who cannot meet those specifications do not have to go through the process of answering the bid. If a particular system is specified to meet a certain function, vendors should have the opportunity to suggest alternative systems with equivalent or better specifications.

The purchase of radiation therapy equipment is usually a shared responsibility between the radiation oncologist, the physicist, and the hospital administrator. The physicist's role is primarily to write technical specifications although most participate in the whole decision process.

The specifications are written in a suitable format so that the vendors can respond to them item by item. Because the vendors' responses are legally binding, clarification should be sought if response to a particular item is not clear. Also, if a specification in a company's brochure falls short of a desired specification, negotiations may be carried out with the vendor to improve the specification in question. Many improvements in the accelerator technology have occurred as a result of customer demand for better specifications.

Certain specifications in regard to beam characteristics and acceptance criteria require carefully stated definitions and methods of measurement. The specifications should clearly spell out these details, especially when conflicting definitions or criteria exist in the literature. As far as possible, the specifications should follow national or international terminology and guidelines unless a special need exists to justify deviations from the accepted standards.

17.6. ACCEPTANCE TESTING

Unless the vendor has agreed to a written set of specifications, the customer has no recourse but to go along with the vendor's acceptance test procedures. These procedures are set up by the company to demonstrate that the product meets the specifications contained in its brochures and satisfies the legal requirements of equipment safety.

If a set of bid specifications was agreed on before the machine was purchased, then the vendor is obligated to satisfy all the specifications and criteria contained in the purchase contract. In practice, the vendor first performs all the tests in accordance with the company's procedure manual. Any deviations or additions stipulated in the bid specifications are then addressed to complete the acceptance testing process.

As a general rule, acceptance testing is required on any piece of equipment that is used in conjunction with patient treatments. Whereas formal testing procedures have been developed for major equipment (linear accelerators, simulators, brachytherapy sources, etc.), these have to be improvised for other equipment. The guiding principle is that any equipment to be used for patients must be tested to ensure that it meets its performance specifications and safety standards.

A. Linear Accelerator

A linear accelerator is a sophisticated piece of equipment that requires several months for installation, acceptance testing, and commissioning. Whereas installation is carried out by the vendor personnel, the acceptance testing and commissioning are the responsibility of the institution's physicist. Patient treatments do not begin until the unit has been commissioned, that is, the machine tested to be acceptable and sufficient data have been acquired to permit treatment planning and dose calculations for patient treatments.

A.1. Radiation Survey

As soon as the installation has reached a stage at which a radiation beam can be generated, the physicist is called on to perform a preliminary radiation survey of the treatment facility (Chapter 16). The survey is evaluated to ensure that during the testing of the machine the exposure levels outside the room will not exceed permissible limits, considering the dose rate output, machine on time, use factors, and occupancy factors for the surrounding areas. A preliminary calibration of the machine output (cGy/MU) is needed to determine the expected dose levels as a function of machine output (MU/min).

After completion of the installation, a formal radiation protection survey is carried out, including the measurement of head leakage; area survey, and tests of interlocks, warning lights, and emergency switches. The survey is evaluated for conditions that are expected to exist in the clinical use of the machine, for example, workload, use factors, and occupancy factors.

A.2. Jaw Symmetry

One of the methods of checking jaw symmetry is with a machinist's dial indicator (Fig. 17.2). With the gantry pointing horizontally and the jaws open to a large field, the feeler of the dial indicator is made to touch the face of one of the jaws and the indicator's reading is noted. The collimator is then rotated through 180 degrees and the reading is taken with the feeler now resting on the opposite jaw. A leveling device is used to set the collimator angles for these measurements. The symmetry error is one-half of the difference between the two readings of the dial indicator. The procedure is repeated for the second set of jaws. The symmetry error of the collimator jaws is typically less than 1 mm.

A.3. Coincidence

Collimator Axis, Light Beam Axis, and Cross-hairs
With a graph paper taped on the table and the gantry vertical, turn on the field light to obtain a rectangular field. Mark the edges of the light field, intersection of the diagonals, and the position of the cross-hair images. Rotate the collimator through 180 degrees and check the coincidence of (a) the light field edges and (b) the intersection of diagonals and the position of cross-hair images. If significant misalignment exists, the field light and cross-hairs should be adjusted to bring about the desired coincidence.

Light Beam with X-ray Beam
Place a ready pack film on the table at the source-to-axis distance (SAD). With the collimator angle set at 0 degrees, obtain a rectangular or square light field and mark the edges with a radiopaque object or a ballpoint pen by drawing lines on the film jacket with sufficient pressure to scratch the emulsion. The film orientation and the collimator angle are noted. A plastic sheet, thick enough to provide maximum electronic buildup, is placed over the film without disturbing its position. This is done to eliminate the perturbing influence of

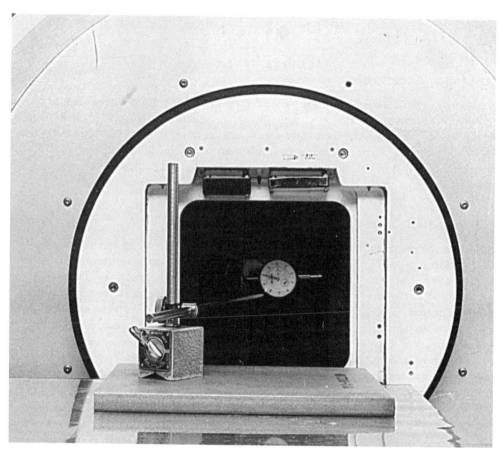

FIG. 17.2. Determination of jaw symmetry with the machinist's dial indicator. The feeler of the dial indicator is shown to rest on the right jaw.

the incident electron contamination. The film is exposed to obtain an optical density in the linear range of its sensitometric curve, usually around 1. Two more exposures at collimator angles of ±90 degrees are made using fresh areas of the same film or on a second film. The film is processed in an automatic rapid processor.

The alignment between the x-ray beam edges (corresponding to an optical density of 50% relative to that on central axis) and the light beam marks can be checked visually or by cross-beam optical density profiles. A typical alignment film is shown in Fig. 17.3. For acceptance testing, the above process should be repeated at 0 degrees, 90 degrees, 180 degrees, and 270 degrees angulation of the gantry.

According to the AAPM guidelines, the alignment between the light beam and the x-ray beam should be within ±3 mm (2). However, a more stringent requirement of ±2 mm can be maintained without difficulty with the modern linear accelerators.

A.4. Mechanical Isocenter

Mechanical isocenter is the intersection point of the axis of rotation of the collimator and the axis of rotation of the gantry. Due to heavy weight, the gantry frame may flex during rotation. This may cause the axis of the gantry rotation to miss the axis of the collimator rotation, thereby creating an uncertainty in the position of the isocenter.

Collimator Rotation

Attach a piece of graph paper on a flat surface of a plastic sheet and mark an intersection point of two graph lines (center point). Using the distance measuring rod attached to the accessory mount, place the center point of the graph at the assumed isocenter (point P).

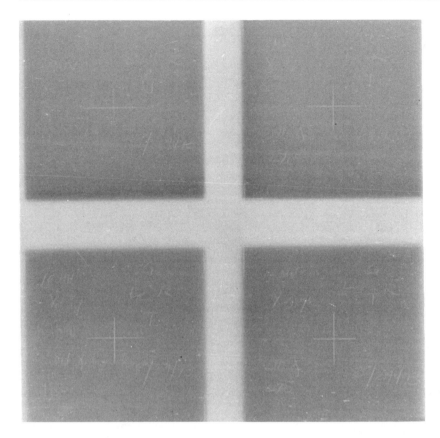

FIG. 17.3. Films to measure coincidence between light beam and radiation beam. Light field borders appear as scratch marks as the corner edges of the radiation field.

Reverse the distance rod and attach an adjustable pointer device with a sharp point, called the center finder or wiggler, to its distal end (Fig. 17.4A).[1] Starting with a 0-degree angle, rotate the collimator to + 90 degrees and note the maximum displacement of the wiggler tip from point P in the X and Y directions. Tap the wiggler point to move it in the X direction through half the distance from point P and then tap the plastic sheet to bring point P under the wiggler tip. Repeat the procedure for the Y axis. Rotate the collimator to ±90 degrees and repeat the whole procedure. By iterative adjustment of the wiggler tip and point P, the displacement of the wiggler tip from point P can be minimized as the collimator is rotated. For an acceptable alignment, the isocenter should stay within a 2-mm-diameter circle when the collimator is rotated through its full range of rotation.

Gantry Rotation

With the wiggler point positioned at the isocenter as determined previously, another horizontal rod with a fine point is held in a ring stand so that the two points coincide as best as possible (Fig. 17.4B). The stand for the horizontal rod should rest on the couch near its end so that there is no possibility of gantry collision with the couch or the apparatus. By moving the gantry through 360 degrees, the displacement between the wiggler point and the horizontal rod point is visually noted and measured. The tolerance of the isocenter motion with full gantry rotation is ±1 mm.

A.5. Radiation Isocenter

Collimator

With the gantry vertical, place a ready pack film flat on the tabletop at the SAD. Open the upper jaws of the collimator wide open and close the lower jaws to obtain a narrow

---

[1] A center finder or wiggler is available from LS Starrett Co., Athol, Massachusetts.

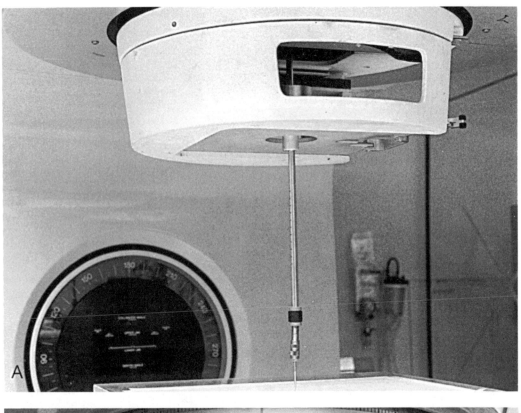

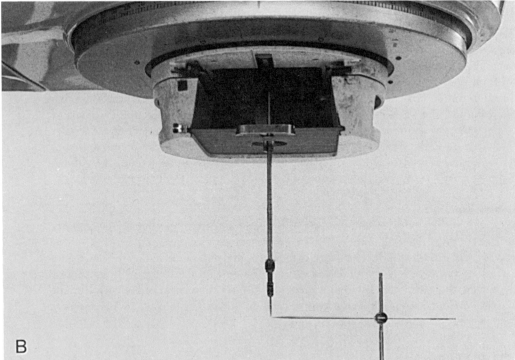

FIG. 17.4. Determination of mechanical isocenter. **A:** Collimator rotation. **B:** Gantry rotation. See text for details.

slit of minimum possible width. Place build-up sheet on top of the film. By rotating the collimator through a number of different angles, the film is exposed to obtain an optical density of about 1. The interval between angles should be such that six to seven exposures can be made to cover full rotation of the collimator without overlaps. Using a new film, repeat the above process with the lower jaws open and the upper jaws closed to a narrow slit.

The processed films will show star patterns, with a dark central region (Fig. 17.5A). By using a ballpoint pen or another film marker with a fine point, lines may be drawn through the middle of the slit images to define more clearly the intersection point(s) of the slit images. For an acceptable result, all the lines should intersect or pass within a 2-mm-diameter circle.

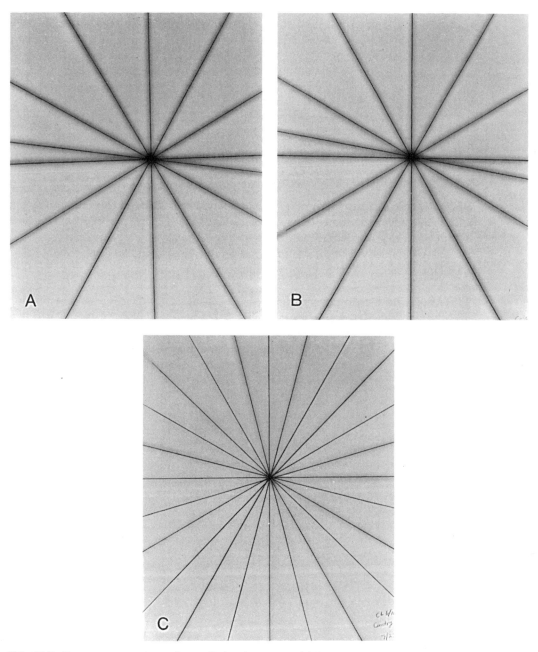

FIG. 17.5. Star pattern to determine radiation isocenter of **(A)** collimator rotation, **(B)** table rotation, and **(C)** gantry rotation.

Treatment Table

Place a film on the tabletop at the SAD. Open the upper collimator jaws wide and close down the lower jaws to a narrow slit. Place a buildup sheet on top of the film. Make six to seven exposures on the same film with the table rotated through a series of different angles to cover the full range of couch rotation. Some exposures may have to be staggered to avoid overlap of images.

A star pattern (Fig. 17.5B) on the processed film should ideally show all the slit images intersecting at one point, the radiation isocenter. Acceptable specification requires that all the lines should intersect or pass within a 2-mm-diameter circle. Stricter specification may be required for a unit designated for stereotactic radiosurgery.

Gantry

A ready pack film, sandwiched between two plastic sheets (e.g., acrylic or clear polystyrene), is placed on the table so that the plane of the film is perpendicular to the plane of couch top and contains the beam central axis for all gantry angles. Create a slit of beam parallel to the gantry axis of rotation. Make 12 exposures on the same film with the gantry rotated between exposures. To avoid overlaps, the first six exposures may be made at 30-degree intervals, the next one at 45 degrees beyond, and the subsequent exposures successively 30 degrees apart.

The gantry star pattern (Fig. 17.5C) should show the lines intersecting or passing within a 2-mm-diameter circle centered around the presumed radiation isocenter.

A.6. Multiple Beam Alignment Check

When a patient is treated with more than one beam, misalignment between beams can occur due to any of the causes discussed previously. Lutz et al. (17) have recommended a test procedure that can detect simultaneously three general causes of beam misalignment: (a) focal spot displacement; (b) asymmetry of collimator jaws, and (c) displacement in the collimator rotation axis or the gantry rotation axis. This method is called the split-field test.

The split-field test consists of double-exposing a film (sandwiched between buildup sheets) to two fields, 180 degrees apart. As shown schematically in Fig. 17.6, a square field is first exposed from above with half the field (region 2) blocked and then exposed from below to expose region 2 with region 1 blocked. Relative shift of the two images is indicative of

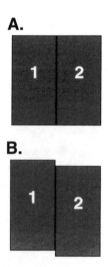

FIG. 17.6. Schematic illustration of Lutz et al. (17) method of determining alignment between opposing fields. **A:** Perfect alignment. **B:** Misalignment.

the misalignment of the parallel-opposed beams. A similar test can be performed between any two beams rotated through 180 degrees.

If beam misalignment is shown by the above test, one can then proceed to investigate the cause of misalignment by checking individually the alignment of the radiation isocenter with the axis of the collimator or gantry rotation as described previously.

A.7. X-ray Beam Performance

Energy

Measurement and specification of photon beam energy have been discussed in Chapter 7. The most practical method of specifying clinical beam energy is by the depth-dose distribution. A central axis depth-dose curve measured with a suitable ion chamber in a water phantom can be compared with published data to specify the energy. The following considerations are relevant to making such a determination.

1. The ion chamber internal diameter should be small (less than 3 mm) to minimize displacement correction (Chapter 8). For a larger diameter chamber, the depth-dose curve should be shifted to the left (toward the source) by $0.6r$, where r is the radius of the chamber.
2. In comparing depth-dose distribution with published data, care must be exercised in regard to the reference depth used in the definition of percent depth dose. To avoid ambiguity, it is preferable to compare depth dose ratios for depths beyond the depth of dose maximum (d_{max}) rather than the absolute values of the percent depth dose. Suitable depths for comparing depth dose ratios are 10 and 20 cm.

The reference depth-dose data used for comparison must be reliable. Data published by national or international organizations are preferable in this regard. The depth-dose data published in the *British Journal of Radiology* (18) is commonly used for specifying energy, although some prefer the method of ionization ratio as a measure of energy and using the data given in the TG-21 protocol (19). Either method is acceptable.

The acceptance criteria is usually specified in terms of depth-dose variance for a 10×10-cm field size, 100-cm SSD, and 10-cm depth. A difference of $\pm 2\%$ in the depth-dose ratio or ionization ratio from the published values is acceptable, considering the fact that this comparison is just for nominal energy designation only. The depth-dose data for clinical use is not the published data but the one that is actually measured for the given accelerator. A small uncertainty in the nominal beam energy designation is not important as long as calibration and the clinically used depth-dose data are based on accurately measured energy parameters (e.g., TG-51 data).

Field Flatness

Field flatness for photon beams has been traditionally defined as the variation of dose relative to the central axis over the central 80% of the field size (reference region) at a 10-cm depth in a plane perpendicular to the central axis (Fig. 17.7A). A dose variation of $\pm 3\%$ is considered acceptable (20).

The AAPM Task Group 45 (14) specifies flatness in terms of maximum percentage variation from average dose across the central 80% of the full width at half maximum (FWHM) of the profile in a plane transverse to the beam axis. This variation or flatness F is mathematically given by:

$$F = \frac{M - m}{M + m} \times 100\% \qquad (17.1)$$

where M and m are the maximum and minimum dose values in the central 80% of the profile.

The above definitions of field flatness do not distinguish between the dose variation produced by the flattening filter and that due to the penumbra. Whereas flatness can be altered by the flattening filter, the dose variation in the penumbra region is governed

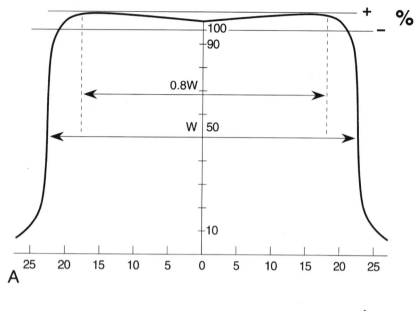

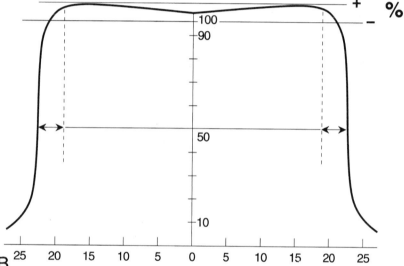

FIG. 17.7. Alternate definitions of photon field flatness. **A:** Flatness is measured within a region bounded by 80% of the field width *(W)*. **B:** Flatness is measured within a region bounded by lines drawn a certain distance (e.g., 2 cm) inside from the field edges. Depth of measurement is specified at 10 cm.

primarily by the geometric and transmission penumbra, photon scatter, and electron scatter. The flatness criteria should, therefore, reflect the effect of the flattening filter and not the penumbra, which is basically unalterable.

Boyer (21) has suggested that the x-ray beam field flatness should be specified to exclude the penumbral effects. The reference region of flatness should be defined with lines at a specified distance from the field edges instead of a certain percentage of the field size (Fig. 17.7B). Typical flatness at a 10-cm depth within the region extending up to 2 cm from the field edge is +3% to −5% (21).

Definitions that specify field flatness and symmetry with respect to average profile values create ambiguity and clinical inconsistency. Because beams are calibrated at the central axis, it is more logical to characterize dose variation relative to the central axis.

In the light of the above discussion, there is a need for a national or international group to examine the prevailing definitions of field flatness and recommend a criterion that checks the effectiveness of the flattening filter, excluding the penumbra. In the meantime, the flatness definition given by Equation (17.1) may be used with the acceptable limit being within ±3%.

For acceptance testing, flatness should be checked for the maximum field size at least at two depths: 10 cm and d_{max}. Whereas the flatness criteria is applied to the profile at a

10-cm depth, the profile at d_{max} should be examined for the extent of peripheral hot spots, or "horns." These horns should not exceed 105%. For bigger horns, an accessory filter may have to be designed to reduce them when using large fields (22).

In addition to the profiles along the principal axes of the field, diagonal scans should be obtained to check field flatness. Typically, the diagonal flatness is +4% to −6% in the reference region, extending up to 2.8 cm from the 50% isodose curve in a plane perpendicular to the central axis and at a 10-cm depth (21).

Field Symmetry

The cross-beam profiles obtained for flatness also can be used for symmetry. The profile plot may be folded at the field center and the two halves of the profiles compared. In the reference region, the dose should not differ more than 2% at any pair of points situated symmetrically with respect to the central ray.

A.8. Electron Beam Performance

Energy

Specification and measurement of electron beam energy are discussed in Chapter 14 as well as in the AAPM TG-25 protocol (23). The depth-dose or depth ionization curve for a broad beam measured with a suitable ion chamber in a water phantom gives the practical or extrapolated range, Rp. The most probable energy $(E_p)_o$ is given by Equation 14.4. $(E_p)_o$ should be within about ± 0.5 MeV of the nominal energy shown on the accelerator control panel.

For a routine check of electron beam energies, film can be used to determine Rp as well as other parameters such as R_{100}, R_{90}, R_{80}, and R_{50}. Computer-driven densitometers are commercially available that can analyze these parameters, including the most probable and mean energies.

Flatness and Symmetry

The flatness and symmetry specifications of electron beams are given in the AAPM TG-25 report (23) and also are discussed in Chapter 14. Again, film dosimetry is quite useful in analyzing flatness and symmetry on a routine basis.

A.9. Monitor Chambers

Linearity of monitor chambers is an important requirement and should be checked as a function of dose rate and for special operating conditions such as total body irradiation, total skin irradiation, and arc rotation. Long-term stability check of monitor chambers forms a major part of the quality assurance program.

A.10. Wedges

Wedge isodose distribution for a 10×10-cm field may be used to check wedge angle (Chapter 11). The measured wedge angles should be within ± 2 degrees of the values specified. This uncertainty in nominal wedge angles is acceptable because wedge filters are always planned using isodose distribution determined for the given wedge.

A.11. Miscellaneous Checks

1. Isocenter shift with couch motion up and down should not exceed ± 2 mm.
2. Optical distance indicators should be accurate within ± 2 mm.
3. Field size indicators should be accurate within ± 2 mm.
4. Gantry angle and collimator angles should be accurate within 1 degree.
5. Laser lights should be aligned with the isocenter within ± 2 mm.
6. Tabletop sag with lateral or longitudinal travel under a distributed weight (similar to patient) of 180 lbs. should not exceed 2 mm.

7. The tennis racket insert for the couch should not sag more than 0.5 cm under the above stated conditions.

8. Other ancillary devices provided with the accelerator should be checked in accordance with the vendor's specifications or as specified in the purchase contract.

B. Simulator

Acceptance testing of a simulator may be divided into two parts: (a) checking of the geometric and spatial accuracies and (b) performance evaluation of the x-ray generator and the associated imaging system. The first part is similar to the acceptance testing of a linear accelerator. The second part deals with the simulator performance like a diagnostic x-ray and fluoroscopic unit.

Several publications have discussed the specifications of treatment simulators and the required testing procedures (24–27). A comprehensive review of the subject has been provided (28). The quality assurance for the x-ray generator and the imaging system has been discussed by the NCRP (29). Specifications and acceptance test procedures may also be available from vendors (30).

Because the simulators are designed to mimic the treatment machines, for example, linear accelerators, their geometric accuracy should be comparable with these machines. Ideally, the simulator should be at least as accurate as the treatment machine in localizing treatment fields. However, differences between the simulator port and the treatment port may arise because of the differences in the treatment tables or accessories. To minimize these differences, it is preferable to have a simulator with the same table design and the accessory holders as the treatment machines.

Table 17.5 is the list of acceptance tests recommended by the British Institute of Radiology. The suggested tolerances for various parameters are the same as or better than their equivalent for linear accelerators as recommended by the IEC (31).

TABLE 17.5. TREATMENT SIMULATOR TOLERANCES

Parameter	IEC Tolerance for Electron Accelerators	BIR Proposed Tolerance for Simulators
Illumination of light field indication		
1. Average illuminance at the normal treatment distance	40 lux	40 lux
Reproducibility		
2. The difference between the maximum and minimum x-ray field size for repeated settings of the same numerical field indication	2 mm	1 mm
3. The maximum distance between any light field edge and x-ray field edge for repeated settings of the same numerical field indication	2 mm	1 mm
Numerical indication of field size		
4. The maximum difference in mm or percentage of field dimension between the numerical field indication and the dimensions of the x-ray field at the normal treatment distance		
5 cm × 5 cm to 20 cm × 20 cm	3 mm	2 mm
Greater than 20 cm × 20 cm	1.5%	1%
Light field indication		
5. The maximum distance along the major axes in mm or percentage of field dimension between the light beam edge and the x-ray field edge at the normal treatment distance		
5 cm × 5 cm to 20 cm × 20 cm	2 mm	1 mm
Greater than 20 cm × 20 cm	1%	0.5%
6. The maximum distance along the major axes between the light beam edge and the x-ray field edge at 1.5 normal treatment distance		
5 cm × 5 cm to 20 cm × 20 cm	4 mm	2 mm
Greater than 20 cm × 20 cm	2%	1%
7. The maximum distance between the centers of the x-ray field and the light field at the normal treatment distance	2 mm	1 mm

(continued)

TABLE 17.5. (*continued*)

Parameter	IEC Tolerance for Electron Accelerators	BIR Proposed Tolerance for Simulators
8. The maximum distance between the centers of the x-ray field and the light field at 1.5 times the normal treatment distance	4 mm	2 mm
Geometry of field delineators		
9. The maximum deviation from parallelity of opposing edges	0.5°	0.5°
10. The maximum deviation from orthogonality of adjacent edges	0.5°	0.5°
Indication of x-ray beam axis		
11. Maximum deviation of the indication of the radiation beam axis from the radiation beam axis		
Over −25 cm from the normal treatment distance (NTD) or the working range of the indicator, beam entry	2 mm	1 mm
12. Over NTD to NTD +50 cm or working range, beam exit	3 mm	2 mm
Displacement of the x-ray beam axis from the isocenter		
13. Maximum displacement of the x-ray beam axis from the radiation isocenter	2 mm	1 mm
Indication of the isocenter		
14. Maximum displacement from the radiation isocenter of any device mounted on the machine for indicating the position of the isocenter	2 mm	1 mm
Indication of distance along the x-ray beam axis		
15. Maximum difference between the indicated distance and the actual distance from isocenter	2 mm	1 mm
16. Maximum difference between the indicated distance and the actual distance from the x-ray target	5 mm	2 mm
17. Maximum difference between the indicated distance and the actual distance between the isocenter and the image plane	N/A	2 mm
Zero position of rotational scales		
Maximum difference between the zero position indicated by the rotational scale and the intended zero position		
18. Rotation of gantry	0.5°	0.5°
19. Rotation of diaphragm housing	0.5°	0.5°
20. Isocenter rotation of the table	0.5°	0.5°
21. Rotation of the tabletop	0.5°	0.5°
22. Pitch of the table	0.5°	0.5°
23. Roll of the table	0.5°	0.5°
Opposing fields		
24. Maximum angular deviation between axes of opposed x-ray fields	1°	1°
Movements of the patient table		
25. Maximum horizontal displacement of the table for a change in height of 20 cm when loaded with 30 kg distributed over 1 m and when loaded with 135 kg distributed over 2 m, both weights acting through the isocenter	2 mm	2 mm
26. Maximum displacement of the axis of isocenter rotation of the table from the radiation isocenter	2 mm	1 mm
Parallelism of table rotation axes		
27. Maximum angle between the isocenter rotation of the table and the axis of rotation of the tabletop	0.5°	0.5°
Longitudinal rigidity of the table		
28. Maximum difference in table height near isocenter between 30 kg load retracted position and 135 kg load extended position	5 mm	5 mm
Lateral rigidity of the table (a)		
29. Maximum angle of lateral tilt from horizontal of the plane of the tabletop	0.5°	0.5°
Lateral rigidity of the table (b)		
30. Maximum deviation of the height of the table as the table is laterally displaced	5 mm	5 mm
X-ray tube		
31. Maximum focal spot size for at least one focal spot	N/A	0.3 mm × 0.3 mm
32. Maximum shift of image at the isocenter for change of focal spot	N/A	0.5 mm

From Treatment Simulators. *Br J Radiol* 1989;[Suppl. 23], with permission.

C. Brachytherapy

The purpose of acceptance testing of brachytherapy equipment is to ensure that the sources and the associated equipment meet the user's specifications. The results of these tests should be carefully evaluated and documented for future reference.

C.1. Intracavitary Sources and Applicators

The following procedures are recommended to evaluate intracavitary sources and manual afterloading applicators.

Source Identity

Physical length, diameter, serial number, and color-coding of all sources should be checked. Whereas source dimensions may be checked by physical measurement or by radiography, the serial number and color-coding can be checked by visual inspection.

Source Uniformity and Symmetry

An autoradiograph of a brachytherapy source reveals distribution of activity as well as active length (Fig. 15.2). The symmetry of the source loading within the capsule may be ascertained by taking a simulator radiograph of the source but leaving it on the film for an appropriate length of time to obtain an autoradiograph. The superposition of the autoradiograph and transmission radiograph provides the required information on source symmetry relative to the physical ends of the sources.

All sources should be checked for source uniformity and symmetry. In addition, one randomly chosen source from each group of designated strength may be autoradiographed to obtain isooptical density curves. This will document symmetry of dose distribution around these sources.

Source Calibration

All sources should be individually calibrated to check source strength specified by the vendor. Methods of source calibration were discussed in section 15.2. A well ionization chamber (e.g., a dose calibrator) is convenient for these calibration checks. A standard source of the same radionuclide and construction having a calibration traceable to NIST is required for these measurements. If the disagreement between the vendor and the user calibration is within $\pm 5\%$, the vendor calibration should be used unless the user's calibration is deemed more accurate than the vendor's. In the latter case, the user's methodology and results of calibration must be fully documented and justification provided for not using the vendor's calibration. Differences larger than $\pm 5\%$ are not acceptable and would require recalibration by the vendor and issuance of a new calibration certificate.

Applicator Evaluation

Applicators for intracavitary application are constructed to hold the sources in a specified geometry. Some applicators (e.g., Fletcher-Suit) have strategically placed lead or tungsten shields to reduce the dose to the rectum and the bladder. Acceptance testing of these applicators is essential to ensure proper source placement and protection of critical structures by the shields.

The internal structure of applicators may be examined by orthogonal radiographs using a 4- or 6-MV x-ray beam. Dummy sources may be inserted to check the position of sources in the applicator. The position of shields should be compared with the vendor's drawings. Mechanical functions such as the ease of source loading and removal should also be checked before accepting the applicators.

C.2. Interstitial Sources

Sources for interstitial implant in the form of needles (e.g., cesium-137) can be tested in the same way as the intracavitary sources described above. For calibration checks, needles of the same radionuclide and construction should be used to obtain a calibration factor for the well ionization chamber. All sources should be individually checked before commissioning into clinical use.

Short-lived interstitial sources in the form of seeds, wires, or seed-loaded ribbons can be tested by visual inspection (behind a leaded glass window) and calibration can be checked with a dose calibrator, as described in the previous section. For a batch of a large number of sources (e.g., ^{192}Ir ribbons), a randomly selected sample of three or four ribbons of a given strength should be checked for calibration. A standard seed of the same kind (with calibration traceable to the NIST) should be used to calibrate the well ionization chamber. Because ribbons of different lengths are used, the ion chamber response should be corrected as a function of ribbon length. These correction factors can be established by using the standard seed and measuring chamber response as a function of seed position in the well ionization chamber.

The calibration check of ^{125}I seeds is difficult because of the low energy of the emitted photons. Unless suitable equipment is available for checking ^{125}I seed calibration, the institution may accept the vendor's calibration. However, the vendor's calibration methodology should be reviewed to ensure that the calibration is performed with an appropriate instrument with a calibration factor traceable to NIST. The vendor's calibration service may be checked by obtaining a repeat calibration of a seed by NIST or an ADCL.

D. Remote Afterloaders

Acceptance procedures for remote afterloading equipment have been discussed by several investigators (32–35) and reviewed by Glasgow et al. (36). The procedures may be broadly divided into (a) operational testing of the afterloading unit, (b) radiation safety check of the facility, (c) checking of source calibration and transport, and (d) checking of treatment planning software. Although the details are presented by Glasgow et al., some of the recommendations are listed in Table 17.6. Most of the acceptance test

TABLE 17.6. ACCEPTANCE TESTING PROCEDURES FOR REMOTE AFTERLOADERS

Functional performance
a. *Console functions.* Main power, battery power, source on/off, door open/close, etc.
b. *Source control.* Source dwell time and source retraction at the end of preset time, unplanned interruption or emergency shutoff
c. *Battery voltage.* Adequacy of battery voltage under load conditions and functional performance under battery power
d. *Timer.* Timer accuracy and end-time effects
e. *Decay correction.* Accuracy of computer-calculated decay corrections
f. *Multichannel indexer.* Proper source sequencing and channel selection
g. *Backup systems.* Proper functioning during simulated power failures or air pressure losses (for pneumatically driven devices)
h. *Radiation detectors.* Proper functioning as specified

Facility check and survey
a. *Door interlocks.* Source retracts when the door is opened; the unit does not start until the door is closed and the interlock is reset
b. *Radiation warning lights.* Proper functioning to indicate radiation on/off condition
c. *Patient viewing and communication.* Proper functioning of closed-circuit TV and the intercommunication system
d. *Radiation survey.* Exposure rates outside the radiation facility should meet the NRC regulations and the leakage radiation rates around the unit should be acceptable (see chapter 16)

Source calibration and transport
Check of source specifications, leak testing, calibration, transport to the applicators, autoradiograph of simulated source positions, and isodose distribution to determine dose anisotropy

procedures consist of testing the unit for its functional performance and safety features, usually covered in the operator's manual. These can be simply carried out by activating various functions and observing the results. The accuracy of source localization and calibration can be checked using procedures that are more or less similar to those used for conventional brachytherapy. Considerations specific to remote afterloaders are discussed below.

D.1. Source Positioning

Source position accuracy can be checked by taking radiographs of dummy sources in the applicators with their positions marked on a ready pack film and combining with autoradiographs of the radioactive sources in the same applicators. The position of dummy sources and radioactive sources should correspond within ± 1 mm.

Special test devices have been designed to test source positioning by autoradiography (34,35,37). Figure 17.8A shows a test phantom designed by Aldrich and Samant (37). The system consists of an acrylic plate with channels drilled to hold the treatment catheters. Lead sheets of dimensions 20 × 20 × 0.8 mm are accurately set into one surface at a regular spacing of 20 mm. The phantom is placed on a ready pack XV2 film with lead sheets facing the film. The sources are programmed to stop every 10 mm for intervals suitable for autoradiography. The autoradiograph thus obtained shows source positions together with

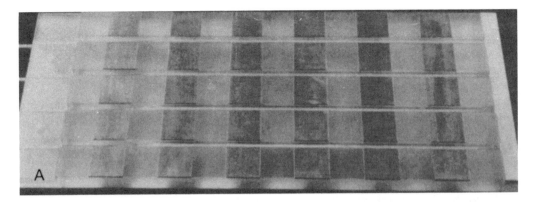

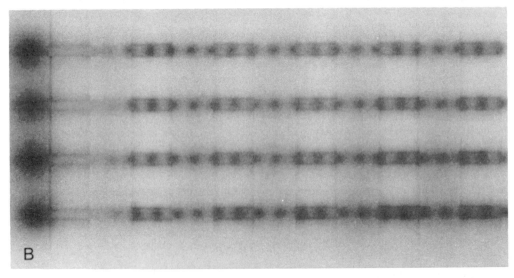

FIG. 17.8. Quality control test for HDR remote afterloaders. **A:** Test phantom to check the accuracy of source positioning. **B:** Autoradiograph of the test phantom showing dwell positions. (From Aldrich JE, Samant S. A test phantom for HDR daily quality control. *Activity* 1992;6:82, with permission.)

fiducial markers provided by the edges of lead sheets (Fig. 17.8B). An accuracy of ± 1 mm in the source positions is acceptable.

D.2. Source Calibration

The LDR sources in remote afterloading units can be calibrated in a well ionization chamber as described by the AAPM Report 13 (2) and in Chapter 15 of this book. The well ionization chamber must bear a calibration for the same kind and specification of source as the given LDR source.

For the calibration of HDR sources, the well ionization chamber must be capable of measuring large currents associated with these sources. Goetsch et al. (38) have described such a chamber for use with ^{192}Ir HDR sources. Calibration of well-type ionization chambers suitable for calibrating HDR sources is available at some ADCLs (University of Wisconsin and K&S Associates, Inc.).

A cylindrical lead insert for a conventional well-ionization chamber (e.g., dose calibrator) has also been used to reduce the ionization current from an HDR source to a measurable value (36). It is important to check the accuracy of such a system by an independent calibration.

Cylindrical ion chambers (e.g., Farmer-type or larger volume, depending on source strength) can be used to calibrate LDR and HDR sources using a free-air geometry (Chapter 15). The ion chamber must be fitted with an appropriate build-up cap and bear a calibration for photon energies emitted by the radionuclide. Goetsch et al. (39) have described an interpolative method of obtaining exposure calibration factor for the chamber. For ^{192}Ir, the calibration factor is obtained by interpolating between factors for ^{137}Cs and 250 kVp x-rays. Ezzell (40) has described a method of interpolating chamber factors for ^{60}Co with a build-up cap and 250 kVp without a cap to obtain chamber factor for ^{192}Ir. Until NIST develops a direct method of chamber calibration with ^{192}Ir, the AAPM (36) recommends this interpolative technique.

17.7. COMMISSIONING

Most equipment is ready for clinical use after acceptance testing. However, some equipment requires additional data before it can be used in conjunction with patient treatments. For example, a linear accelerator cannot be used for patient treatments until it has been calibrated and all the beam data and necessary parameters for treatment planning have been obtained. These data are then input into a treatment-planning computer in accordance with the software requirements. The computer-generated dose distributions are checked against measured data and/or manually calculated distributions. After all the necessary beam data have been acquired and adopted to the treatment-planning system, the machine can be released or *commissioned* for clinical use.

Commissioning of a linear accelerator is the responsibility of the medical physicist. The machine should not be used for patient treatments until the physicist has declared it commissioned. Because of different beam modalities and energies, it may not be possible to commission the machine in one step. For example, commissioning may be done for photon beams while data are being acquired on electron beams. However, because commissioning takes long periods for machine use and apparatus set-up, it is better not to release the machine for clinical use until all the commissioning has been completed.

A. Linear Accelerator

Table 17.7 gives a list of typical data that are required for commissioning a linear accelerator. Details of various measurement procedures have been discussed in the previous chapters.

TABLE 17.7. COMMISSIONING DATA FOR A LINEAR ACCELERATOR

Data	Description
Calibration	Dose per monitor unit calibration of all modalities and energies according to current protocol
Depth dose	Central axis depth-dose distribution for all modalities and energies, sufficient number of field sizes to allow interpolation of data and all available electron cones
Profiles	Transverse, longitudinal, and diagonal dose profiles for all modalities and energies at d_{max} for electrons and selected depths for photons (e.g., d_{max}, 5, 10, and 20 cm); all cones for electrons and selected field sizes for photons (e.g., 5 × 5, 10 × 10, and 40 × 40 cm)
Isodose distribution	Isodose curves for all modalities and energies, all cones for electrons and selected field sizes for photons (e.g., 5 × 5, 10 × 10, 40 × 40 cm), all wedge filters for selected field sizes (e.g., 5 × 5, 10 × 10, maximum)
Output factors	$S_{c,p}$, S_c, and S_p factors as a function of field size for all photon energies: output factors for all electron energies, cones, and standard inserts; tray transmission factors and wedge transmission factors
Off-axis ratios	A table of off-axis ratios for all photon energies as a function of distance from central axis; these data may be obtained from dose profiles for a 5 × 40-cm field at selected depths (e.g., d_{max}, 5, 10, 20 cm)
Inverse square law	Verification of inverse square law for all photon energies, virtual source position for all electron energies, and effective SSD for all electron energies and cones
Tissue-phantom ratios	Direct measurement of TPRs/TMRs for all photon energies and selected field sizes (e.g. 5 × 5, 10 × 10, 40 × 40 cm) and depths (5, 10, 30 cm) for verification of values calculated from percent depth doses
Surface and buildup dose	For all photon energies and selected field sizes (5 × 5, 10 × 10, 30 × 30, and 40 × 40 cm), percent surface dose for all electron energies for a 10 × 10-cm cone
Treatment-planning system	Beam data input, generation, and verification of central axis percent depth dose and tissue-phantom/tissue-maximum ratio tables; sample isodose curves (e.g. 5 × 5, 10 × 10, maximum) for unwedged, wedged, asymmetric and blocked fields; sample isodose curves for multiple field plans using rectangular and elliptical contours; electron beam depth dose data, isodose curves for all cones and sample isodose curves on rectangular and circular contours
Special dosimetry	Data for special techniques such as total body irradiation, total skin irradiation, stereotactic radiosurgery, intraoperative electron therapy, etc.

Commissioning is complete only after the beam data have been input into the treatment-planning computer and the computer-generated dose distributions have been checked.

A.1. Central Axis Depth-dose Tables

The percent depth dose and TPR/TMR tables may be prepared manually by interpolation of the measured data or generated by the computer. The measured and the computer-generated depth-dose distributions for all clinically used depths and field sizes should agree within ±2% (preferably ±1%).

A.2. Isodose Curves

The measured and computer-generated isodose curves should agree within ±2% in the central part of the field (e.g., up to about 1 cm inside the field edge) and within about 2 mm in the penumbra region (e.g., between 90% and 20% decrement lines). The same criteria apply to the wedge isodose curves, except that the computer algorithms usually are not as accurate near the thin edges of the wedges. Also, some algorithms may not accurately calculate the beam-hardening correction, which needs to be applied as a function of depth and field size.

A.3. Monitor Unit Calculations

Calculation of monitor units to deliver a certain dose at a point at depth on the central axis (e.g., isocenter) requires a number of dosimetric quantities measured as part of commissioning. A final check of the formalism (Chapter 10) should be made to ascertain that doses can be accurately delivered at a point for a given energy, field size, and depth. It is important to establish the accuracy of the relationship between calibration and the dose to be delivered at any point in the patient.

B. Treatment-planning Computer System

Acceptance testing and commissioning of the treatment-planning computer system have been discussed by a few investigators (41–45). Procedures have been described for testing both hardware and software. The hardware tests include, but are not limited to, checking the accuracy and linearity of input digitizers, output plotters, and printers. The software tests pertain to checking the accuracy of dose distributions for a selected set of treatment conditions against measured distributions or manual calculations.

Another important aspect of commissioning of a treatment-planning computer is the algorithm verification—its accuracy, precision, limitations, and special features. It is imperative for the user to understand the algorithm as it pertains to beam generation, normalization, beam weights, contour corrections, field blocking, off-axis distribution, asymmetric collimation, tissue heterogeneities, wedged beams, blocked wedged beams, etc. It is the responsibility of the medical physicist to oversee proper use of the system and interpretation of the treatment plan.

Brachytherapy software commissioning includes testing of the linear source and seed programs. Dose distributions around individual sources should be generated and compared with published tables. An agreement of ± 2% in dose rates and published tables is acceptable, excluding anisotropy or extreme oblique filtration conditions. Special attention should be directed to the units of source strength, filtration, tissue attenuation, source anisotropy, and other relevant features of the program that affects the accuracy of dose distribution or the interpretation of the treatment plan. Multiple source distributions should be checked by manual calculations for typical intracavitary and interstitial implant conditions.

17.8. PERIODIC QUALITY ASSURANCE

A periodic quality assurance program is designed to maintain the system within its acceptable performance standards. The program is usually designed to conduct tests similar to acceptance testing on a regular basis. The type and frequency of testing is dictated primarily by the probability of occurrence of a particular performance error, its clinical impact, and the time required for performing the test. Because the amount of testing required to make the equipment absolutely error-proof is unlimited, practical and logistic considerations play an important part in designing a periodic QA program. The guiding principle is to follow national or international standards if they exist. If formal standards do not exist, the institution should design its own program by consulting relevant literature, manufacturer's manuals, and other equipment users. Moreover, a QA program should be reviewed on a regular basis (e.g., annually) to incorporate ideas from new protocols, the user's experience, and the experience of other users.

A. Linear Accelerator

Periodic quality assurance for linear accelerator has been discussed by the AAPM (2,8). Institutions should carry out this program at the recommended frequency to maintain conformity with the national standards. Some tests or their frequency may have to be

TABLE 17.8. PERIODIC QA OF LINEAR ACCELERATORS

Frequency	Procedure	Tolerance[a]
Daily	**Dosimetry**	
	X-ray output constancy	3%
	Electron output constancy[b]	3%
	Mechanical	
	Localizing lasers	2 mm
	Distance indicator (ODI)	2 mm
	Safety	
	Door interlock	Functional
	Audiovisual monitor	Functional
Monthly	**Dosimetry**	
	x-ray output constancy[c]	2%
	Electron output constancy[c]	2%
	Backup monitor constancy	2%
	x-ray central axis dosimetry parameter (PDD, TAR) constancy	2%
	Electron central axis dosimetry parameter constancy (PDD)	2 mm at therapeutic depth
	x-ray beam flatness constancy	2%
	Electron beam flatness constancy	3%
	x-ray and electron symmetry	3%
	Safety interlocks	
	Emergency off switches	Functional
	Wedge, electron cone interlocks	Functional
	Mechanical checks	
	Light/radiation field coincidence	2 mm or 1% on a side[d]
	Gantry/collimator angle indicators	1°
	Wedge position	2 mm (or 2% change in transmission factor)
	Tray position	2 mm
	Applicator position	2 mm
	Field size indicators	2 mm
	Cross-hair centering	2 mm diameter
	Treatment couch position indicators	2 mm/1°
	Latching of wedges, blocking tray	Functional
	Jaw symmetry[e]	2 mm
	Field light intensity	Functional
Annual	**Dosimetry**	
	x-ray/electron output calibration constancy	2%
	Field size dependence of x-ray output constancy	2%
	Output factor constancy for electron applicators	2%
	Central axis parameter constancy (PDD, TAR)	2%
	Off-axis factor constancy	2%
	Transmission factor constancy for all treatment accessories	2%
	Wedge transmission factor constancy[f]	2%
	Monitor chamber linearity	1%
	x-ray output constancy vs gantry angle	2%
	Electron output constancy vs gantry angle	2%
	Off-axis factor constancy vs gantry angle	2%
	Arc mode	Mfrs. specs.
	Safety interlocks	
	Follow manufacturers test procedures	Functional
	Mechanical checks	
	Collimator rotation isocenter	2 mm diameter
	Gantry rotation isocenter	2 mm diameter
	Couch rotation isocenter	2 mm diameter
	Coincidence of collimetry, gantry, couch axes with isocenter	2 mm diameter
	Coincidence of radiation and mechanical isocenter	2 mm diameter
	Table top sag	2 mm
	Vertical travel of table	2 mm

[a]The tolerances listed in the tables should be interpreted to mean that if a parameter either: (1) exceeds the tabulated value (e.g., the measured isocenter under gantry rotation exceeds 2 mm diameter); or (2) that the change in the parameter exceeds the nominal value (e.g., the output changes by more than 2%), then an action is required. The distinction is emphasized by the use of the term constancy for the latter case. Moreover, for constancy, percent values are ± the deviation of the parameter with respect its nominal value; distances are referenced to the isocenter or nominal SSD.
[b]All electron energies need not be checked daily, but all electron energies are to be checked at least twice weekly.
[c]A constancy check with a field instrument using temperature/pressure corrections.
[d]Whichever is greater. Should also be checked after change in light field source.
[e]Jaw symmetry is defined as difference in distance of each jaw from the isocenter.
[f]Most wedges' transmission factors are field size and depth dependent.
From AAPM. Comprehensive QA for radiation oncology: report of the AAPM Radiation Therapy Committee Task Group 40. *Med Phys* 1994;21:581–618, with permission.

modified to take into account certain unique characteristics of a given accelerator. However, these modifications should be made with the intention of improving the QA program rather than cutting corners.

All QA measurements must be entered in log books. This is important not only in following machine performance over the years but also because it is a legal record that documents the operational health of the machine for any time in which patients were treated.

A procedure must be in place to deal with incidents in which significant deviation in the machine performance is noted. For example, if output calibration (dose/MU) changes

TABLE 17.9. PERIODIC QA OF COBALT-60 UNITS

Frequency	Procedure	Tolerance[a]
Daily	Safety	
	Door interlock	Functional
	Radiation room monitor	Functional
	Audiovisual monitor	Functional
	Mechanical	
	Lasers	2 mm
	Distance indicator (ODI)	2 mm
Weekly	Check of source positioning	3 mm
Monthly	Dosimetry	
	Output constancy	2%
	Mechanical checks	
	Light/radiation field coincidence	3 mm
	Field size indicator (collimator setting)	2 mm
	Gantry and collimator angle indicator	1°
	Cross-hair centering	1 mm
	Latching of wedges, trays	Functional
	Safety interlocks	
	Emergency off	Functional
	Wedge interlocks	Functional
Annual	Dosimetry	
	Output constancy	2%
	Field size dependence of output constancy	2%
	Central axis dosimetry parameter constancy (PDD/TAR)	2%
	Transmission factor constancy for all standard accessories	2%
	Wedge transmission factor constancy	2%
	Timer linearity and error	1%
	Output constancy vs gantry angle	2%
	Beam uniformity vs gantry angle	3%
	Safety interlocks	
	Follow test procedures of manufacturers	Functional
	Mechanical checks	
	Collimator rotation isocenter	2 mm diameter
	Gantry rotation isocenter	2 mm diameter
	Couch rotation isocenter	2 mm diameter
	Coincidence of collim., gantry, couch axis with isocenter	2 mm diameter
	Coincidence of radiation and mechanical isocenter	2 mm diameter
	Table top sag	2 mm
	Vertical travel of table	2 mm
	Field-light intensity	Functional

[a]The tolerances listed in the tables should be interpreted to mean that if a parameter either: (1) exceeds the tabulated value (e.g., the measured isocenter under gantry rotation exceeds 2 mm diameter); or (2) that the change in the parameter exceeds the nominal value (e.g., the output changes by more than 2%), then an action is required. The distinction is emphasized by the use of the term constancy for the latter case. Moreover, for constancy, percent values are ± the deviation of the parameter with respect to its nominal value; distances are referenced to the isocenter or nominal SSD. From AAPM. Comprehensive QA for radiation oncology: report of the AAPM Radiation Therapy Committee Task Group 40. *Med Phys* 1994;21:581–618, with permission.

TABLE 17.10. PERIODIC QA OF SIMULATORS

Frequency	Procedure	Tolerance[a]
Daily	Localizing lasers	2 mm
	Distance indicator (ODI)	2 mm
Monthly	Field size indicator	2 mm
	Gantry/collimator angle indicators	1°
	Cross-hair centering	2 mm diameter
	Focal spot-axis indicator	2 mm
	Fluoroscopic image quality	Baseline
	Emergency/collision avoidance	Functional
	Light/radiation field coincidence	2 mm or 1%
	Film processor sensitometry	Baseline
Annual	Mechanical checks	
	Collimator rotation isocenter	2 mm diameter
	Gantry rotation isocenter	2 mm diameter
	Couch rotation isocenter	2 mm diameter
	Coincidence of collimator, gantry, couch axes and isocenter	2 mm diameter
	Table top sag	2 mm
	Vertical travel of couch	2 mm
	Radiographic checks	
	Exposure rate	Baseline
	Table top exposure with fluoroscopy	Baseline
	Kvp and mAs calibration	Baseline
	High and low contrast resolution	Baseline

[a]The tolerances mean that the parameter exceeds the tabulated value (e.g., the measured isocenter under gantry rotation exceeds 2 mm diameter).
From AAPM. Comprehensive QA for radiation oncology: report of the AAPM Radiation Therapy Committee Task Group 40. *Med Phys* 1994;21:581–618, with permission.

suddenly, this should be investigated thoroughly before calibration pots are adjusted to bring the machine into correct calibration. Checks with another dosimeter system and/or by another physicist may be necessary to verify the change. Changes in output calibration can also occur due to detuning of the machine or changes in beam flatness. All these factors should be checked before adjusting the calibration. If the calibration change is unusually large (beyond an occasional drift), the matter should be thoroughly investigated and discussed with the manufacturer. Monitor chambers could get unsealed, which could cause calibration to change. In short, the QA program must be designed so that significant changes in machine performance receive prompt attention and investigation to determine the cause of the malfunction.

Table 17.8 is based on the AAPM recommended list of various tests, the frequency with which they should be performed and the acceptable limit of variation. The annual *full* calibration should include output calibration in accordance with the current protocol, central axis depth dose curves for selected field sizes, beam profiles at selected depths and field sizes, output factors, check of inverse square law, tray factors, wedge factors, and other parameters that are not covered in the tests on a more frequent basis.

B. Cobalt-60 Unit

Quality assurance of cobalt-60 teletherapy should be similar to that of a linear accelerator except that some aspects of the QA are mandated by the Nuclear Regulatory Commission (46). Table 17.9 contains the NRC requirements as well as recommendations by the AAPM. Greater details on this subject are provided by the American National Standards Institute (ANSI) (47).

As discussed in Chapter 16, the NRC requires full calibration of a teletherapy unit: (a) before the first medical use of the unit; (b) whenever spot-check measurements differ by more than 5% from the output at the last full calibration, corrected for radioactive decay;

(c) following replacement of the source or relocation of the unit; (d) following repairs that could affect the source exposure assembly; and (e) at intervals not exceeding 1 year.

The NRC requirements for full calibration checks include (a) output being within $\pm 3\%$ for the range of field sizes and distances used clinically, (b) coincidence of radiation and light fields, (c) uniformity of radiation field and its dependence on the orientation of the radiation field, (d) timer constancy and linearity over the range of use, (e) on-off error, and (f) accuracy of all distance measuring and localization devices in medical use.

C. Simulator

Geometric accuracy of a simulator must be comparable with that of the linear accelerator. Therefore, the simulator is subjected to the same QA checks as the accelerator except for the checks related to the image quality of the former and the dosimetry of the later. A formal periodic QA program for simulators has been proposed by the AAPM (8), which contains specific recommendations on the subject (Table 17.10).

REFERENCES

1. ACR. *Physical aspects of quality assurance.* Reston, VA: American College of Radiology, 1990.
2. AAPM. Physical aspects of quality assurance in radiation therapy. Report No. 13. Colchester, VT: AIDC, 1984.
3. ACMP. Radiation control and quality assurance in radiation oncology: a suggested protocol. Report No. 2. Reston, VA: American College of Medical Physics, 1986.
4. Hank GE, Herring DF, Kramer S. The need for complex technology in radiation oncology: correlations of facility characteristics and structure with outcome. *Cancer* 1985;55:2198.
5. Peters LJ. Departmental support for a quality assurance program. In: Starkschall G, Horton J, eds. *Quality assurance in radiotherapy physics.* Madison, WI: Medical Physics, 1991:105.
6. ISCRO. Radiation oncology in integrated cancer management: report of the Inter-Society Council for Radiation Oncology. Reston, VA: American College of Radiology, 1991.
7. ACR. Quality assurance program in radiation oncology. Reston, VA: American College of Radiology, 1989.
8. AAPM. Comprehensive QA for radiation oncology: report of the Radiation Therapy Task Group 40. *Med Phys* 1994;21:581–618.
9. AAPM. Essentials and guidelines for hospital-based medical physics residency training programs. Report No. 36. Colchester, VT: AIDC, 1990.
10. Khan FM. Residency training for medical physicists. *Med Phys* 1991;18:339.
11. Khan FM. Residency training for medical physicists. *Int J Radiat Oncol Biol Phys* 1992;24:853.
12. AAPM. The roles, responsibilities, and status for the clinical medical physicist. Colchester, VT: AIDC, 1986.
13. AAPM. The role of a physicist in radiation oncology. Report No. 38. Colchester, VT: AIDC, 1993.
14. Nath R, Biggs PJ, Bova FJ, et al. AAPM code of practice for radiotherapy accelerators: report of AAPM Radiation Therapy Task Group No. 45. *Med Phys* 1994;21:1093–1121.
15. ICRU. Determination of absorbed dose in a patient irradiated by beams of x or gamma rays in radiotherapy procedures. Report No. 24. Washington, DC: International Commission on Radiation Units and Measurements, 1976.
16. ICRU. Use of computers in external beam radiotherapy procedures with high energy photons and electrons. Report No. 42. Washington, DC: International Commission on Radiation Units and Measurements, 1988.
17. Lutz WR, Larsen RD, Bjärngard BE. Beam alignment tests for therapy accelerators. *Int J Radiat Oncol Biol Phys* 1981;7:1727.
18. Central axis depth dose data for use in radiotherapy. *Br J Radiol* 1983;[suppl 17].
19. AAPM. A protocol for the determination of absorbed dose from high energy photons and electron beams. *Med Phys* 1983;10:741.
20. NCRP. Dosimetry of x-ray and gamma ray beams for radiation therapy in the energy range of 10 keV to 50 MeV. Report No. 69. Bethesda, MD: National Council on Radiation Protection and Measurements, 1981.
21. Boyer AL. QA foundations in equipment specifications, acceptance testing, and commissioning. In: Starkschall G, Horton J, eds. *Quality assurance in radiotherapy physics.* Madison, WI: Medical Physics, 1991:5.
22. Boge RJ, Tolbert DD, Edland RW. Accessory beam flattening filter for the Varian Clinac-4 linear accelerator. *Radiology* 1975;115:475.
23. Khan FM, Doppke K, Hogstrom KR, et al. Clinical electron-beam dosimetry. Report of the AAPM Radiation Therapy Committee Task Group No. 25. *Med Phys* 1991;18:73.

24. McCullough EC, Earl JD. The selection, acceptance testing, and quality control of radiotherapy simulators. *Radiology* 1979;131:221.

25. Connors SG, Battista JJ, Bertin RJ. On technical specifications of radiotherapy simulators. *Med Phys* 1984;11:341.

26. IEC. Functional performance characteristics of radiotherapy simulators. Draft Report. Geneva: International Electrotechnical Commission, Subcommittee 62C, 1990.

27. Suntharalingam N. Quality assurance of radiotherapy localizer/simulators. In: Starkschall G, Horton J, eds. *Quality assurance in radiotherapy physics.* Madison, WI: Medical Physics, 1991:61.

28. Bomford CK, et al. Treatment simulators. *Br J Radiol* 1989;[suppl 23]:1–49.

29. NCRP. Quality assurance for diagnostic imaging equipment. Report No. 99. Bethesda, MD: National Council on Radiation Protection and Measurements, 1988.

30. *Customer acceptance test procedure for Ximatron C-series.* Palo Alto, CA: Varian Associates, 1990.

31. IEC. Medical electron accelerators, functional performance, characteristics. Geneva: International Electrotechnical Commission, Subcommittee 62C, 1988.

32. Grigsby PW. Quality assurance of remote afterloading equipment at the Mallinckrodt Institute of Radiology. *Selectron Brachytherapy* 1989;1:15.

33. Flynn A. Quality assurance check on a MicroSelection-HDR. *Selectron Brachytherapy* 1990;4:112.

34. Jones CH. Quality assurance in brachytherapy using the Selectron LDR/MDR and MicroSelectron-HDR. *Selectron Brachytherapy* 1990;4:48.

35. Ezzell GA. Acceptance testing and quality assurance of high dose rate afterloading systems. In: Martinez AA, Orton CG, Mould RF, eds. *Brachytherapy HDR and LDR.* Columbia, MD: Nucletron, 1990:138.

36. AAPM. Remote afterloading technology. Report No. 41. Colchester, VT: AIDC, 1993.

37. Aldrich JE, Samant S. A test phantom for HDR daily quality control. *Activity* 1992;6:82.

38. Goetsch SJ, Attix FH, DeWerd LA, et al. A new re-entrant ionization chamber for the calibration of Ir-192 HDR sources. *Int J Radiat Oncol Biol Phys* 1992;24:167.

39. Goetsch SJ, Attix FH, Pearson DW, et al. Calibration of ^{192}Ir high dose rate afterloading systems. *Med Phys* 1991;18:462.

40. Ezzell GA. Evaluation of calibration technique for a high dose rate remote afterloading iridium-192 source. *Endocuriether Hyperthermia Oncol* 1990;6:101.

41. Rosenow UF, Dannhausen HW, Lubbert K, et al. Quality assurance in treatment planning: report from the German Task Group. In: Bruinvis IAD, Van der Giessen PH, van Kleffens HJ, et al., eds. *Proceedings of the ninth international conference on the use of computers in radiotherapy.* Silver Spring, MD: IEEE Computer Society, 1987.

42. Jacky J, White CP. Testing a 3-D radiation therapy planning program. *Int J Radiat Oncol Biol Phys* 1990;18:253.

43. Curran B, Starkschall G. A program for quality assurance of dose planning computers. In: Starkschall G, Horton J, eds. *Quality assurance in radiotherapy physics.* Madison, WI: Medical Physics, 1991:207.

44. Van Dyk J, Barnett R, Cygler J, et al. Commissioning and QA of treatment planning computers. *Int J Radiat Oncol Biol Phys* 1993;26:261–273.

45. Fraas BA. Quality assurance for 3-D treatment planning. In: Mackie TR, Palta JR, eds. *Teletherapy: present and future.* Madison, WI: Advanced Medical Publishing 1996:253–302.

46. NRC. Code of federal regulations. 10 CFR Part 0–50. Washington, DC: U.S. Government Printing Office, 1993.

47. American National Standards Institute. Guidelines for maintaining cobalt-60 and cesium-137 teletherapy equipment. ANSI N449.1–1974. New York: ANSI, 1974.

18

TOTAL BODY IRRADIATION

Total body irradiation (TBI) with megavoltage photon beams is most commonly used as part of the conditioning regimen for bone marrow transplantation which is used in the treatment of a variety of diseases such as leukemia, aplastic anemia, lymphoma, multiple myeloma, autoimmune diseases, inborn errors of metabolism, and so on. The role of TBI is to destroy the recipient's bone marrow and tumor cells, and to immunosuppress the patient sufficiently to avoid rejection of the donor bone marrow transplant. Usually the patient undergoes a chemotherapy conditioning program before the TBI and bone marrow transplant. Although chemotherapy alone can be used as a conditioning regimen, addition of TBI is considered beneficial for certain diseases and clinical conditions. For example, TBI allows the delivery of a homogeneous dose to the entire body including "sanctuary areas" where chemotherapy may not be effective. Also, selected parts of the body (e.g., lungs, kidneys, head) can be shielded, if desired.

18.1. TECHNIQUES AND EQUIPMENT

Numerous techniques have been used to deliver TBI. Details of some of the commonly used techniques and the associated dosimetry are discussed in the literature (1–5). The choice of a particular technique depends on the available equipment, photon beam energy, maximum possible field size, treatment distance, dose rate, patient dimensions, and the need to selectively shield certain body structures. An anteroposterior (AP/PA) technique generally provides a better dose uniformity along the longitudinal body axis but the patient positioning, other than standing upright, may pose problems. Bilateral TBI (treating from left and right) can be more comfortable to the patient if seated or laying down supine on a TBI couch, but presents greater variation in body thickness along the path of the beam. Compensators are required to achieve dose uniformity along the body axis to within +10%, although extremities and some noncritical structures may exceed this specification.

A. Beam Energy

Lower energy megavoltage beams (e.g., cobalt-60) have been used to deliver TBI, especially for protocols involving low dose rate of 5 to 10 cGy/min. A review of these techniques and the modifications required to achieve large homogeneous fields with these machines is summarized in the AAPM Report No. 17 (3). Because linear accelerator is the most commonly used equipment for radiation therapy, current TBI techniques have been adopted for linacs. The choice of photon beam energy is dictated by patient thickness and the specification of dose homogeneity. In addition to the thickness variation along the axis of the patient, the patient diameter along the path of beam also affects dose uniformity, depending upon beam energy. As discussed in Chapter 11, Section 11.5A, the thicker the patient, the higher is the beam energy required to produce acceptable dose uniformity for parallel-opposed fields. A term *tissue lateral effect* has been used to describe the situation in

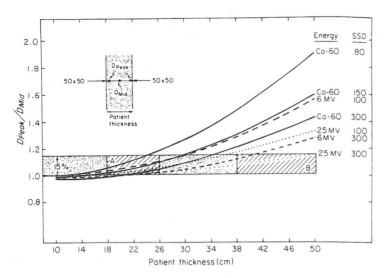

FIG. 18.1. A plot of the ratio of dose at d_{max} to that at the midplane as a function of patient thickness for a number of beam energies. The shaded region represents a 15% spread in the ratio. Regions A and B represent the range of adult patient thickness in the AP and lateral directions, respectively. SSD, source-to-surface distance in centimeters. (From American Association of Physicists in Medicine. The physical aspects of total and half body photon irradiation. AAPM Report No. 17. Colchester, VT: AIDC, 1986, with permission.)

which lower energy or a thicker patient treated with parallel-opposed beams can give rise to an excessively higher dose to the subcutaneous tissues compared with the midpoint dose. Figure 18.1 shows that the ratio of the maximum dose to the midline dose is a function of energy and patient thickness when parallel-opposed beams are used. Not considering the initial dose build-up effect, it is seen that higher the beam energy, greater is the dose uniformity for any thickness patient. If the maximum thickness of the patient parallel to the beam central axis is less than 35 cm and source-to-surface dose (SSD) is at least 300 cm, a 6-MV beam can be used for parallel-opposed TBI fields without increasing the peripheral dose to greater than 110% of the midline dose. For patients of thickness greater than 35 cm, energies higher than 6 MV should be used to minimize the tissue lateral effect.

B. Initial Dose Build-up

Surface or skin dose in megavoltage beams is substantially less than the dose at the point of maximum dose (D_{max}), as has been discussed in Chapter 13, Section 13.3. The dose build-up characteristics depend on many factors such as energy, field size, SSD, and beam angle relative to the surface. Dose build-up data obtained at normal SSDs (e.g., 100 cm) does not apply accurately at TBI distances (e.g., 400 cm) because of the longer distance and the intervening air (1). However, most TBI protocols do not require skin sparing. Instead, a bolus or a beam spoiler is specified to bring the surface dose to at least 90% of the prescribed TBI dose. A large spoiler screen of 1- to 2-cm thick acrylic is sufficient to meet these requirements, provided the screen is placed as close as possible to the patient surface.

C. Patient Support/Positioning Devices

Patient support and positioning devices are designed to implement a given treatment technique. Important criteria include patient comfort, stability, and reproducibility of set-up and treatment geometry that allows accurate calculation and delivery of dose in accordance with the TBI protocol. The following techniques are currently in use at the University of Minnesota and are presented here as examples. The associated equipment have been designed to meet various protocol criteria, based principally on two techniques: AP/PA and bilateral.

C.1. Bilateral Total Body Irradiation

A technique involving left and right lateral opposing fields with the patient seated on a couch in a semi-fetal position was designed by Khan et al. (1). Basic treatment geometry is

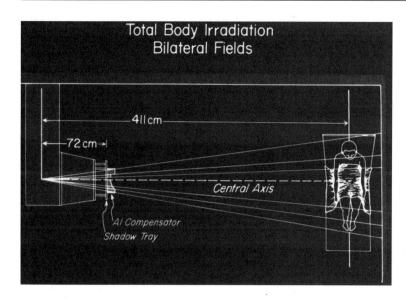

FIG. 18.2. Schematic diagram illustrating patient set-up geometry for the bilateral TBI technique. (From Khan FM, Williamson JF, Sewchand W, et al. Basic data for dosage calculation and compensation. *Int J Radiat Oncol Biol Phys* 1980;6:745–751, with permission.)

illustrated in Fig. 18.2. A special TBI couch allows the patient to be seated comfortably with the back supported and legs semi-collapsed as seen in Fig. 18.3. The arms are positioned laterally to follow the body contour and placed in contact with the body at the mid AP-thickness level. Care is taken to assure that the arms shadow the lungs instead of the spinal column located posteriorly. The patient set-up is recorded in terms of distances measured between external bony landmarks as shown in Fig. 18.4. The source-to-body axis distance is measured by a sagittal laser light installed in the ceiling to mark the TBI distance. The laser light also helps to position the patient's sagittal axis at right angles to the beam's central axis.

Lateral body thickness along the patient axis varies considerably in the bilateral TBI technique. To achieve dose uniformity within approximately +10% along the sagittal axis of the body, compensators are designed for head and neck, lungs (if needed), and legs. The reference thickness for compensation is the lateral diameter of the body at the level of umbilicus (not including the arms), assuming that the protocol specifies dose prescription to be at the midpoint at the level of umbilicus. Compensators can be designed out of any material, but at the University of Minnesota they are custom-made out of aluminum. A special tray and clamps are used to hold these compensators in place (Fig. 18.5). Field light

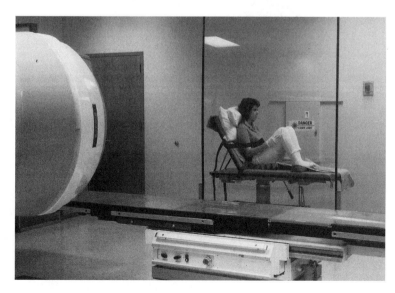

FIG. 18.3. Photograph demonstrating patient set-up on the TBI couch for the bilateral technique.

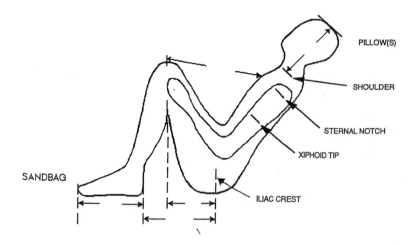

FIG. 18.4. Patient positioning measurements. (From Khan FM, Kim TH. Total body irradiation. In: Paliwal BR, Griem ML, eds. *Syllabus: a categorical course in radiation therapy.* Oakbrook, IL: Radiological Society of North America, 1986:111–116, with permission.)

is used to cast a shadow of the compensator onto the patient's body. Alignment is checked using shadows of positioning pegs on the compensators and the patient's reference bony landmarks.

C.2. AP/PA Total Body Irradiation

The patient is irradiated anteroposteriorly by parallel-opposed fields while positioned in a standing upright position at the TBI distance. This technique was developed at the Memorial Sloan Kettering Hospital in New York (6) and adopted at the University of Minnesota. Details of the technique and the modifications made to it to accommodate shielding of specific organs such as lungs, kidneys, and brain, are described by Dusenbery and Gerbi (5). The principle of the technique is that the standing TBI allows shielding of certain critical organs from photons and boosting of superficial tissues in the shadow of the blocks with electrons. For example, dose to the lungs can be reduced using lung blocks of about one half-value thickness and the chest wall under the blocks can be boosted with electrons of appropriate energy. For a special group of patients treated for inborn error of metabolism such as Hurler's syndrome, adrenoleukodystrophy and metachromatic leukodystrophy, TBI can be delivered AP/PA with the head turned sideways and the brain

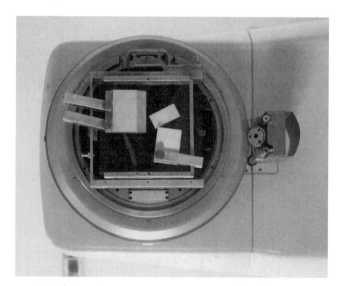

FIG. 18.5. Photograph of TBI compensators in actual use. Compensation pieces are mounted on the TBI tray inserted into head of the machine.

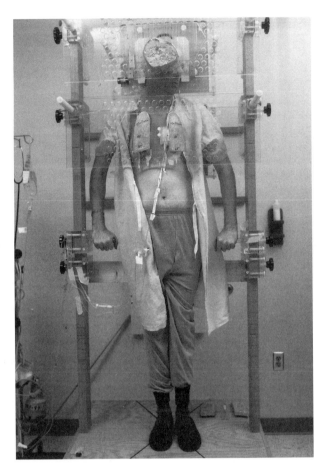

FIG. 18.6. Patient in the standing TBI position with the head turned sideways for shielding of the brain. A 5-HVL cerrobend block is mounted on an acrylic plate attached to the TBI stand. (From Dusenbery KE, Gerbi BJ. Total body irradiation in conditioning regimens for bone marrow transplantation. In: Levitt SH, Khan FM, Potish RA, et al., eds. Philadelphia: Lippincott Williams & Wilkins, 1999:499–518, with permission.)

shielded with five half-value layer blocks. The shielded skull area is then boosted with electrons of appropriate energy to spare the brain.

The AP/PA technique can also be adopted for treating small children in the reclining position. The patient is treated in the supine and posterior positions while laying down on a low-height couch, with the couch top only a few inches off the floor. The shielding blocks are placed on top of an acrylic box tray at a short distance from the patient's surface. The tray, which is about 1 cm thick, also acts as a beam spoiler to build up the skin dose to at least 90% of the prescription dose when treated with parallel-opposed TBI fields. Figures 18.6 and 18.7 show AP/PA technique for standing and reclining TBI, respectively.

D. Dosimetry Data

Details of machine calibration, dosimetry, and monitor unit calculation for TBI have been discussed in the literature (1–5). A direct output calibration of the machine for TBI may be performed by measuring dose per monitor unit using a 0.6 cm³ Farmer type ionization chamber placed in a water phantom of dimensions approximately 40 × 40 × 40 cm³. The position of the chamber is fixed at the TBI distance (source-to-body axis distance). The collimator is opened to its maximum size and the chamber depth is varied by moving the chamber and the phantom while keeping the source-to-chamber distance

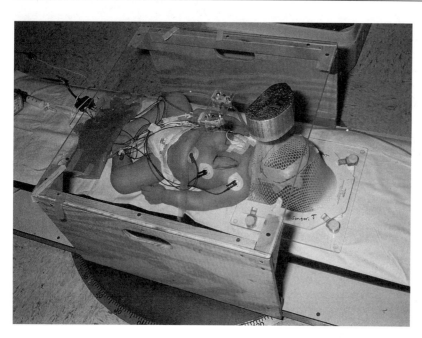

FIG. 18.7. Pediatric patient in the reclining TBI position on the floor. The legs are placed in the "frog legged" position to cover the entire patient in the radiation field with adequate margins. Brain-sparing shielding block is placed on top of an acrylic tray to shadow the central part of the skull with the head turned sideways.

constant (= TBI distance). A table of output factors (dose per MU) is generated as a function of depth that can be used to calculate monitor units for a patient of given midline depth at the prescription point. It is assumed in this case that the patient is dosimetrically equivalent to the phantom, which is not a bad approximation considering the fact that tissue maximal ratios (TMRs) for large fields (e.g., >30 × 30 cm) are not very sensitive to field dimensions.

Alternative to direct output factor measurements, is the calculation formalism based on TMRs, S_c, S_p, and the inverse square law factor (see Chapter 10). The basic equation to calculate dose per monitor unit (D/MU) is:

$$D/MU = k \cdot TMR(d, r_e) \cdot S_c(r_c) \cdot S_p(r_e) \cdot (f/f')^2 \cdot OAR(d) \cdot TF \qquad (18.1)$$

where D is dose in cGy, k is 1 cGy/MU under reference calibration conditions, TMR is the tissue-maximum ratio at depth d and field size equivalent to the patient (r_e), S_c is the collimator scatter factor for the field size projected at isocenter (r_c), S_p is the phantom scatter factor for the patient-equivalent field size (r_e), f is the source-to-calibration point distance, f' is the source-to-patient axis distance at the prescription point, OAR is off-axis ratio at depth d, and TF is the transmission factor for the block tray, beam spoiler or any other absorber placed between the machine diaphragm and the patient.

The equivalent field at the point of calculation means that it is dosimetrically equivalent to the patient in terms of scatter. In theory one could determine equivalent field by doing Clarkson integration (see Chapter 9) of a scatter function (e.g., scatter-air ratio, SAR, or scatter-maximum ratio, SMR) at the point of calculation in the patient and comparing it with the average scatter function calculated at the same depth for a square field in a water phantom. Such calculations done for a standard Rando phantom exposed to a TBI field have been reported in the literature (7) and are presented in Table 18.1. For example, for the umbilicus point, the Rando phantom-equivalent field is 28 × 28 cm on the average. Although patient dimensions vary, scatter factors are not too sensitive to field size variation for large fields. Therefore, it is reasonable to use a fixed equivalent field size for TBI. A 40 × 40 cm field for large patients and a 30 × 30 cm field for pediatric patients seem to be reasonable approximations (within approximately ±2% of dose accuracy).

The TMR data obtained under standard conditions (at isocenter) must be checked for its validity at the TBI distance. In addition, the inverse square law factor must also be verified for the TBI distance. Alternatively, D/MU calculated by Equation 18.1 using standard TMRs, S_c, S_p and inverse square law factors may be compared with directly

TABLE 18.1. EQUIVALENT FIELD AT VARIOUS POINTS OF CALCULATION IN A RANDO PHANTOM IRRADIATED WITH TBI FIELD USING DIFFERENT BEAM ENERGIES

Photon Energy	Side of Equivalent Square (cm)				
	Head	Neck	Chest	Umbilicus	Hips
Co-60	17	22	31	30	28
4 MV	16	20	30	29	23
6 MV	18	23	29	27	26
10 MV	17	22	33	27	26
18 MV	>18	>18	>18	>18	>18
Mean	17	22	31	28	26
Lateral dimension	15	12–16	31	27	31
Equivalent length	19	30	31	29	20

From Kirby HT, Hanson WF, Cates DA. Verification of total body photon irradiation dosimetry techniques. *Med Phys* 1988;15:364, with permission.

measured output factors (D/MU) at the TBI distance. If the difference is within +2%, Equation 18.1 may be used for TBI as it is used for regular isocentric treatments. Larger differences should be investigated and, if necessary, directly measured output factors at the TBI distance should be used.

E. Compensator Design

Most TBI protocols require dose homogeneity along the body axis to be within +10%. This requirement cannot be met without the use of compensators. General principles of compensator design have been discussed in Chapter 12. Compensator design for TBI is complicated because of large variation in body thickness, lack of complete body immobilization, and internal tissue heterogeneities. Considering only the lung inhomogeneity and change in body thickness, compensators can be designed to deliver the dose within acceptable uniformity.

The design of TBI compensators is discussed in the literature (1,3,8). The thickness of compensator required along a ray-line depends on the tissue deficit compared to the reference depth at the prescription point, material of the compensator (e.g., its density), distance of the compensator from the point of dose compensation, depth of the point of dose compensation, field size, and beam energy (see Chapter 12). Because the compensator is designed to be dosimetrically equivalent to a bolus (of thickness equal to the tissue deficit) but placed at a distance from the skin surface, the bolus-equivalent thickness of the compensator is reduced to compensate for reduction in scatter reaching the point of dose compensation. The required thickness of a tissue-equivalent compensator that gives the same dose at the point of interest as would a bolus of thickness equal to the tissue deficit, is called the thickness ratio (τ) (9). The τ depends on many variables but for TBI an average value of 0.70 provides a good approximation for all beam energies and compensation conditions (1). The overall dosimetric accuracy of a compensator is approximately +5% considering all variables (1,9).

The thickness of a compensator, t_c, at any point in the field is given by:

$$t_c = TD \cdot (\tau / \rho_c) \qquad (18.2)$$

where TD is the tissue deficit and ρ_c is the density of the compensator. Equation 18.2 gives compensator thickness based on tissue deficit at a given point but does not take into account cross-beam profile or off-axis ratio.

An alternative method of determining compensator thickness, t_c, at any point in the field is based on the following equations (3):

$$I / I_o = [T(A_R, d_R) / T(A, d)] \cdot OAR_d \qquad (18.3)$$

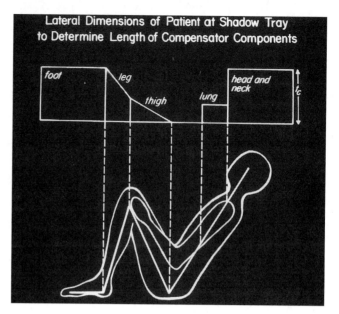

FIG. 18.8. Schematic diagram showing areas of compensation. (From Khan FM, Williamson JF, Sewchand W, et al. Basic data for dosage calculation and compensation. *Int J Radiat Oncol Biol Phys* 1980;6:745–751, with permission.)

and

$$I/I_o = \exp(-\mu_{\text{eff}} t_c) \tag{18.4}$$

where I_o and I are the doses administered before and after the compensator is added, $T(A_R, d_R)$ and $T(A,d)$ are the tissue-phantom ratios or TMRs for the reference body section and the section to be compensated for equivalent fields A_R and A at midline depths d_R and d, OAR_d is the off-axis ratio at depth d relative to the prescription point, and μ_{eff} is the effective linear attenuation coefficient for the compensator material measured under TBI conditions.

Depending on the tissue deficits encountered in a particular TBI technique (AP/PA or bilateral), compensator material should be selected so that the compensator is not too bulky or of too high a density that small errors in machining would amount to large errors in dose. Because of these and other practical considerations, aluminum compensators are used at the University of Minnesota. The compensators are designed in two dimensions (varying in thickness only along the sagittal body axis) and are held in the beam by clamps attached to a compensator tray (Figs. 18.5, 18.8).

Compensators can be designed not only to take into account tissue deficit but also tissue inhomogeneities such as lungs. In the latter case, a bulk density correction is used to calculate radiologic path length through the inhomogeneity.

F. In Vivo Patient Dosimetry

After a particular TBI technique has been established and commissioned for clinical use, it is recommended that an in vivo dosimetry check be performed on the first 20 or so patients. Thermoluminescent dosimeter (TLD) capsules or chips, surrounded by suitable build-up bolus, may be placed on the patient skin at strategic locations and doses measured for the actual treatments given. TLD results should be compared with expected doses, calculated by summing entrance and exit doses at the location of the TLDs and taking into account thickness variation, compensation, and off-axis ratios at the depth of TLDs. An agreement of +5% between the calculated and measured doses is considered reasonably good. An overall dose uniformity of +10% is considered acceptable for most protocols.

G. Total Body Irradiation Program Implementation

The use of TBI in conjunction with bone marrow transplantation involves numerous protocols, specifying many different regimens: single fraction with low dose rate, single fraction with high dose rate, fractionated TBI, hyperfractionated TBI, AP/PA technique, bilateral technique, use of compensators or no compensators, blocking of critical organs or no blocking, and so on. Each of these procedures involve special equipment or treatment aids, custom dosimetry, and rigorous quality assurance. Before embarking on a TBI program, institutions must design a careful plan of implementation. One of the most important part of this plan should be to form a TBI team, including radiation oncologist, medical physicist, medical dosimetrist, and radiation therapist. Key members of this team should visit another institution that has an active TBI program, to learn all aspects of the TBI procedure, down to the most minute details such as patient measurements, patient set-up, dosimetry, quality assurance procedures, and worksheets specifically designed for TBI. General TBI principles are presented in this chapter along with selected references in the literature for further details. But aside from acquiring pertinent knowledge from the literature, it is emphasized that the TBI team needs practical training, which may be obtained at another institution with a well-established TBI program.

REFERENCES

1. Khan FM, Williamson JF, Sewchand W, et al. Basic data for dosage calculation and compensation. *Int J Radiat Oncol Biology Phys* 1980;6:745–751.
2. Glasgow GP. The dosimetry of fixed, single source hemibody and total body irradiators. *Med Phys* 1982;9:311–323.
3. American Association of Physicists in Medicine. The physical aspects of total and half body photon irradiation. AAPM Report No. 17. Colchester, VT: American Institute of Physics, c/o AIDC, 1986.
4. Khan FM, Kim TH. Total body irradiation. In: Paliwal BR, Greim ML, eds. *Syllabus: a categorical course in radiation therapy treatment planning*. Oak Brook, IL: Radiological Society of North America, 1986:111–116.
5. Dusenbery KE, Gerbi BJ. Total body irradiation in conditioning regimens for bone marrow transplantation. In: Levitt SH, Khan FM, Potish RA, et al., eds. *Technological basis of radiation therapy*. Philadelphia: Lippincott Williams & Wilkins, 1999:499–518.
6. Shank B, Chu FCH, Dinsmore R, et al. Hyperfractionated total body irradiation for bone marrow transplantation: results in seventy leukemia patients with allogeneic transplants. *Int J Radiat Oncol Biol Physics* 1983;9:1607–1611.
7. Kirby TH, Hanson WF, Cates CA. Verification of total body photon irradiation dosimetry techniques. *Med Phys* 1988;15:364–369.
8. Galvin JM, D'Angio GJ, Walsh G. Use of tissue compensators to improve the dose uniformity for total body irradiation. *Int J Radiat Oncol Biol Phys* 1980;6:767–771.
9. Khan FM, Moore VC, Burns DJ. The construction of compensators for cobalt teletherapy. *Radiology* 1970;96:187.

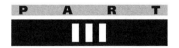

PART III

MODERN RADIATION THERAPY

19

THREE-DIMENSIONAL CONFORMAL RADIATION THERAPY

19.1. INTRODUCTION

By three-dimensional conformal radiotherapy (3-D CRT), we mean treatments that are based on 3-D anatomic information and use dose distributions that conform as closely as possible to the target volume in terms of adequate dose to the tumor and minimum possible dose to normal tissue. The concept of conformal dose distribution has also been extended to include clinical objectives such as maximizing tumor control probability (TCP) and minimizing normal tissue complication probability (NTCP). Thus, the 3-D CRT technique encompasses both the physical and biologic rationales in achieving the desired clinical results.

Although 3-D CRT calls for optimal dose distribution, there are many obstacles to achieving these objectives. The most major limitation is the knowledge of the tumor extent. Despite the modern advances in imaging, the clinical target volume (CTV) is often not fully discernible. Depending on the invasive capacity of the disease, what is imaged is usually not the CTV. It may be what is called the gross tumor volume (GTV). Thus, if the CTVs drawn on the cross-sectional images do not fully include the microscopic spread of the disease, the 3-D CRT loses its meaning of being conformal. If any part of the diseased tissue is missed or seriously underdosed, it will inevitably result in failure despite all the care and effort expended in treatment planning, treatment delivery, and quality assurance. From the TCP point of view, accuracy in localization of CTV is more critical in 3-D CRT than in techniques that use generously wide fields and simpler beam arrangements to compensate for the uncertainty in tumor localization.

In addition to the difficulties in the assessment and localization of CTV, there are other potential errors that must be considered before planning 3-D CRT. Patient motion, including that of tumor volume, critical organs and external fiducial marks during imaging, simulation, and treatment, can give rise to systematic as well as random errors that must be accounted for when designing the planning target volume (PTV). If sufficient margins have been allowed for in the localization of PTV, the beam apertures are then shaped to conform and adequately cover the PTV (e.g., within 95% to 105% isodose surface relative to prescribed dose). In the design of conformal fields to adequately treat the PTV, consideration must be given to the cross-beam profile, penumbra, and lateral radiation transport as a function of depth, radial distance, and tissue density. Therefore, sufficient margins must be given between the PTV outline and the field boundary to ensure adequate dose to PTV at every treatment session.

Even if the fields have been optimally designed, biologic response of the tumor and the normal tissues needs to be considered in achieving the goals of 3-D CRT. In other words, the optimization of a treatment plan has to be evaluated not only in terms of dose distribution (e.g., dose volume histograms) but also in terms of dose-response characteristics of the given disease and the irradiated normal tissues. Various models involving TCP and NTCP have been proposed, but the clinical data to validate these models are scarce.

Until more reliable data are available, caution is needed in using these concepts to evaluate treatment plans. This is especially important in considering dose-escalation schemes that invariably test the limits of normal tissue tolerance within or in proximity to the PTV.

Notwithstanding the formidable obstacles in defining and outlining the true extent of the disease, the clinician must follow an analytic plan recommended by the International Commission on Radiation Units and Measurements (ICRU) (1). Various target volumes (GTV, CTV, PTV, etc.) should be carefully designed considering the inherent limitations or uncertainties at each step of the process. The final PTV should be based not only on the given imaging data and other diagnostic studies but also the clinical experience that has been obtained in the management of that disease. Tightening of field margins around image-based GTV, with little attention to occult disease, patient motion, or technical limitations of dose delivery, is a misuse of 3-D CRT concept that must be avoided at all cost. It should be recognized that 3-D CRT is not a new modality of treatment, nor is it synonymous with better results than successful and well-tested conventional radiation therapy. Its superiority rests entirely on how accurate the PTV is and how much better the dose distribution is. So, instead of calling it a new modality, it should be considered as a superior tool for treatment planning with a potential of achieving better results.

19.2. TREATMENT-PLANNING PROCESS

The main distinction between treatment planning of 3-D CRT and that of conventional radiation therapy is that the former requires the availability of 3-D anatomic information and a treatment-planning system that allows optimization of dose distribution in accordance with the clinical objectives. The anatomic information is usually obtained in the form of closely spaced transverse images, which can be processed to reconstruct anatomy in any plane, or in three dimensions. Depending on the imaging modality, visible tumor, critical structures, and other relevant landmarks are outlined slice-by-slice by the planner. The radiation oncologist draws the target volumes in each slice with appropriate margins to include visible tumor, the suspected tumor spread, and patient motion uncertainties. This process of delineating targets and relevant anatomic structures is called *segmentation.*

The next step is to follow the 3-D treatment-planning software to design fields and beam arrangements. One of the most useful features of these systems is the computer graphics, which allow *beam's-eye-view* (BEV) visualization of the delineated targets and other structures. The term BEV denotes display of the segmented target and normal structures in a plane perpendicular to the central axis of the beam, as if being viewed from the vantage point of the radiation source. Using the BEV option, field margins (distance between field edge and the PTV outline) are set to cover the PTV dosimetrically within a sufficiently high isodose level (e.g., ≥95% of the prescribed dose). Ordinarily a field margin of approximately 2 cm is considered sufficient to achieve this, but it may need further adjustments depending on the given beam profile and the presence of critical structures in the vicinity of the PTV.

Nonetheless, it is important to remember that each beam has a physical penumbra (e.g., region between 90% and 20% isodose level) where the dose varies rapidly and that the dose at the field edge is approximately 50% of the dose at the center of the field. For a uniform and adequate irradiation of the PTV, the field penumbra should lie sufficiently outside the PTV to offset any uncertainties in PTV.

Optimization of a treatment plan requires not only the design of optimal field apertures, but also appropriate beam directions, number of fields, beam weights, and intensity modifiers (e.g., wedges, compensators, dynamic multileaf collimators, etc.) In a forward-planning system, these parameters are selected iteratively or on a trial-and-error basis and therefore, for a complex case, the whole process can become very labor intensive if a high degree of optimization is desired. In practice, however, most planners start with a standard technique and optimize it for the given patient using 3-D treatment-planning tools such as BEV, 3-D dose displays, non-coplanar beam options, intensity modulation, and dose-volume histograms. The time required to plan a 3-D CRT treatment depends on the complexity of a given case, experience of the treatment-planning team, and the speed of the treatment-planning system. The final product, the treatment plan, is as good as its individual components, namely, the quality of input patient data, image segmentation, image registration, field apertures, dose computation, plan evaluation, and plan optimization.

A. Imaging Data

Anatomic images of high quality are required to accurately delineate target volumes and normal structures. Modern imaging modalities for treatment planning include computed tomography (CT), magnetic resonance imaging (MRI), ultrasound (US), single photon emission tomography (SPECT), and positron emission tomography (PET). Although CT and MRI are the most commonly used procedures, other modalities offer special advantages in imaging certain types of tumors. A brief review of image characteristics of these modalities is presented to elucidate particular advantages and limitations with regard to their use in treatment planning.

A.1. Computed Tomography

As discussed in Chapter 12, a CT image is reconstructed from a matrix of relative linear attenuation coefficients measured by the CT scanner. The matrix typically consists of $1,024 \times 1,024$ picture elements, called pixels. Each pixel is a measure of relative linear attenuation coefficient of the tissue for the scanning beam used in the CT scanner. By appropriate calibration of the CT scanner using phantoms containing tissue substitutes (CT phantoms), a relationship between pixel value (CT numbers) and tissue density can be established. This allows pixel by pixel correction for tissue inhomogeneities in computing dose distributions.

One of the important features of 3-D treatment planning is the ability to reconstruct images in planes other than that of the original transverse image. These are called the *digitally reconstructed radiographs* (DRRs). An example is shown in Fig. 19.1. To obtain high-quality DRRs, not only images of high contrast and resolution are required, the slice thickness must also be sufficiently small. A slice thickness of 2 to 10 mm is commonly used depending on the need, for example, thinner slices for tumor localization or high-quality DRRs and thicker slices for regions outside the tumor volume. The *spiral* or *helical* CT scanners allow continuous rotation of the x-ray tube as the patient is translated through the scanner aperture. This substantially reduces the overall scanning time and therefore allows acquisition of a large number of thin slices required for high-quality CT images and the DRRs.

Besides high-image-quality CT scanning, treatment planning requires special considerations such as patient positioning, immobilization, and external markings that are visible in the images. For treatment planning, the CT couch must be flat and the patient must be set up in the same position as for actual treatment. Immobilization devices are essential for 3-D CRT and should be the same as those for CT as used in the treatment. Fiducial points marked on the patient skin or masks should be visible in the CT images by using radiopaque markers such as plastic catheters.

Because CT images can be processed to generate DRRs in any plane, conventional simulation may be replaced by *CT simulation*. A CT simulator is a CT scanner equipped with some additional hardware such as laser localizers to set up the treatment isocenter, a flat table or couch insert, and image registration devices. A computer workstation with special software to process a CT data, plan beam directions and generate BEV DRRs, allows CT simulation films with the same geometry as the treatment beams. For a practical detail of CT simulation, the reader is referred to Coia et al. (2).

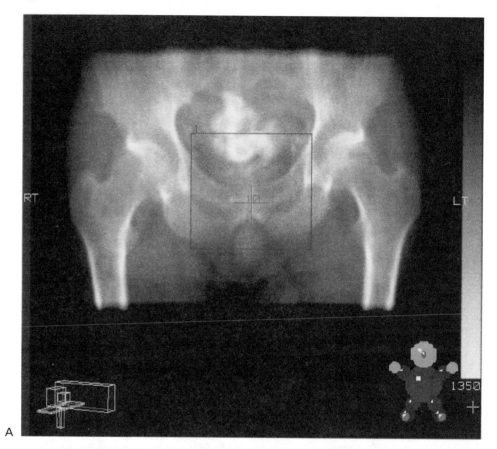

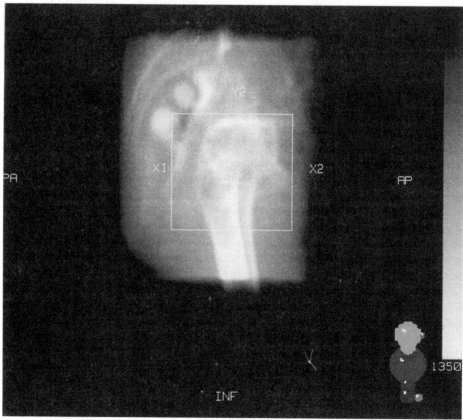

FIG. 19.1. An example of digital reconstructed radiographs created from transverse computed tomography scans. Image **A** is frontal and image **B** is lateral.

A.2. Magnetic Resonance Imaging

Principles of MRI are discussed in Chapter 12. In treatment planning, MRI images may be used alone or in conjunction with CT images. In general, MRI is considered superior to CT in soft tissue discrimination such as CNS tumors and abnormalities in the brain. Also, MRI is well suited to imaging head and neck cancers, sarcomas, the prostate gland, and lymph nodes. On the other hand, it is insensitive to calcification and bony structures, which are best imaged with CT. Although important differences exist between CT and MRI image characteristics, the two are considered complementary in their roles in treatment planning.

The most basic difference between CT and MRI is that the former is related to electron density and atomic number (actually representing x-ray linear attenuation coefficients) while the latter shows proton density distribution. Although the best spatial resolution of both modalities is similar (~1 mm), MRI takes much longer than CT and, therefore, is susceptible to artifacts from patient movement. On the advantageous side, MRI can be used to directly generate scans in axial, sagittal, coronal, or oblique planes.

One of the most important requirements in treatment planning is the geometric accuracy. Of all the imaging modalities, CT provides the best geometric accuracy and, therefore, CT images are considered a reference for anatomic landmarks, when compared with the other modality images.

Functional MRI (fMRI) also has potential to be useful in treatment planning by showing physiologic activity as it happens and, therefore, may be useful in outlining of the target volumes and critical structures for highly conformal radiation therapy such as in the brain.

B. Image Registration

The term *registration* as applied to images connotes a process of correlating different image data sets to identify corresponding structures or regions. Image registration facilitates comparison of images from one study to another and fuses them into one data set that could be used for treatment planning. For example, computer programs are now available that allow image fusing, for example, mapping of structures seen in MRI onto the CT images. Various registration techniques include point-to-point fitting, interactively superimposing images in the two data sets, and surface or topography matching. An example of image fusion of a CT and MRI study is shown in Fig. 19.2 (see color insert). For further discussion on image registration, the reader is referred to Kessler et al. (3), Pelizzari et al. (4), and Austin-Seymour et al. (5).

C. Image Segmentation

The term image segmentation in treatment planning refers to slice-by-slice delineation of anatomic regions of interest, for example, external contours, targets, critical normal structures, anatomic landmarks, etc. The segmented regions can be rendered in different colors and can be viewed in BEV configuration or in other planes using DRRs. Segmentation is also essential for calculating dose-volume histograms (DVHs) for the selected regions of interest.

Image segmentation is one of the most laborious but important processes in treatment planning. Although the process can be aided for automatic delineation based on image contrast near the boundaries of structures, target delineation requires clinical judgment, which cannot be automated or completely image-based. Nor should it be delegated to personnel other than the physician in charge of the case, the radiation oncologist. Figure 19.3 (see color insert) shows an example of a segmented image for prostate gland treatment planning.

D. Beam Aperture Design

After image segmentation has been completed, the treatment planner gets to the task of selecting beam direction and designing beam apertures. This is greatly aided by the BEV

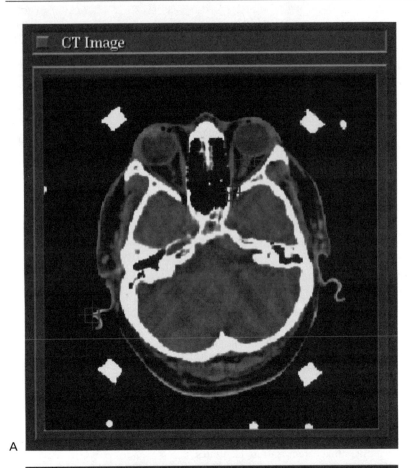

A

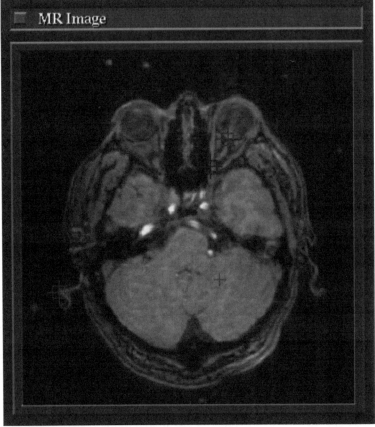

B

FIG. 19.2. An example of fusion between CT **(A)** and MR **(B)** images. Three points of correlation were selected for fusion. Split slice image **(C)** shows correlation at the interface of two images. Fused image **(D)** (see color insert) shows slice overlay with CT as red and MR as green.

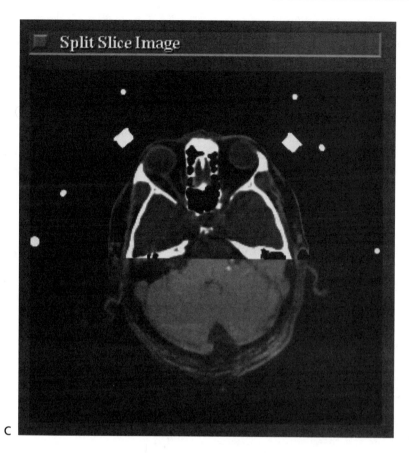

C

FIG. 19.2. (*continued*)

capability of the 3-D treatment-planning system. Targets and critical normal structures made visible in different colors through segmentation can be viewed from different directions in planes perpendicular to the beam's central axis. Beam directions that create greater separation between targets and critical structures are generally preferred unless other constraints such as obstructions in the path of the beam, gantry collision with the couch or patient, etc., preclude those choices. BEV capability, combined with DRRs, is a powerful tool in selecting beam directions and shaping fields around the target.

Beam apertures can be designed automatically or manually depending on the proximity of the critical structures and the uncertainty involved in the allowed margins between the CTV and PTV. In the automatic option, the user sets a uniform margin around the PTV. A nonuniform margin requires manual drawing of the field outline. A considerable give and take occurs between target coverage and sparing of critical structures in cases where the spaces between the target and critical structures are tight, thus requiring manual design of the beam apertures. In simpler cases, automatic margins may be assigned between the PTV and field edges, taking into account the field penumbra and the required minimum isodose coverage of the PTV. Generally, a 2-cm margin between PTV and the field edge assures better than 95% isodose coverage of the PTV but this must be ascertained through actual computation of the dose distribution. Figure 19.4 (see color insert) shows examples of BEV of beam apertures and dose distributions in transverse, sagittal, and coronal planes. The sagittal and coronal images are derived from DRRs.

E. Field Multiplicity and Collimation

Three-dimensional treatment planning encourages the use of multiple fields because targets and critical structures can be viewed in the BEV configuration individually for each field. Multiplicity of fields also removes the need for using ultra high-energy beams (>10 MV) which are required when treating thoracic or pelvic tumors with only two parallel-opposed fields. In general, greater the number of fields, less stringent is the requirement on beam energy because the dose outside the PTV is distributed over a larger volume. The 3-D treatment planning also allows non-coplanar beam direction, that is, the beam central axis lies in a plane other than the transverse plane of the patient. Non-coplanar beam directions can be useful in certain cases, for example, brain tumors, head and neck and other regions where a critical structure can be avoided by choosing a non-coplanar beam direction. To use a non-coplanar beam, the couch is rotated ("kicked") through a specified angle, making sure that it will not collide with the gantry.

Using a large number of fields (greater than four) creates the problem of designing an excessive number of beam shaping blocks and requiring longer set-up times as each block is individually inserted into the accessory mount and verified for correct placement of the field on the patient. Carrying so many heavy blocks, patient after patient, creates a nuisance for therapists who have to guard against dropping a block accidentally or using a wrong block.

A good alternative to multiple field blocking is the use of a multileaf collimator (MLC) (Chapter 13). MLCs can be used with great ease and convenience to shape fields electronically. A field drawn on a simulator film or a BEV print out can be digitized to set the MLC setting. BEV field outlines can also be transmitted electronically to the accelerator to program the MLC. Because MLC fields can be set at the control console as programmed, a large number of fields can be treated efficiently and reproducibly.

Combination of MLCs and independent jaws provides almost unlimited capability of designing fields of any shape. Custom designed blocks are still useful, however, in treating small fields (unless mini-MLCs with ultra small step size are available), mid-field blocking ("island" blocks), or complex field matching. Thus, in 3-D conformal radiation therapy, where the use of shaped multiple-fields is the norm, MLC provides a logistic solution to the problem of designing, carrying, and storing a large number of heavy blocks. For further details on MLC use and characteristics, the reader is referred to Boyer (6).

F. Plan Optimization and Evaluation

Criteria for an optimal plan include both the biologic and the physical aspects of radiation oncology. By definition, an optimal plan should deliver tumoricidal dose to the entire tumor and spare all the normal tissues. These goals can be set, but are not attainable in the absolute terms. To achieve quantitative biologic endpoints, models have been developed involving biologic indices such as tumor control probability (TCP) and normal tissue complication probability (NTCP). Clinical data required to validate these models are scarce and, therefore, currently most evaluations are carried out on the basis of physical endpoints, namely, dose distribution within the specified target volumes and dose to organs designated as critical. Discussion of biologic models is beyond the scope of this book. The reader is referred to Kutcher and Jackson (7) for a review. Physical aspects of plan optimization and evaluation are discussed below.

F.1. Isodose Curves and Surfaces

Traditionally treatment plans are optimized iteratively by using multiple fields, beam modifiers (e.g., wedges and compensators, etc.), beam weights, and appropriate beam directions. Dose distributions of competing plans are evaluated by viewing isodose curves in individual slices, orthogonal planes (e.g., transverse, sagittal, and coronal), or 3-D isodose surfaces. The latter represent surfaces of a designated dose value covering a volume. An isodose surface can be rotated to assess volumetric dose coverage from different angles. Figure 19.5 (see color insert) is an example of isodose curves displayed in orthogonal planes and an isodose surface just covering the target volume. One of the major advantages of 3-D treatment planning is the display of dose distribution, which can be manipulated with ease to show volumetric dose coverage in individual slices, orthogonal planes, or as 3-D isodose surfaces.

The dose distribution is usually normalized to be 100% at the point of dose prescription (see ICRU) (1) so that the isodose curves represent lines of equal dose as a percentage of the prescribed dose. For a treatment plan involving one or more "boosts" (increased dose to certain parts of the target, usually the GTV), a composite isodose plan is useful, which can again be displayed by isodose distribution in individual slices, orthogonal planes, or as isodose surfaces.

F.2. Dose-volume Histograms

Display of dose distribution in the form of isodose curves or surfaces is useful not only because it shows regions of uniform dose, high dose, or low dose but also their anatomic location and extent. In 3-D treatment planning, this information is essential but should be supplemented by dose-volume histograms (DVH) for the segmented structures, for example, targets, critical structures, etc. A DVH not only provides quantitative information with regard to how much dose is absorbed in how much volume but also summarizes the entire dose distribution into a single curve for each anatomic structure of interest. It is, therefore, a great tool for evaluating a given plan or comparing competing plans.

The DVH may be represented in two forms: the cumulative integral DVH and the differential DVH. The cumulative DVH is a plot of the volume of a given structure receiving a *certain dose or higher* as a function of dose (Fig. 19.6) (see color insert). Any point on the cumulative DVH curve shows the volume that receives the indicated dose or higher. The differential DVH is a plot of volume receiving a dose within a specified dose interval (or dose bin) as a function of dose. As seen in Fig. 19.6E (see color insert), the differential form of DVH shows the extent of dose variation within a given structure. For example, the differential DVH of a uniformly irradiated structure is a single bar of 100% volume at the stated dose. Of the two forms of DVH, the cumulative DVH has been found to be more useful and is more commonly used than the differential form.

19.3. DOSE COMPUTATION ALGORITHMS

Semi-empirical methods suitable for the calculation of dose at a point in a patient have been discussed in Chapter 10. Corrections for contour irregularity and tissue heterogeneity were also presented in Chapter 12. Some elements of these methods have been adopted into dose computation algorithms in some of the commercially available computer treatment-planning systems. Modern treatment planning systems have upgraded the software additionally for 3-D data input and processing, dose calculation, and special 3-D graphics. Some 3-D treatment-planning systems continue to use basically two-dimensional dose computation algorithms (calculation of dose distribution in a given slice being unaffected by changes in tissue composition in the adjacent slices) but rendered into three dimensions through interpolation. In the case of tissue heterogeneities, it is assumed that the adjacent slices are identical in the tissue composition to the slice in which the dose is being calculated. This assumption is obviously wrong but is not as bad as it sounds. Lateral scatter from adjacent slices is usually a second order effect except for situations in which small fields are used to treat tumors or structures surrounded by lung or large air cavities. On the other hand, by assuming the same composition for the adjacent slices, simpler algorithms can be used that greatly speed up the dose computation process. However, in 3-D CRT, where non-coplanar beams are often used and dose distributions are evaluated in multiple planes or volumes, it is essential that the dose calculation algorithm has acceptable accuracy (within $\pm 3\%$ for homogeneous and $\pm 5\%$ for heterogeneous tissues such as lung). Because plan optimization is an iterative process, speed of calculation is of paramount importance. Therefore, the best computational algorithm is the one in which accuracy and speed are well balanced.

Dose calculation algorithms for computerized treatment planning have been evolving since the middle of the 1950s. In broad terms the algorithms fall into three categories:

(a) correction-based, (b) model-based, and (c) direct Monte Carlo. Either one of the methods can be used for 3-D treatment planning, although with a varying degree of accuracy and speed. However, the model-based algorithms and the direct Monte Carlo are becoming more and more the algorithms of the future. This is because of their ability to simulate radiation transport in three dimensions and therefore, more accurately predict dose distribution under conditions of charged particle disequilibrium, which can occur in low-density tissues such as lung and heterogeneous tissue interfaces. Although currently they are plagued by slow speed, this limitation is fast disappearing with the ever-increasing speed and data storage capacity of modern computers.

A. Correction-based Algorithms

These algorithms are semi-empirical. They are based primarily on measured data (e.g., percent depth doses and cross-beam profiles, etc.) obtained in a cubic water phantom. Various corrections in the form of analytic functions or factors are applied to calculate dose distributions in a patient. The corrections typically consist of a (a) attenuation corrections for contour irregularity; (b) scatter corrections as a function of scattering volume, field size, shape and radial distance; (c) geometric corrections for source to point of calculation distance based on inverse square law; (d) attenuation corrections for beam intensity modifiers such as wedge filters, compensators, blocks, etc.; and (e) attenuation corrections for tissue heterogeneities based on radiologic path length (unit-density equivalent depth).

Correction-based algorithms represent a variety of methods ranging from those that simply interpolate measured depth-dose data to specially formulated analytic functions that predict the various correction factors under specified conditions. The dose at any point is usually analyzed into primary and scattered components, which are computed separately and then summed to obtain the total dose. Equations 9.31 and 10.14 are examples of calculations that measured quantities such as percent depth doses, TARs, TMRs, etc., and the Clarkson's method (see Chapter 9) of dose integration for any shaped field. Contour corrections and tissue heterogeneity corrections are discussed in Chapter 12. These methods can be used for manual calculations as well as made part of a correction-based computer algorithm for the calculation of absorbed dose at a point in a patient.

As pointed out previously, the accuracy of correction-based algorithms is limited for 3-D heterogeneity corrections in lung and tissue interfaces especially in situations where electronic equilibrium is not fully established.

B. Model-based Algorithms

A model-based algorithm computes dose distribution with a physical model that simulates the actual radiation transport. Because of its ability to model primary photon energy fluence incident at a point and the distribution of energy subsequent to primary photon interaction, it is able to simulate the transport of scattered photon and electrons away from the interaction site. A class of model-based algorithms, called convolution-superposition, has been under development since the mid 1980s (8–11). An example of such methods is discussed below. For a literature review the reader in referred to Mackie et al. (12,13).

B.1. Convolution-superposition Method

A convolution-superposition method involves a convolution equation that separately considers the transport of primary photons and that of the scatter photon and electron emerging from the primary photon interaction. The dose $D(\vec{r})$ at a point $\vec{r}$ is given by:

$$D(\vec{r}) = \int \frac{\mu}{\rho} \Psi_p(\vec{r}') A(\vec{r} - \vec{r}') d^3\vec{r}'$$

$$= \int T_p(\vec{r}') A(\vec{r} - \vec{r}') d^3\vec{r}' \tag{19.1}$$

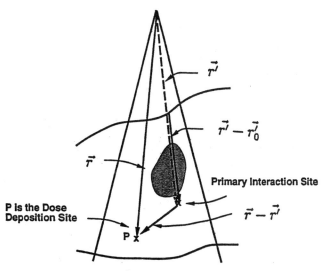

FIG. 19.7. Geometry of photon interaction and radiation transport from the site of interaction. (From Mackie TR, personal communication.)

where μ/ρ is the mass attenuation coefficient, $\Psi_p(\vec{r}')$ is the primary photon energy fluence, and $A(\vec{r} - \vec{r}')$ is the convolution kernel (a matrix of dose distribution deposited by scatter photons and electrons set in motion at the primary photon interaction site). Figure 19.7 shows the geometry of the radiation transport. The product of mass attenuation coefficient and the primary energy fluence is called *terma*, $T_p(\vec{r}')$, which stands for total energy released per unit mass. Terma is analogous to kerma, which represents the kinetic energy released per unit mass in the form of electrons set in motion by photons (see Chapter 8). Kernel is the dose matrix generated per unit terma at the interaction site. The product of terma and the dose kernal when integrated (convolved) over a volume gives the dose $D(\vec{r})$ as given in Equation 19.1.

The convolution kernel, $A(\vec{r} - \vec{r}')$, can be represented by a dose spread array obtained by calculation or by direct measurement. The most commonly used method is the Monte Carlo which simulates interactions of a large number of primary photons and determines dose deposited in all directions by electrons and scattered photons originating at the primary photon interaction site. Figure 19.8 shows a ^{60}Co kernel for water generated by a Monte Carlo program (EGS4 Monte Carlo code). Examination of dose distribution in the kernel indicates that the dose deposition by the kernel is forward peaked, as expected for a megavoltage photon beam.

Modeling of primary photon transport and the calculation of dose kernel for a linear accelerator x-ray beam requires the knowledge of photon energy spectrum. Again, Monte Carlo may be used to calculate the energy spectrum of a linac beam. Mohan and Chui (14) used EGS4 code to calculate energy spectrum of linac x-ray beams. Such spectra can be used both for the transport of primary photons and the generation of a dose kernel by the Monte Carlo method. Thus, the Monte Carlo generated energy spectrum and the kernel are essential ingredients of the convolution equation to compute dose at any point in the patient. One of the important tasks of commissioning a treatment-planning system that uses a convolution equation such as Equation 19.1 is to modify (tweak) the Monte Carlo generated energy spectrum in order to fit the modeled beam with the measured depth dose distribution and cross-beam dose profiles as a function of field size and depth.

A convolution equation when modified for radiological path length (distance corrected for electron density relative to water) is called the convolution-superposition equation:

$$D(\vec{r}) = \int T_p(\rho_{\vec{r}'} \cdot \vec{r}') \, A(\rho_{\vec{r}-\vec{r}'} \cdot (\vec{r} - \vec{r}')) \, d^3\vec{r}' \qquad (19.2)$$

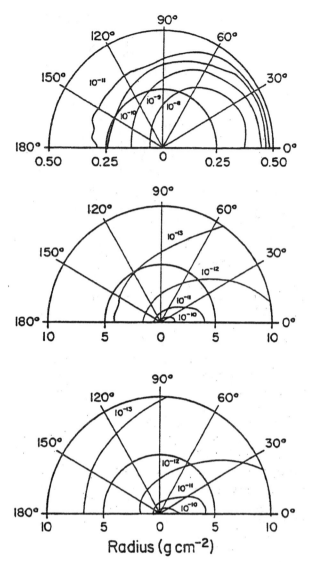

FIG. 19.8. Cobalt-60 dose kernels for water computed with Monte Carlo simulation. The isovalue lines are in units of cGyMeV^{-1} photon^{-1}. *Top:* primary contribution by electrons set in motion by primary photons. *Middle:* the first-scatter contribution. *Bottom:* the sum of primary and scatter contributions. (From Mackie TR, Bielajew AF, Rogers DWO, et al. Generation of photon energy deposition kernels using the EGS4 Monte Carlo Code. *Phys Med Biol* 1988;33:1–20, with permission.)

where $\rho_{\vec{r}'} \cdot \vec{r}'$ is the radiologic path length from the source to the primary photon interaction site and $\rho_{\vec{r}-\vec{r}'} \cdot (\vec{r} - \vec{r}')$ is the radiologic path length from the site of primary photon interaction to the site of dose deposition. The dose kernel $A(\rho_{\vec{r}-\vec{r}'} \cdot (\vec{r} - \vec{r}'))$ can be calculated by using range scaling by electron density of the Monte Carlo generated kernel in water. Figure 19.9 shows that the kernel obtained with the range scaling method compares well with that generated by Monte Carlo directly for the heterogeneous medium.

B.2. Direct Monte Carlo

The Monte Carlo technique consists of a computer program (MC code) that simulates the transport of millions of photons and particles through matter. It uses fundamental laws of physics to determine probability distributions of individual interactions of photons

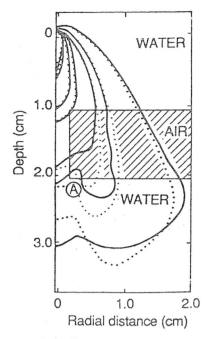

FIG. 19.9. Comparison of Monte Carlo-generated 6-MeV primary photon kernel in a water phantom containing a ring of air. The *continuous line* is a kernel computed expressly for the heterogeneous situation. The *dashed line* is a kernel modified for the heterogeneous phantom using range scaling. (From Woo MK, Cunningham JR. The validity of the density scaling method in primary electron transport for photon and electron beams. *Med Phys* 1990;17:187–194, with permission.)

and particles. The larger the number of simulated particles (histories), the greater the accuracy of predicting their distributions. However, as the number of simulated particles is increased, the computational time becomes prohibitively long. So the challenge in writing an MC code is that of being able to use a relatively small sample of randomly selected particles to predict the average behavior of the particles in the beam. The dose distribution is calculated by accumulating (scoring) ionizing events in bins (voxels) that give rise to energy deposition in the medium. It is estimated that the transport of a few hundred million to a billion histories will be required for radiation therapy treatment planning with adequate precision.

A number of MC codes has been used in radiation transport simulation and, more recently, in treatment planning: Electron Gamma Shower version 4 (EGS4) (15), ETRAN/ITS (16), Monte Carlo N-particle (MCNP) (17), PENELOPE (18) and PEREGRINE (developed at Lawrence Livermore National Laboratory) (19). For a detailed review and bibliography of MC codes, the reader is referred to (20,21).

Notwithstanding inordinate amounts of computational times, Monte Carlo is the most accurate method of calculating dose distribution in a patient. Sample plans done with Monte Carlo simulation has shown significant gains in accuracy of dose calculation, especially at interfaces of heterogeneous tissues and in lung where particle disequilibrium can occur under certain conditions. With the continuing advancement in computer technology and computation algorithms, it now seems probable that the Monte Carlo methodology will be implemented for routine treatment planning in the not too distant future.

REFERENCES

1. ICRU. Prescribing, recording, and reporting photon beam therapy. Report No. 50. Bethesda, MD: International Commission on Radiation Units and Measurements, 1993.

2. Coia LR, Schutheiss TE, Hanks GE, eds. *A practical guide to CT simulation.* Madison, WI: Advanced Medical Publishing, 1995.
3. Keller ML, Pitluck S, Petti P, et al. Integration of multimodality imaging data for radiotherapy treatment planning. *Int J Radiat Oncol Biol Phys* 1991;21:1653–1667.
4. Pelizzari CA, Chen GTY, Spelbring DR, et al. Accurate three-dimensional registration of PET, CT, and MR images of the brain. *J Comput Assist Tomogr* 1989;13:20–27.
5. Austin-Seymour M, Chen GTY, Rosenman J, et al. Tumor and target delineation: current research and future challenges. *Int J Radiat Oncol Biol Phys* 1995;33:1041–1052.
6. Boyer AL. Basic applications of a multileaf collimator. In: Mackie TR, Palta JR, eds. *Teletherapy: present and future.* College Park, MD: American Association of Physicists in Medicine, 1996.
7. Kutcher GJ, Jackson A. Treatment plan evaluation. In: Khan FM, Potish RA, eds. *Treatment planning in radiation oncology.* Baltimore: Williams & Wilkins, 1998.
8. Mackie TR, Scrimger JW, Battista JJ. A convolution method of calculating dose for 15 MV x-rays. *Med Phys* 1985;12:188–196.
9. Boyer AL, Mok EC. A photon dose distribution model employing convolution calculations. *Med Phys* 1985;12:169–177.
10. Mohan R, Chui C, Lidofsky L. Differential pencil beam dose computation model for photons. *Med Phys* 1986;13:64–73.
11. Ahnesjo A, Andreo P, Brahme A. Calculation and application of point spread functions for treatment planning with high energy photon beams. *Acta Oncol* 1987;26:49–56.
12. Mackie TR, Reckwerdt P, McNutt T, et al. Photon beam dose computation. In: Mackie TR, Palta JR, eds. *Teletherapy: present and future.* College Park, MD: American Association of Physicists in Medicine, 1996.
13. Mackie TR, Helen HL, McCullough EC. Treatment planning algorithms. In: Khan FM, Potish RA, eds. *Treatment planning in radiation oncology.* Baltimore: Williams & Wilkins, 1998.
14. Mohan R, Chui C. Energy and angular distributions of photons from medical linear accelerators. *Med Phys* 1985;12:592–597.
15. Nelson WR, Hirayama H, Rogers DWO. *The ESG4 code system.* Stanford Linear Accelerator Center Report SLAC-265, Stanford, CA: SLAC, 1985.
16. Berger MJ, Seltzer SM. ETRAN, Monte Carlo code system for electron and photon transport through extended media. Documentation for RSIC Computer Package CCC-107. Oak Ridge, TN: Oak Ridge National Laboratory, 1973.
17. Hendricks JS. A Monte Carlo code for particle transport. *Los Alamos Scientific Laboratory Report* 1994;22:30–43.
18. Salvat F, Fernandez-Vera JM, Baro J, et al. J. PENELOPE, An algorithm and computer code for Monte Carlo simulation of electron-photon showers. Barcelona: Informes Técnicos Ciemat, 1996.
19. Walling R, Hartman Siantar C, Albright N, et al. Clinical validation of the PEREGRINE Monte Carlo dose calculation system for photon beam therapy. *Med Phys* 1998;25:A128.
20. Rogers DWO, Bielajew AF. Monte Carlo techniques of electron and photon transport for radiation dosimetry. In: Kase KR, Bärngard BE, Attix FH, eds. *The dosimetry of ionizing radiation.* San Diego: Academic Press, 1990:427–539.
21. Li JS, Pawlicki T, Deng J, et al. Validation of a Monte Carlo dose calculation tool for radiotherapy treatment planning. *Phys Med Biol* 2000;45:2969–2969.

INTENSITY-MODULATED RADIATION THERAPY

20.1. INTRODUCTION

In the traditional external beam photon radiation therapy, most treatments are delivered with radiation beams that are of uniform intensity across the field (within the flatness specification limits). Occasionally, wedges or compensators are used to modify the intensity profile to offset contour irregularities and/or produce more uniform composite dose distributions such as in techniques using wedges. This process of changing beam intensity profiles to meet the goals of a composite plan is called intensity modulation. Thus, the compensators and wedges may be called as intensity modulators, albeit much simpler than the modern computer-controlled intensity modulation systems such as dynamic multileaf collimators.

The term intensity-modulated radiation therapy (IMRT) refers to a radiation therapy technique in which nonuniform fluence is delivered to the patient from any given position of the treatment beam to optimize the composite dose distribution. The treatment criteria for plan optimization are specified by the planner and the optimal fluence profiles for a given set of beam directions are determined through "inverse planning." The fluence files thus generated are electronically transmitted to the linear accelerator, which is computer-controlled, that is, equipped with the required software and hardware to deliver the intensity-modulated beams (IMBs) as calculated.

The clinical implementation of IMRT requires at least two systems: (1) a treatment-planning computer system that can calculate nonuniform fluence maps for multiple beams directed from different directions to maximize dose to the target volume while minimizing dose to the critical normal structures, and (2) a system of delivering the nonuniform fluences as planned. Each of these systems must be appropriately tested and commissioned before actual clinical use.

20.2. INTENSITY-MODULATED RADIATION THERAPY PLANNING

The principle of IMRT is to treat a patient from a number of different directions (or continuous arcs) with beams of nonuniform fluences, which have been optimized to deliver a high dose to the target volume and acceptably low dose to the surrounding normal structures. The treatment-planning program divides each beam into a large number of beamlets and determines optimum setting of their fluences or weights. The optimization process involves inverse planning in which beamlet weights or intensities are adjusted to satisfy predefined dose distribution criteria for the composite plan.

A number of computer methods have been devised to calculate optimum intensity profiles (1–10). These methods, which are based on inverse planning, can be divided into two broad categories:

(i) Analytic methods. These involve mathematical techniques in which the desired dose distribution is inverted by using a back projection algorithm. In effect, this is a reverse of a computed tomography (CT) reconstruction algorithm in which two-dimensional images are reconstructed from one-dimensional intensity functions. If one assumes that the dose distribution is the result of convolutions of a point-dose kernel and kernel density, then the reverse is also possible, namely, by deconvolving a dose kernel from the desired dose distribution, one can obtain kernel density or fluence distribution in the patient. These fluences can then be projected onto the beam geometry to create incident beam intensity profiles.

One problem with analytical methods is that, unlike CT reconstruction, exact analytical solutions do not exist for determining incident fluences that would produce the desired dose distribution without allowing negative beam weights. The problem can be circumvented by setting negative weights to zero but not without penalty in terms of unwanted deviations from the desired goal. So some algorithms have been devised to involve both analytical and iterative procedures.

(ii) Iterative methods. Optimization techniques have been devised in which beamlet weights for a given number of beams are iteratively adjusted to minimize the value of a cost function, which quantitatively represents deviation from the desired goal. For example, the cost function may be a least square function of the form:

$$C_n = \left[\left(\frac{1}{N} \right) \sum_r W(\vec{r})(D_o(\vec{r}) - D_n(\vec{r}))^2 \right]^{0.5} \tag{20.1}$$

where C_n is the cost at the nth iteration, $D_o(\vec{r})$ is the desired dose at some point $\vec{r}$ in the patient, $D_n(\vec{r})$ is the computed dose at the same point, $W(\vec{r})$ is the weight (relative importance) factor in terms of contribution to the cost from different structures and the sum is taken over a large N number of dose points. Thus, for targets the cost is the root mean squared difference between the desired (prescribed) dose and the realized dose. For the designated critical normal structures, the cost is the root mean squared difference between zero dose (or an acceptable low dose value) and the realized dose. The overall cost is the sum of the costs for the targets and the normal structures, based on their respective weights.

The optimization algorithm attempts to minimize the overall cost at each iteration until the desired goal (close to a predefined dose distribution) is achieved. A quadratic cost function such as that given by Equation 20.1 has only one minimum. However, when optimizing beam weights for all the beams from different directions to reach a global minimum, the same cost function exhibits multiple local minima. Therefore, in the iteration process occasionally it is necessary to accept a higher cost to avoid "trapping" in local minima. An optimization process, called simulated annealing (3,10) has been devised that allows the system to accept some higher costs in pursuit of a global minimum.

Simulated annealing takes its name from the process by which metals are annealed. The annealing process for metals involves a controlled process of slow cooling to avoid amorphous states, which can develop if the temperature is allowed to decrease too fast. In the analogous process of simulated annealing, the decision to accept a change in cost is controlled by a probability function. In other words, If $\Delta C_n < 0$, the change in the variables is always accepted. But if $\Delta C_n > 0$ the change is accepted with an acceptance probability, P_{acc}, given by:

$$P_{\text{acc}} = \exp - (\Delta C_n / \kappa T_n) \tag{20.2}$$

where $\Delta C_n = C_n - C_{n-1}$, κT_n is analogous to thermal energy at iteration n (it has the same dimensions as ΔC_n), T_n may be thought of as temperature and κ as Boltzmann constant.[1] At the start of simulated annealing, the "thermal energy" is large, resulting in a larger probability of accepting a change in variables that gives rise to a higher cost. As

---

[1] Boltzmann constant is derived from the theory of expansion of gasses.

the optimization process proceeds, the acceptance probability decreases exponentially in accordance with Equation 20.2 and thus drives the system to an optimal solution. The process is described by Web (10) as being analogous to a skier descending from a hilltop to the lowest point in a valley.

The patient input data for the inverse planning algorithm is the same as that needed for forward planning, as discussed in Chapter 19. Three-dimensional image data, image registration, and segmentation are all required when planning for IMRT. For each target (PTV) the user enters the plan criteria: maximum dose, minimum dose, and a dose-volume histogram. For the critical structures, the program requires the desired limiting dose and a dose-volume histogram. Depending on the IMRT software, the user may be required to provide other data such as beam energy, beam directions, number of iterations, etc., before proceeding to optimizing intensity profiles and calculating the resulting dose distribution. The evaluation of an IMRT treatment plan also requires the same considerations as the "conventional" 3-D CRT plans, namely, viewing isodose curves in orthogonal planes, individual slices, or 3-D volume surfaces. The isodose distributions are usually supplemented by dose-volume histograms.

After an acceptable IMRT plan has been generated, the intensity profiles (or fluence maps) for each beam are electronically transmitted to the treatment accelerator fitted with appropriate hardware and software to deliver the planned intensity-modulated beams. The treatment-planning and delivery systems must be integrated to ensure accurate and efficient delivery of the planned treatment. Because of the "black box" nature of the entire process, rigorous verification and quality assurance procedures are required to implement IMRT.

20.3. INTENSITY-MODULATED RADIATION THERAPY DELIVERY

Radiation therapy accelerators normally generate x-ray beams that are flattened (made uniform by the use of flattening filters) and collimated by four moveable jaws to produce rectangular fields. Precollimation dose rate can be changed uniformly within the beam but not spatially, although the scanning beam accelerators (e.g., Microtron) have the capability of modulating the intensity of elementary scanning beams. To produce intensity-modulated fluence profiles, precalculated by a treatment plan, the accelerator must be equipped with a system that can change the given beam profile into a profile of arbitrary shape.

Many classes of intensity-modulated systems have been devised. These include compensators, wedges, transmission blocks, dynamic jaws, moving bar, multileaf collimators, tomotherapy collimators, and scanned elementary beams of variable intensity. Of these, only the last five allow dynamic intensity modulation. Compensators, wedges, and transmission blocks are manual techniques that are time consuming, inefficient, and do not belong to the modern class of IMRT systems. Dynamic jaws are suited for creating wedged shaped distributions but are not significantly superior to conventional metal wedges. Although a scanning beam accelerator can deliver intensity-modulated elementary beams (11), the Gaussian half-width of the photon "pencil" at the isocenter can be as large as 4 cm and therefore does not have the desired resolution by itself for full intensity modulation. However, scanning beam may be used together with a dynamic MLC to overcome this problem and provide an additional degree of freedom for full dynamic intensity modulation. The case of dynamic MLC with upstream fluence modulation is a powerful but complex technique that is currently possible only with scanning beam accelerators such as microtrons (12).

For linear accelerators it seems the computer-controlled MLC is the most practical device for delivering intensity-modulated beams (IMB). Competing with this technology are the tomotherapy-based collimators—one embodied by the MIMiC collimator of the NOMOS Corporation and the other designed for a tomotherapy machine under construction at the University of Wisconsin.

A. Multileaf Collimator as Intensity Modulator

A computer-controlled multileaf collimator is not only useful in shaping beam apertures for conventional radiotherapy it can also be programmed to deliver IMRT. This has been done in three different ways:

A.1. Multisegmented Static Fields Delivery

The patient is treated by multiple fields and each field is subdivided into a set of subfields irradiated with uniform beam intensity levels. The subfields are created by the MLC and delivered in a stack arrangement one at a time in sequence without operator intervention. The accelerator is turned off while the leaves move to create the next subfield. The composite of dose increments delivered to each subfield creates the intensity modulated beam as planned by the treatment planning system. This method of IMRT delivery is also called "step-and-shoot" or "stop-and-shoot." The theory of creating subfields and leaf-setting sequence to generate the desired intensity modulation has been discussed by Bortfeld et al. (13). The method is illustrated in Fig. 20.1 for one-dimensional intensity modulation in which a leaf-pair takes up a number of static locations and the radiation from each static field thus defined is delivered at discrete intervals of fluence (shown by dotted lines). In this example ten separate fields have been stacked in a leaf-setting arrangement known as the "close-in" technique (Fig. 20.2A). Another arrangement called the "leaf-sweep" is also shown (Fig. 20.2B). The two arrangements are equivalent and take the same number of cumulative monitor units. In fact, if N is the number of subfields stacked, it has been shown that there are $(N!)^2$ possible equivalent arrangements (14). The two-dimensional intensity modulation is realized as a combination of multiple subfields of different sizes and shapes created by the entire MLC.

The advantage of step-and-shoot method is the ease of implementation from the engineering and safety points of view. A possible disadvantage is the instability of some accelerators when the beam is switched "off" (to reset the leaves) and "on" within a fraction of a second. The use of a gridded pentode gun could overcome this problem as it allows monitoring and termination of dose within about one-hundredth of a monitor unit, MU. However, not all manufacturers have this type of electron gun on their linear accelerators.

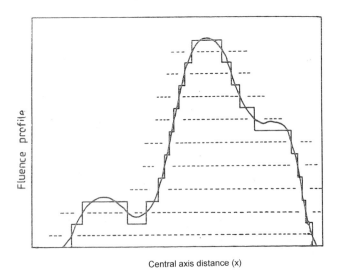

Central axis distance (x)

FIG. 20.1. Generation of one-dimensional intensity-modulation profile. All left leaf settings occur at positions where the fluence is increasing and all right leaf settings occur where the fluence is decreasing. (From Web S. *The physics of conformal radiotherapy.* Bristol, UK: Institute of Physics Publishing, 1997:131, with permission.)

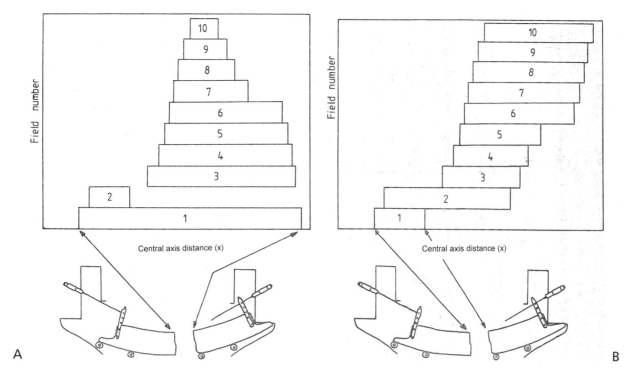

FIG. 20.2. Ten separate fields are stacked to generate the beam profile shown in Fig. 20.1. Multileaf collimator leaves are shown schematically below the fields; **(A)** leaf setting as "close-in" technique; **(B)** leaf settings as "leaf-sweep" technique. (From Web S. *The physics of conformal radiotherapy.* Bristol, UK: Institute of Physics Publishing, 1997:132, with permission.)

A mixed mode of IMB delivery, called "dynamic-step-and-shoot," has also been used. In this method the radiation is "on" all the time, even when the leaves are moving from one static subfield position to the next. This technique has the advantage of blurring the incremental steps in the delivery of static subfields (15).

Bortfeld et al. (13) have demonstrated that relatively small number of steps (10 to 30 to cover a 20-cm wide field) can be used to deliver an intensity-modulated profile with an accuracy of 2% to 5%. A nine-field plan could be delivered in less than 20 minutes, including extra time allowed for gantry rotation (13). Figure 20.3 is an example of intensity-modulated fluence profile generated by the step-and-shoot method and compared with calculated and measured dose.

A.2. Dynamic Delivery

In this technique the corresponding (opposing) leaves sweep simultaneously and unidirectionally, each with a different velocity as a function of time. The period that the aperture between leaves remains open (dwell time) allows the delivery of variable intensity to different points in the field. The method has been called by several names: the "sliding window," "leaf-chasing," "camera-shutter," and "sweeping variable gap."

The leaves of a dynamic MLC are motor driven and are capable of moving with a speed of greater than 2 cm per second. The motion is under the control of a computer, which also accurately monitors the leaf positions. The problem of determining leaf velocity profiles has been solved by several investigators (12,16,17). The solution is not unique but rather consists of an optimization algorithm to accurately deliver the planned intensity-modulated profiles under the constraints of maximum possible leaf velocity and minimum possible treatment time.

The basic principle of dynamic collimation is illustrated in Fig. 20.4. A pair of leaves defines an aperture with the leading leaf 2 moving with velocity $V_2(x)$ and the trailing leaf 1

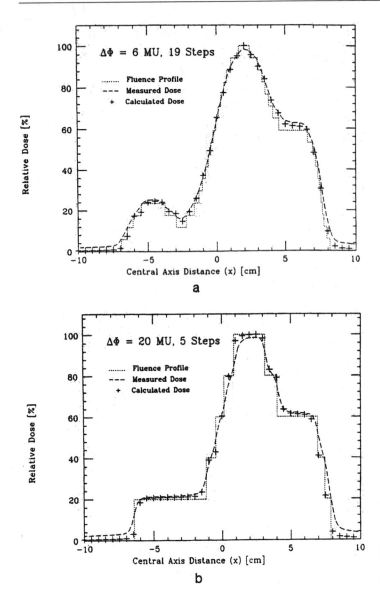

FIG. 20.3. Comparison of calculated fluence, measured dose, and calculated dose for the intensity modulated profile generated by step-and-shoot method. (From Bortfeld TR, Kahler DL, Waldron TJ, et al. X-ray field compensation with multileaf collimators. *Int J Radiat Oncol Biol Phys* 1994;28:723–730, with permission.)

with velocity $V_1(x)$. Assuming that the beam output is constant with no transmission through the leaves, penumbra or scattering, the profile intensity $I(x)$ as a function of position x is given by the cumulative beam-on times, $t_1(x)$ and $t_2(x)$, in terms of cumulative MUs that the inside edges of leaves 1 and 2, respectively, reach point x, that is:

$$I(x) = t_1(x) - t_2(x) \tag{20.3}$$

Differentiating Equation 20.3 with respect to x gives:

$$\frac{dI(x)}{dx} = \frac{dt_1(x)}{dx} - \frac{dt_2(x)}{dx} \tag{20.4}$$

or

$$\frac{dI(x)}{dx} = \frac{I}{V_1(x)} - \frac{I}{V_2(x)} \tag{20.5}$$

To minimize the total treatment time, the optimal solution is to move the faster of the two leaves at the maximum allowed speed, V_{max} and modulate the intensity with the slower leaf. If the gradient of the profile $dI(x)/dx$ is zero, then according to Equation 20.5, the two speeds are equal and should be set to V_{max}. If the gradient is positive, then the speed of leaf 2 is higher than that of leaf 1 and therefore it is set equal to V_{max}; and if the

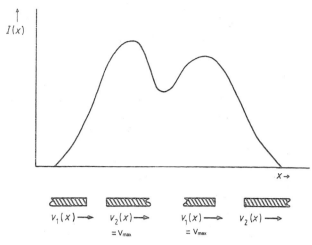

FIG. 20.4. Illustration of dynamic multileaf collimator motion to generate intensity-modulated profile. A pair of leaves with the leading leaf 2 moving with velocity $V_2(x)$ and the trailing leaf 1 with velocity $V_1(x)$. In the rising part of the fluence profile, leaf 2 moves with the maximum speed V_{max} and in the falling part of the fluence, leaf 1 moves with V_{max}. (Adapted from Web S. *The physics of conformal radiotherapy.* Bristol, UK: Institute of Physics Publishing, 1997:104.)

gradient is negative then the speed of leaf 1 is set equal to V_{max}. Once the speed of the faster leaf is set to V_{max}, the speed of the slower leaf can be uniquely determined from Equation 20.5, that is:

$$\left.\begin{array}{l} V_2(x) = V_{max} \\[2mm] V_1(x) = \dfrac{V_{max}}{1 + V_{max}(dI(x)/dx)} \end{array}\right\} \text{ when } \frac{dI(x)}{dx} \geq 0 \qquad (20.6)$$

and

$$\left.\begin{array}{l} V_1(x) = V_{max} \\[2mm] V_2(x) = \dfrac{V_{max}}{1 - V_{max}(dI(x)/dx)} \end{array}\right\} \text{ when } \frac{dI(x)}{dx} < 0 \qquad (20.7)$$

In summary, the DMLC algorithm is based on the following principles:

(i) if the gradient of the intensity profile is positive (increasing fluence), the leading leaf should move at the maximum speed and the trailing leaf should provide the required intensity modulation;

(ii) if the spatial gradient of the intensity profile is negative (decreasing fluence), the trailing leaf should move at the maximum speed and the leading leaf should provide the required intensity modulation.

A.3. Intensity-modulated Arc Therapy

Yu et al. (14) have developed an intensity-modulated arc therapy (IMAT) technique that uses the MLC dynamically to shape the fields as well as rotate the gantry in the arc therapy mode. The method is similar to the step-and-shoot in that each field (positioned along the arc) is subdivided into subfields of uniform intensity, which are superimposed to produce the desired intensity modulation. However, the MLC moves dynamically to shape each subfield while the gantry is rotating and the beam is on all the time. Multiple overlapping arcs are delivered with the leaves moving to new positions at a regular angular interval, for example, 5 degrees. Each arc is programmed to deliver one subfield at each gantry angle. A new arc is started to deliver the next subfield and so on until all the planned arcs and their

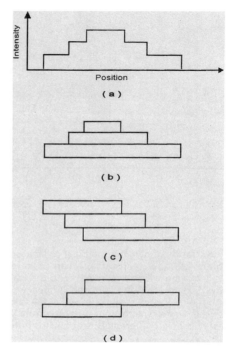

FIG. 20.5. Stacking of three subfields using multiple arcs. Different decomposition patterns are possible but only three are shown **(b, c, d)** to generate profile shown in **(a)**. (From Yu CX. Intensity modulated arc therapy: a new method for delivering conformal radiation therapy. In: Sternick ES, ed. *The theory and practice of intensity modulated radiation therapy.* Madison, WI: Advanced Medical Publishing, 1997:107–120, with permission.)

subfields have been delivered. The magnitude of the intensity step per arc and the number of arcs required depend on the complexity of the treatment. A typical treatment takes three to five arcs and the operational complexity is comparable to conventional arc therapy (18).

The IMAT algorithm divides the two-dimensional intensity distribution (obtained through inverse treatment planning) into multiple one-dimensional intensity profiles to be delivered by pairs of opposing leaves. The intensity profiles are then decomposed into discrete intensity levels to be delivered by subfields in a stack arrangement using multiple arcs as shown in Fig. 20.5. The leaf positions for each subfield are determined based on the decomposition pattern selected. As discussed earlier, there are $(N!)^2$ possible decomposition patterns for an N-level profile (to be delivered by N arcs) of only one peak. For example, a simple case of one-dimensional profile with three levels (Fig. 20.5A), there are $(3!)^2 = 36$ different decomposition patterns of which only three are shown (Fig. 20.5B–D). The decomposition patterns are determined by a computer algorithm, which creates field apertures by positioning left and right edges of each leaf pair. For efficiency, each edge is used once for leaf positioning. From a large number of decomposition patterns available, the algorithm favors those in which the subfields at adjacent beam angles require the least distance of travel by the MLC leaves.

As discussed earlier, the superimposition of subfields (through multiple arcs) creates the intensity modulation of fields at each beam angle. Whereas a one-dimensional profile is generated by stacking of fields defined by one leaf pair, the two-dimensional profiles are created by repeating the whole process for all the leaf pairs of the MLC.

B. Tomotherapy

Tomotherapy is an IMRT technique in which the patient is treated slice by slice by intensity-modulated beams in a manner analogous to CT imaging. A special collimator is designed to generate the IMBs as the gantry rotates around the longitudinal axis of

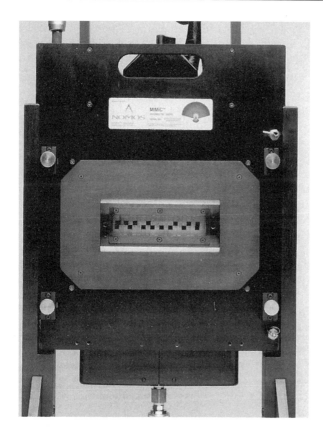

FIG. 20.6. Multileaf intensity-modulating collimator consisting of a long transverse slit aperture with two banks of 20 leaves each. (From Curran B. Conformal radiation therapy using a multileaf intensity modulating collimator. In: Sternick ES, ed. *The theory and practice of intensity modulated radiation therapy.* Madison, WI: Advanced Medical Publishing, 1997:75–90, with permission.)

the patient. In one device the couch is indexed one to two slices at a time and in the other the couch moves continuously as in a helical CT. The former was developed by the NOMOS Corporation[2] and the latter by the medical physics group at the University of Wisconsin.[3]

B.1. The Peacock System

The NOMOS collimator device is called the multileaf intensity-modulating collimator (MIMiC) and is used in conjunction with a treatment planning system, PEACOCKPLAN. The MIMiC and the PECOCKPLAN together are known as the PEACOCK system. Other important accessories include a special indexing table called the CRANE, a patient-fixation device called the TALON and an ultrasound based target localization system called the BAT (all NOMOS products are named after birds).

Multileaf Intensity-modulating Collimator

The MIMiC collimator consists of a long transverse slit aperture provided with two banks of 20 leaves each (Fig. 20.6). Each leaf can be moved independently and can provide an opening (at isocenter) of either (1 cm × 1 cm) or (1 cm × 2 cm). Each bank can therefore treat 1- or 2-cm thick slices of tissue 20 cm in diameter; because there are two such banks,

[2] NOMOS Corporation, Sewickley, Pennsylvania.
[3] University of Wisconsin, Madison, Wisconsin.

a 2- or 4-cm slice of tissue can be treated at one time. For extending the length of treatment volume beyond 4 cm, the couch is moved to treat the adjacent slices. This gives rise to field junctions, which is of concern in MIMiC-based IMRT.

The MIMiC leaves are made of tungsten and approximately 8 cm thick in the direction of the beam. The transmitted intensity through a leaf is approximately 1% for 10-MV x-rays. The leaf interfaces are multi-stepped to limit interleaf leakage to within 1%. Each leaf can be switched in 100 to 150 milliseconds, thus allowing a rapid change in beam apertures as the gantry rotates. Considering the number of possible field apertures at each gantry angle and the number of intensity steps that can be delivered at each gantry position, it is possible to create more than 10^{13} beam configurations for each arc (19). Thus the intensity modulation of beams can be finely controlled by the MIMiC technology.

A potential problem with MIMiC-based IMRT is the possibility of mismatch between adjacent slice pairs needed to treat a long target volume. Carol et al. (20) have studied the problem and shown that perfectly matched slices gave rise to 2% to 3% dose inhomogeneity across the junction. However, even a 2-mm error in indexing the couch resulted in dose inhomogeneity of the order of 40%. NOMOS solved this problem by designing accurate table indexing and patient fixation devices.

Crane

Because of the potential field matching problems in the use of MIMiC for treating adjacent slice pairs along the length of the patient, it is imperative to move the couch with extreme accuracy. A special indexing table called the CRANE has been designed by NOMOS, which is capable of moving the couch longitudinally with a 300-lb weight to distances of 0.1 to 0.2 mm. With such accuracy it is possible to reduce the junctional dose inhomogeneity to within ±3% (20).

Talon

Because of the stringent matchline requirements, NOMOS supplies an invasive head fixation system called the TALON. The device is attachable to the CT or the treatment unit couch and fixes the head position by the insertion of two bone screws into the inner table of the skull. Once the bone screws have been inserted, the TALON can be removed or reattached quickly as needed. An evacuated headrest can also be used to assist in repositioning at each treatment session.

For further details on the PEACOCK system of IMRT the reader is referred to reference 19.

B.2. Helical Tomotherapy

Mackie et al. (21) have proposed a method of IMRT delivery in which the linac head and gantry rotate while the patient is translated through the doughnut-shaped aperture in a manner analogous to a helical CT scanner. In this form of tomotherapy, the problem of inter-slice matchlines is minimized because of the continuous helical motion of the beam around the longitudinal axis of the patient.

A schematic diagram of the tomotherapy unit proposed by Mackie et al. is shown in Fig. 20.7. The linear accelerator is mounted on a CT-like gantry and rotates through a full circle. At the same time the patient couch is translated slowly through the aperture, thus creating a helical motion of the beam with respect to the patient. The unit is also equipped with a diagnostic CT scanner for target localization and treatment planning. The unit is able to perform both the diagnostic CT and the megavoltage CT.

The intensity-modulation of the fan beam is created by a specially designed collimator: a temporally modulated MLC consisting of a long, narrow slit with a set of multiple leaves at right angles. The leaves can be moved dynamically under computer control, in and out of the slit aperture to define a one-dimensional profile of the IMB as with the MIMiC. The major difference between the MIMiC-based tomotherapy and the helical tomotherapy is that in the former case the patient couch is stationary while the gantry rotates to treat each slice pair at a time and in the latter case the patient is translated continuously along

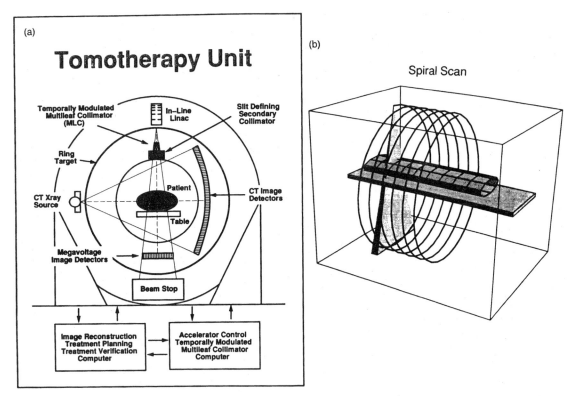

FIG. 20.7. A schematic diagram of the tomotherapy unit. (From Mackie TR, Holmes T, Swerdloff S, et al. Tomotherapy: a new concept for the delivery of conformal radiotherapy using dynamic collimation. *Med Physics* 1993;20:1709–1719, with permission.)

with the gantry rotation. The field match problems are thus minimized in the helical tomotherapy.

20.4. COMMISSIONING OF INTENSITY-MODULATED RADIATION THERAPY

IMRT is an integrated planning and delivery system of intensity-modulated beams, which are optimized to create highly conformal dose distributions for the treatment of planning target volume. Its clinical implementation requires careful testing of its component systems: the IMRT treatment-planning system (TPS) and the intensity-modulated beam (IMB) delivery system. In general, this will involve acquisition and input of appropriate beam data into the computer as required by the TPS algorithm, mechanical checks of the IMB delivery system and dosimetric verification of selected IMBs and IMRT plans. Some of the tests are repeated at scheduled intervals as part of a quality assurance program.

As a matter of principle, national or international protocols should be followed with regard to commissioning and QA. However, in the absence of established protocols, the user is advised to work closely with the equipment manufacturer as well as review the relevant literature to design appropriate programs. Many of the essential tests are devised by manufacturers who are more than willing to assist the physicist in acceptance testing and commissioning because it is in their interest to ensure safe operation and use of the equipment. The final approval for clinical application is the responsibility of the physicist and the physician in charge.

Although the commissioning and QA procedures will vary depending upon the IMRT system to be implemented, (e.g., step-and-shoot, sliding window, IMAT, tomotherapy) the critical issue is the confirmation that the approved treatment of a patient is delivered safely and with acceptable accuracy. The following discussion pertains to the sliding window IMRT technique, as an example.

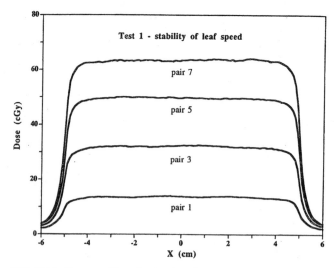

FIG. 20.8. Dose profiles obtained with test 1 to check the stability of leaf speed. (From Chui CS, Spirou S, LoSasso T. Testing of dynamic multileaf collimation. *Med Phys* 1996;23:635–641, with permission.)

A. Mechanical Testing of Dynamic Multileaf Collimator

To assure accurate delivery of IMBs with the dynamic multileaf collimator (DMLC), it is essential that the speed, acceleration, and position of leaves are controlled precisely and accurately as planned by the TPS. Chui et al. (22) have recommended the following five tests as a check of the mechanical accuracy of DMLC, which is fundamental to the accurate delivery of IMBs.

A.1. Stability of Leaf Speed

Individual pairs of opposed leaves should be tested for stability of their speed. This can be accomplished by instructing the opposed leaf pairs to move at different but constant speeds. If the leaf speeds are stable, the generated intensity profiles will be uniform. Figure 20.8 shows dose profiles generated by different leaf pairs which were made to move at different speeds. The profiles are measured using film placed perpendicular to central axis and at a depth greater than that of maximum dose in a phantom. Any fluctuations (over and above the film variation or artifacts) should indicate instability of leaf motion.

A.2. Dose Profile Across Adjacent Leaves

The film obtained with the test described above may be scanned in the direction perpendicular to leaf motion. Since the intensity within the width of each leaf is uniform, the intensity profile across the leaf pairs is expected to be a step function indicating different speeds or intensity levels for each leaf pair. However, the dose profile measured in a phantom will show a wavy pattern as seen in Fig. 20.9. The smearing of the intensity steps is caused by lateral scatter of photons and electrons in the phantom.

In this test one should look for any irregularity in the expected dose profile pattern in the direction perpendicular to the path of leaf motion.

A.3. Leaf Acceleration and Deceleration

In a normal delivery of intensity-modulated beams with DMLC, leaves are instructed to move at different speeds from one segment of the field to another. Discontinuities in

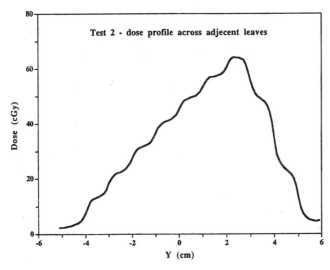

FIG. 20.9. Dose profile resulting from test 2 to check dose profile between adjacent leaves. The exposed film is scanned across the leaves in the direction perpendicular to the leaf motion. Due to the spread of secondary electrons and scattered photons, there is no flat dose region within the width of the leaves. (From Chui CS, Spirou S, LoSasso T. Testing of dynamic multileaf collimation. *Med Phys* 1996;23:635–641, with permission.)

planned intensity profiles could possibly occur as a result of acceleration or deceleration of leaves due to inertia. The extent of any such problem may be determined by repeating the test in A.1 and intentionally interrupting the beam several times. As the beam is turned off, the leaves decelerate to stop. Similarly, when the beam is resumed, the leaves accelerate to reach their normal speed. Dosimetric consequences of leaf acceleration and deceleration can thus be observed in the form of discontinuities in dose profiles at the points of beam interruption. Figure 20.10 shows no fluctuation beyond normal uncertainty in film dosimetry.

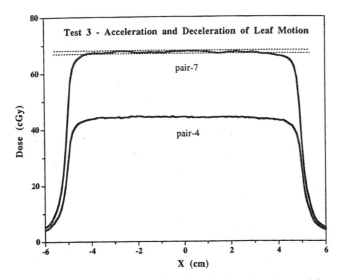

FIG. 20.10. Dose profiles resulting from leaf acceleration and deceleration (test 3). A dose variation of ± 1% is shown by dashed lines. (From Chui CS, Spirou S, LoSasso T. Testing of dynamic multileaf collimation. *Med Phys* 1996;23:635–641, with permission.)

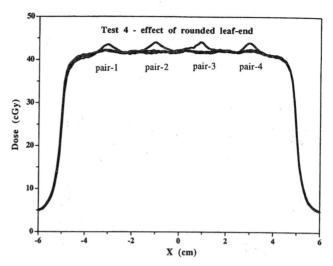

FIG. 20.11. Dose profile resulting from test 4 to check positional accuracy and the effect of rounded leaf end. A hot spot of approximately 5% in dose is seen in all profiles. (From Chui CS, Spirou S, LoSasso T. Testing of dynamic multileaf collimation. *Med Phys* 1996;23:635–641, with permission.)

A.4. Positional Accuracy of Leaves

To test the positional accuracy of leaves, the left and right leaves of an opposed pair are made to travel at the same speed but with a time lag between them. Each leaf is instructed to stop at the same position for a fixed duration of beam-on time and then continues its motion as before. Different pairs are instructed to stop at different positions. The uniformity of dose profiles in this case will indicate accurate leaf positioning. If any of the leaves were to under-travel or over-travel, there would be a hot spot or cold spot created depending upon if a gap or overlap occurred between the opposing leaves at the stoppage points. The MLC designed with rounded ends will naturally give rise to hot spots because of extra radiation leakage at the match positions. Thus the presence of hot or cold spots in dose profiles indicates positional inaccuracy except for the normal hot spots caused by the rounded ends of the leaves. Figure 20.11 shows the results indicating hot spots due to rounded ends but none due to positional errors.

A.5. Routine Mechanical Check

An overall check of the mechanical accuracy of DMLC has also been recommended (22), which may be incorporated into a routine QA program (e.g., daily or on the day of DMLC use). The test is similar to A.4 except that the stop positions of the opposing leaves are shifted with respect to each other to create a 1-mm gap. As a result, a hot spot appears at the gap positions. Driving all the leaves in fixed steps (e.g., 2 cm) and creating 1-mm-wide gaps at the stop positions will give rise to a pattern of straight dark lines on an irradiated film as shown in Fig. 20.12. Any variation in the location or the width of the dark lines would indicate positional error of a leaf. This can be assessed by visual inspection of the film image. The precision of this procedure is approximately 0.2 mm, which is approximately the tolerance allowed in the leaf calibration.

B. Dosimetric Checks

A series of dosimetric checks have been recommended by LoSasso et al. (23) specifically for the "sliding window" technique. These include measurements of MLC transmission, transmission through leaf ends, head scatter, and dose distribution in selected intensity modulated fields.

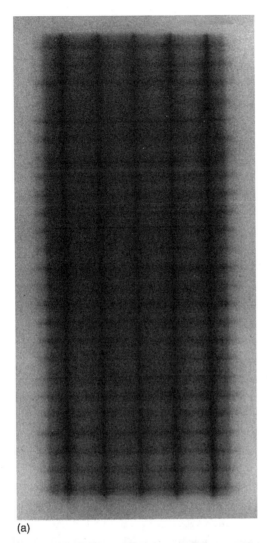

(a)

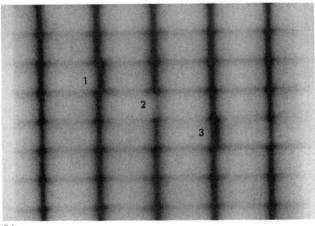

(b)

FIG. 20.12. Routine mechanical check (test 5). All 26 pairs produce dark lines on film at equally placed positions. If there is a
positional error in any leaf, the location or width of the dark lines
would differ from the other pairs. **A:** Normal condition with no
discernible positional error. **B:** Shift of dark lines caused by an in-
tentional error of 1mm introduced in three leaf pairs. (From Chui
CS, Spirou S, LoSasso T. Testing of dynamic multileaf collimation.
Med Phys 1996;23:635–641, with permission.)

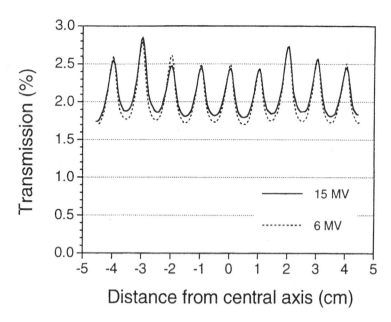

FIG. 20.13. The midleaf and interleaf transmission measured with film at isocenter. Transmission is the ratio of dose with the multileaf collimator blocked to that with the field open. Field size = 10 × 10 cm² and depth = 15cm. (From LoSasso T, Chui CS, Ling CC. Physical and dosimetric aspects of a multileaf collimation system used in the dynamic mode for implementing intensity-modulated radiotherapy. *Med Phys* 1998;25:1919–1927, with permission.)

B.1. Multileaf Collimator Transmission

Transmission through the MLC may be determined by measuring dose/MU in a phantom with the MLC closed and dividing it by dose/MU measured with the MLC open. Because the measurements are relative, the ratio of detector responses is equated to the ratio of doses. Because of the difference through the leaf and interleaf transmissions, the reading should be averaged with the detector (e.g., ion chambers) at different positions under the leaves. A film may also be used provided its response is corrected for the sensitometric curve determined for the given beam energy and depth in the phantom. Figure 20.13 shows the results obtained for a Varian MLC. It is seen that the MLC transmission varies between 1.7% at midleaf to 2.7% between leaves. An average transmission of 2% may be assumed in this case for the purpose of treatment planning calculations.

Several manufacturers offer MLCs with rounded leaf ends. This is done to maintain a constant geometric penumbra at different leaf positions in the beam. As an example, Fig. 20.14 shows the views of a Varian MLC from the side and from the front. Each leaf is 6-cm thick and has a rounded end. The central 3 cm of the end is circular with an 8.0-cm radius of curvature. The rest of end is straight at an angle of 11.3 degrees relative to the vertical axis. It has also been suggested that the effect of rounded leaf edges may be approximated in the treatment planning algorithm as an offset of leaves by 1 mm (23).

The leakage between the adjacent leaves is minimized by designing the leaves so that their sides partially overlap, that is, one side of the leaf protrudes outwards ("tongue") and the other recesses inward ("groove") so that the central parts of the adjacent leaves fit like a jigsaw puzzle. This overlap of the leaves reduces the extent of radiation leakage through interleaf gaps, which are necessary for leaf motion relative to each other. This so called "tongue and groove" effect gives rise to higher radiation leakage than that through middle body of the leaves but less than what it would be if the leaf sides were designed plane-faced. As shown earlier, interleaf transmission with the "tongue and groove" is between 2.5% to 2.7% (Fig. 20.13).

B.2. Head Scatter

Definition and measurement of collimator or head scatter factor (S_c) has been discussed in Chapter 10. If the MLC in the linac head is installed closer to the patient surface than the collimator jaws (as in Varian accelerators) the S_c factor depends predominately on the jaw opening and not on the MLC opening. In the use of static MLC in conventional radiotherapy, S_c for a given jaw opening is affected very little by the MLC setting for fields

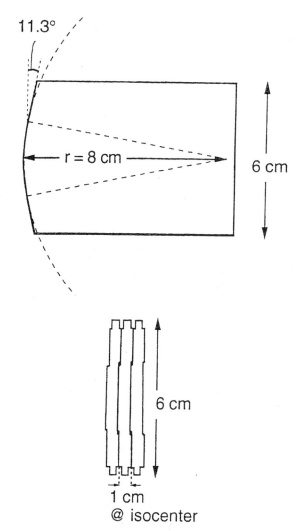

FIG. 20.14. Views of the leaves (*top*) from the side and (*bottom*) from the front. (From LoSasso T, Chui CS, Ling CC. Physical and dosimetric aspects of a multileaf collimation system used in the dynamic mode for implementing intensity modulated radiotherapy. *Med Phys* 1998;25:1919–1927, with permission.)

larger than 4×4 cm. However, as the MLC aperture is reduced to much smaller openings, S_c factor could drop significantly (e.g., by 5% for a 1×1 cm field). The reduction is caused by the MLC aperture approaching the geometric penumbra (radiation source has a finite size). On the other hand, if the MLC is located above the collimator jaws, the head scatter would be affected more by the MLC setting than the jaw opening. In either case, the treatment-planning algorithm must account for the S_c factors depending upon the MLC geometry and the IMRT technique used.

In the sliding window technique with the Varian DMLC, typically 1- to 4-cm wide moving gaps are used. The overall effect of the head scatter as a percentage of the target dose is minimal. A comparative influence of head scatter, MLC transmission, and the rounded edge transmission is shown in Fig. 20.15. As part of the commissioning procedure, these data should be measured and accounted for in the TPS.

B.4. Treatment Verification

After basic checks have been made with regard to the mechanical and dosimetric accuracy of DMLC, the following checks are needed to verify relative dose distribution as well as absolute dose delivered by DMLC for selected fields and treatment plans:

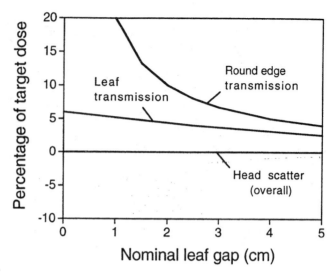

FIG. 20.15. Relative contribution of multileaf collimator transmission through midleaf, rounded edge and overall head scatter. (From LoSasso T, Chui CS, Ling CC. Physical and dosimetric aspects of a multileaf collimation system used in the dynamic mode for implementing intensity modulated radiotherapy. *Med Phys* 1998;25:1919–1927, with permission.)

Sliding Aperture Field. Using a film placed perpendicular to central axis and at a suitable depth in a phantom (e.g., 10 cm), dose distribution for a 10 × 10 cm field generated by a sliding MLC aperture (e.g., 5-mm wide) may be compared with a 10 × 10 cm static field. Absolute dose may also be verified by comparing optical densities (related to dose through a film sensitrometic curve measured at the same depth) or by an ion chamber in a water phantom.

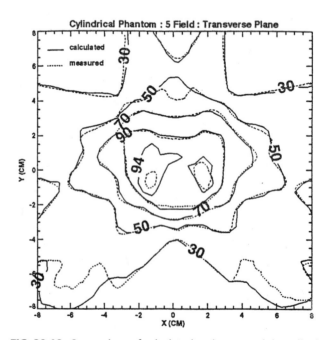

FIG. 20.16. Comparison of calculated and measured dose distribution with corrections for multileaf collimator transmission and head scatter. (From LoSasso T, Chui CS, Ling CC. Physical and dosimetric aspects of a multileaf collimation system used in the dynamic mode for implementing intensity modulated radiotherapy. *Med Phys* 1998;25:1919–1927, with permission.)

TABLE 20.1. IMRT QUALITY ASSURANCE PROGRAM[a]

Frequency	Procedure	Tolerance
Before first treatment	Individual field verification, plan verification	3% (point dose), other per clinical significance
Daily	Dose to a test point in each IMRT field	3%
Weekly	Static field vs. sliding window field dose distribution as a function of gantry and collimator angles	3% in dose delivery
Annually	All commissioning procedures: stability of leaf speed, leaf acceleration and deceleration, multileaf collimator transmission, leaf positional accuracy, static field vs. sliding window field as a function of gantry and collimator angles, standard plan verification	3% in dose delivery, other per clinical significance

[a] As an example for a "sliding window" IMRT program.

Individual IMRT fields generated by the treatment planning system can be verified by film dosimetry in a cubic phantom at a suitable depth (e.g., 10 cm). Commercial systems are available which allow side-by-side comparison of calculated vs. measured dose distributions. Exposed films are scanned into the computer, which has the software to convert optical densities into dose by using an appropriate sensitometric curve. The calculated and measured dose distributions are compared side by side or by viewing the differences between the two.

Multiple Field Plan. A multiple field IMRT plan may be generated in a cubic or cylindrical phantom and the dose distribution as well as absolute dose may be verified using film or an ion chamber. Alternatively, an IMRT plan of a particular patient (e.g., prostate plan) may be set up on a cylindrical or a cubic phantom to compare the calculated vs. measured distribution. Figure 20.16 is an example of such a comparison.

C. Quality Assurance

After the IMRT technique has been commissioned it is essential to set up a quality assurance program to maintain original accuracies, tolerances, and specifications of the system. Because of the complexity of the IMRT beams and the difficulty of verifying treatment doses by manual calculations, it is generally recommended to do plan verification and pretreatment checks in addition to the periodic testing of the system. A few of these tests are listed in Table 20.1, which are recommended until superseded by national/international QA protocols.

Plan verification procedure is discussed in section B.2 above. This check should be performed before the first treatment is delivered. In the daily pre-treatment check, each IMRT field should be spot-checked in a phantom by measuring dose to a test point. Detector systems that are routinely used for daily linac output constancy check or in vivo patient dose monitoring (e.g., ion chamber matrix, diode system) can also be used for this measurement.

20.5. DOSE CALCULATION ALGORITHMS

Dose calculation algorithms for IMRT are basically the same as those for standard 3-D treatment planning (see Chapter 19) except for the dynamic features of multileaf collimation. In-air fluence distribution is first calculated based on the time (or MUs) a point is exposed to in the open part of the MLC window and the time it is shielded by the leaves. For simplicity, the calculated fluence may be represented by a step function, having full intensity in the open and only transmitted intensity in the shielded part of the field. Refinements are added by taking into account leaf-edge penumbra (e.g., offset for rounded edges), interleaf transmission (e.g., "tongue and groove" effect) and head scatter as a function of MLC aperture and jaw position.

A. In-air Fluence Distribution

The in-air photon fluence information for an intensity-modulated beam is imbedded in a computer file, which specifies the position of each leaf and jaw at any instant of time. The algorithm reconstructs the fluence distribution by integrating an output function, which is dependent on whether the point is in the open portion of the field or under the MLC, for example,

$$\Psi(x, y) = \int I_{air}(t) \, T(x, y, t) \, dt \qquad (20.8)$$

where $\Psi(x, y)$ is the photon energy fluence in air at a point (x, y) and $I_{air}(x, y, t)$ is the beam intensity or energy fluence rate at time t; $T(x, y, t)$ is the leaf transmission factor at any time t, being unity when the point is in the open portion of the field and a transmission fraction when under a jaw or leaf.

B. Depth-dose Distribution

Once the photon energy fluence distribution incident on the patient has been calculated, any of the methods discussed in Chapter 19 may be used to compute depth-dose distribution. Because the size and shape of the beam apertures are greatly variable and field dimensions of 1 cm or less may be frequently required to provide intensity modulation, the most commonly used methods of dose calculation in IMRT are the pencil beam and the convolution-superposition. Monte Carlo techniques are also under development but are considered futuristic at this time because of their limitation on computation speed.

C. Monitor Unit Calculations

Manual calculations of monitor units for IMRT is difficult, if not impossible. Reliance is usually made on the TPS to calculate monitor units, following the same algorithm as used in the calculation of depth-dose distribution. Some additional data (e.g., S_C, S_P, TMRs, reference dose/MU) specific to the accelerator and the algorithm may be required but the MU calculations are performed internally by the TPS in parallel with dose calculations. This practice seems contrary to the long-standing principle that the monitor units must be calculated or checked independently of the TPS. IMRT, however, is given an exception because of its complexity, caused primarily by intensity modulation. The user is encouraged to develop or acquire an independent MU calculation system, if available commercially. The latter will require rigorous commissioning of its own before it could be used as a check on the TPS. Nonetheless, it is incumbent on the user to verify MUs either by independent calculations or by phantom measurements. These checks are part of patient-specific quality assurance and should be conducted in addition to the initial commissioning of IMRT (even though commissioning includes experimental verification of MU calculations by the TPS under benchmark conditions).

In view of the facts that the IMRT treatment planning system is like a "black box," that manual calculations are impractical and that patient-specific dosimetry is labor intensive, the need for independent MU calculation cannot be overemphasized. A few reports (24,25) have addressed this problem but commercial software needs to be developed as an adjunct to the TPS to provide an independent verification of MUs.

Methods of calculating MUs to deliver a certain dose are inverse of the methods used in the calculation of dose when a patient is irradiated with a given beam weight or fluence. Although doses in a TPS are calculated as relative distributions, the normalizing conditions used by the algorithm can be related to the calibration conditions to provide MUs. In IMRT, because beam intensity within the field is modulated (beam profile is no longer uniform), pencil beam or convolution-superposition algorithms are the methods of choice for dose calculations. However, they are not suitable for manual calculation of monitor units. It is more practical to write a separate computer program, which simplifies these or other models and applies them more transparently to the problem of monitor unit calculation. Basic principles of this approach are presented below as examples.

C.1. Finite-size Pencil Beam

Instead of generating an infinitesimally small pencil beam analytically, it is possible to measure a finite-size pencil beam (FSPB) experimentally. The latter consists of measured depth-dose distribution and profiles for a small field size (e.g., 1×1 cm^2). In the FSPB dose calculation formalism, a given intensity modulated field is divided into finite-size elements (1×1 cm^2) and the dose from all the FSPBs is integrated, taking into account the relative weight for the total fluence for each pencil beam. The following equation summarizes the relationship between monitor units (MU) and dose $D_i(P)$ at a point P at depth d contributed by the nth FSPB:

$$D_i(P) = k \cdot \text{MU} \cdot \text{TMR}(d) \cdot S_{C,P} \cdot T_i \cdot \text{ISF} \cdot \text{OAR}_i(d) \qquad (20.9)$$

where K is the calibration factor of the accelerator (dose/MU under reference conditions); TMR (d) is the tissue-maximum ratio at depth d for the FSPB; $S_{C,P}$ is the output factor at the reference depth of maximum dose for the FSPB relative to the calibration field size (10×10 cm^2); T_i is the transmission factor (T_i is a small fraction when P is under the leaf and is equal to unity when P is in the open); ISF is the inverse square law factor to account for change in distance from the source to point P versus the distance from the source to the reference point of calibration; and OAR$_i$ (d) is the off-axis ratio at point P relative to the central axis of FSPB$_i$. It should be noted that the above equation is similar to the one used for traditional radiation therapy beams (see Chapter 10). Total dose at point P is calculated by summing the contribution of all FSPBs to the point P.

The above method of calculating dose distribution has been used by a commercially available TPS, CORVUS[4]. Details of the algorithm have been published by Sternick et al. (26). Because the method involves convolution of FSPBs and many other corrections related to patient contours and the specific IMB collimator, it is not possible to adopt it as such for manual calculations. However, with a few reasonable approximations, a simpler computer program can be written to provide an independent verification of monitor units. Such a program has been developed by Kung et al. (25) and is briefly discussed below.

Kung et al.'s method is based on the concept of modified Clarkson integration (see Chapter 9) in which the Clarkson integration is carried out over annular sectors instead of pie sectors. A given IMRT field is divided into concentric circles, centered at central axis. It is assumed that the fluence contributed to central axis from subfields located at radius r is the same as would be by uniformly irradiated subfields of averaged fluence at radius r. In other words, fluence or MUs delivered to subfields at radius r can be averaged to calculate their contribution to scattered dose along central axis, because of the azimuthal symmetry.

Details of monitor units to be delivered to subfields are contained in the DMLC file. Composite of weighted MUs of each subfield gives a fluence map in terms of MU(x, y). Average fluence, $\overline{\text{MU}}(r)$, at the circumference of a circle of radius r is given by:

$$\overline{\text{MU}}(r) = \frac{1}{2\pi} \int_{\text{circle}} \text{MU}(x, y) \, d\theta \qquad (20.10)$$

---

[4] Produced by NOMOS Corporation, Sewickley, Pennsylvania.

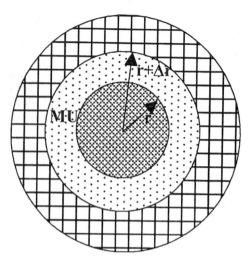

FIG. 20.17. Schematic of modified Clarkson method in which integration is carried out over annular sectors. The dose contributed by an annulus (dotted) is the difference between the doses from the circular fields of radii $r + \Delta r$ and r. (Redrawn from Kung JH, Chen GTY, Kuchnir FK. A monitor unit verification calculation in intensity modulated radiotherapy as a dosimetry quality assurance. *Med Phys* 2000;27:2226–2230.)

The contribution of scattered D_s to central axis at depth from an annulus between radii r and $r + \Delta r$, uniformly irradiated by $\overline{MU}(r)$, is given by:

$$D_s(d, \text{annulus}) = K \cdot \overline{MU}(r) \cdot S_C \cdot [S_P(r + \Delta r) \cdot \text{TMR}(r + \Delta r)$$
$$- S_P(r) \cdot \text{TMR}(r)] \cdot \text{ISF} \qquad (20.11)$$

where K is the dose/MU under reference conditions of calibration, S_C is the head scatter (corresponding to jaw opening, ignoring MLC scatter); S_P and TMR (defined in Chapter 10) correspond to a circular field of radius r which can be derived from equivalent rectangular field data (see Chapter 9); and ISF is the inverse squarer law factor, defined earlier.

Total dose, $D(d)$, at the center of an annulus is the sum of primary dose D_P, and scattered dose; D_S.

$$D(d) = D_P(d) + D_S(d) \qquad (20.12)$$

Referring to Fig. 20.17, D_P is calculated from $\overline{MU}(0)$, which is obtained by averaging $MU(x, y)$ over a small central circular area (e.g., $r = 1$ cm).

$$D_P = K \cdot \overline{MU}(0) \cdot S_C \cdot S_P(0) \cdot \text{TMR}(0) \cdot \text{ISF} \qquad (20.13)$$

The total scattered dose at central axis, D_S, is calculated by Clarkson integration over all annuli:

$$D_S = K \cdot S_C \cdot \text{ISF} \Sigma \overline{MU}(r)[S_P(r + \Delta r) \cdot \text{TMR}(r + \Delta r) - S_P(r) \cdot \text{TMR}(r)] \qquad (20.14)$$

Kung et al. (25) have tested the above algorithm for a number of IMRT cases and found an agreement within $\pm 3\%$ with CORVUS.

C.2. Convolution Algorithms

The convolution method involves radiation transport in which primary interactions are calculated separately from the interaction of secondary particles (charged particles and scattered photons). The dose in a phantom is calculated by convolving the terma distribution with dose kernels (see Chapter 19). The convolution dose engine basically calculates dose per unit energy fluence. Since the incident energy fluence is proportional to MUs, the dose can be scaled to give dose/MU.

A suitable formalism for the calculation of monitor units using convolution algorithm could be based on dose per unit energy fluence. For example, the basic equation used by ADAC Pinnacle[5] treatment planning system is of the form:

$$\text{MU} = \frac{D_d}{K \cdot \text{ND} \cdot S_C \cdot \text{ISF}} \tag{20.15}$$

where D_d is the prescribed dose at depth d and ND is the normalized dose factor. ND is the ratio of dose per unit energy fluence at the prescription point to the dose per unit energy fluence at the reference point of calibration.

It can be shown that for a normally incident beam in a water phantom, ND $=$ TMR $\times S_p$. Let C denote the field size defined by collimator jaws; C_o be the reference field size (10×10 cm^2); and Ψ be the photon energy fluence.

By definition, at the prescription point:

$$\text{ND} = \frac{D_d(C)}{\Psi(C)} \cdot \frac{\Psi(C_o)}{D_{d_m}(C_o)} \tag{20.16}$$

or,

$$\text{ND} = \frac{D_d(C)}{D_{d_m}(C)} \cdot \frac{D_{d_m}(C)}{D_{d_m}(C_o)} \cdot \frac{\Psi(C_o)}{\Psi(C)} \tag{20.17}$$

From the definitions of TMR, S_C, S_p and $S_{C,p}$ (see Chapter 10), Equation 20.17 becomes:

$$\text{ND} = \text{TMR} \cdot S_{C,p} \cdot \frac{1}{S_C} \tag{20.18}$$

or,

$$\text{ND} = \text{TMR} \cdot S_p \tag{20.19}$$

Thus the MU calculation formalism based on dose per unit energy fluence is consistent with the traditional system using TMR, S_C, S_p, etc. The advantage of using dose per unit energy fluence is that the MUs are calculated simultaneously with dose computation by the convolution dose engine for which the raw output is the dose per unit energy fluence.

Mackie et al. (27) have suggested calibration of the accelerator in terms of incident energy fluence per monitor unit $\Psi(P)/\text{MU}$ at a defined point P (e.g., reference point of calibration). If D_{meas} is the measured dose in a water phantom at P and D_{calc} is the calculated dose (by convolution algorithm) at the same point in a simulated water phantom, under the same irradiation conditions, then the energy fluence calibration factor is given by:

$$\frac{\Psi(P)}{\text{MU}} = \frac{D_{\text{meas}}/\text{MU}}{D_{\text{calc}}/\Psi(P)} \tag{20.20}$$

The computed dose per incident energy fluence $D(x, y, z)/\Psi(P)$ at any point can thus be converted to dose per monitor unit $D(x, y, z)/\text{MU}$ using the energy fluence calibration factor given by Equation 20.20:

$$D(x, y, z)/\text{MU} = [D(x, y, z)/\Psi(P)] \cdot \Psi(P)/\text{MU} \tag{20.21}$$

As discussed earlier, for a conventional radiotherapy beam, monitor units calculated by convolution algorithms can be verified by using traditional concepts of TMRs and measured

---

[5] ADAC Laboratories, Milpitas, California.

output factors. In IMRT, where the fields are irradiated with intensity-modulated beams, the traditional formalisms break down unless the field is subdivided into elementary fields of uniform intensity but different fluences. A method like the modified Clarkson integration could then be applied using TMRs and output factors for the reference elementary beam, as described earlier. Since manual verification is still difficult, the need for independent computer codes cannot be avoided.

20.6. CLINICAL APPLICATION

IMRT can be used for any treatment for which external beam radiation therapy is an appropriate choice. The basic difference between conventional radiotherapy (including 3-D CRT) and IMRT is that the latter provides an extra degree of freedom, that is, intensity modulation, in achieving dose conformity. Especially targets of concave shape surrounding sensitive structures can be treated conformly with steep dose gradients outside the target boundaries—a task that is almost impossible to accomplish with conventional techniques. Figure 20.18 (see color insert) is an example of such a target.

For localized lesions in any part of the body, IMRT compares well with or exceeds the capabilities of other techniques or modalities. In treating brain lesions, IMRT can generate dose distributions comparable to those obtained with stereotactic radiation therapy using x-ray knife or gamma knife. Figure 20.19 (see color insert) shows a few examples of head and neck tumors. Additionally, IMRT is not limited by target size or its location.

IMRT can also compete well with proton beam therapy for all disease sites, albeit with some subtle differences radiobiologically but not so subtle differences cost wise. The price of IMRT capability is only a small fraction of that of a proton beam facility.

Superficial disease sites (e.g., parotid, neck nodes, chest wall), often treated with electrons, can also be treated with IMRT as effectively, if not better. However, practical considerations may preclude sometimes the use of IMRT for cases where electrons offer a technically simpler option, e.g., skin cancers, total skin irradiation, superficial breast boost, etc.

IMRT is comparable to brachytherapy in dose conformity but it is a different modality radiobiologically. So the choice between IMRT and brachytherapy should be based not only on the technical or dosimetric considerations, but also on the radiobiologic properties of brachytherapy versus external beam. For example, treatment of prostate with seed implants has a different rationale than it is for IMRT although dose conformity is comparable in terms of dose fall off beyond the prostate volume. Radiobiology of the two modalities is obviously different because of differences in dose homogeneity and dose rate or fractionation (e.g., continuous vs. fractionated dose delivery).

Of all the sites suitable for IMRT, the prostate gland has received the greatest attention because of the greater degree of dose conformity that can be achieved compared to the conventional techniques, including 3-D conformal (Fig. 20.20) (see color insert). However, it is debatable whether a higher degree of dose conformity correlates with better treatment outcome or if it is a sufficient rationale for dose escalation. The reader should bear in mind that dose conformity is a "double-edged sword," with more normal tissue sparing on the one hand and greater possibility of target miss on the other. As discussed earlier in conjunction with 3-D CRT (see Chapter 19), an image-based treatment plan cannot fully account for (a) the true extent of clinical target volume, (b) accurately applicable TCP and NTC, and (c) natural motion of target volume and organs at risk. Because of these unavoidable uncertainties, too much emphasis on dose conformity can backfire, resulting in inadequate target coverage or increase in normal tissue complication especially when following aggressive dose-escalation schemes. The reader is referred to Levitt and Khan (28) for a cautionary note on conformal radiotherapy and dose escalation in the prostate gland.

IMRT is an elegant treatment planning and delivery technique. It allows practically unlimited control over shaping of dose distribution to fit tumors of complex shape while sparing critical normal tissues in close proximity. Undoubtedly, the IMRT is the ultimate tool in external beam radiation therapy and is expected to supersede other techniques including 3-D CRT and stereotactic radiation therapy. However, it should be recognized that technical precision alone in dose planning and delivery does not ensure superior clinical results. Of equal or greater importance are the design of PTV, localization of organs at risk, patient immobilization, and on-line portal imaging. In short, the success of IMRT when indicated does not depend on *if* it is applied but rather *how* it is applied.

REFERENCES

1. Brahme A. Optimization of stationary and moving beam radiation therapy techniques. *Radiother Oncol* 1988;12:129–140.
2. Källman P, Lind B, Ekloff A, et al. Shaping of arbitrary dose distribution by dynamic Multileaf collimation. *Phys Med Biol* 1988;33:1291–1300.
3. Web S. Optimization of conformal dose distributions by simulated annealing. *Phys Med Biol* 1989;34:1349–1370.
4. Bortfeld TR, Burkelbach J, Boesecke R, et al. Methods of image reconstruction from projections applied to conformation therapy. *Phys Med Biol* 1990;35:1423–1434.
5. Rosen II, Lane RG, Morrill SM, et al. Treatment planning optimization using linear programming. *Med Phys* 1991;18:141–152.
6. Convery DJ, Rosenbloom ME. The generation of intensity-modulated fields for conformal radiotherapy by dynamic collimation. *Phys Med Biol* 1992;37:1359–1374.
7. Mohan R, Mageras GS, Baldwin B, et al. Clinically relevant optimization of 3D conformal treatments. *Med Phys* 1992;933–944.
8. Holmes T, Mackie TR. A filtered back projection dose calculation method for inverse treatment planning. *Med Phys* 1994;21:303–313.
9. Mageras GS, Mohan R. Application of fast simulated annealing to optimization of conformal radiation treatment. *Med Phys* 1993;20:639–647.
10. Web S. *The physics of conformal radiotherapy.* Bristol, UK: IOP Publishing, 1997.
11. Lind B, Brahme A. Development of treatment technique for radiotherapy optimization. *Int J Imaging Sys Technol* 1995;6:33–42.
12. Spirou SV, Chui CS. Generation of arbitrary intensity profiles by combining the scanning beam with dynamic Multileaf collimation. *Med Phys* 1996;23:1–8.
13. Bortfeld TR, Kahler DL, Waldron TJ, et al. X-ray field compensation with multileaf collimators. *Int J Radiat Oncol Biol Phys* 1994;28:723–730.
14. Yu CX. Intensity modulated arc therapy with dynamic Multileaf collimation: an alternative to tomotherapy. *Phys Med Biol* 1995;40:1435–1449.
15. Yu CX, Symons M, Du MN, et al. A method for implementing dynamic photon beam intensity modulation using independent jaws and a Multileaf collimator. *Phys Med Biol* 1995;40:769–787.
16. Stein J, Bortfeld T, Dörshel B, et al. Dynamic x-ray compensation for conformal radiotherapy by dynamic collimation. *Radiother Oncol* 1994;32:163–173.
17. Svensson R, Källman P, Brahme A. Analytical solution for the dynamic control of Multileaf collimators. *Phys Med Biol* 1994;39:37–61.
18. Yu CX. Intensity modulated arc therapy: a new method for delivering conformal radiation therapy. In: Sternick ES, ed. *The theory and practice of intensity modulated radiotherapy.* Madison, WI: Advanced Medical Publishing, 1997:107–120.
19. Curran B. Conformal radiation therapy using a multileaf intensity modulating collimator. In: Sternick ES, ed. *The theory and practice of intensity modulated radiotherapy.* Madison, WI: Advanced Medical Publishing, 1997:75–90.
20. Carol MP, Grant W, Bleier AR, et al. The field-matching problem as it applies to the Peacock three-dimensional conformal system for intensity modulation. *Int J Radiat Oncol Biol Phys* 1996;183–187.
21. Mackie TR, Holmes T, Swerdloff S, et al. Tomotherapy: a new concept for the delivery of conformal radiotherapy using dynamic collimation. *Med Phys* 1993;20:1709–1719.
22. Chui CS, Spirou S, LoSasso T. Testing of dynamic multileaf collimation. *Med Phys* 1996;23:635–641.
23. LoSosso T, Chui CS, Ling CC. Physical and dosimetric aspects of a Multileaf collimation system used in the dynamic mode for implementing intensity modulated radiotherapy. *Med Phys* 1998;25:1919–1927.
24. Boyer A, Xing L, Ma C-M, et al. Theoretical considerations of monitor unit calculations for intensity modulated beam treatment planning. *Med Phys* 1999;26:187–195.

25. Kung JH, Chen GTY, Kuchnir FK. A monitor unit verification calculation in intensity modulated radiotherapy as a dosimetry quality assurance. *Med Phys* 2000;27:2226–2230.
26. Sternick ES, Carol MP, Grand W. Intensity-modulated radiotherapy. In: Khan FM, Potish RA, eds. *Treatment planning in radiation oncology.* Baltimore: Williams & Wilkins, 1998:187–213.
27. Mackie TR, Rechwerdt P, McNutt T, et al. Photon beam dose computations. In: Mackie TR, Palta JR, eds. *Teletherapy: present and future.* Madison, WI: Advanced Medical Publishing, 1996:103–135.
28. Levitt SH, Khan FM. The rush to judgment: does the evidence support the enthusiasm over three-dimensional conformal radiation therapy and dose escalation in the treatment of prostate cancer? *Int J Radiat Oncol Biol Phys* 2001;51:871–879.

21

STEREOTACTIC RADIOSURGERY

21.1. INTRODUCTION

Stereotactic radiosurgery (SRS) is a single fraction radiation therapy procedure for treating intracranial lesions using a combination of a stereotactic apparatus and narrow multiple beams delivered through noncoplanar isocentric arcs. The same procedure when used for delivering multiple dose fractions is called stereotactic radiotherapy (SRT). Both techniques involve three-dimensional imaging to localize the lesion and delivering treatment that concentrates the dose in the target volume and spares as much as possible the normal brain. A high degree of dose conformity is a hallmark of SRS, which is generally achieved by using appropriate circular beams to fit the lesion, optimizing arc angles and weights and using multiple isocenters or dynamically shaping the field during arc rotations with mini (or micro) multileaf collimators.

Accuracy of beam delivery is another hallmark of SRS. It is strictly controlled by a specially designed stereotactic apparatus, which is used through all steps of the process: imaging, target localization, head immobilization, and treatment set-up. Because of the critical nature of brain tissue, elaborate quality assurance procedures are observed. The best achievable mechanical accuracy in terms of isocenter displacement from the defined center of target image is 0.2 mm ± 0.1 mm, although a maximum error of ± 1.0 mm is commonly accepted in view of the unavoidable uncertainties in target localization.

The term radiosurgery was coined by a neurosurgeon Lars Leksell in 1951 (1). He developed the procedure in the late 1940s to destroy dysfunctional loci in the brain using orthovoltage x-rays and particle accelerators. His later work involved the use of a specially designed cobalt unit, called the gamma knife. Currently there are three types of radiation used in SRS and SRT: heavy-charged particles, cobalt-60 gamma rays, and megavoltage x-rays. Of these, the most commonly used modality is the x-rays produced by a linear accelerator. In analogy to gamma knife, the linac-based SRS unit may be called x-ray knife. Although the clinical differences between the gamma knife and x-ray knife are insignificant, the cost of the former is about ten times that of the latter; both are substantially cheaper than a heavy particle accelerator. Of course, most of the radiation generators used for SRS are also used for other radiotherapy procedures with the exception of gamma knife, which is dedicated solely for SRS.

21.2. STEREOTACTIC RADIOSURGERY TECHNIQUES

Two SRS techniques are described in this chapter: linac-based x-ray knife, and gamma knife. Greater details are provided on the most frequently used system, the x-ray knife, while a brief review is given on the gamma knife for general information. Extensive literature exists on SRS techniques. The reader is referred to AAPM Report No. 54 (2) for review and pertinent bibliography.

A. X-ray Knife

The linac-based SRS technique consists of using multiple noncoplanar arcs of circular (or dynamically shaped) beams converging on to the machine isocenter, which is stereotactically placed at the center of imaged target volume. A spherical dose distribution obtained in this case can be shaped to fit the lesion more closely by manipulating several parameters: selectively blocking parts of the circular field, shaping the beams-eye-aperture dynamically with a multileaf collimator, changing arc angles and weights, using more than one isocenter and combining stationary beams with arcing beams. Optimization of some of these parameters is carried out automatically by the treatment-planning software.

A.1. Stereotactic Frame

There are basically two linac-based SRS systems: pedestal-mounted frame and couch-mounted frame. The frame in this case refers to an apparatus called stereotactic frame, which is attachable to the patient's skull as well as to the couch or pedestal. This provides a rigidly fixed frame of coordinates for relating the center of imaged target to isocenter of treatment. Several frames have been developed for general stereotactic applications and some of these have been adopted for SRS. The most noteworthy of the SRS frames are: Leksell, Riechert-Mundinger, Todd-Wells, and Brown-Robert-Wells (BRW). These have been described in detail by Galloway and Maciunas (3). Only the BRW frame will be discussed in this chapter.

Figure 21.1 shows the basic stereotactic system with the BRW frame, computed tomography (CT) localizer, angiographic localizer and a device for fixing the frame to the patient support table. The BRW frame has three orthogonal axes: anterior, lateral, and axial (Fig. 21.2). The three axes intersect at the center of the circular frame and the origin is defined 80 mm from the top surface of the ring.

The CT localizer frame is equipped with nine fiducial rods, which appear as dots in the transaxial slice image. Since the location of these points in the frame space is precisely known, any point in the image can be defined in terms of the frame coordinates. A patient docking device couples the frame to the accelerator through the patient support system (pedestal or couch-mount bracket). The origin of the frame is aligned with the linac isocenter to within 0.2 to 1.0 mm, depending on the system (pedestal-mounted systems tend to be more accurate than the couch mounted ones).

The angiographic localizer frame consists of four plates and attaches to the BRW head ring. Each plate is embedded with four lead markers, which act as fiducial markers for the angiographic images.

The MRI localizer is a slightly modified version of the CT localizer and is compatible with magnetic resonance imaging (MRI). It has fiducial rods whose locations are precisely known with respect to the BRW frame, thus allowing the localization of any point within the MRI image.

A special relocatable head ring, called the Gill-Thomas-Cosman (GTC), has been designed for fractionated SRT (Fig. 21.3). It uses a bite block system, headrest bracket and Velcro straps attached to the BRW frame.

A.2. Linac Isocentric Accuracy

An essential element of SRS procedure is the alignment of stereotactic frame coordinates with the linac isocenter (point of intersection of the axes of rotation of the gantry, collimator and couch). Acceptable specification of linac isocentric accuracy requires that the isocenter (mechanical as well as radiation isocenter) remains within a sphere of radius 1.0 mm with any combination of gantry, collimator, and couch rotation. The same specification holds good for a linac used for SRS, with an added stipulation that the stereotactically determined target isocenter is coincident with the linac isocenter within ± 1.0 mm (2). Tests required to check the linac specifications and its isocentric accuracy are described in the AAPM

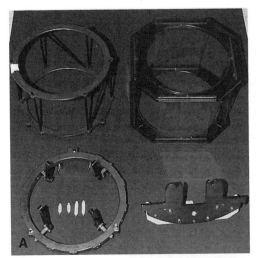
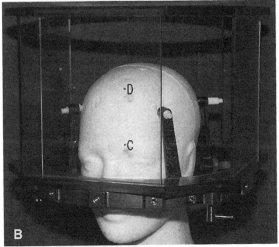
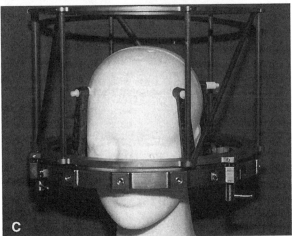

FIG. 21.1. Basic stereotactic system showing **(A)** (starting clockwise from upper right) CT localizer, angiographic localizer, patient-positioning mount and head ring with posts and pins; **(B)** angiographic localizer; and **(C)** CT localizer. (From Bova FJ, Meeks SL, Friedman WA. Linac radiosurgery: system requirements, procedures, and testing. In: Khan FM, Potish RA, eds. *Treatment planning in radiation oncology.* Baltimore: Williams & Wilkins, 1998:215–241, with permission.)

Reports 40 and 45 (2,4). These recommendations, which are also discussed in Chapter 17, form the basis of linac QA required for SRS.

A.3. Stereotactic Accuracy

The BRW frame system includes a verification device called the phantom base (Fig. 21.4). It has identical coordinates (anteroposterior, lateral, and vertical) to those of the BRW frame. As a standalone device, it provides an absolute frame of reference for stereotactic coordinates of the entire system: BRW frame, patient support system, and the localizer systems for CT, MRI, and angiography. The accuracy of phantom base should be carefully maintained because it serves as a reference standard for all other steps in the stereotactic localization process. Gerbi et al. (5) have constructed a simple and mechanically rugged device to routinely test the accuracy of the phantom base.

Lutz et al. (6) have described a procedure of using the phantom base to check the alignment of radiation isocenter with the target point defined by the coordinates set on the BRW pedestal. This test is performed by setting the target point (treatment isocenter) coordinates on the phantom base. The tip of the phantom base pointer is matched to the tip of the transfer pointer. The tapered tip of the transfer pointer is then replaced with

Post support   Positional label

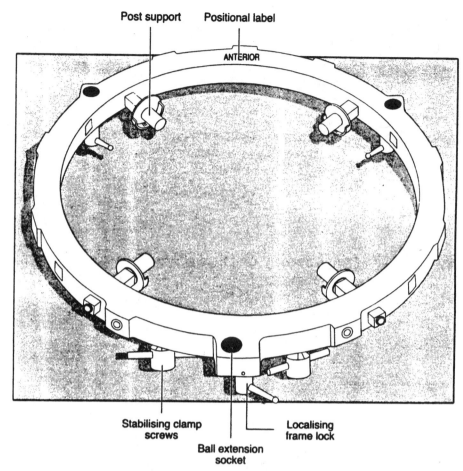

Stabilising clamp
screws

Ball extension
socket

Localising
frame lock

FIG. 21.2. Schematic drawing of BRW frame. (From Cho KH, Gerbi BJ, Hall WA. Stereotactic radiosurgery and radiotherapy. In: Levitt SH, Khan FM, Potish RA, et al., eds. *Technological basis of radiation therapy.* Philadelphia: Lippincott Williams & Wilkins, 1999:147–172, with permission.)

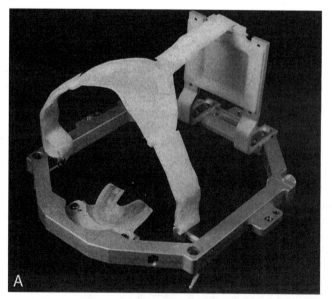
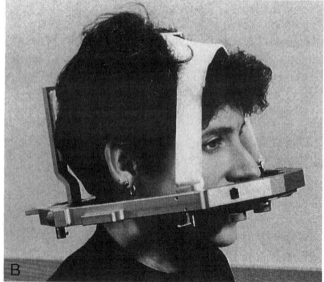

FIG. 21.3. **A:** The GTC relocatable head ring with bite block and Velcro straps. **B:** The GTC head ring worn by the patient. (From Cho KH, Gerbi BJ, Hall WA. Stereotactic radiosurgery and radiotherapy. In: Levitt SH, Khan FM, Potish RA, et al., eds. *Technological basis of radiation therapy.* Philadelphia: Lippincott Williams & Wilkins, 1999:147–172, with permission.)

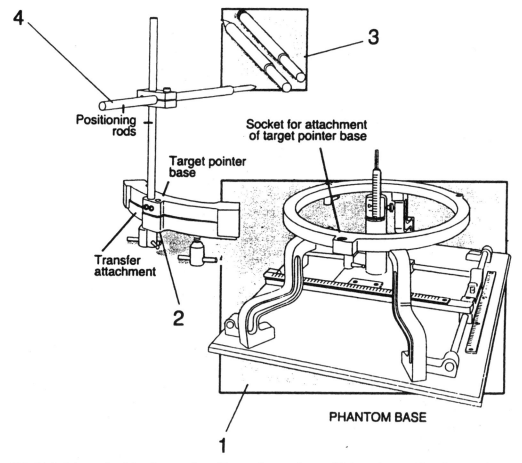

FIG. 21.4. Schematic of the phantom base (1), transfer attachment (2), interchangeable pointer, and target ball devices (3), and the transfer pointer assembly (4). (From Cho KH, Gerbi BJ, Hall WA. Stereotactic radiosurgery and radiotherapy. In: Levitt SH, Khan FM, Potish RA, et al., eds. *Technological basis of radiation therapy.* Philadelphia: Lippincott Williams & Wilkins, 1999:147–172, with permission.)

a tungsten ball, thus assuring that its center is located exactly at the tapered tip position (Fig. 21.5A). The transfer pointer (also known as target simulator) is then attached to the pedestal (also known as independent support stand [ISS]) whose coordinates are set to the same BRW coordinates as those set on the phantom base. A series of port films of the tungsten ball is taken at a number of gantry and couch angle combinations (Fig. 21.5B). Figure 21.5C shows the results for eight gantry-table combinations. Concentricity of the ball image within the circular field is analyzed with special magnifying eyepiece containing a fine scale. This test can indicate alignment to within ± 0.1 mm.

In the couch-mounted system, the tip of the phantom pointer is aligned with the intersection point of the wall-mounted lasers. After a precise alignment, the tapered tip is replaced with the tungsten ball. The center of this sphere simulates the target point within the patient's brain. Verification films are then taken for a number of gantry-and couch-angle combinations. This test assures that the target point, the radiation isocenter, and the intersection point of the wall-mounted lasers are aligned regardless of the gantry or table position.

A.4. Overall Accuracy

Before the SRS system is declared ready for patient treatments, the entire radiosurgery procedure should be tested for geometric accuracy (2). This can be accomplished by using a suitable head phantom with imageable hidden targets. The test phantom and the targets

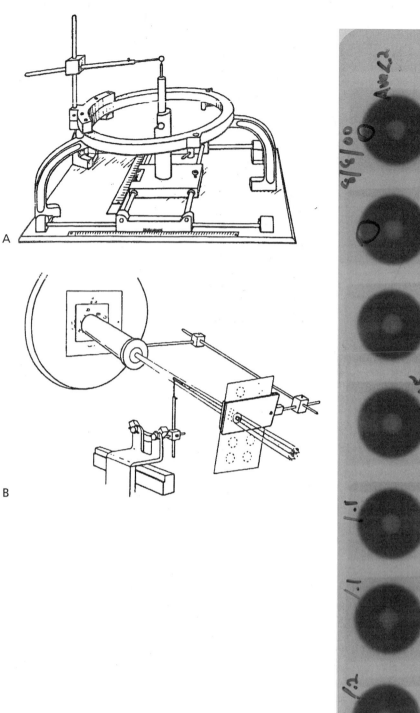

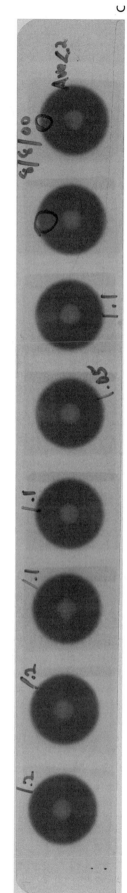

FIG. 21.5. A: Schematic of target simulator (steel ball) attached to the BRW phantom base. **B:** Target simulator mounted on the pedestal to verify target alignment with radiation isocenter as a function of table and gantry angles. **C:** Port films of the tungsten ball for eight gantry-ball combinations. (Figure 21.5A,B are reproduced from Lutz W, Winston KR, Maleki N. A system for stereotactic radiosurgery with a linear accelerator. *Int J Radiat Oncol Biol Phys* 1988;14:373, with permission.)

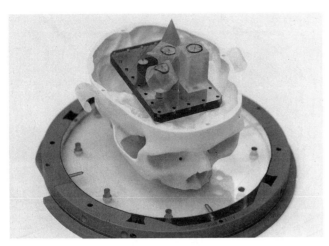

FIG. 21.6. A head phantom used for the verification of CT and MRI scanners. (From Cho KH, Gerbi BJ, Hall WA. Stereotactic radiosurgery and radiotherapy. In: Levitt SH, Khan FM, Potish RA, et al., eds. *Technological basis of radiation therapy.* Philadelphia: Lippincott Williams & Wilkins, 1999:147–172, with permission.)

must be compatible with the imaging modality used. One such test phantom for CT and MRI is commercially available and is shown in Fig. 21.6. The phantom contains test objects: a cube, sphere, cone and cylinder. The top center point of each of these objects is identified in the CT and MRI images and the BRW coordinates are reconstructed by the treatment-planning software. The comparison of these coordinates with the known coordinates of these points in the phantom gives the geometric accuracy. The analysis can be extended step by step to the entire SRS process.

If the change in individual coordinates is denoted by Δ, the localization error, LE, is given by:

$$\text{LE} = \left[(\Delta \text{AP})^2 + (\Delta \text{Lat})^2 + (\Delta \text{Vert})^2 \right]^{0.5} \tag{21.1}$$

Lutz et al. have analyzed localization accuracy in the "treatment" of 18 hidden targets in a test phantom and reported average errors of $1\cdot3 \pm 0.5$ mm and 0.6 mm ± 0.2 mm, respectively, for CT and plane film angiography.

The geometric accuracy of target localization for MRI is not as good as for CT or angiography. However, MRI is a superior diagnostic tool for many types of brain lesions. Moreover, it is often desirable to use all of the three imaging modalities for improved target localization. Special software is commercially available which allows correlation between CT, MRI, and angiography using automatic image fusion (see Chapter 19).

A.5. Beam Collimation

SRS or SRT is normally used for small lesions requiring much smaller fields than those for conventional radiation therapy. In addition, the geometric penumbra (which is inversely proportional to source-to-diaphragm distance, see Equation 4.2 in Chapter 4) must be as small as possible. A tertiary collimation system for SRS is therefore designed to bring the collimator diaphragm closer to the surface. This has been achieved, for example, by using 15-cm-long circular cones made of Cerrobend lead, encased in stainless steel. The cones are mounted below the x-ray jaws, which provide a square opening larger than the inside diameter of the cone, but small enough to prevent radiation escape from the sidewalls of the cone. A range of cone diameters from 5 mm to 30 mm is needed for treating SRS lesions. A few cones of larger diameter may also be available for treating larger lesions with SRT.

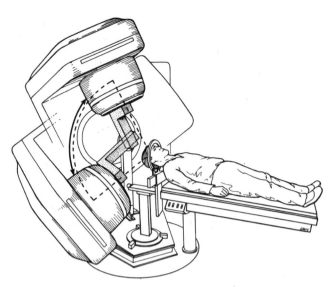

FIG. 21.7. Schematic of patient treatment set-up showing gantry positions and ISS subgantry to maintain isocenter accuracy independent of the linac isocenter accuracy. (From Friedman WA, Bova FJ. The University of Florida radiosurgery systems. *Surg Neurol* 1989;32:334, with permission.)

As stated previously, attachment of long cones below the x-ray jaws extends the SDD, thus reducing the geometric penumbra. The cones are mounted with their central axes aligned with the beam central axis. As a result the radiation isocenter of the beam remains centered within the cone opening and follows the same deviation (less than $\pm$ 1 mm) as allowed with gantry rotation.

Isocentric accuracy of the accelerator gantry and the attached cones have been improved by the design of a special ISS subgantry at the University of Florida[1] (Fig. 21.7). The cone is rigidly attached to the subgantry and, therefore, its isocenter remains fixed as defined by the subgantry rotation. The top end of the cone is attached to the accelerator gantry through a gimbal bearing with a sliding mount, which couples the linac gantry with the ISS subgantry. The isocentric stability is thus governed by the rotation of the ISS subgantry rather than that of the linac gantry, although a slight misalignment may exist between the mechanical isocenters of the two gantries. Because the isocenter of the ISS subgantry is more stable (because it is lighter) than that of the accelerator gantry, the accuracy of this system is better than that of the couch-mounted systems and, in fact, comparable to the accuracy achievable with a gamma knife (e.g., better than 0.5 mm).

As mentioned earlier, the SRS fields can be shaped with multileaf collimators (MLC). BrainLab[2] has designed a micro-multileaf collimator specifically for SRS, which shapes the field to fit the beams-eye-view outline of the target as the gantry rotates to deliver the treatment. The treatment-planning software shapes the MLC dynamically at each angle to achieve conformity to the outlined target as well adjust arc weights to optimize dose distribution.

B. Gamma Knife

The gamma knife delivers radiation to a target lesion in the brain by simultaneous irradiation with a large number of isocentric gamma ray beams. In a modern unit 201 cobalt-60 sources are housed in a hemispherical shield (central body) and the beams are collimated to focus on a single point at a source-to-focus distance of 40.3 cm (Fig. 21.8). The central beam is tilted through an angle of 55 degrees with respect to the horizontal plane. The

[1] Commercially available from Elekta Oncology Systems, Inc., Norcross, Georgia.
[2] BrainLab, Inc., Glen Court, Moorestown, New Jersey.

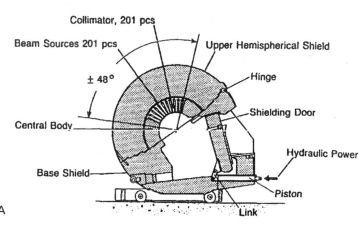
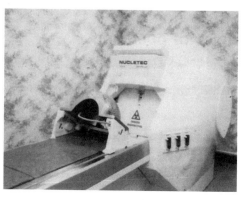

FIG. 21.8. **A:** Cross-sectional view of the gamma knife unit. **B:** Picture of the Leksell gamma unit. (Figure 21.8A is reproduced from Wu A, Maitz AH, Kalend AM, et al. Physics of gamma knife approach on convergent beams in stereotactic radiosurgery. *Int J Radiat Oncol Biol Phys* 1990;18:941, with permission. Figure 21.8b is reproduced courtesy of Elekta Instruments, Stockholm, Sweden.)

sources are distributed along two hemispherical arcs: one in the longitudinal plane and the other in the transverse plane of the treatment unit. The lower half of the housing contains a shielded entrance door. The opening and closing of the door as well as movement of the patient treatment table in and out of the unit are controlled by a hydraulic system.

Beam channels machined in the central body provide the primary collimation of individual gamma ray beams. Further collimation is achieved by one of four interchangeable helmets with collimator channels aligned with the central body channels. The central axes of all 201 beams intersect at the focus with a mechanical precision of ±0.3 mm. Micro switches control the alignment of helmet channels with the central body channels with a positioning accuracy of ±0.1 mm. Each helmet is characterized by its channel diameter that produces a circular field opening of 4, 8, 14, or 18 mm at the focus point. Selected channels can be blocked with plugs to shield the eyes or to optimize the dose distribution. The plugs are made of 6-cm-thick tungsten alloy.

Treatment target in the brain is localized with the Leksell's stereotactic frame attached to the patient's skull and by performing imaging studies, such as CT, MRI or angiography. After the target pint coordinates with respect to the Leksell's stereotactic frame have been determined through treatment planning, the frame is positioned in the helmet by setting these coordinates and fixing the frame to the trunnions of the helmet. This brings the target point to the focal point of the unit. The process can be repeated if there are multiple target points (e.g., to shape the dose distribution) or if more than one target is to be treated in the brain.

As stated previously, there are no significant clinical differences between gamma knife and x-ray knife treatments. However, gamma knife can only be used for small lesions because of its field size limitation (maximum diameter of 18 mm), although several isocenters can be placed within the same target to expand or shape dose distribution. For treating multiple isocenters or targets, gamma knife is more practical than the x-ray knife because of its simplicity of set-up. For the same reasons, gamma knife can produce a more conformal dose distribution than that possible with x-ray knife unless the latter is equipped with special field-shaping collimators such as the dynamic MLC. On the other hand the x-ray knife is far more economical because it is linac-based. Besides, the linac can be used for all kinds of radiation therapy techniques including SRS, SRT, intensity-modulated radiation therapy, and conventional radiation therapy.

21.3. DOSIMETRY

Typically there are three quantities of interest in SRS dosimetry: central axis depth distribution (% depth dose or TMRs), cross-beam profiles (off-axis ratios), and output factors

($S_{c,p}$ or dose/MU). Measurement of these quantities is complicated by two factors: detector size relative to the field dimensions and a possible lack of charged particle equilibrium. In either case, the detector size must be as small as possible compared to the field size.

For the measurement of central axis depth dose, an essential criterion is that the sensitive volume of the detector must be irradiated with uniform electron fluence (e.g., within ± 0.5%). Because in a small circular field the central axis area of uniform intensity does not extend beyond a few mm in diameter, this puts a stringent requirement on the detector diameter. For a crossbeam profile measurement, the detector size is again important because of the steep dose gradients at the field edges. The dosimeter, in such a case, must have high spatial resolution to accurately measure field penumbra, which is critically important in SRS.

Several different types of detector systems have been used in SRS dosimetry: ion chambers, film, thermoluminescent dosimeters, and diodes. There are advantages and disadvantages to each of these systems. For example, ion chamber is the most precise and the least energy-dependent system but usually has a size limitation; film has the best spatial resolution but shows energy dependence and a greater statistical uncertainty (e.g., ± 3%); thermoluminescent dosimeters show little energy dependence and can have a small size in the form of chips but suffer from the same degree of statistical uncertainty as the film; and diodes have small size but show energy dependence as well as possible directional dependence. Thus the choice of any detector system for SRS dosimetry depends on the quantity to be measured and the measurement conditions.

A. Cross-beam Profiles

The effect of detector size on the accuracy of beam profiles has been investigated by Dawson et al. (7) and Rice et al. (8). It has been shown that with a detector size of 3.5 mm diameter, the beam profiles of circular fields in the range of 12.5 to 30.0 mm in diameter can be measured accurately within 1 mm. Because cross-beam profiles involve relative dose measurement (doses are normalized to central axis value) and there is little change in the photon energy spectrum across small fields, diodes and film are the detectors of choice.

Beam profiles at various depths can be measured with a film (e.g., Kodak X-OMAT V) sandwiched parallel to central axis between slabs of a unit-density phantom (e.g., polystyrene or solid water) as discussed in Chapter 14. Because in film dosimetry, spatial resolution is governed primarily by the densitometer aperture, it is recommended that the aperture size be 1 mm or less. Digital film scanners are commercially available with special dosimetry software that allows the input of film sensitometric data and other corrections to convert optical density to dose.

B. Depth-dose Distribution

Measurement of central axis depth dose in a small field requires that the detector dimensions should be small enough so that it lies well within the central uniform area of the beam profile. For field sizes of diameter 12.5 mm or greater, it has been shown that the central axis depth dose can be measured correctly with a parallel plate ionization chamber of diameter not exceeding 3.0 mm (10). Smaller diameter chambers will be required for smaller field sizes.

Film or diodes can also be used for central axis depth dose distribution, especially for very small field sizes. Because the proportions of scattered photons of lower energy increases with depth, energy-dependence of the film or diodes must be taken into account. Depth dependent correction factors can be determined by comparing film or diode curves with ion chamber curves using larger fields (e.g., 30 to 50 mm diameter).

Although TMRs can be measured directly, they can be calculated from percent depth doses as discussed in Chapter 10.

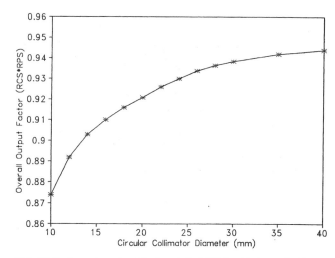

FIG. 21.9. Sample output factors (cGy/MU) for 10 through 40 mm diameter cones. The x-ray jaws were set at 8 × 8 cm. (From Friedman WA, Bova FJ. The University of Florida radiosurgery systems. *Surg Neurol* 1989;32:334, with permission.)

C. Output Factors

Output factors ($S_{c,p}$) for small fields pose the same kinds of problems as for beam profiles and depth-dose measurements. Detector size in relation to the field size is the critical parameter. It has been shown that for fields of diameter 12.5 mm and larger, cylindrical or parallel-plate chambers of 3.5 mm diameter allow the output factors to be measured accurately to within 0.5% (8). Figure 21.9 shows an example of output factors as a function of field size.

For ultra-small fields (the diameter of 10 mm or less), film, TLDs or diodes are the most appropriate detectors for profile, depth dose and output factor measurements. Because of their small size, these systems offer high spatial resolution, which is of paramount importance in such measurements. However, they should be properly calibrated against ion chambers using a large enough field size for ion chambers dosimetry (e.g., 3 to 5 cm diameter).

21.4. DOSE CALCULATION ALGORITHM

Any of the dose calculation methods discussed in Chapters 10 and 19 can be adopted for SRS dose calculations. The approximate spherical geometry of the human head and homogeneity of tissue density greatly simplify the demands on a dose calculation algorithm. One of the simplest methods of beam modeling is based on tissue-maximum ratios, off-axis ratios, exponential attenuation, output factors and inverse-square law. The beam data are acquired specifically for the beam energy and circular fields, used in SRS, as discussed previously.

The patient surface contour geometry is defined three-dimensionally by CT scans. The multiple arc geometries are simulated by stationary beams separated by angles of 5 to 10 degrees. The choice of dose calculation grid has been discussed by Niemierko and Goitein (11). They have shown that a 2-mm grid spacing produces a dose uncertainty of 1% to 2%, compared to 3% to 4% uncertainty with a 4-mm grid spacing. Of course, the overall accuracy depends on the accuracy of all dose calculation parameters, beam modeling, interpolation routines, grid size, positional accuracy, etc.

The CT and MRI scans for treatment planning are obtained with a slice separation typically between 3 and 10 mm. Greater resolution is required for target definition. So a smaller slice separation of 1 to 3 mm is used to scan the lesion and the critical structures in its close vicinity. Target volumes are outlined slice by slice in the CT images and correlated with MRI scans and angiograms through fusion techniques.

Calculated dose distributions are overlaid on individual CT, MRI, or angiographic images. Volumetric displays in the form of isodose surfaces are also useful. Dose volume histograms (DVH) of the target and normal structures complement the isodose display.

21.5. QUALITY ASSURANCE

Stereotactic radiosurgery or radiotherapy is a special procedure, which requires careful commissioning followed by a rigorous quality assurance program to maintain its original accuracy specifications. Several QA protocols pertinent to SRS have been published (2,4). These protocols should provide guidelines for an institution to design its QA program.

Quality assurance involves both the clinical and physical aspects of SRS. The physics part may be divided into two categories: treatment QA and routine QA. The former involves checking or double-checking of the procedures and treatment parameters pertaining to individual patients; and the latter is designed to periodically inspect the hardware and software performance to ensure compliance with original specifications.

A. Treatment Quality Assurance

Patient treatment involves many steps and procedures. It is highly desirable that detailed checklists are prepared to documents these steps in a proper sequence. The objective of the checklist should be to ensure procedural accuracy at each step of the way and to minimize the chance of a treatment error.

Major components of treatment QA consist of checking (a) stereotactic frame accuracy including phantom base, CT/MRI/angiographic localizer, pedestal or couch mount; (b) imaging data transfer, treatment plan parameters, target position, monitor unit calculations; (c) frame alignment with gantry and couch eccentricity, congruence of target point with radiation isocenter, collimator setting, cone diameter, couch position, patient immobilization and safety locks; and (d) treatment console programming of beam energy, monitor units, arc angles, etc.

Examples of treatment QA checklists have been published (2) that may be used as rough guides. It should be realized that the SRS QA program involves health professionals in different departments. Therefore, personnel coordination is important for successful implementation of a QA program.

B. Routine Quality Assurance

A routine QA program is designed to check the hardware/software performance of SRS equipment on a scheduled frequency basis. For the linear accelerator, the relevant QA protocol is the AAPM Report No. 40 (4). For the SRS apparatus, the routine QA schedule is recommended by the AAPM Report No. 54 (2).

A QA program for the gamma knife must be compliant with the NRC regulations. An example program, implemented at the University of Pittsburgh is published in the AAPM Report 54.

21.6. CLINICAL APPLICATIONS

Stereotactic radiosurgery was originally developed for the treatment of benign lesions of the brain such as arteriovenous malformations (AVM), meningiomas, and acoustic neuromas. Its use has been extended to treat many malignant tumors such as gliomas and brain metastases. More recently SRS has also been used to treat functional disorders, for example, trigeminal neuralgia and movement disorders. Fractional SRT is now commonly being used

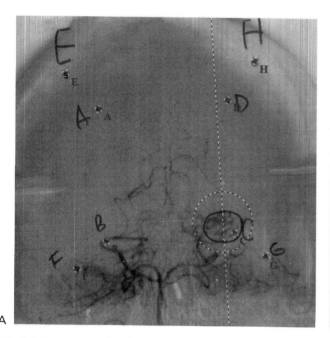
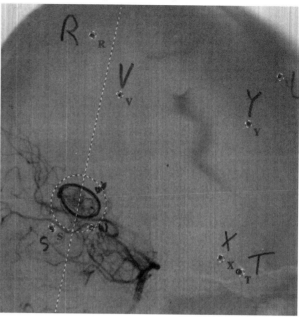

FIG. 21.10. An example of stereotactic radiosurgery treatment of arteriovenous malformation. **(A)** Anterior angiographic view of nidus; **(B)** lateral view of nidus; **(C)** beam arrangement using five noncoplanar arcs (see color insert); isodose region (color wash) corresponding to 90% of the maximum dose is shown in anterior view **(D)** and lateral view **(E)** (see color insert).

to treat malignant brain tumors, especially those in proximity to critical structures such as brain stem and optic pathways. For overviews of clinical rationale, the reader is referred to McKenzie et al. (12), Luxton et al. (13), and Cho et al. (9).

Radiobiologic principles of SRS are currently not well understood. However, attempts have been made to rationalize the delivery of a single large fraction of dose to a small-circumscribed lesion (e.g., less than 4 cm in diameter) in the brain. Because the intended effect is to cause thrombosis in the case of AVM and reproductive cell death in the case of a tumor, the potential benefits of fractionated radiation therapy are not considered in SRS. However, in the case of malignant tumors treated with SRT, the well-established principles of radiobiology, namely repair, reoxygenation, redistribution and repopulation (i.e., "4 R's") are considered just as important as in conventional radiation therapy. Accordingly, the fractionation schemes are similar depending on the tumor volume and the radiobiologic characteristics of the disease.

Dose distribution achievable with SRS is highly conformal. This is made possible by tertiary collimation (i.e., cones) and the use of multiple non-coplanar arcs. Because in single-fraction radiosurgery, no attempt is made to spare normal tissue within the target volume, dose conformity is essential to minimize irradiation of the normal brain outside the target. Tight margins between the target and the prescription isodose are made possible by rigid immobilization of the patient and the stereotactic accuracy of the SRS procedure. In the fractionated SRT of malignant tumors, same considerations apply to the design of target volume (e.g., planning target volume) as in three-dimensional conformal radiation therapy. Figures 21.10–21.11 (see color insert) show selected examples of cases treated with SRS and SRT.

REFERENCES

1. Leksell L. The stereotactic method and radiosurgery of the brain. *Acta Chir Scand* 1951;102:316–319.
2. AAPM. *Stereotactic radiosurgery.* Report No. 54. Woodbury, NY: American Institute of Physics, 1995.
3. Galloway RL, Maciunas RJ. Stereotactic neurosurgery. *Biomedical Engineering* 1990;18:181.

4. AAPM. Comprehensive QA for radiation oncology: report of the AAPM Radiation Therapy Committee Task Group 40. *Med Phys* 1994;21:581–618.

5. Gerbi BJ, Roback DM, Humphery SD, et al. Maintaining accuracy in radiosurgery. *Int J Radiat Oncol Biol Phys* 1995;32:1199–1203.

6. Lutz WA, Winston KR, Maleki N. A system for stereotactic radiosurgery with a linear accelerator. *Int J Radiat Oncol Biol Phys* 1988;14:373.

7. Dawson DJ, Schroeder NJ, Hoya JD. Penumbral measurements in water for high-energy x-rays. *Med Phys* 1986;13:101–104.

8. Rice KR, Hansen JL, Svensson GK, et al. Measurement of dose distribution in small beams of 6MV x-rays. *Phys Med Biol* 1987;32:1087–1099.

9. Cho KH, Gerbi BJ, Hall WA. Stereotactic radiosurgery and radiotherapy. In: Levitt SH, Khan FM, Potish RA, et al., eds. *Technological basis of radiation therapy.* Philadelphia: Lippincott Williams & Wilkins, 1999:147–172.

10. Bjarngard BE, Tsai JS, Rice RK. Doses on central axis of narrow 6-MV x-ray beams. *Med Phys* 1990;17:794.

11. Niemierko A, Goitein M. The influence of the size of the grid used for dose calculation on the accuracy of dose estimation. *Med Phys* 1989;16:239.

12. McKenzie MR, Southami L, Podgorsak EB, et al. Photon radiosurgery: a clinical review. *Canadian J Neurol Sci* 1992;19:212.

13. Luxton G, Zbigniew P, Jozsef G, et al. Stereotactic radiosurgery: principles and comparison of treatment methods. *Neurosurgery* 1993;32:241.

HIGH DOSE RATE BRACHYTHERAPY

22.1. INTRODUCTION

Most of the clinical experience in brachytherapy has been obtained using low dose rate (LDR) implants, that is, with prescription dose rate on the order of 0.5 to 2 cGy/min. ICRU Report 38 (1) classifies high dose rate (HDR) as 20 cGy/min or higher. With the introduction of remote afterloading technology, it is possible to deliver HDR brachytherapy safely and more precisely than possible with the classical LDR brachytherapy. Although LDR brachytherapy can also be delivered using remote afterloading devices, logistic problems of prolonged treatment and patient hospitalization make LDR less attractive than HDR.

As discussed in Chapter 15, the principal advantage of HDR over LDR is that it permits treatments on an outpatient basis. For that reason, it is well suited for treating large patient populations. Greater control over dose distribution is another major advantage, which is being explored as a tool for delivering highly conformal dose to well-localized tumors, for example, as a boost or primary treatment for prostate cancer. Although the role of HDR in brachytherapy is not yet fully established, all indications point toward its widespread use as a sole procedure or in conjunction with external beam. If the current trends continue, it is quite possible that HDR will replace all brachytherapy techniques in the not too distant future.

22.2. HIGH DOSE RATE UNIT

A. Remote Afterloader

A HDR remote afterloading unit contains a single source of high activity ($\sim$10 Ci or 370 GBq). Although cobalt-60 and cesium-137 have been used in the past, iridium-192 is the most commonly used radioisotope in HDR. For HDR brachytherapy, ^{192}Ir is the best choice because of its higher specific activity (allows smaller source for the same activity) and lower photon energy (requires less shielding). A disadvantage, on the other hand, is its shorter half-life, necessitating source replacement every 3 to 4 months.

The ^{192}Ir source used in HDR is a small line source welded to the end of a flexible drive cable. The cable with the source attached at the end is also called source wire. The dimensions of the source vary between 0.3 to 0.6 mm in diameter and 3.5 to 10 mm in length, depending on the HDR model. The source wire, when not extended, is stored in a shielded safe of the HDR unit (Fig. 22.1). In compliance with the NRC regulations (2), the leakage radiation levels outside the unit do not exceed 1 mR/h at a distance of 10 cm from the nearest accessible surface surrounding the safe with the source in the shielded position.

The HDR unit is equipped with several channels and an indexer system to direct the source to each channel. In one of the models,[1] channels are provided on a rotating turret

---

[1] VariSource, Varian Oncology Systems, Palo Alto, California.

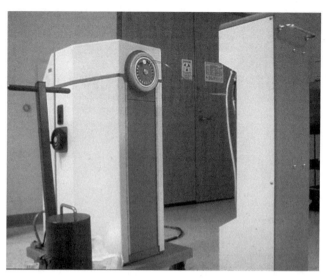

FIG. 22.1. A picture of Varian high dose rate unit (VariSource).

in which any channel can be aligned with the source wire path. Applicators or catheters implanted in the patient are connected to the channels by catheters called transfer tubes or transfer guides. Before the active source wire is extended for treatment, a dummy wire is extended to verify that the path is clear of any obstruction.

The source wire (or dummy wire) can be advanced or retracted through individual channels, transfer tubes and applicators by a remote computer controlled drive mechanism consisting of stepper motors. The positioning of the source at the programmed dwell positions in the applicators is accomplished in precise increments by the stepper motors. The positioning accuracy of the source is specified at ± 1 mm. The dose control precision is provided by a 0.1-second dwell time resolution.

A number of safety systems are provided for the HDR. For example, interlocks prevent initiation of treatment if the door is open or the applicator is not attached or the connections between a programmed channel, the transfer tube and the applicator are not secure. Backup batteries are provided to take over operation in case of power failure. A manual source retraction mechanism is available to withdraw the source into the storage safe if it gets stuck and cannot be retracted by the emergency switch. The treatment is aborted if the system detects blockage or excessive friction during source transit.

B. High Dose Rate Applicators

Brachytherapy applicators used for low dose rate implants can also be used for HDR. For example, some of the most commonly used applicators, for a variety of HDR applications, are:

Fletcher-Suit or Fletcher-Suit-Delclos. These applicators are used for the treatment of gynecological malignancies of the uterus, cervix and pelvic side walls. The applicator set typically consists of three rigid intrauterine tandems, with curvature of 15-, 30-, and 45-degree angles, and a pair of ovoids or colpostats with shields in place to reduce dose to rectum and bladder.

Vaginal Cylinder. These are acrylic cylinders having a variety of diameters and axially drilled holes to accommodate a stainless steel tandem. Coupling catheters for attachment to the transfer tubes and marker wires to fit the length of the tandem are provided in the set. The applicator is suitable for treating tumors in the vaginal wall.

Rectal Applicator. Acrylic cylinders of different diameters are designed to treat superficial tumors of the rectum. Selective shielding is incorporated to spare normal tissue. Coupling catheters and marker wires are provided in the HDR set.

Intraluminal Catheter. Suitable diameter catheters of various lengths are available for treating intraluminal disease such as endobronchial carcinoma.

Nasopharyngeal Applicators. These applicators are used for treating nasopharyngeal tumors with HDR. The applicator set includes tracheal tube, catheter, and a nasopharyngeal connector.

Besides the above examples, HDR applicators and catheters are available for virtually every type of application deemed suitable for intravitary brachytherapy.

Interstitial Implants. Hollow, stainless steel needles are implanted into the tumor following standard brachytherapy rules of implant (see Chapter 15) and closed ended catheters are inserted to accommodate the HDR source wire. Marker wires are used to plan the dwell positions of the source as with the other HDR applicators. Examples of interstitial implants are prostate gland, breast, and some head and neck tumors.

C. Facility Design

C.1. Shielding

The HDR unit must be housed in an adequately shielded room. The shielding and safety requirements are mandated by the Nuclear Regulatory Commission (2). The HDR treatment room can be designed as a dedicated facility (e.g., "HDR suite") or adopted from an existing ^{60}Co or linac room. In either case, the shielding must satisfy or exceed the NRC requirements.

The shielding calculations are based on the dose limits specified by the NRC in 10 CFR 20.1301 (for individual members of the public) and 10CFR 20.1201 (for occupational personnel). The NRC annual effective dose equivalent limits follow the NCRP guidelines (see Table 16.5). These are summarized as follows:

Public: 0.1 rem (1mSv) in 1 year for continuous or frequent exposures; or 0.5 rem (5mSv) in 1 year for infrequent exposure. In the case of HDR the limit for infrequent exposure, namely, 0.5 rem in 1 year is more relevant.

Occupational: 5 rems (50mSv) in 1 year.

In addition to the annual limits, the NRC requires that the dose in any unrestricted area must not exceed 2 mrem (20 mSv) *in any 1 hour.* The underlined words mean that with the workload and use factor applied, the dose received in an unrestricted area shall not exceed 2 mrem in any 1 hour.

The methods of calculating primary and secondary barriers are the same as discussed for megavoltage beams in Chapter 16. Equations 16.4, 16.6, and 16.10 are valid also for HDR room design, provided appropriate factors related to ^{192}Ir source are used. These factors include: average photon energy = 0.38 MeV, tenth-value layer (TVL) = 5.8 inches of concrete (density 2.35 g cm^{-3}) and exposure rate constant = 4.69R cm^2/mCi − h. The following examples illustrate the method of barrier thickness calculation or evaluation of an existing barrier.

Example 1

Calculate barrier thickness at a distance of 5 feet from the HDR source to protect a controlled area.

Because the HDR source, ^{192}Ir, requires less shielding than a megavoltage teletherapy unit and can be assumed isotropic (same intensity in all directions) in the context of shielding design, it is reasonable to construct all barriers of the same thickness. Additionally, as a conservative measure, one could design all barriers as primary, for a maximum transmission of 2 mrems in any 1 hour. Or, even more conservatively, a limit of 2 mrem/h (instantaneous dose rate) could be adopted.

Assuming that, from radiation protection point of view in this case, 1R $\cong$ 1cGy $\cong$ 1 rem, the dose equivalent rate ($\dot{H}$) at a distance of 5 feet from the source is given by (inverse square law):

$$\dot{H} = \frac{(10{,}000\text{mCi})(4.69 \times 1{,}000 \text{ mrem cm}^2/\text{mCi} - \text{h})}{(5 \text{ ft} \times 30.5 \text{ cm/ft})^2} = 2{,}000 \text{ mrem/h}$$

If B is the barrier transmission factor required to reduce $\dot{H}$ to 2 mrem/h, then:

$$B = 10^{-3}$$

If n is the number of TVLs required for shielding.

$$\left(\frac{1}{10}\right)^n = 10^{-3}$$

or

$$\left(\frac{1}{10}\right)^n = \left(\frac{1}{10}\right)^3$$

or

$$n = 3$$

Since TVL = 5.8 inches of concrete (3),

$$\text{barrier thickness} = 3 \times 5.8 \text{ inches}$$
$$= 17.4 \text{ inches}$$

Thus an HDR suite in this case would have all barriers (walls, floor, and ceiling) of thickness about 18 inches of concrete provided a minimum clearance, 5 ft in this case, between the source and the area to be protected is assured. These shielding requirements could be reduced if a larger clearance is maintained and realistic workload and occupancy factors are applied.

If no maze is provided to prevent direct incidence of radiation beam at the door, the door must be shielded (e.g., with lead lining) for a transmission equivalent to that of 18 inches of concrete or 3 TVLs. Because the TVL for ^{192}Ir gamma rays in lead is 2 cm (3), the equivalent lead thickness must be $2 \times 3 = 6$ cm. A better alternative is to provide a maze or add a shielded partition between the source and the door.

Example 2

What is the door shielding required if a maze is provided for an HDR suite, with source to wall (facing the door) distance of 15 ft and maze length of 10 ft?

With the maze wall thickness of 18 inches of concrete, the transmitted dose incident at the door would be 2 mrem/h or less. The dose due to scatter off the wall facing the inside of the door can be calculated as follows:

Assuming average reflection coefficient (α) of 2×10^{-2} per m^2 for ^{192}Ir (4) and the area of scatter at the facing wall to be 5m^2, the dose rate ($\dot{H}_s$) at the inside of the door due to scattering would be:

$$\dot{H}_s = \frac{(10{,}000\text{mCi})(4.69 \times 1{,}000 \text{ mrem cm}^2/\text{mCi} - \text{h})(2 \times 10^{-2}/\text{m}^2)5\text{m}^2}{(10 \text{ ft} \times 30.5 \text{ cm/ft})^2(15 \text{ ft} \times 30.5 \text{ cm/ft})^2}$$

$$= 2.4 \times 10^{-4} \text{ mrem/h}$$

which is negligible. Thus, no shielding is required for the door if an appropriate maze is provided in an HDR suite.

Example 3

Evaluate the shielding of an existing 6 MV linear accelerator for HDR use.

Transmitted dose for each existing barrier can be calculated using inverse square law and TVL for ^{192}Ir gamma rays, as discussed above. For example, if a secondary barrier for a 6-MV room is 40 inches of concrete and the minimum distance between the source and the area to be evaluated for protection is 10 ft, then the effective dose equivalent rate ($\dot{H}$) in the area can be calculated as below:

$$B = \left(\frac{1}{10}\right)^{40/5.8} = 1.27 \times 10^{-7}$$

$$\dot{H} = \frac{(10{,}000\,\text{mCi})(4.69 \times 1{,}000\ \text{mrem cm}^2/\text{mCi} - \text{h}) \times 1.27 \times 10^{-7}}{(10\ \text{ft} \times 30.5\ \text{cm/ft})^2}$$

$$= 6.4 \times 10^{-5}\ \text{mrem/h}$$

which is negligible. Similar calculations have shown that rooms designed with adequate shielding for megavoltage teletherapy units are more than adequate for HDR shielding (5).

Whether it is a dedicated HDR suite or an existing teletherapy vault, the shielding adequacy of the facility must be documented before applying for an HDR license. Since most institutions use existing teletherapy rooms to house HDR units, a shielding evaluation report must be submitted with the license application as required by the NRC.

C.2. Safety Features

Safety requirements for a dedicated HDR vault or an existing teletherapy room adopted for HDR, are mandated by the NRC (2). These include: electrical interlock system that retracts the source when the door is opened and does not allow resumption of the treatment unless the door is closed and the interlock is reset; mechanism to ensure that only one device can be placed in operation at a given time if the HDR is installed in an existing teletherapy room; inaccessibility of console keys to unauthorized persons; a permanent radiation monitor capable of continuous monitoring of the source status; continuous viewing and intercom systems to allow for patient observation during treatment; and restricted area controls such as signs, locks, visible/audible alarms, door warning lights indicating "Radiation On," etc.

22.3. LICENSING REQUIREMENTS

Purchasers of HDR units must apply for a license or license amendment with the appropriate regulatory agency. In the United States, it is the Nuclear Regulatory Commission (NRC) or the state if it is an Agreement State. The licensing requirements for LDR brachytherapy were discussed in Chapter 16, Section 16.10. Essential items included (a) applicant's qualifications (education, training, experience) and a description of personnel training program (initial as well as periodic); (b) administrative requirements: ALARA program, radiation safety officer, radiation safety committee and a written quality management program; and (c) technical requirements: calibration and survey instruments, leak testing and inventory of sources, conditions for patient release, post treatment survey of patients, and posting of radiation signs. If the applicant already has an LDR brachytherapy license, an amendment must be requested for the remote afterloading device by listing license conditions specific to the use of that device.

The information required specifically for HDR licensing is contained in the NRC document (2). A typical license application includes the following information:

1. Source description (radionuclide, manufacturer's name and model number, maximum activity, maximum number of sources to be possessed at the facility at any given time and the physical construction of the source).
2. Manufacturer's name and model of the HDR unit.
3. Intended use (cancer treatment in humans using interstitial, intracavitary, intraluminal brachytherapy, etc.)
4. Authorized users (physicians) and authorized physicist(s), verifying that they meet educational and experience qualifications set forth in 10CFR 35.940 and 10CFR 35.961, respectively.

5. An outline of initial training of authorized users and device operators (didactic training plus a minimum of 8 hours of "hands on" device operation training.)
6. Description of radiation detection and survey instruments to be used.
7. A floor plan of the facility, identifying room(s), doors, windows, conduits, density and thickness of shielding materials of walls, floors and ceiling and distances to the adjacent inhabitable areas with indication of whether the areas are restricted or unrestricted.
8. Shielding calculations to show that the adjacent areas comply with the regulatory standards.
9. Area security and safety features (Section 22.2C.2)
10. Calibration procedures and frequency, leak test procedures and frequency and the qualifications of those performing these tests.
11. Quality assurance program, including pretreatment or daily quality assurance procedures and periodic testing (e.g., monthly, quarterly, annually).
12. Training and frequency of retraining of individual operators (e.g., annually or every 2 years).
13. Training or certification of individuals performing source changes (normally vendor representative).
14. Personnel radiation monitoring program.
15. Emergency procedures, postings, locations.
16. Disposal arrangements of decayed sources (usually by return to vendor).
17. Operating procedures and manuals, their availability to personnel and location.
18. Inspection and servicing of HDR equipment at intervals not to exceed one year, by the manufacturer or a person licensed by NRC/Agreement State. Records of inspection and service to be maintained for the durations of the license for guidance.

    Note: Requirements of License application may change from time to time. The applicant should consult the most current NRC document.

A. High Dose Rate Quality Management Program

As a condition for awarding an HDR license, the NRC requires a written quality management program (QMP) as it does for the LDR brachytherapy. General requirements of such a program were discussed in Chapter 16, Section 16.10B. An HDR QMP includes general as well as specific tests to assure safe application of the HDR procedure. The program is designed by the institution and must be submitted as part of the license application. A sample HDR QMP is described below.

A.1. Written Directive

A written directive (prescription) must be provided by the "authorized physician user" that includes the name and hospital number of the patient, the HDR source material, the dose per fraction, the total dose, and the site of administration.

A.2. Patient Identification

The identity of the patient must be verified by two independent methods as the individual named in the written directive. This may be accomplished by asking the patient his/her name and confirming the name by comparison with the patient's identification bracelet or hospital identification card.

A.3. Treatment Plan Verification

The "authorized physician" and the "authorized physicist" must check the treatment plan to ensure that (i) the plan parameters (e.g., source specification, source strength, source position, dose per fraction, total dose) are correct and in accordance with the written directive; (ii) the treatment parameters generated by the plan for input into the HDR device (e.g., channel numbers, source positions, dwell times) are correct; and (iii) the dose distribution agrees with an independent (e.g., manual) spot check within reasonable limits (e.g., $\pm 5\%$).

A.4. Pre-treatment Safety Checks

Pre-treatment safety checks of the HDR equipment must be performed on any day that the HDR procedure is schedules. A sample is provided in section 22.3B.

A.5. Treatment Delivery

Prior to the initiation of treatment, the "authorized operator" (authorized medical physicist, dosimetrist or radiation therapist) must verify that the name of the patient, the dose, the site of administration and the times for each dwell locations are in agreement with the written directive and the approved treatment plan.

A.6. Post-treatment Survey

Immediately after each treatment, a survey of the afterloading device and the patient must be performed to assure that the source has been returned to the fully shielded position. The survey will include connectors and applicator apparatus, the full length of the catheter guide tube, and the external surface of the device to ensure that the source is fully retracted. The patient shall be surveyed over the body surface near the treatment site before removing the patient from the treatment room.

A.7. Source Replacement and Calibration Check

Vendor will conduct source replacement and perform source and performance checks following installation. A copy of this report will be on file. Calibration of the source will be performed by "authorized physicist" before first patient treatment.

A.8. Recording

The operator administering the treatment will record and initial the treatment after completion. Following the treatment, he/she will assemble and file records of the prescription, patient identification, and treatment delivery, and post-treatment surveys. The records for each treatment along with a completed checklist will be kept on file. These records will be maintained in an auditable form for a minimum of 3 years.

A.9. Supervision

During all patient treatments, both the "authorized physician user" and the "authorized medical physicist" will be physically present. Physical presence, for this purpose, is defined as within audible range of normal human speech.

A.10. Recordable Event or Misadministration

Any unintended deviation from the written directive will be identified and evaluated in terms of a "recordable event" or a "misadministration." Definitions of these terms and the required actions are the same as for the LDR brachytherapy, discussed in Chapter 16, Section 16.10B.

A.11. Periodic Reviews

(a) Brachytherapy cases will be reviewed at intervals no greater than 12 months by an "authorized physician" and/or an "authorized physicist." A representative number of cases, corresponding to lot tolerance defective of 2%, using the acceptance sampling table of 10CFR 32.110, will undergo this review which will consist of checking that the delivered radiation dose was in accordance with the written directive and plan of treatment.

If a recordable event or misadministration is uncovered during the periodic review, the number of cases to be reviewed will be expanded to include all cases for that calendar year.

(b) The QMP will be reviewed on an annual basis to determine the effectiveness of the program and to identify actions to make the program more effective.

(c) A written summary of this annual review will be submitted to the Radiation Safety Officer and the Radiation Safety Committee for review and final approval.

(d) Any modification made to the QMP will be reported to the appropriate NRC Regional Office (or the state if governed by Agreement State) within 30 days after modification has been made. Ministerial changes authorized under 19 CFR35 will not require the notification of the NRC.

B. Pre-treatment Safety Checks

The HDR pre-treatment safety checks are performed before treatment on any day that the HDR procedure is to be carried out. A sample is provided below for an HDR unit installed in a 6-MV linear accelerator room.

1. Verify that the double pole-double throw HDR door interlock switch is turned to the HDR position. Then verify that the 6-MV linac console cannot be activated. Activate the HDR console ON.
2. Check radiation monitor in the treatment room for proper operation with a dedicated check source, which is located in HDR afterloader storage room. This check will verify expected reading within $\pm 20\%$ as well as activation of the warning light.
3. The two video monitors (one with a long view and the other for close up) at the HDR console will be viewed to verify proper visualization by the cameras in the treatment room. The two-way audio communication will be checked by one person in the room at the location of the patient and the other at the console.
4. Turn on HDR afterloader and position for test. Verify that all lights/status indicators are operational.
5. Clear any personnel in room, and close treatment door as you leave. Verify that the door warning light is operational and console lights/status indicators are operational. Test console printer operation.
6. Activate HDR test run from console. Verify that the door warning light indicates "Radiation On." Verify that the door interlock terminates treatment by opening door during test run. Re-close the door and verify that the HDR unit cannot be turned on without resetting the HDR activation button.
7. If the door interlock malfunctions, the HDR unit will be locked in the "off" position and not used until the door interlock system is restored to proper operation.
8. Check mechanical integrity of all applicators, source guide tubes, and connectors to be used in this treatment by visual inspection and/or radiographics.
9. Check "Quick-Connect" sensor by placing an incorrectly seated catheter "Quick-Connect" with catheter into the HDR turret. Using dummy wire check that treatment is prevented.
10. Results of these tests will be recorded on the morning checklist.

C. High Dose Rate Operating Procedures

The NRC requires HDR operating procedures to be submitted as part of the license application (Item 17, Section 22.3). The procedures must be available to personnel at a suitable location. Depending on the particular device, the operating procedures are written to guide the operator step-by-step in the safe operation of the equipment and treatment delivery. The following is a generic sample, which may be adopted with appropriate modifications to suit the available equipment and personnel.

1. The HDR unit will be stored in a storage space provided in the designated shielded room (e.g., 6-MV linear accelerator room). The storage area will be locked when the unit is unattended. The door key will be available only to the authorized operator(s).
2. Pre-treatment safety checks will be performed on the day of the treatment (section 22.3B).
3. Only the patient under treatment will be in the treatment room during activation of the HDR unit for treatment. Patient identification will be verified by two independent means.
4. The following pre-treatment checks are to be performed before initiating HDR treatment:
   a. Verify that the source activity and calibration date are correct on the printouts;
   b. Verify the correct patient file name in the case of multiple patient files on the same disk;
   c. Verify that the printout matches the one shown on the afterloader printout;
   d. The planned dwell times should be verified before initiating treatment;
   e. Ensure that in multiple-channel treatments each catheter is connected to the correct machine channel. Catheters should be marked and verified that the treatment plan and the afterloader match as far as which catheter is which;
   f. Verify correctness of patient information on printouts;
   g. Verify dwell positions with catheter measurements;
   h. Ensure that all catheters are fully seated into the machine connectors, with the connector plunger fully extended;
   i. Before positioning the active source into the patient treatment catheter, the dummy source wire will be run into each treatment catheter to verify that the catheter is not blocked or kinked. The HDR afterloader will not run the active source into the catheter if the dummy wire encounters resistance.
5. For each catheter channel run, check total source dwell time using manual timer and verify that the manual timer measurement agrees with the total programmed dwell time.
6. Treatment planning computer disk with the plan data stored for each patient's treatment will be labeled with the corresponding patient's name and identification number. If these disks are reused, they will be re-labeled in accordance with the manufacturer's instructions.
7. Immediately after each use of the HDR device, the physicist will ensure the source has been returned to the full-shielded position and will perform a survey of the device and the patient. The survey will include the patient, connectors, applicators, full length of guide tubes, and the external surface of the device to ensure that the source is fully retracted.
8. The post-treatment survey will be recorded on an appropriate survey form and the report maintained for a period of at least 3 years.
9. If the radiation monitor or post-treatment patient survey indicated that the source is not fully retracted to a shielded position in the device, personnel (authorized physician and physicist) will immediately implement the applicable emergency procedures (posted at the HDR console and in the treatment room) (see section D). If other emergencies occur during HDR treatment (e.g., electrical power loss, applicator dislodge, timer failure) authorized HDR personnel will immediately implement the applicable emergency procedure.
10. No treatment procedure will be continued for which a de-coupled or jammed source cannot be removed expeditiously from the patient and placed in the shielded container available in the room.
11. During all patient treatments using HDR device, both the authorized physician and

the medical physicist must be physically present. Physical presence, for this purpose, is defined as within audible range of normal human speech.

D. Emergency Procedures

One of the licensing requirements (Item 15, Section 22.3) is the submission of emergency procedures, postings, and locations. The following emergency procedures are presented as samples (assuming a particular HDR unit, Varisource). Appropriate emergency equipment, for example, two pairs of long-handled forceps, shielded container, heavy duty cable cutters, pair of long-handled scissors, portable survey meter and stop watch or timer, must be available at all times.

D.1. Improper Source Retraction

If the room monitor or afterloader console indicates that the active source wire has failed to retract, proceed as follows:

(a) Enter the room with a portable survey meter and observe the emergency hand wheel. If the hand wheel is not turning, and radiation is present: turn the wheel clockwise through eight revolutions, or until the independent radiation monitor no longer detects radiation. If radiation is still detected, proceed to procedure (b).

    If the hand wheel is turning, and radiation is present, proceed to procedure (b).

(b) Remove all applicators/catheters from the patient without disconnection at any point and place them in the shielded container. The removal of applicators/catheters is accomplished by cutting any external sutures, physically removing the entire applicator/catheter apparatus and placing it in the shielded container provided. Surgical tools for removal of the sutures are located in the HDR treatment room.

(c) In all cases above, remove the patient from the immediate area, survey the patient, and if it is safe to do so, evacuate the patient from the room and lock the room. Post a warning sign: "This room must remain locked. HDR source exposed. Do not enter." Notify all emergency contacts listed below (e.g., Radiation Safety Officer, vendor). Estimate and record the additional dose to the patient. Also estimate and record any exposure to hospital staff.

D.2. Electrical Power Loss

(a) In case of power loss during treatment, the afterloader unit has an uninterrupted power supply (UPS) that enables all systems to continue operation for up to 30 minutes. This will enable completion of any HDR treatment in progress at the time of AC power failure.

(b) If both AC power and UPS system fail to operate, the HDR afterloader unit is equipped with an emergency backup source retract battery that will automatically retract the source into the storage position and if a patient is being treated, will record the date and time at which the patient treatment is interrupted.

(c) If all the AC, UPS and emergency backup source retract battery all fail at the same time, the operator must follow the emergency manual source retraction procedure (section 22.3 D.1). For any of the above emergency occurrences the HDR operator must notify the emergency call list posted at the HDR console.

D.3. Applicator Dislodging

In the event that the applicator dislodges from the patient during an HDR treatment, or a source guide tube becomes dislodged, the following emergency steps must be taken:

(a) Activate HDR emergency off button at control console.

(b) If the source fails to retract, follow emergency manual source retraction procedure (section 22.3 D.1).
(c) Immediately notify individuals on Emergency call list posted at HDR console.

D.4. Timer Failure

In the event that the HDR treatment timer fails to operate or terminate the treatment, the following steps must be taken:

(a) Activate HDR emergency OFF button at control console.
(b) Stop manual timer at time that emergency OFF button retracts source (this manual timer is started at the beginning of every HDR treatment).
(c) If this emergency OFF button fails to retract the source, follow the emergency manual source retraction procedure (section 22.3 D.1).
(d) Immediately call persons on emergency call list posted at HDR console.

22.4. HIGH DOSE RATE SOURCE CALIBRATION

As discussed in Chapter 15, the strength of a brachytherapy source may be specified in terms of activity, exposure rate at a specified distance, equivalent mass of radium, apparent activity, or air kerma strength. The American Association of Physicists in Medicine (AAPM) recommends air kerma strength (S_k). In practice, S_k is determined from exposure rate ($\dot{X}$) measured in free air at a distance of 1 m from the source. The relationship between S_k and $\dot{X}$ has been derived in section 15.2.

If $\dot{X}$ is measured in R/h at a distance of 1 m, then Equation 15.6 gives:

$$S_k = 8.76 \times 10^3 \, \dot{X} (\mathrm{m}^2 \mu \mathrm{Gy/h}) \qquad (22.1)$$

The National Institute of Standards and Technology (NIST) has established air kerma (or exposure) calibration standards for the LDR brachytherapy sources, for example, radium, ^{60}Co, ^{137}Cs, and ^{192}Ir. The NIST calibrates a working standard of each source type and construction with spherical graphite thimble chambers of known volume using open-air geometry. Because the air volume in the chamber cavity is precisely known, and the chamber is irradiated under conditions of electronic equilibrium, exposure rate can be measured in accordance with its definition (1R = 2.58×10^{-4} C/kg air). For lower energy LDR brachytherapy sources (e.g., ^{125}I, ^{103}Pd), the NIST has developed a wide-angle free-air ionization chamber that is capable of measuring radiation from a 2π area of the source (6). The NIST also uses a spherical re-entrant (well) chamber for calibrating brachytherapy sources. The calibration factors for these chambers are maintained by comparative measurements with a spherical thimble chamber used in open-air geometry or the wide-angle free-air chamber, depending upon the source type.

Secondary calibration laboratories such as the Accredited Dosimetry Calibration Laboratories (ADCLs) provide calibration of re-entrant well ionization chambers for commonly used brachytherapy sources. They can also provide calibration of standard sources. The ADCL calibrations are "directly traceable" to NIST because ADCLs possess reference class chambers or standard sources that are calibrated by the NIST. For the users to have their source calibrations traceable to NIST, they should get their well chamber calibrated by an ADCL or acquire an ADCL calibrated standard source of a given type and design to calibrate the well chamber. Unlike the LDR sources, the NIST has no standard, as of yet, for calibrating HDR sources. Goetsch et al (7) have described a method of calibrating a thimble-type chamber for ^{192}Ir HDR sources by interpolation of its response to ^{137}Cs gamma rays and 250 kVp (medium filter) x-rays. To ensure electronic equilibrium, a wall plus cap thickness of 0.3 g/cm^2 is recommended for all measurements. An open-air geometry is used at distances ranging from 10 to 40 cm from the source in a low scatter environment. Because the thimble chamber bears a NIST exposure calibration for ^{137}Cs and 250 kVp x-rays, this interpolative method can be considered as directly traceable to NIST.

A. Re-entrant Chamber

Calibration of ^{192}Ir HDR sources with a thimble chamber using open-air geometry is a time-consuming procedure and is not suitable for routine calibrations. The nuclear medicine well-type chamber ("dose calibrator"), which is commonly used for routine calibration of LDR sources (section 15.2B), is also not suitable for calibrating HDR sources, because of its overly large sensitive volume and, consequently, too high a sensitivity. A well-type re-entrant chamber of smaller volume has been designed specifically for ^{192}Ir HDR sources (8).

The University of Wisconsin re-entrant ion chamber[2] is filled with air and communicates to the outside air through a vent hole. The active volume of the chamber is approximately 245 cm^3, which for HDR measurements is just large enough to give an optimum ionization current to be measured accurately with most clinical electrometers. A thin-walled aluminum tube is fitted on the axis of the chamber, which allows the insertion of HDR source catheter until the end of it touches the bottom. The thickness of aluminum between the source and the ion-collecting volume of the chamber exceeds 0.3 g/cm^2, as required for attaining electronic equilibrium with ^{192}Ir gamma rays. The bias voltage applied to the chamber is about 300 V, which gives ionic collection efficiency of better than 99.96% for measuring a 6.5 Ci, ^{192}Ir source.

The HDR-specific re-entrant chamber is calibrated by an ADCL using calibrated thimble chambers in an open-air geometry, as discussed previously. A yearly calibration of this chamber by the ADCL is recommended. The constancy of its calibration may be checked routinely (e.g., before each use) by means of a strontium-90–yttrium-90 opthalmic applicator, which can be positioned reproducibly at the top of the well when the central tube assembly is removed.

The ionization current reading of a re-entrant chamber is dependent on the position of the source in the well. If the source is positioned at the maximum reading point, the chamber response is typically constant within ± 5 mm of the maximum reading position. For example, if a source catheter is inserted in the well chamber (all the way), the HDR source may be programmed to dwell at maximum reading positions to obtain multiple readings. The mean maximum reading may thus be determined to check the source strength.

The calibration factor for the chamber is given in terms of air kerma strength per unit reading. Measurements can be of either charge or current. In the current mode of measurement,

$$S_k = I \times C_{T,P} \times N_{el} \times N_C \times A_{ion} \times P_{ion}, \tag{22.2}$$

where S_k is the air kerma strength of the source, I is the current reading, $C_{T,P}$ is the correction for temperature and pressure, N_{el} is the electrometer calibration factor, N_C is the chamber calibration factor, A_{ion} is the ion recombination correction factor at the time of chamber calibration, and P_{ion} is the ion recombination correction at the time of source calibration. In the integrate mode, charge can be measured for a given interval or dwell time. Equation 22.2 can be used to determine S_k, where I is the integrated charge measured per unit time and N_C is the chamber calibration factor in terms of air kerma strength per unit charge. For a routine calibration of the HDR source, it is preferable to use the current mode of measurement because it is free of the source transit effect.

---

[2] Commercially available at Standard Imaging, Middleton, Wisconsin.

22.5. TREATMENT PLANNING

A. Simulation

The HDR treatment planning process starts with the patient preparation and placement of applicators, catheters or needles, depending upon the procedure. The physician places the implant devices in the treatment area, normally under local anesthesia, for example, gynecologic applicators with palpation and visual inspection, prostate template with ultrasound, endobronchial tube with bronchoscopy guidance. The patient is then simulated using an isocentric x-ray unit such as a C-arm or a simulator. Marker wires are inserted into the applicators all the way to the closed ends. Orthogonal radiographs are obtained to localize the applicators and the marker wires. These radiographs allow the radiation oncologist to plan the treatment segment and dwell locations in relation to the distal end of the applicator. Next, the total length of the catheter required for source travel is determined. This is accomplished by connecting the transfer guide tube to the applicator and passing a measurement wire through the catheter to the distal end. A measurement clip is attached to the wire at the point where it exits the free end of the guide tube. The wire is then removed and inserted into a calibration ruler until the measurement clip is at the zero end of the ruler. The catheter length is determined by reading the tip of the measurement wire within the catheter against the ruler graduation.

The simulation films are carefully labeled with patient name, date, catheter identification and length, magnification factor and marker seeds consecutively from the distal end of each catheter. Regions of interest including anatomical structures where dose contribution is to be calculated are drawn on the films.

B. Computer Planning

B.1. Orthogonal Radiography-based

The computer planning session starts with the input of patient and simulation data. Orthogonal films are scanned into the computer and the target volumes as well as organs at risk are outlined on the images. Selected dose specification points are marked and can be used to optimize dose distributions according to constraints.

Most optimization methods consist of obtaining desired doses at a number of points designated by the planner. The codes are written to search for dwell times to deliver the desired doses at the selected points as closely as possible. Several analytic techniques of optimization have been discussed in the literature including least squares minimization (9), linear programming (10), simulated annealing (11), and others (12,13). It should be realized that although these techniques are capable of meeting the specified dose constraints, not all result in the same dose distribution or the same set of dwell times.

Treatment plans are iteratively optimized and evaluated by viewing isodose curves in different planes. Because the applicators do not necessarily lie in planes parallel to those of the orthogonal films, it is important that appropriate planes of calculation are chosen for dose specification. For example, in a tandem and ovoid case, the frontal plane of calculation should be rotated to coincide with the plane that contains the length of the tandem (or the initial straight part of a curved tandem) and bisects the vaginal sources. In the lateral view, the plane of calculation should again include the length of the tandem, with the vaginal sources lying anterior and posterior to that plane.

After physician's review and approval, the plan is printed out with all the input and output data including planned source positions and dwell times. A floppy diskette is prepared to export the plan to the HDR afterloader computer.

B.2. Three-dimensional Image-based

Traditionally, computer treatment planning of brachytherapy has been based on orthogonal radiography. Although dose distribution is calculated in three dimensions and can be displayed in any plane, it cannot be viewed three-dimensionally relative to the patient anatomy. With the advent of three-dimensional (3-D) imaging by means of computed tomography (CT), magnetic resonance (MR), and ultrasounds (US), it is now possible to perform full-fledged 3-D treatment planning of brachytherapy implants. Software has been developed that allows slice-by slice delineation of targets, applicators, and organs at risk. The structures can be reconstructed three-dimensionally and viewed in any plane with the overlaid isodose curves. Treatment plans can be evaluated by viewing isodose curves, isodose surfaces, or dose-volume histograms.

A number of papers have been published on 3-D treatment planning of brachytherapy (14–16) although most of these programs pertain to LDR brachytherapy including permanent seed implants for the treatment of prostate cancer. Software for 3-D treatment planning of HDR implants is under active development and should be commercially available in the very near future.

C. Dose Computation

Dose distribution around a linear ^{192}Ir source used in HDR afterloaders can be calculated using a number of methods such as Sievert integral, TG-43 formalism or Monte Carlo. As discussed in Chapter 15, the TG-43 formalism (17) has advantages over the Sievert integral approach in that the effects of various physical factors on dose distribution are considered separately and that the dosimetric quantities involved can be individually measured or calculated using Monte Carlo. TG-43 is especially suitable for sources of complex design or those in which filtration effects of the source or its encapsulation cannot be accurately modeled analytically.

Basic data for a number of commercial HDR sources have been measured or calculated using TG-43 and Monte Carlo (18–21). Along and away tables, dose rate constant, radial dose function, and anisotropy function for these sources have been published. However, a given HDR treatment-planning system may or may not incorporate these data. For example, some systems are based on the Sievert integral or even a point source approximation, ignoring oblique filtration through the source or its anisotropy. The user of these systems must be aware of the accuracy limitations of such algorithms.

Even if a system uses TG-43 formalism based on measured data or Monte Carlo, it may lack full implementation. For example, some TG-43 based systems use an average anisotropy factor instead of the anisotropy function as a function of angle. Commercial HDR sources exhibit significant anisotropy along the axis, e.g., in the range of 35% to 60% depending on the source model (19,21). It should be pointed out that even the LDR steel-clad ^{192}Ir seed shows axial anisotropy of 19% to 23% (17).

Tables have been published that give dose rate distribution as a function of distance away and along the available HDR sources (19,21). These Monte Carlo data can be used as the basis of a dose computation algorithm or as quality assurance of treatment planning systems for afterloaders that use these sources. Alternatively, TG-43 formula (Equation 15.16) may be used with factors measured or calculated specifically for the given HDR source. These factors for the above-mentioned sources have been calculated using Monte Carlo codes (19,21).

D. Plan Verification

Independent verification of a computer plan is an essential part of HDR quality assurance. Some of these checks consist of verifying the accuracy of input data such as dose prescription, catheter lengths, dwell times, current source strength, etc. Others involve independent spot checks of dose calculation, manually or by a second computer program. Verification of the dose at the prescription point (or another suitable point) within ± 5% is considered reasonable, considering the severe dose gradients encountered in brachytherapy.

A number of manual methods of checking HDR computer calculations have been discussed in the AAPM Task Group No. 59 (22). The reader is referred to these for review and possible adoption in the quality assurance program. One of the simplest methods consists of using inverse square law. The dose is calculated at the prescription point or at a point in its close vicinity, provided the distance of the point of calculation from the dwell positions (center of source) is at least twice the active length of the source. As discussed in section 15.3A.1, at these distances inverse square law can be assumed without significant loss of accuracy.

For a point source of ^{192}Ir, the TG-43 formula (see Equation 15.6) reduces to:

$$\dot{D}(r) = \Lambda\, S_k \frac{g(r)}{r^2} \Phi_{an} \qquad (22.3)$$

where $\dot{D}(r)$ is the dose rate at a distance r in the medium, Λ is the dose rate constant for the source, $g(r)$ is the radial dose function and Φ_{an} is the average anisotropy factor. As a further approximation in a manual check, $g(r)$ and Φ_{an} can each be equated to unity. Then Equation 22.3 simplifies to:

$$\dot{D}(r) = \Lambda\, S_k / r^2 \qquad (22.4)$$

In practice, r is measured from the center of the source at each dwell position. Dose rates calculated by Equation 22.4 at the various dwell positions are multiplied by the corresponding dwell times and summed to give the total dose.

In the use of Equation 22.4, care must be taken regarding units. If S_k is given in units of air kerma strength (U) ($1U = $ cGy cm^{2}h^{-1} in air), then Λ must be in terms of dose rate in the medium (water) per unit air kerma strength (cGy h^{-1}U^{-1}). If S_k is given in units of apparent activity (mCi), then Λ must be in units of cGy h^{-1} mCi^{-1}.

In order to assess agreement with the computer output, the value of Λ used in Equation 22.4 should be the same as used by the computer program. The following Λ values have been calculated for two of the commercially available HDR sources using Monte Carlo codes: VariSource (Varian Oncology Systems), $\Lambda = 1.044$cGy h^{-1}U^{-1} [21]; microSelectron (Nucletron), $\Lambda = 1.115$cGy h^{-1}U^{-1} [19].

22.6. QUALITY ASSURANCE

A quality assurance (QA) program is a set of policies and procedures to maintain the quality of patient care. Whereas the standards of quality are set collectively by the profession, a QA program is designed to follow these standards as closely as possible and minimize the occurrence of treatment mistakes caused by equipment malfunction or human error. The design of such a program for HDR starts with the license application. The United States Nuclear Regulatory Commission requires the licensee to meet certain standards including personnel education and training, operating procedures, equipment safety checks, radiation monitoring, emergency procedures, recording and maintenance of treatment data and reporting of any misadministration. A policy and guidance directive for the HDR brachytherapy license has been published by the NRC [2], which provides a template for designing a quality management program acceptable to the NRC (or Agreement State). A summary review of the NRC requirements was presented earlier in section 22.3. It should be understood that all tests and procedures written in the license application are legally binding and therefore, represent minimum QA standards. These standards should be augmented by QA tests and procedures recommended by professional organizations, national or international.

The AAPM has published several documents on quality assurance in radiation therapy. For HDR, the reader is referred to TG-59 [22]. Additional reports, TG-56 [23] and TG-40 [24], are also useful and should be consulted. It should be realized that because of the broad range of HDR afterloader designs a universal set of QA tests has not been formulated. It is expected that each institution will design its own QA program, which addresses the characteristics of the specific equipment, NRC requirements and treatment standards set for the program.

The AAPM recommends QA tests at three frequencies: daily, quarterly, and annually (23). Unless HDR treatments are given every day, it is sufficient to perform "daily QA" tests only on days when patients are treated. These tests are described in section 22.3. The quarterly QA essentially consists of source calibration and a more thorough review of equipment function. The quarterly interval coincides with the frequency with which HDR sources are replaced. The annual QA is a comprehensive review of all equipment, procedures, and patient records, approaching the thoroughness of initial acceptance testing/commissioning of the system.

22.7. CLINICAL APPLICATIONS

HDR brachytherapy can be used essentially for any cancer that is suitable for LDR brachytherapy. The most common uses of HDR are in the treatment of endobronchial

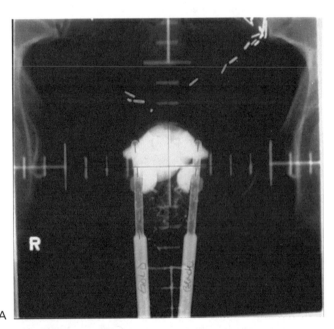

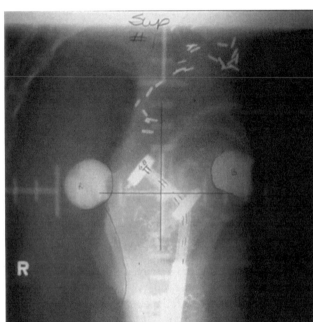

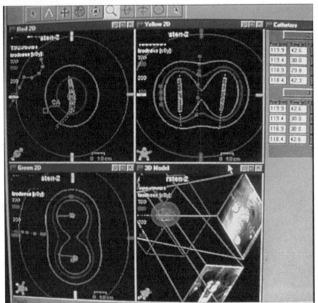

FIG. 22.2. A: Anteroposterior view of ovoids in a simulator radiograph. **B:** Lateral view of ovoids. **C:** Isodose distribution shown in three orthogonal views.

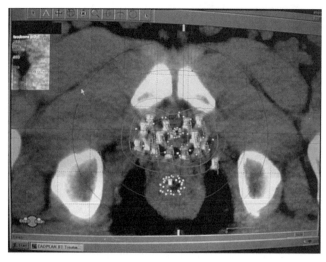

FIG. 22.3. Prostate gland high dose rate implant shown in a transverse computed tomography slice.

obstruction by lung cancer, postoperative treatment of endometrial carcinoma (vaginal cuff irradiation), and localized prostate cancer. The use of HDR in the treatment of cervical carcinoma is not as common because clinically it is not expected to outperform the LDR treatment in terms of disease control or survival. However, HDR does offer theoretical advantages of better dose distribution for the target volume and greater sparing of the bladder and rectum than possible with the LDR. Although HDR is not yet a well-established procedure for treating cervix cancer, it has the potential to replace LDR for practical reasons if not clinical.

Figure 22.2 shows an example of HDR use in the treatment of endometrial cancer with familiar isodose distribution around ovoids. The shape of the isodose curves can be optimized by adjusting dwell times as discussed earlier. Figure 22.3 is an example of HDR prostate implant using ultrasound for guidance. This procedure is discussed in Chapter 23. For further review of clinical applications of HDR, the reader is referred to reference 24.

REFERENCES

1. ICRU. Dose and volume specifications for reporting intracavitary therapy. ICRU Report No. 38. Bethesda, MD: International Commission on Radiation Units and Measurements, 1985.
2. NRC. Policy and guidance directive, FC-86–4; Revision 1: Information required for licensing remote afterloading devices. Nuclear Regulatory Commission. Washington, DC: U.S. Government Printing Office, 1993.
3. NCRP. Protection against radiation from brachytherapy sources. NCRP Report No. 40. Washington DC: National Council on Radiation Protection and Measurements, 1972.
4. NCRP. Structural shielding design and evaluation for medical use of x-rays and gamma rays of energies up to 10 MeV. NCRP Report No. 49. Washington, DC: National Council on Radiation Protection and Measurements, 1976.
5. Klein EE, Grisby PW, Williamson JF, Meigooni AS. Pre-installation empirical testing of room shielding for high dose rate remote afterloaders. *Int J Radiat Oncol Biol Phys* 1993;27:927–931.
6. Weaver JT, Loftus TP, Loevinger R. NBS measurement services: calibration of gamma-ray-emitting brachytherapy sources. National Bureau of Standards (NIST) special publication no. 250–19. Gaithersburg, MD: National Bureau of Standards, 1988.
7. Goetsch SJ, Attix FJ, Pearson DW, et al. Calibration of ^{192}Ir high-dose rate afterloading systems. *Med Phys* 1991;462–467.
8. Goetsch SJ, Attix FH, DeWerd LA, et al. A new well ionization chamber for the calibration of iridium-192 high dose rate sources. *Int J Radiat Oncol Biol Phys* 1992;24:167–170.
9. Anderson LL. Plan optimization and dose evaluation in brachytherapy. *Semin Radiat Oncol* 1993;3:290–300.
10. Renner WD, O'Conner TP, Bermudez NM. An algorithm for generation of implant plans for high-dose rate irradiators. *Med Phys* 1990;17:35–40.

11. Sloboda RS. Optimization of brachytherapy dose distribution by simulated annealing. *Med Phys* 1992;19:955–964.

12. Van der Laars R, Prius TPE. Introduction to HDR brachytherapy optimization. In: Mould RF, Battermann JJ, Martinez AA, et al., eds. *Brachytherapy from radium to optimization.* Veenendaal, The Netherlands: Nucletron Corporation, 1994.

13. Ezzel GA, Luthermann RW. Clinical implementation of dwell time optimization techniques for single stepping-source remote applicators. In: Williamson J, Thomadsen B, Nath R, eds. *Brachytherapy physics.* Madison, WI: Medical Physics Publishing, 1994.

14. McShan DL, Ten Haken RK, Fraas BA. 3-D treatment planning: IV. Integrated brachytherapy planning. In: Bruimvis IAD, et al., eds. Proceedings of the Ninth International Conference: the use of computers in radiation therapy. Scheveningen, The Netherlands. North-Holland: Elsevier Science Publishers BV, 1987:249–252.

15. Schoeppel SL, Lavigne ML, Mantel MK, et al. Three dimensional treatment planning of intercavity gynecologic implants analysis of ten cases and implications for dose specification. *Int J Radiat Oncol Biol Phys* 1993;28:277–283.

16. Weeks KJ. Brachytherapy object-oriented treatment planning based on three dimensional image guidance. In: Thomadsen B, ed. *Categorical course in brachytherapy physics.* Oak Brook, IL: Radiological Society of North America, 1997:79–86.

17. Nath R, Anderson LL, Luxton G, et al. Dosimetry of interstitial brachytherapy sources: recommendations of the AAPM Radiation Therapy Committee Task Group No. *43. Med Phys* 1995;22:209–234.

18. Muller-Runkel R, Cho SH. Anisotropy measurements of a high dose rate Ir-192 source in air and polystyrene. *Med Phys* 1994;21:1131–1134.

19. Williamson JF, Li Z. Monte Carlo aided dosimetry of the microselection pulsed and high dose-rate ^{192}Ir sources. *Med Phys* 1995;22:809–819.

20. Mishra V, Waterman FM, Suntharalingam N. Anisotropy of an iridium 192 high dose rate source measured with a miniature ionization chamber. *Med Phys* 1997;24:751–755.

21. Wang R, Sloboda RS. Monte Carlo dosimetry of the VariSource high dose rate ^{192}Ir source. *Med Phys* 1998;25:415–423.

22. Kubo HD, Glasgow GP, Pethel TD, et al. High dose-rate brachytherapy treatment delivery: report of the AAPM Radiation Therapy Committee Task Group No. 59. *Med Phys* 1998;25:375–403.

23. Nath R, Anderson LL, Meli JA, et al. Code of practice for brachytherapy physics: AAPM Radiation Therapy Committee Task Group No. 56. *Med Phys* 1997;24:1557–1598.

24. Stitt JA, Thomadsen BR. Clinical applications of low dose rate and high dose rate brachytherapy. In: Levitt SH, Khan FM, Potish RA, et al., eds. *Technological basis of radiation therapy.* Philadelphia: Lippincott Williams & Wilkins, 1999:210–219.

PROSTATE IMPLANTS

23.1. INTRODUCTION

Treatment options for carcinoma of the prostate include radical prostatectomy (e.g., nerve-sparing surgical procedure), external photon beam irradiation and brachytherapy implantation. The selection of a particular procedure or a combination of procedures depends on established prognostic factors such as stage, grade, and pre-treatment prostate-specific antigen (PSA) concentration. In general, surgery is indicated if the tumor is confined to the prostate gland with no extension through the capsule or into the seminal vesicles. Implants are used for early stage cancers, either alone or in conjunction with external beam radiation therapy. However, patients with extensive tumors (TNM stage T3 and T4) are not good candidates for implantation.

Except as general information, clinical aspects of prostate gland cancer and its treatment are beyond the scope of this book. The reader is referred to a wealth of information on this subject in the medical literature. In this chapter we will discuss the physical and technologic aspects of prostate gland implants using radioactive seeds and high-dose-rate brachytherapy.

23.2. SEED IMPLANTS

Two types of seed implants have been used for prostate gland: a temporary implant and a permanent implant. The temporary implants involve radioisotopes of relatively long half-life and sufficient dose rate to deliver the prescribed target dose in 3 to 4 days. The sources are removed at the end of that period. In the permanent implant the radioisotope either has a short half-life (e.g., gold-198) or emits photons of low enough energy that the radiation from the patient poses no significant hazard to persons in the surrounding environment. The sources are left in the patient forever and the prescribed dose is delivered during complete decay of the sources. Of these two types of seed implants, the permanent implants are gaining more popularity and will be discussed in greater detail.

A. Permanent Implants

Permanent implants with iodine-125 or palladium-103 are used in the treatment of early stage prostate cancer as the sole modality or in combination with external beam radiation therapy. The target volume for implantation in either case is the prostate gland itself, with minimal margins allowed to account for uncertainty of prostate localization.

Whitmore and Hilaris pioneered prostatic implantation with ^{125}I seeds in the early 1970s at Memorial-Sloan Kettering Cancer Center. They used retropubic approach, which entailed a major surgical procedure. The treatment results were disappointing and so, by the mid-1980s, the retropubic technique was abandoned.

The modern technique of implantation, which began in the 1980s, consists of transperineal approach in which ^{125}I or ^{103}Pd seeds are inserted into the prostate gland with the guidance of transrectal ultrasonography and perineal template. The procedure is nonsurgical and performed on an outpatient basis. The implant is done in an approved operating room with the patient requiring a spinal anesthetic.

A.1. Volume Study

Localization of prostate by a series of transverse ultrasound images constitutes a volume study. The patient is placed in the dorsal lithotomy position and the transrectal ultrasound probe (5- to 6-MHz transducer) is securely anchored. The probe is moved precisely to obtain transverse images of the prostate gland from base to apex at 5-mm intervals. A grid is superimposed on each image to represent template coordinates. The prostate gland is visualized on each of the transverse images and the implantation target is drawn to encompass the prostate. The sagittal image is also obtained to measure the length of the gland from the base to the apex. This provides a double check of the number of transverse images and the number of seeds required for the central needle.

Prior to the volume study, evaluation is made from computed tomography (CT) scans of the prostate gland size and the pubic arch in relation to the prostate. If the pubic arch is too narrow it would prevent the needles from reaching the target. In the case of a large gland and significant pubic arch interference, the patient may need hormonal therapy for a few months to shrink the gland to allow for an adequate implant. Some radiation oncologists prefer hormonal therapy in most cases to reduce the gland size to minimize technical problems of implantation.

A.2. Treatment Planning

A treatment-planning system specifically designed for prostate gland implants allows the target outlines from the volume study to be digitized into the computer. The implant is planned with an interseed spacing of 1 cm (center to center) and a needle spacing of 1 cm. The computer software allows the placement of seeds in the template grid in each of the ultrasound image. Individual seeds can be added or deleted iteratively to optimize isodose coverage of the target volume. Seed strength can be adjusted to deliver a prescribed minimum peripheral dose (MPD) which is the isodose surface just covering the prostate target volume. Before the availability of computer dosimetry, seed strength and the required number of seeds were determined by the method of dimension averaging used in conjunction with a precalculated nomogram (1). The modern computer programs allow the use of any seed strength as well as fine adjustment of this parameter to obtain the desired MPD. Typical seed strengths required are on the order of 0.3 mCi for ^{125}I (MPD = 144Gy) and 1.7 mCi for ^{103}Pd (MPD = 125Gy).

Based on the approved computer plan, a worksheet is prepared specifying the number of needles, seeds in each needle and the template coordinates. Figure 23.1 (see color insert) shows an example of pre-implant treatment plan for ^{125}I along with the dose-volume histogram and statistics.

Post-implant dosimetry may also be performed using CT scans to assess stability of the implant after swelling of the prostate gland has gone down. A major problem with permanent seed implants is the usual disagreement between the pre-implant and post-implant dose distributions. Hot and cold spots can develop as a result of source movement with time (Fig. 23.2) (see color insert), leaving one to wonder if the prescribed dose was delivered to the target accurately with a pattern of dose distribution as originally planned.

Another equally serious problem is that of source anisotropy. Because of the low gamma ray energy emitted and the design of the source in which radiation is severely attenuated along the length of the seed, cold spots of greater than 50% (reduction in dose) exist at the ends (see Figs. 15.4 and 15.6). This anisotropy in dose distribution however, is more of a problem if the sources are aligned permanently end to end with each other along straight lines. A certain degree of randomness that naturally develops after implantation reduces the overall anisotropy effect in a prostate gland implant.

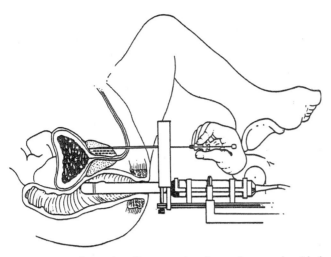

FIG. 23.3. Schematic diagram showing ultrasound-guided transperineal template implant procedure. (From Grim PD, Blasko JC, Ragde H. *Atlas of the Urologic Clinics of North America* 1994;2: 113–125, with permission.)

The seed anisotropy has been significantly reduced by a newly designed ^{125}I source (model L S-1 BrachySeed manufactured by DRAXIMAGE Inc.[1]). Dosimetric Characteristics of this source have been discussed by Nath and Yue (2).

A.3. Implant Procedure

The implant procedure is carried out as an outpatient treatment in an operating room with the patient in the dorsal lithotomy position under spinal anesthesia. Figure 23.3 shows the implantation apparatus consisting of a transrectal ultrasound probe and a template to guide specifically designed sterile 18-gauge, 21-cm long needles. The needles are preloaded with the planned number of seeds and spacers and placed in a needle holder at appropriate template coordinates. The needle loading procedure is performed behind an L-shaped leaded glass barrier. Each needle is equipped with a plunger and the tip is sealed with bone wax to keep the seeds in place until implantation.

The needles are inserted one at a time into the prostate using the ultrasound and template guidance. In each case, using sagittal images and distance measurements from the hub of the needle to the template, it is ascertained that the needle tip is at the correct plane and depth. After verifying the needle position, the needle is slowly withdrawn while the plunger is held stationary. This action results in the injection of the seeds and the spacers into the tissues along the track of the withdrawing needle. Each ultrasound image is carefully reviewed to assess the position of the seeds. Final verification of the implant is made with anteroposterior fluoroscopy. Extra seeds are available for implantation if cold spots are identified. Cystoscopy is performed at the conclusion of the procedure to retrieve any stray seeds in the bladder or the urethra.

For further technical details of the operative technique and implant procedure, the reader is referred to Grim et al. (3,4).

A.4. Radiation Protection

The AAPM code of practice for brachytherapy (5) is a comprehensive document on the physics and quality assurance of brachytherapy procedures. Before implementing a prostate

---

[1] DRAXIMAGE, Inc., 16751, Route Transcandienne, Kirkland (Quebec), Canada.

implant program, one should consult this document together with the relevant Nuclear Regulatory Commission regulations. The basic requirement for releasing a permanent implant patient from the hospital is that the total exposure to any other individual from the released patient does not exceed 0.5 rem over the life of the implant. This condition is easily met with a prostate implant using ^{125}I or ^{103}Pd seeds. Low energy radiation is locally absorbed within the patient, posing little risk to surrounding organs or people. However, patients are instructed at the time of discharge to observe certain precautions. For example, they are advised not to have prolonged physical contact with pregnant women or young children for a period of 2 months, to abstain from sexual activity for 2 weeks, and to use condoms during intercourse for the first few weeks in case a seed is discharged into the vagina.

During the implant procedure, a medical physicist or dosimetrist assisting in the procedure also assures that the total number of seeds is accounted for at all times. A thin window GM tube or a scintillation counter is available to locate any dropped or misplaced seed. Personnel are not allowed to leave the operating room without being surveyed to prevent accidental transport of any seed outside the room. At the conclusion of the procedure, the trash, the room, and the personnel are surveyed for any misplaced seed.

B. Temporary Implants

Temporary prostate gland implants have almost exclusively used iridium-192. The treatment is given mainly as a boost to external beam therapy (6–8). Traditionally, these implants have been carried out at the time of laparotomy and pelvic-node sampling. The needles are implanted intraoperatively with the guidance of a transperineal template. Iridium seeds in plastic ribbons are afterloaded into the needles and left in place for about 3 days. Usually 10 to 15 needles are required for the implant. The patient is hospitalized and bed-bound for the duration of the implant, requiring analgesia.

Current refinements in the temporary implantation technique include ultrasound guidance, avoiding open laparotomy. However, patient hospitalization is still required with the attendant radioprotection problems for personnel administering postoperative care.

23.3. DOSIMETRY

A. Calibration

Brachytherapy sources are calibrated by the vendor before shipment and bear a calibration certificate with stated limits of uncertainty, usually 10%. Although vendor calibrations are, in most cases, traceable to the National Institute of Standards and Technology (NIST), the user is advised to check the calibration values of a sample of sources from the batch as a matter of quality assurance. Agreement within $\pm 5\%$ with the vendor calibration is acceptable, in which case the vendor values may be used for patient dose calculations. In case of a larger disagreement, the user must resolve the difference with the vendor and if unsuccessful, use the in-house calibration, with full documentation of the procedure used.

The NIST uses large-volume ion chambers in a open-air geometry to calibrate ^{192}Ir sources and free-air ionization chamber for ^{125}I (9,10). The stated uncertainties in these calibrations are on the order of 2%. The NIST calibration techniques require considerable attention to detail and are not practical for routine use.

The most suitable method of routine calibration of brachytherapy sources is the well ionization or re-entrant chamber. As discussed in section 15.2B, a nuclear medicine dose calibrator may be converted into a brachytherapy well chamber by placing a source-holding tube along the axis of the chamber. The chamber response, however, depends significantly on the energy of radiation, source construction, and source position along the chamber axis. It is therefore essential that the well chamber bears a NIST-traceable calibration specifically for the type of source to be calibrated.

The well chamber calibration for given types of sources may be obtained from the Accredited Dose Calibration Laboratories (ADCLs) which maintain traceability with the NIST. Alternatively, the chamber may be calibrated in-house by using a standard source of the same type, which has been calibrated by an ADCL. The standard source should not only be the same Radionuclide but also have the same construction or model. In addition, the calibration geometry (source position along the chamber axis) should be the same for the standard source as for the source to be calibrated. If different source positions are intended appropriate corrections should be determined as a function of source position.

B. Dose Computation

Dose distribution around ^{125}I, ^{103}Pd, or ^{192}Ir is not isotropic. Analytical methods of dose calculations such as Sievert integral are not suitable for these sources because of complexity in source construction, filtration, and low energy of the emitted radiation. The AAPM Task Group 43 or simply TG-43 formalism (11) gets around this problem by parametrizing the dose distribution around a specific source type in terms of actual measurements or detailed Monte Carlo calculations. The general TG-43 equation (Equation 15.16) for the calibration of dose at a point $P(r,\theta)$ which includes anisotropy effects, is as follows:

$$\dot{D}(r, \theta) = \Lambda\, S_k \frac{G(r, \theta)}{G(1, \pi/2)} g(r)\, F(r, \theta) \tag{23.1}$$

where $\dot{D}(r, \theta)$ is the dose rate at point P in a medium (e.g., water), Λ is the dose rate constant, S_k is the air kerma strength of the source, G is the geometry factor, g is radial dose function and F is the anisotropy function. These quantities are defined in Chapter 15.

In order to use Equation 23.1 rigorously for an implant, the seed orientation must be known and fixed. In prostate gland implants, although seeds are placed along straight lines with known coordinates, their post-implant orientation becomes somewhat randomized and variable with time. It is therefore acceptable to treat these seeds as point sources in a dose calculation formalism. For a point source, Equation 23.1 reduces to:

$$\dot{D}(r) = \Lambda\, S_k \frac{g(r)}{r^2} \overline{\Phi}_{an} \tag{23.2}$$

where $\overline{\Phi}_{an}$ is the average anisotropy factor. Current values of Λ, $g(r)$ and $\overline{\Phi}_{an}$ for prostate implant sources are given in Tables 23.1 to 23.3.

A treatment-planning system for prostate gland implants usually has the reference data (Λ, $g(r)$ and $\overline{\Phi}_{an}$) stored for a number of commercially available seeds. It is the responsibility of the user to assure that these data pertain to the type of sources to be implanted and represent currently accepted values (e.g., published in peer-reviewed literature).

TABLE 23.1. RECOMMENDED DOSE RATE CONSTANTS IN A WATER MEDIUM

Seed	cGy hr^{-1} U^{-1}
^{192}Ir	1.12
Iron clad	
^{125}I model 6702	0.93
^{125}I model 6711	0.88
^{103}Pd model 200	0.74

From Nath R, Anderson LL, Luxton G, et al. Dosimetry of interstitial brachytherapy sources: recommendations of the AAPM Radiation Therapy Committee Task Group no. 43. *Med Phys* 1995;22:209–234, with permission.

TABLE 23.2. RADIAL DOSE FUNCTIONS, $g(r)$

Distance Along Transverse Axis (cm)	Radial Dose Function, $g(r)$			
	^{103}Pd	^{126}I Model 6711	^{125}I Model 6702	^{192}Ir
0.5	1.29	1.04	1.04	0.994
1.0	1.00	1.00	1.00	1.00
1.5	0.765	0.926	0.934	1.01
2.0	0.576	0.832	0.851	1.01
2.5	0.425	0.731	0.760	1.01
3.0	0.310	0.632	0.670	1.02
3.5	0.224	0.541	0.586	1.01
4.0	0.165	0.463	0.511	1.01
4.5	0.123	0.397	0.445	1.00
5.0	0.0893	0.344	0.389	0.996
5.5		0.300	0.341	0.985
6.0		0.264	0.301	0.972
6.5		0.233	0.266	0.957
7.0		0.204	0.235	0.942
7.5				0.927
8.0				0.913
8.5				0.900
9.0				0.891

From Nath R, Anderson LL, Luxton G, et al. Dosimetry of interstitial brachytherapy sources: recommendations of the AAPM Radiation Therapy Committee Task Group no. 43. *Med Phys* 1995;22: 209–234, with permission.

B.1. Total Dose

As the sources decay with a half-life $T_{1/2}$, the dose rate decreases exponentially with time t as:

$$\dot{D} = \dot{D}_0 e^{-0.693\, t/T_{1/2}} \tag{23.3}$$

where $\dot{D}$ is the dose rate (dD/dt) and $\dot{D}_0$ is the initial dose rate as given by Equation 23.2. The cumulated dose D_c in time t is obtained by integrating Equation 23.3:

$$D_c = \dot{D}_0(1.44\, T_{1/2})(1 - e^{0.693\, t/T_{1/2}}) \tag{23.4}$$

which is the same as Equation 15.28, since $1.44\, T_{1/2}$ is the average life (T_{av}). For a permanent implant, the total dose D_{total} is delivered after complete decay of the sources (i.e., $t \gg T_{1/2}$).

TABLE 23.3. ANISOTROPY FACTORS, $\phi_{an}(r)$, AND ANISOTROPY CONSTANTS, $\overline{\phi}_{an}$, FOR INTERSTITIAL SOURCES

Distance, r (cm)	Anisotropy Factors, $\phi_{an}(r)$			
	^{103}Pd	^{125}I Model 6711	^{125}I Model 6702	^{192}Ir
1	0.921	0.944	0.968	0.991
2	0.889	0.936	0.928	0.947
3	0.820	0.893	0.897	0.970
4	0.834	0.887	0.942	0.989
5	0.888	0.884	0.959	0.998
6		0.880	0.891	0.949
7		0.901	0.907	0.965
8				0.955
9				0.974
Anisotropy constants $\overline{\phi}_{an}$	0.90	0.93	0.95	0.98

From Nath R, Anderson LL, Luxton G, et al. Dosimetry of interstitial brachytherapy sources: recommendations of the AAPM Radiation Therapy Committee Task Group no. 43. *Med Phys* 1995;22: 209–234, with permission.

In that case, Equation 23.4 reduces to:

$$D_{\text{total}} = 1.44 \, \dot{D}_0 \, T_{1/2}$$

or

$$D_{\text{total}} = \dot{D}_0 \, T_{\text{av}} \qquad\qquad (23.5)$$

Example 1

A prostate gland implant with ^{125}I seeds delivered an initial dose rate of 0.07 Gy/h to the prostate gland. What will be the dose delivered after (a) 1 month and (b) after complete decay of the sources?

$$\text{Half-life of } ^{125}\text{I} = 59.4 \text{ days}$$
$$\text{Average life} = 1.44 \times 59.4 = 85.54 \text{ days}$$
$$= 2{,}052.9 \text{ h}$$
$$\dot{D}_0 = 0.07 \text{ Gy/h}$$

From Equation 23.4:

$$D_c = 0.07 \times 2{,}052.9(1 - e^{-0.693 \times 30/59.4})$$
$$= 42.44 \text{ Gy}$$

From Equation 23.5:

$$D_{\text{total}} = 0.07 \times 2{,}052.9 = 143.7 \text{ Gy}$$

The initial minimum dose rate in a prostate gland implant is very low (e.g., approximately 7 cGy/h) and approximately 30% of the prescribed dose is delivered in the first month.

EXAMPLE 2

Repeat Example 1 for ^{103}Pd implant with an initial dose rate of 0.21 Gy/h.

$$\text{Half-life of } ^{103}\text{Pd} = 16.97 \text{ days}$$
$$\text{Average life} = 1.44 \times 16.97 = 24.44 \text{ days}$$
$$= 586.5 \text{ h}$$
$$\dot{D}_0 = 0.21 \text{ Gy/h}$$

From Equation 23.4:

$$D_c = 0.21 \times 586.5(1 - e^{-0.693 \times 30/16.97})$$
$$= 87 \text{ Gy}$$

From Equation 23.5:

$$D_{\text{total}} = 0.21 \times 586.5 = 123.2 \text{ Gy}$$

For respective prescribed doses, the dose rate for a ^{103}Pd implant is typically about three times that for an ^{125}I implant. In the case of ^{103}Pd, because of its shorter half-life, the bulk of the prescribed dose (approximately 70%) is delivered in the first month.

23.4. HIGH DOSE RATE IMPLANTS

Prostate cancer is a slowly progressive disease. Consequently, the superiority of one treatment technique over another cannot be established in a short time (e.g., 5 to 10 years).

Although the results with seed implants are so far encouraging, caution is needed to interpret these results because of the relative short time of the studies and the many competing causes of failure in these patients. In addition, the clinical impact of dose inhomogeneity (caused by seed displacement and anisotropy) and extremely low dose rate (LDR) in a permanent implant is not well understood. However, the ability of brachytherapy to concentrate the dose in the tumor and spare surrounding normal tissues is well recognized. High-dose-rate (HDR) brachytherapy has that advantage and, in addition, offers better control of dose homogeneity and dose conformity compared to LDR brachytherapy.

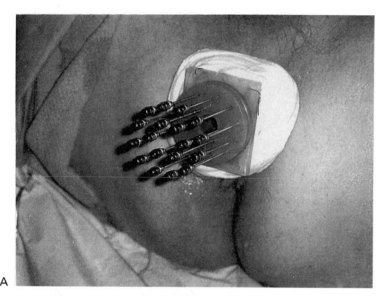

A

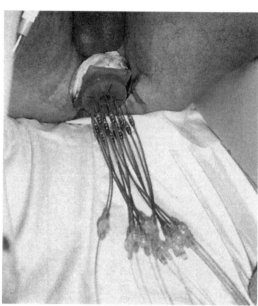

B

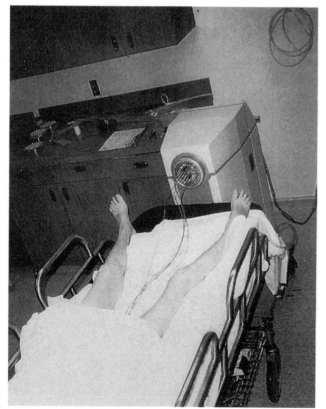

C

FIG. 23.4. Prostate implant procedure using ultrasound-guided HDR procedure showing **(A)** implant needles in place; **(B)** flexible adapters screwed into guide needles; and **(C)** flexible adapters connected to the HDR remote afterloaders. (From Syed AMN, Puthawala AA, Barth N, et al. High dose rate brachytherapy treatment of the prostate: preliminary results. *Journal of Brachytherapy Intl* 1997;13:315–331, with permission.)

A. Procedure

The HDR prostatic implant procedure using transrectal guidance is similar to the LDR brachytherapy with ^{192}Ir (12). The patient is placed in a lithotomy position and receives epidural anesthesia. A transrectal ultrasound probe is used to evaluate the prostate gland. Coronal and sagittal images allow the determination of prostate volume. A prostate gland template is sutured transperineally and HDR guide needles are implanted into the prostate gland with ultrasound guidance (Fig. 23.4a). Ten to fifteen needles are usually required to cover the prostate gland. The bladder is filled with Hypaque and dummy source wires are loaded into the guide needles to obtain intraoperative x-ray localization radiographs. The patient is sent to the recovery room and subsequently simulated to obtain orthogonal films for HDR treatment planning.

Treatment-planning algorithms for HDR have been discussed in Chapter 22. These programs are based on either orthogonal films or CT data. Dwell times of the source in each needle are calculated to provide optimized dose distribution. CT-based treatment planning provides full three-dimensional dose distributions including slice-by-slice isodose curves, isodose surfaces, and dose-volume histograms.

After the treatment plan has been optimized and approved, the guide needles are connected to the HDR afterloader through adapters and transfer catheters (Fig. 23.4B,C). The treatment is delivered as planned. After conclusion of the treatment, the transfer catheters are disconnected from the adapters and the patient is sent to his room.

Although dose fractionation with HDR is not yet well established, the total dose typically ranges from 10 to 25 Gy (minimum isodose surface) given in three to four fractions. This dose is given in addition to the 45 Gy of external beam radiation therapy.

REFERENCES

1. Hilaris BS, Nori D, Anderson LL. *Atlas of brachytherapy.* New York: MacMillan, 1988.
2. Nath R, Yue N. Dosimetric characterization of a newly designed encapsulated interstitial brachytherapy source of iodine-125-model LS-1 BrachySeed. *Appl Radiat Isot* 2001;55:813–821.
3. Grim PD, Blasko JC, Ragde H. Ultrasound-guided transperineal implantation of iodine-125 and palladium-103 for the treatment of early-stage prostate cancer. *Atlas of the Urologic Clinics of North America* 1994;2:113–125.
4. Porter AT, Blasko JC, Grimm PD, et al. Brachytherapy for prostate cancer. *CA Cancer J Clin* 1995;45:165–178.
5. Nath R, Anderson LL, Meli JA, et al. Code of practice for brachytherapy physics: AAPM Radiation Therapy Committee Task Group No. 56. *Med Phys* 1997;24:1557–1598.
6. Tansey LA, Shanberg AM, Syed AMN, et al. Treatment of prostatic cancer by pelvic lymphadenectomy, temporary iridium-192 implant and external irradiation. *Urology* 1983;21:594–598.
7. Syed AMN, Puthawala AA, Tansey LA, et al. Temporary interstitial irradiation in the management of carcinoma of the prostate: "current status of a new approach." *Int Med Spec* 1984;5:146–161.
8. Syed AMN, Puthawala A, Austin P, et al. Temporary iridium-192 implant in the management of carcinoma of the prostate. *Cancer* 1992;69:2515–2524.
9. Weaver JT, Loftus TP, Loevinger R. NBS measurement services: calibration of gamma-ray emitting brachytherapy sources. National Bureau of Standards (NIST) special publication no. 250–19. Gaithersburg, MD: National Bureau of Standards, 1988.
10. Loftus TP. Standardizing of 125-I seeds used for brachytherapy. *J Res Natl Bureau Stand* 1984;89:295–303.
11. Nath R, Anderson LL, Luxton G, et al. Dosimetry of interstitial brachytherapy sources: recommendations of the AAPM Radiation Therapy Committee Task Group No. 43. *Med Phys* 1995;22:209–234.
12. Syed AMN, Puthawala AA, Barth N, et al. High dose rate brachytherapy in the treatment of carcinoma of the prostate: preliminary results. *J Brachytherapy Int* 1997;13:315–331.

INTRAVASCULAR BRACHYTHERAPY

24.1. INTRODUCTION

Coronary artery disease is most commonly treated using bypass surgery or percutaneous transluminal coronary angioplasty (PTCA). A major problem with PTCA, however, is the high incidence of restenosis and recurrence of artery blockage at the site of treatment. Restenosis is usually arbitrarily defined as a narrowing of the lumen by 50% or greater in diameter compared to the adjacent normal appearing segments. Although the occurrence of restenosis is significantly reduced by the implantation of coronary stents, the restenosis rate following balloon angioplasty in randomized trials is 30% to 40% (1).

Most restenosis after angioplasty or stenting is caused by thrombosis or blood clotting at the PTCA site, which can be prevented partially by using anti-clotting drugs. However, another process, which begins within days after angioplasty, is the neointimal growth of tissues prompted by the wound healing process following tissue injury by angioplasty. This component of restenosis cannot be prevented by anticoagulants or stents.

Intraluminal irradiation of coronary and peripheral arteries together with balloon angioplasty and/or stent implantation significantly lowers the rate of neointimal formation, thereby reducing the rate of restenosis to well below 10% (2). Radiation kills cells and inhibits the growth of neointimal tissues in a manner similar to its effect on benign diseases such as keloids and heterotopic bone formation. Basic radiation biology and vascular pathology are discussed by several authors (3–5).

24.2. TREATMENT VOLUME

A. Arterial Anatomy

The arteries carry blood from the heart to various parts of the body. The main artery, the aorta, is the largest blood vessel (2 to 3 cm in diameter) and carries blood from the left ventricle of the heart to the branching arteries and capillaries in all the body organs and tissues, including the heart muscle. The coronary arteries are blood vessels lying on the outer surface of the heart and the peripheral arteries supply blood to other organs and tissues. The luminal diameter of arteries ranges from 3 to 5 mm initially and tapers slowly through their path length. Within this range, the peripheral arteries tend to be of larger diameter than the coronary arteries. The minimum normal artery diameter required for angioplasty and stenting is approximately 3 mm.

The inside of the arteries is lined with a layer of cells called endothelium. Next to the endothelium is the connective tissue layer, the intima, followed by layers of elastic membrane, smooth muscle cells, and elastic tissues. The outermost layer of the arteries is called adventitia, made up chiefly of collagenous fiber.

B. Angioplasty and Restenosis

The arteries can be partially blocked due to atherosclerosis or plaque formation. Reduction of their lumen diameter compromises the flow of blood and the delivery of oxygen to the body tissues. As an alternative to a major surgical procedure such as bypass surgery, balloon angioplasty is used to dilate the lumen diameter. This stretching action often ruptures the internal elastic lamina of the wall and causes fissures in the medial layers. The acute risk of angioplasty procedure is thrombosis that can be controlled by drugs, as mentioned previously. The more protracted risk, however, is that of restenosis by neointimal hyperplasia. This process involves growth of new tissues in the cracks and crevices of the arterial wall caused by angioplastic injury. Although implantation of stent angioplasty reduces the overall rate of restenosis by approximately 50%, it does not prevent neointimal growth and may, in fact, stimulate the process.

C. Target Volume

Target volume for vascular brachytherapy is confined to the region of angioplasty. Typically, it is 2 to 5 cm in length of artery and 0.5 to 2 mm in thickness of arterial wall. Occasionally, these dimensions may be exceeded depending on the location and extent of the disease. With 3 to 5 mm of luminal diameter, the radial range of treatment may extend as far as to about 5 mm from the center of the artery.

Because of the severity of inverse square fall-off of radiation at short distances, transluminal irradiation with intravascular brachytherapy produces highly conformal dose distribution, delivering a high dose to the arterial wall while sparing surrounding normal vessels or myocardium. Again, because of the predominance of inverse square law effect, penetrating power of radiation, depending on energy and modality, is not critically important, except with regard to dose rate or duration of implant and radiation protection of personnel involved with the procedure. Beta particle sources, in general, give higher dose rates and provide greater radiation protection compared to the gamma ray sources.

The depth of dose prescription for intracoronary irradiation is recommended by the American Association of Physicists in Medicine (AAPM) (6) to be 2 mm from the center of the source and for the peripheral arteries 2 mm beyond the average lumen radius. For each case, dose distribution in at least three planes perpendicular to the catheter and along its length should be determined. In addition, average, maximum, and minimum doses within the target volume should be reported (6).

24.3. IRRADIATION TECHNIQUES

Intravascular brachytherapy techniques may be classified into two categories: temporary implants (sealed sources or liquid-filled balloons) and permanent implants (radioactive stents). Each method has its advantages and limitations, but the catheter-based sealed source is the most commonly used method of treatment. It is the preferred method because of its better control of dose delivery. A variety of β and γ-ray sources have been used for endovascular therapy although the choice of one modality over the other is yet not clearly established. The pros and cons of a few sources and devices are discussed below.

A. Radiation Sources

Typical dosimetric requirements of a temporary intravascular implant are: (a) to deliver a target dose of 15 to 20 Gy to a 2- to 3-cm length of the arterial wall involved at a radial distance of about 2 mm from the source center; (b) to minimize the dose to tissues outside the region of angioplasty; and (c) to take as little a time as possible for completion of the procedure, that is, provide target dose rates on the order of 5 Gy/min or greater. These requirements suggest the suitability of high-energy β-sources such as strontium-90, yttrium-90, and phosphorus-32 or high activity γ-sources such as iridium-192. The latter could be a high dose rate (HDR) afterloading unit with the source dimensions small enough to allow intravascular brachytherapy.

The β-sources have several advantages over γ-sources: higher specific activity, higher dose rate, longer half-life, and greater radiation safety for the patient as well as personnel.

TABLE 24.1. POSSIBLE ISOTOPES FOR INTRALUMINAL BRACHYTHERAPY

Isotope	Emission	Maximum Energy (keV)	Average Energy (keV)	Half-Life	Activity Required
Ir-192	Gamma	612	375	74 d	1.0 Ci (37 GBq)
Iodine-125	X ray	35	28	60 d	3.8 Ci (140.6 GBq)
Palladium-103	X ray	21	21	19 d	3.9 Ci (144.3 GBq)
Phosphorus-32	Beta−	1,710	690	14 d	40.0 mCi (1,480 MBq)
Strontium/yttrium-90	Beta−	2,270	970	28 y	30.0 mCi (1,110 MBq)
Tungsten/rhenium-188	Beta−	2,130	780	69 d	35.0 mCi (1,295 MBq)
Vanadium-48	Beta+	690	230	16 d	1.0 μCi (37 Bq) stent

From Amols HI. Physics and dosimetry of intravascular brachytherapy. In: Thomadsen B, ed. *Categorical course in brachytherapy physics.* Oak Brook, IL: Radiological Society of North America, 1997, with permission.

The major disadvantage of β-sources, however, is the extremely rapid radial dose fall-off within the target region; γ-sources such as ^{192}Ir provide relatively more uniform target dose, governed primarily by the inverse square law fall-off with distance, but require high activity to yield reasonably high dose rate (≥ 5 Gy/min). Consequently, radiation protection problems with such sources become more significant. Although the HDR afterloaders using gamma sources could provide sufficiently high dose rate, they would require expensive shielding of the catheterization laboratories.

Table 24.1 contains a list of possible isotopes that have been or could be used for intravascular brachytherapy. The last column shows the activities required to obtain a dose rate of 5 Gy/min to a 2 cm length of a vessel at a radial distance of 2 mm from the source center. It is seen that the γ-sources, because of lower specific activity, require much higher activities than the β-sources for a catheter-based intravascular procedure. On the other hand, a permanent radioactive stent using ^{48}V requires only 1 μCi to produce the same dose rate.

Although dose rate per unit-activity favors β-emitters, radial dose distribution is better for the γ-sources, if it is assumed that the dose uniformity across the target volume is radiobiologically beneficial. This assumption has not been clinically validated but it seems logical, based on experience in conventional radiation therapy. Figure 24.1 compares radial dose distribution as a function of radial distance for some of the sources listed in Table 24.1. Nath and Liu (7) have studied radial dose function (g) for point sources of photons and electrons using Monte Carlo simulation. Their data show that from the point of view of adequate depth of penetration for intravascular brachytherapy, photon sources above 20 keV and electron sources above 1.0 MeV are acceptable.

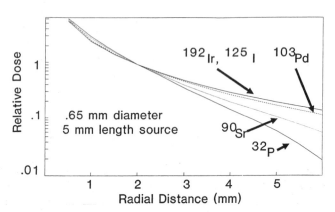

FIG. 24.1. Radial dose fall off with distance for a number of sources. Doses are normalized to 1.0 at a radial distance of 2.0 mm. (From Amols HI, Zaider M, Weinberger J, et al. Dosimetric considerations for catheter-based beta and gamma emitters in the therapy of neointimal hyperplasia in human coronary arteries. *Int J Radiat Oncol Biol Phys* 1996;36:913–921, with permission.)

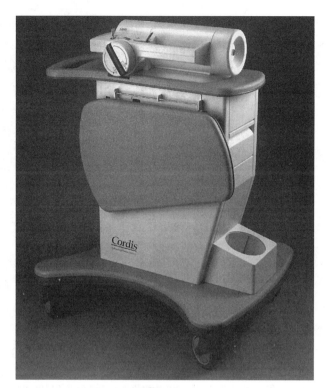

FIG. 24.2. The Cordis CHECKMATE system showing delivery device on a cart. (From Ali NM, Kaluza GL, Raizner AE. Catheter-based endovascular radiation therapy devices. *Vasc Radiother Monitor* 2000;2:72–81, with permission.)

B. Radiation Delivery Systems

Irradiation of blood vessels to prevent restenosis following angioplasty has been carried out using external beam as well as brachytherapy. Current trends favor catheter-based endovascular brachytherapy devices. While research continues to develop new sources and delivery techniques, a number of systems have become available commercially. Of these the U.S. Food and Drug Administration has approved only a few for clinical use. A brief review of some of the available devices is presented below. For more detailed product information and specifications, the reader is referred to the respective company literature.

B.1. Cordis CHECKMATE

The Cordis CHECKMATE System[1] consists of three components: (a) a nylon ribbon containing an array of ^{192}Ir seeds, (b) a delivery catheter, and (c) a ribbon delivery device. The Iridium seeds are 3 mm in length and 0.5 mm in diameter. The interseed spacing is 1mm and the outer diameter of the nylon ribbon containing the seeds is 1mm. The number of seeds in a ribbon can be altered to provide source lengths of 19 to 80 mm. Each ^{192}Ir seed has an activity of about 33 mCi, thus making it possible to keep the treatment time within 15 to 25 minutes. The ribbon delivery device is mounted on a cart (Fig. 24.2) and uses a hand-crank mechanism to advance the ribbon into a closed-end delivery catheter.

Although the ^{192}Ir source provides better dose homogeneity because of the lower depth-dose gradient (ratio of surface-to-adventitial dose), its higher activity and gamma ray energy raise radiation protection concerns for personnel. Longer irradiation times and non-centering of the delivery catheter are other disadvantages of this device.

---

[1] www.cordis.com.

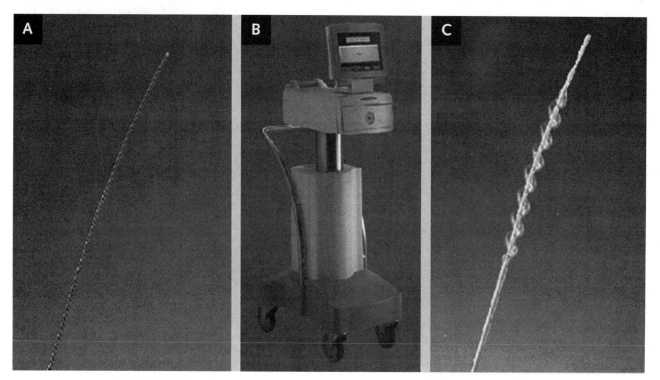

FIG. 24.3. Guidant GALILEO system: **(A)** source wire; **(B)** source delivery unit; and **(C)** spiral centering catheter. (From Ali NM, Kaluza GL, Raizner AE. Catheter-based endovascular radiation therapy devices. *Vasc Radiother Monitor* 2000;2:72–81, with permission.)

B.2. Guidant GALILEO

The Guidant GALILEO System[2] uses a β-source, ^{32}P, for intravascular brachytherapy. The ^{32}P source is hermetically sealed in the distal 27-mm tip of a flexible 0.018-inch nitinol wire. A spiral centering balloon catheter (Fig. 24.3), which centers the source wire, is flexible to navigate through the arteries and also has perfusion capabilities to limit myocardial ischemia during the procedure. The source delivery unit is an automatic afterloader device that can be controlled from a remote location to advance and retract the source wire. A treatment-planning system is provided to calculate dwell times required to deliver the prescribed dose.

The major advantages of the system are the centering capability of the delivery catheter, automation of the afterloader, and availability of the treatment-planning system. The disadvantage is the rapid dose fall-off radially, which is a characteristic of all the β-sources.

B.3. Novoste Beta-Cath

The Novoste Beta-Cath System[3] uses β-sources of ^{90}Sr/^{90}Y isotope. It is a manual afterloader device with a catheter-based delivery system. The system consists of two main components: (a) a transfer device for housing and hydraulic delivery of a radiation source train, and (b) a delivery catheter to transport the source train.

The delivery catheter (Fig. 24.4) has three lumens. The first lumen is used for travel of the guidewire. The second lumen is for transport of the source train consisting of sealed

---

[2] www.guidant.com.
[3] www.novoste.com.

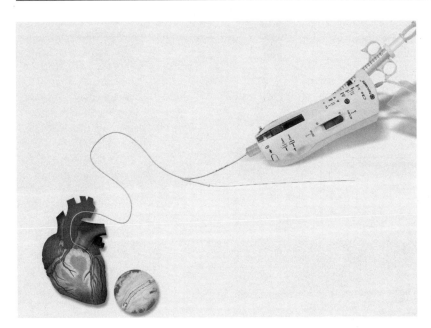

FIG. 24.4. Novoste Beta-Cath system with source train and transfer device. (Courtesy of Novoste: www.novoste.com.)

cylindrical seeds of ^{90}Sr/^{90}Y. The source train is delivered to the distal end of the delivery catheter by applying manual hydraulic pressure through a syringe, which contains sterile water and is attached to the transfer device. The third lumen, which is also attached to the transfer device, is designed to provide an opposite hydraulic pressure for returning the source train back into the storage position of the transfer device.

Major advantages of the Novoste system is its use of the ^{90}Sr/^{90}Y source, which is one of the highest energy β-emitters with a long half-life (28 years). Other advantages include high dose rate (treatment time approximately 5 minutes), patient and personnel safety, and simplicity of the handheld transfer device. The major disadvantage is the lack of a catheter-centering device, which could result in extreme dosimetric hot and cold spots within the target volume.

B.4. β-Emitting Liquid-filled Balloon

An alternative to catheter-based wires and seeds is to inflate the balloon dilation catheter with β-emitting radioactive liquid. The advantages of a liquid-filled balloon are inherent source centering and dose uniformity to the vessel wall. Several β-emitting isotopes such as ^{32}P, ^{90}Y, and ^{188}Re, which can be obtained in a liquid radiopharmaceutical preparation, may be used in this technique.

The major disadvantages of liquid-filled balloons include: (a) higher ratio of surface/adventitial dose compared to the catheter based γ-source systems; and (b) the possibility, although remote, of balloon rupture and consequently leakage of radioisotope within the patient. Of the radioisotopes mentioned previously, the rhenium-188 formulation is preferable because of the reduced radiation dose to organs such as colon and thyroid due to its rapid renal elimination in the event of balloon rupture. ^{188}Re also has a favorable maximum β-energy (2.13 MeV).

One of the liquid-filled balloon devices was developed at the Columbia University/Oak Ridge National Laboratory (8). The system uses a liquid preparation of ^{188}Re (^{188}Re-MAG$_3$), which is obtained at high specific activities from a tungsten (^{188}W) generator and delivered into a perfusion angiography balloon. A commercial system (RADIANT[4]) also

---

[4] Progresive Angioplasy Systems, Menlo Park, California.

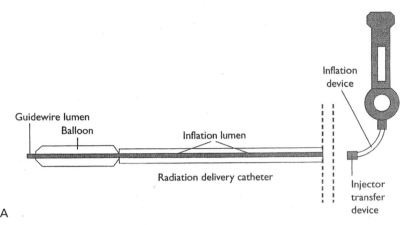

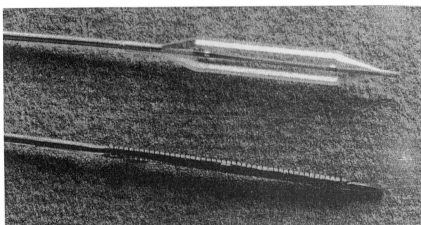

FIG. 24.5. (A) Schematic of RADIANT radiation delivery system; **(B)** PAS RADIANT isolated beta source balloon. *Top,* inflated balloon. *Bottom,* WRAP balloon protective sheath. (From Eigler N, Whiting JS, Makkar R, et al. Isolated liquid beta source balloon radiation delivery system (RADIANT). In: Waksman R, Serruys PW, eds. *Handbook of vascular brachytherapy.* London: Martin Dunitz Ltd, 1998:107–110, with permission.)

uses a ^{188}Re-filled balloon and is similar to conventional balloon PTCA (Fig. 24.5). It may be used before or after stent placement.

B.5. Radioactive Stents

Because permanent stents are frequently used in conjunction with balloon angioplasty, incorporation of radioactivity into the stent has been suggested to make it more effective in preventing restenosis (9–13). ^{32}P, ^{90}Y, and ^{48}V are some of the suitable β-emitting isotopes for impregnation into the stent. The stent is rendered radioactive by activation in a cyclotron or by ion implantation with the radioisotope.

The advantage of a radioactive stent is primarily the combining of two procedures, stenting and irradiation, into one. Proximity of the radioactive source with the vessel walls may be another advantage, although the gridded structure of the stent gives rise to greater dose inhomogeneity at the vessel surface than with a liquid-filled balloon or a catheter-based source. Figure 24.6 shows peaks and valleys of dose distribution for a 1.0-μCi ^{32}P Palmaz-Schatz stent.[5]

The implantation technique of a radioactive stent is the same as that required for a non-radioactive stent. Because of the very low activity (e.g., 0.5 to 5.0 μCi) of the β-radioisotope, the radioactive stent procedure is the safest from the radiation protection point of view. However, the dosimetry is much more complicated than that of the catheter-based systems, as will be discussed later.

---

[5] Isocent, Inc., Belmont, California.

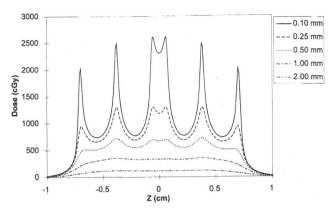

FIG. 24.6. Calculated dose distribution for a 1.0 μCi ^{32}P Palmaz-Schatz stent, 15 mm in length. Dose to tissue is that given in 14.3 days after implant. (From Janicki C, Duggan DM, Coffey CW, et al. Radiation dose from a phosphorus-32 impregnated wire mesh vascular stent. *Med Phys* 1997;24:437–445, with permission.)

24.4. DOSIMETRY

A. Dose Calculation Formalisms

A.1. Catheter-based Gamma Emitters

The AAPM TG-43 formalism (13) is generally applicable to the problem of dose calculation for catheter-based intravascular systems. For a system using photon-emitting sources, the dose D at a point (r, θ) is given by:

$$D(r, \theta) = S_k \Lambda [G(r, \theta)/ G(r_o, \theta_o)]g(r) F(r, \theta) \tag{24.1}$$

where S_k is the air kerma strength, Λ is the dose rate constant, G is the geometry factor, g is the radial dose function, F is the anistrophy factor, and (r_o, θ_o) are the polar coordinates of the reference point.

As discussed in Chapter 15, the reference distance r_o in conventional brachytherapy is 1 cm. For intravascular brachytherapy, the AAPM (6) recommends $r_o = 2$ mm. Equation (24.1) is therefore modified to incorporate this reference point specifically:

$$D(r, \theta) = S_k \Lambda_{r_o} [G(r, \theta)/ G(r_o, \theta_o)]g_{r_o}(r) F(r, \theta) \tag{24.2}$$

where Λ_{r_o} is the dose rate constant at a reference distance of r_o and g_{r_o} is the radial dose function normalized to the reference radial distance r_o.

Depending upon the source dimensions and the location of the point (r, θ), the source may be considered as a line source or a point source. In the case of the point source, Equation 24.2 can be written as an approximation:

$$D(r) \cong S_k \Lambda_{r_o} \frac{r_o^2}{r^2} g_{r_o}(r) \Phi_{\text{an}} \tag{24.3}$$

where Φ_{an} is the average anisotropy factor.

For a uniformly distributed line source, the geometry factor is given by:

$$G(r, \theta) = (\theta_2 - \theta_1)/ Lr \sin \theta \tag{24.4}$$

where L is the active length of the source.

A.2. Catheter-based Beta Emitters

Because the quantity air kerma strength does not apply to beta-emitting sources, the AAPM TG-60 report recommends the following equation for the calculation of dose at a point

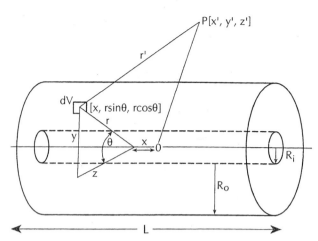

FIG. 24.7. Geometry of dose calculation at a point $P(x', y', z')$ from a balloon catheter with outer diameter R_o, inner diameter R_i and axial length L, uniformly filled with beta-emitting radioisotope. (From Amols HI, Reinstein LE, Weinberger J. Dosimetry of a radioactive coronary balloon dilution catheter for treatment of neointimal hyperplasia. *Med Phys* 1996;23:1783–1788, with permission.)

(r, θ) for the beta sources:

$$D(r, \theta) = D(r_o, \theta_o)[G(r, \theta)/(r_o, \theta_o)]g(r)F(r, \theta) \qquad (24.5)$$

where $D(r_o, \theta_o)$ is the dose rate in water at the reference point (r_o, θ_o). This quantity, $D(r_o, \theta_o)$ may be determined by calibration of the beta source at the reference point of $r_o = 2$ mm and $\theta_o = \pi/2$.

A.3. Radioactive Liquid-filled Balloons

Amols et al. (14) have calculated dose at a point $P(x', y', z')$ from a radioactive liquid-filled balloon (Fig. 24.7) by numeric integration of a Monte Carlo–generated beta dose kernel over the volume of the balloon:

$$D(P) = \int k(r') \cdot (A/V) \cdot dV \qquad (24.6)$$

where $D(P)$ is the dose rate (grays per second) at point P, $k(r)$ = dose kernel (grays per decay), $r'(\text{cm}) = [(x' - x)^2 + (y' - r\sin\theta)^2 + (z' - r\cos\theta)^2]^{1/2}$, A/V = activity per unit volume (becquerels/cm^3), and $dv = r.dr.d\theta.dx$. The integration limits are $-L/2 < x < L/2$, $R_i < r < R_o$ and $0 < \theta < 2\pi$. As seen in Fig. 24.7, the central channel of the catheter contains a lumen of radius R_i to allow passage of the guide wire.

Using a 3-mm diameter and 20-mm long balloon filled with ^{90}Y-chloride solution, Amols et al. (14) verified the calculated dose distribution by measurement with Gaf-Chromic film. The agreement between the measured and calculated radial dose distribution was ±6% at distances of 2.5 to 5.0 mm from the center of the catheter (or 1.0 to 3.5 mm from the surface of the balloon). They used the kernel for ^{90}Y, which had been calculated by Simpkin and Mackie (15).

The dose kernel is defined (15) as "the expectation value of the spatial distribution of the energy deposited in target volumes centered about a point radionuclide source per unit mass of the target volume per decay of the point source." Dose kernels for a number of beta emitters, ^{32}P, ^{67}Cu, ^{90}Y, ^{105}Rh, ^{131}I, ^{153}Sm, and ^{188}Re have been calculated using EGS4 Monte Carlo code (15). Some of these have potential use in intravascular brachytherapy with liquid-filled balloons.

A.4. Radioactive Stents

Dosimetric and radiobiologic characteristics of radioactive stents are complicated because of the gridded structure of the stent and the differences in dose rates delivered by stent versus an acute catheter-based irradiation. Dosimetric evaluation of clinical studies in animals by the AAPM task group (6) revealed "a confusing variety of different dose specifications in radioactive stent implantation." The analysis of a group of cases also showed that the dose delivered per unit-activity for the same radionuclide varied by almost a factor of four. Thus, the user must exercise caution in using stent activities and dosages specified in the clinical studies reported in the literature. The AAPM recommends (6) that "for each type of radioactive stent the three-dimensional dose distributions around stents of various lengths, diameters, and activities should be carefully determined by benchmark dosimetry studies before clinical implementation."

The dosimetric calculations of radioactive stents have been investigated by a number of investigators (16–19). A stent is modeled theoretically as a cylindrical shell of water, immersed in water, with the radioisotope (a β-emitter) uniformly distributed throughout the shell. The source is divided into infinitesimal elements of volume, each representing a point source. The dose distribution of a point source is represented by the dose-point-kernel function $K(\vec{r}, \vec{r}')$, which is defined as the dose at point $\vec{r}$ produced by a point source of unit activity located at $\vec{r}'$. The dose $D(\vec{r}, t)$ at a point $\vec{r}$ outside the stent, accumulated over a time t is calculated by convolution:

$$D(\vec{r}, t) = \int K(\vec{r}, \vec{r}')a(\vec{r}, t)d^3\vec{r}' \qquad (24.7)$$

where $a(\vec{r}, t)$ is the activity volume density. The dose point kernel is derived from Monte Carlo simulation of electron transport in water (15).

For mathematical details of the above or similar algorithms, the reader is referred to Prestwich et al. (16) and Janicki et al. (18).

B. Measurement of Dose Distribution

Dose distribution around intravascular brachytherapy sources is best measured by film dosimetry. Because of the high dose rate and steep dose gradients near the source, the film must have very thin emulsion, slow speed, and high resolution. Radiochromic films meet these requirements and are the detectors of choice for measuring dose distribution around brachytherapy sources in a contact geometry (see Chapter 8).

GafChromic film is tissue equivalent, has a linear sensitometric (optical density vs. dose) response and a large dynamic range (e.g., several grays to obtain an optical density between 0.5 and 2.5). The film does not require processing after irradiation.

In dosimetric measurements, the film is sandwiched in a water equivalent plastic phantom or wrapped around a cylindrical phantom, just like any film dosimetry arrangement. The exposed film is analyzed by a high resolution scanning densitometer (spatial resolution on the order of 0.1 mm). Optical density is converted to dose based on the predetermined sensitometric curve.

C. Calibration

C.1. Catheter-based Gamma Sources

The strength of the gamma-emitter sources is determined by measurement of exposure rate in free-space at 1m using a free-air ionization chamber or a well-type ionization chamber, which bears calibration traceable to the National Institute of Standards and Technology (NIST) for a source of the same type. The air kerma strength, S_k, at distance ℓ is given by:

$$S_k = \dot{x}_\ell(\overline{w}/e)\ell^2 \qquad (24.8)$$

where $\dot{x}_\ell$ is the exposure rate at distance ℓ, and $\overline{w}/e$ is the average energy absorbed per unit charge of ionization in air, assuming energy loss due to bremsstrahlung in air to be negligible (see section 15.2, A.5).

The calibration procedure of gamma-emitting seeds for conventional brachytherapy has been discussed in Chapters 15 and 23. In the case of intravascular sources, the AAPM (6) recommends that the dose rate in water at a distance of 2 mm from the center of the source must be specified. Equation 24.2 may be used to calculate dose rate at the reference point of (2 mm, $\pi/2$). However, at this point, the data for Λ_{ro} and g_{ro} are not available. Amols et al. (20) have used extrapolated values of the line source functions given by the AAPM TG-43 (13) to calculate dose distribution at distances less than 1 cm. For ^{192}Ir source (0.5 mm diameter, 3 mm length), they have compared calculated distributions with those measured with GafChromic film and shown an agreement of $\pm7\%$ at distances of 1.5 to 5.0 mm. Thus, until TG-43 functions are available at distances less than 0.5 cm, the user may use Amols et al.'s calculative or experimental methodology to determine the dose rate at the reference point of (2 mm, $\pi/2$).

C.2. Catheter-based Beta Sources

The strength of beta sources for intravascular brachytherapy is specified in terms of dose rate in water at the reference point (r_o, θ_o). Accordingly, the reference point for calibration of these sources should at $r_o = 2$ mm and $\theta_o = \pi/2$. Soares et al. (21) have described a method of calibrating beta sources using an extrapolation ionization chamber that has a 1-mm diameter collecting electrode (22). The absorbed dose rate at a depth close to 2 mm averaged over a 1-mm diameter area is determined from measurements in a A150 plastic phantom. The absorbed dose to A150 plastic is converted to absorbed dose to water using an appropriate scaling factor and density corrections (21).

C.3. Radioactive Stents

Calibration of a radioactive stent is complicated by the fact that stents are shipped under sterile conditions in acrylic cylinders of wall thickness sufficient to absorb all the beta particles. Activity measurements need therefore be made without disturbing the sterile environment. Although the beta particles are completely absorbed in the acrylic shield, bremsstrahlung x-rays escape. The intensity of these x-rays is proportional to the numbers of beta particles emitted, thus making it possible to infer activity of the radioactive stent by external measurement of bremsstrahlung. This method of assaying stent activity has been discussed by Larson and Mohrbacher (23) and Coffey and Duggan (24).

Relative calibration procedures based on bremsstrahlung measurements are available using a well-type ionization chamber, a NaI(Tr) scintillation counter, or a liquid scintillation counter. However, standards are needed to first calibrate the instrument. NIST offers a reference ^{32}P standard for activity analysis and hopefully more will be forthcoming for users to calibrate their instruments through transfer techniques. Relative calibrations require reference standards of the same radionuclide and construction. Large errors can result if one compares sources of different geometries for relative calibrations.

24.5. QUALITY ASSURANCE

A comprehensive quality assurance (QA) program should assure accurate and safe delivery of intravascular brachytherapy. In addition, it should be designed to satisfy the relevant regulations of the Nuclear Regulatory Commission (NRC) or state if it is designated as an Agreement State. Although several QA reports have been published on the use of conventional brachytherapy (25,26), the report most pertinent to intravascular brachytherapy is the AAPM TG-60 (6). Recommendations of this report are summarized below:

1. Document radiation source properties.
2. Develop protocols for receipt of sources, acceptance testing, and commissioning procedures.
3. Develop guidelines for storage, access, and inventory of sources.
4. Check physical integrity of sealed source; perform leak testing and other essential pretreatment QA procedures, depending on the source or device (e.g., remote afterloader).
5. Verify source activity using in-house equipment such as dose calibrator, re-entrant chamber, etc.
6. Develop methods to properly sterilize sources.
7. Develop protocol for safe transportation of radioactive material.
8. Develop protocol for safe disposal of sources after use.
9. Assure availability of ancillary equipment at the time of the procedure.
10. Develop emergency procedures.
11. Develop roles and responsibilities of each individual involved with the procedure.
12. Develop a prescription form (written directive).
13. Develop dose calculation check/double check procedures.
14. Verify correct choice of sources and treatment parameters for the patient in question.
15. Monitor radiation levels around patient and surrounding areas during treatment.
16. Perform post-treatment radiation survey of the patient and surrounding areas.
17. Provide radiation safety instructions to patients with permanent implants (e.g., radioactive stent) at the time of patient discharge.
18. Develop education and training program for personnel.

REFERENCES

1. Fisherman DL, Leon MB, Bain DS. A randomized comparison of stent placement and balloon angioplasty in the treatment of coronary artery disease. *N Engl J Med* 1994;331:496–501.
2. Waksman R. Radiation for prevention of restenosis: where are we? *Int J Radiat Oncol Biol Phys* 1996;36:959–961.
3. Hall EJ, Miller RC, Brenner DJ. The basic radiobiology of intravascular irradiation. In: Waksman R, ed. *Vascular brachytherapy.* Armonk, NY: Futura, 1999.
4. Fajardo LF, Berthrong M. Vascular lesions following radiation. *Pathol Annu* 1988;23:297–330.
5. Reinhold HS, Fajardo LF, Hopewell JW. The vascular system. In: Altman KI, Lett JT, eds. *Advances in radiation biology,* Vol 14. Relative radiation sensitivities of human organ systems, Part II. San Diego: Academic Press, 1990:177–226.
6. Nath R, Amols H, Coffey C, et al. Intravascular brachytherapy physics: report of the AAPM Radiation Therapy Committee Task Group No. 60. *Med Phys* 1999;26:119–152.
7. Nath R, Lui L. On the depth of penetration of photons and electrons for intravascular brachytherapy. *Med Phys* 1997;24:1358(abst.).
8. Weinburger J, Schiff PB, Trichter F, et al. Results of the Columbia Safety and Feasibility (CURE) trial of liquid isotopes for coronary vascular brachytherapy. *Circulation* 1999;100[suppl 1]:1–75.
9. Fischell TA, Kharma BK, Fischell DR, et al. Low-dose beta particle emission from 'stent' wire results in complete, localized inhibition of smooth muscle cell proliferation. *Circulation* 1994;90:2956–2963.
10. Laird JR, Carter AJ, Kuffs WM, et al. Inhibition of neointimal proliferation with a beta particle emitting stent. *Circulation* 1996;93:529–536.
11. Hehrleim C, Stintz M, Kinscherf R, et al. Pure β-particle emitting stents inhibit neointimal formation in rabbits. *Circulation* 1996;93:641–645.
12. Carter AJ, Laird JR. Experimental results with endovascular irradiation via a radioactive stent. *Int J Radiat Oncol Biol Phys* 1996;36:797–803.
13. Nath R, Anderson L, Luxton G, et al. Dosimetry of interstitial brachytherapy sources: recommendations of the AAPM Radiation Therapy Task Group No. 43. *Med Phys* 1995;22:209–234.
14. Amols HI, Reinstein LE, Weinberger J. Dosimetry of a radioactive coronary balloon dilution catheter for treatment of neointimal hyperplasia. *Med Phys* 1996;23:1783–1788.
15. Simpkin DJ, Mackie TR. EGS4 Monte Carlo determination of the beta dose kernel in water. *Med Phys* 1990;17:179–186.
16. Prestwich WV, Kennet TJ, Kus FW. The dose distribution produced by a ^{32}P-coated stent. *Med Phys* 1995;22:313–320.
17. Prestwich WV. Analytic representation of the dose from a ^{32}P-coated stent. *Med Phys* 1996;23:9–13.
18. Janicki C, Duggan DM, Coffey CW, et al. Radiation dose from a ^{32}P impregnated Palmaz-Schatz wire mesh vascular stent. *Med Phys* 1997;24:437–445.

19. Duggan DM, Coffey CW, Levit S. Dose distribution for a ^{32}P impregnated coronary stent: comparison of theoretical calculations and measurements with radiochromic film. *Int J Radiat Oncol Biol Phys* 1998;40:713–720.

20. Amols HI, Zaider M, Weinberger J, et al. Dosimetric considerations for catheter-based beta and gamma emitters in the therapy of neointimal hyperplasia in human coronary arteries. *Int J Radiat Oncol Biol Phys* 1996;36:913–921.

21. Soares CG, Halpern DG, Wang CK. Calibration and characterization of beta-particle sources for intravascular brachytherapy. *Med Phys* 1998;25:339–346.

22. Soares CG. Calibration of ophthalmic applicators at NIST—a revised approach. *Med Phys* 1991;18:787–193.

23. Larson IL, Mohrbacher DA. Analysis of P-32 labeled solutions using integrated bremsstrahlung radiation. *Radioact Radiochem* 1992;3:4–7.

24. Coffey C, Duggan D. Dosimetric consideration and dose measurement analysis of a P-32 radioisotope stent. In: Waksman R, King S, Crocker IA, et al., eds. *Vascular brachytherapy.* The Netherlands: Nucletron, 1996:207–216.

25. Kutcher GJ, Coia J, Gillin M, et al. Comprehensive QA for radiation oncology: report of AAPM Radiation Therapy Committee Task Group No. 40. *Med Phys* 1994;21:581–618.

26. Nath R, Anderson LL, Meli JA, et al. Code of practice for brachytherapy physics: AAPM Radiation Therapy Committee Task Group No. 56. *Med Phys* 1997;24:1557–1598.

APPENDIX

TABLE A.1. RATIOS OF AVERAGE, RESTRICTED STOPPING POWERS FOR PHOTON BEAMS, $\Delta = 10$ keV

Nominal Accelerating Potential (MV)	$(\overline{L}/\rho)^{med}_{air}$							
	Water	Polystyrene	Acrylic	Graphite	A-150	C-552	Bakelite	Nylon
2	1.135	1.114	1.104	1.015	1.154	1.003	1.084	1.146
^{60}Co	1.134	1.113	1.103	1.012	1.151	1.000	1.081	1.142
4	1.131	1.108	1.099	1.007	1.146	0.996	1.075	1.136
6	1.127	1.103	1.093	1.002	1.141	0.992	1.070	1.129
8	1.121	1.097	1.088	0.995	1.135	0.987	1.063	1.120
10	1.117	1.094	1.085	0.992	1.130	0.983	1.060	1.114
15	1.106	1.083	1.074	0.982	1.119	0.972	1.051	1.097
20	1.096	1.074	1.065	0.977	1.109	0.963	1.042	1.087
25	1.093	1.071	1.062	0.968	1.106	0.960	1.038	1.084
35	1.084	1.062	1.053	0.958	1.098	0.952	1.027	1.074
45	1.071	1.048	1.041	0.939	1.087	0.942	1.006	1.061

Data from Cunningham JR, Schulz RJ. Published in Task Group 21, Radiation Therapy Committee, American Association of Physicists in Medicine. A protocol for the determination of absorbed dose from high energy photon and electron beams. *Med Phys* 1983;10:741, with permission.

TABLE A.2. RATIOS OF MASS STOPPING POWERS AND MASS ENERGY ABSORPTION COEFFICIENTS FOR COBALT-60 γ RAYS[a]

Chamber Wall or Build-up Cap	$(\overline{L}/\rho)^{wall}_{air}$ ($\Delta = 10$ keV)	$(\overline{\mu}_{en}/\rho)^{air}_{wall}$
Polystyrene	1.112	0.928
Acrylic	1.103	0.925
Graphite	1.010	0.999
Water	1.133	0.899
A-150	1.145	0.906
Nylon	1.141	0.910
C-552	1.000	1.000
Bakelite	1.080	0.945

[a]These data apply to ion chambers exposed in air.
From Johns HE, Cunningham JR. *The physics of radiology*. 4th ed. Springfield, IL: Charles C Thomas, 1983, with permission.

TABLE A.3. STOPPING POWER RATIOS, $\left(\dfrac{\bar{L}}{\rho}\right)_{air}^{water}$, FOR ELECTRON BEAMS ($\Delta = 10$ keV)

Depth (g/cm²)	Electron Beam Energy (MeV)																			
	60.0	50.0	40.0	30.0	25.0	20.0	18.0	16.0	14.0	12.0	10.0	9.0	8.0	7.0	6.0	5.0	4.0	3.0	2.0	1.0
0.0	0.902	0.904	0.912	0.928	0.940	0.955	0.961	0.969	0.977	0.986	0.997	1.003	1.011	1.019	1.029	1.040	1.059	1.078	1.097	1.116
0.1	0.902	0.905	0.913	0.929	0.941	0.955	0.962	0.969	0.978	0.987	0.998	1.005	1.012	1.020	1.030	1.042	1.061	1.081	1.101	1.124
0.2	0.903	0.906	0.914	0.930	0.942	0.956	0.963	0.970	0.978	0.988	0.999	1.006	1.013	1.022	1.032	1.044	1.064	1.084	1.106	1.131
0.3	0.904	0.907	0.915	0.931	0.943	0.957	0.964	0.971	0.979	0.989	1.000	1.007	1.015	1.024	1.034	1.046	1.067	1.089	1.112	1.135
0.4	0.904	0.908	0.916	0.932	0.944	0.958	0.965	0.972	0.980	0.990	1.002	1.009	1.017	1.026	1.036	1.050	1.071	1.093	1.117	1.136
0.5	0.905	0.909	0.917	0.933	0.945	0.959	0.966	0.973	0.982	0.991	1.003	1.010	1.019	1.028	1.039	1.054	1.076	1.098	1.122	
0.6	0.906	0.909	0.918	0.934	0.946	0.960	0.967	0.974	0.983	0.993	1.005	1.012	1.021	1.031	1.043	1.058	1.080	1.103	1.126	
0.8	0.907	0.911	0.920	0.936	0.948	0.962	0.969	0.976	0.985	0.996	1.009	1.016	1.026	1.037	1.050	1.067	1.090	1.113	1.133	
1.0	0.908	0.913	0.922	0.938	0.950	0.964	0.971	0.979	0.988	0.999	1.013	1.021	1.031	1.043	1.058	1.076	1.099	1.121		
1.2	0.909	0.914	0.924	0.940	0.952	0.966	0.973	0.981	0.991	1.002	1.017	1.026	1.037	1.050	1.066	1.085	1.108	1.129		
1.4	0.910	0.916	0.925	0.942	0.954	0.968	0.976	0.984	0.994	1.006	1.022	1.032	1.044	1.058	1.075	1.095	1.117	1.133		
1.6	0.912	0.917	0.927	0.944	0.956	0.971	0.978	0.987	0.997	1.010	1.027	1.038	1.050	1.066	1.084	1.104	1.124			
1.8	0.913	0.918	0.929	0.945	0.957	0.973	0.981	0.990	1.001	1.014	1.032	1.044	1.057	1.074	1.093	1.112	1.130			
2.0	0.914	0.920	0.930	0.947	0.959	0.975	0.983	0.993	1.004	1.018	1.038	1.050	1.065	1.082	1.101	1.120	1.133			
2.5	0.917	0.923	0.934	0.952	0.964	0.981	0.990	1.000	1.013	1.030	1.053	1.067	1.083	1.102	1.120	1.131				
3.0	0.919	0.926	0.938	0.956	0.969	0.987	0.997	1.008	1.023	1.042	1.069	1.084	1.102	1.119	1.129					
3.5	0.922	0.929	0.941	0.960	0.974	0.994	1.004	1.017	1.034	1.056	1.085	1.102	1.118	1.128						
4.0	0.924	0.932	0.944	0.964	0.979	1.001	1.012	1.027	1.046	1.071	1.101	1.116	1.126							
4.5	0.927	0.935	0.948	0.969	0.985	1.008	1.021	1.037	1.059	1.086	1.115	1.125	1.127							
5.0	0.929	0.938	0.951	0.973	0.990	1.016	1.030	1.049	1.072	1.101	1.123	1.126								
5.5	0.931	0.940	0.954	0.978	0.996	1.024	1.040	1.061	1.086	1.113	1.125									
6.0	0.934	0.943	0.958	0.983	1.002	1.033	1.051	1.074	1.100	1.121										
7.0	0.938	0.948	0.965	0.993	1.017	1.054	1.075	1.099	1.118	1.122										
8.0	0.943	0.954	0.972	1.005	1.032	1.076	1.098	1.116	1.120											
9.0	0.947	0.960	0.981	1.018	1.049	1.098	1.114	1.118												
10.0	0.952	0.966	0.990	1.032	1.068	1.112	1.116													
12.0	0.962	0.980	1.009	1.062	1.103															
14.0	0.973	0.996	1.031	1.095	1.107															
16.0	0.986	1.013	1.056	1.103																
18.0	1.000	1.031	1.080																	
20.0	1.016	1.051	1.094																	
22.0	1.032	1.070																		
24.0	1.048	1.082																		
26.0	1.062	1.085																		
28.0	1.071																			
30.0	1.075																			

Based on data by Berger M. Published in Task Group 21, Radiation Therapy Committee, American Association of Physicists in Medicine. A protocol for the determination of absorbed dose from high energy photon and electron beams. *Med Phys* 1983;10:741.

TABLE A.4. STOPPING POWER RATIOS, $\left(\dfrac{\bar{L}}{\rho}\right)_{air}^{polystyrene}$, FOR ELECTRON BEAMS ($\Delta$ = 10 keV)

Depth (g/cm²)	60.0	50.0	40.0	30.0	25.0	20.0	18.0	16.0	14.0	12.0	10.0	9.0	8.0	7.0	6.0	5.0	4.0	3.0	2.0	1.0
															Electron Beam Energy (MeV)					
0.0	0.875	0.878	0.887	0.903	0.915	0.929	0.936	0.943	0.950	0.959	0.970	0.975	0.982	0.990	0.999	1.010	1.030	1.049	1.069	1.089
0.1	0.876	0.879	0.888	0.904	0.916	0.930	0.936	0.943	0.951	0.960	0.970	0.977	0.983	0.991	1.000	1.011	1.032	1.052	1.074	1.100
0.2	0.876	0.880	0.889	0.905	0.917	0.931	0.937	0.944	0.952	0.961	0.972	0.978	0.985	0.993	1.002	1.013	1.034	1.056	1.080	1.109
0.3	0.877	0.881	0.890	0.906	0.917	0.931	0.938	0.945	0.953	0.962	0.973	0.979	0.986	0.994	1.004	1.016	1.038	1.061	1.086	1.114
0.4	0.878	0.882	0.891	0.907	0.918	0.932	0.939	0.946	0.954	0.963	0.974	0.980	0.988	0.996	1.007	1.019	1.042	1.066	1.092	1.116
0.5	0.878	0.883	0.892	0.908	0.919	0.933	0.940	0.947	0.955	0.964	0.975	0.982	0.990	0.999	1.009	1.023	1.046	1.071	1.098	
0.6	0.879	0.883	0.893	0.909	0.920	0.934	0.941	0.948	0.956	0.965	0.977	0.984	0.992	1.001	1.012	1.027	1.051	1.076	1.103	
0.8	0.881	0.885	0.894	0.911	0.922	0.936	0.943	0.950	0.959	0.968	0.980	0.983	0.996	1.006	1.019	1.035	1.060	1.087	1.111	
1.0	0.882	0.887	0.896	0.912	0.924	0.938	0.945	0.952	0.961	0.971	0.984	0.992	1.001	1.012	1.026	1.044	1.070	1.096		
1.2	0.883	0.888	0.898	0.914	0.926	0.940	0.947	0.955	0.963	0.974	0.988	0.996	1.006	1.019	1.034	1.054	1.080	1.105		
1.4	0.884	0.889	0.900	0.916	0.927	0.942	0.949	0.957	0.966	0.978	0.992	1.001	1.012	1.026	1.043	1.064	1.089	1.111		
1.6	0.886	0.891	0.901	0.918	0.929	0.944	0.951	0.959	0.969	0.981	0.997	1.007	1.019	1.033	1.052	1.073	1.098			
1.8	0.887	0.892	0.903	0.919	0.931	0.946	0.954	0.962	0.972	0.985	1.002	1.012	1.025	1.041	1.060	1.083	1.106			
2.0	0.888	0.894	0.904	0.921	0.933	0.948	0.956	0.965	0.975	0.989	1.007	1.018	1.032	1.049	1.069	1.092	1.110			
2.5	0.891	0.897	0.908	0.925	0.937	0.954	0.962	0.972	0.984	0.999	1.020	1.034	1.050	1.070	1.091	1.108				
3.0	0.893	0.900	0.911	0.929	0.942	0.959	0.969	0.979	0.992	1.010	1.035	1.051	1.069	1.090	1.105					
3.5	0.896	0.903	0.914	0.933	0.947	0.965	0.975	0.987	1.002	1.023	1.051	1.069	1.088	1.103						
4.0	0.898	0.905	0.917	0.937	0.951	0.971	0.982	0.995	1.013	1.036	1.068	1.086	1.101							
4.5	0.900	0.908	0.920	0.941	0.956	0.978	0.990	1.005	1.024	1.051	1.085	1.099	1.105							
5.0	0.902	0.910	0.923	0.945	0.961	0.985	0.998	1.015	1.037	1.067	1.097	1.103								
5.5	0.904	0.913	0.927	0.949	0.966	0.992	1.008	1.026	1.051	1.081	1.102									
6.0	0.906	0.915	0.930	0.954	0.972	1.000	1.017	1.038	1.065	1.093										
7.0	0.910	0.920	0.936	0.963	0.984	1.018	1.040	1.063	1.089	1.100										
8.0	0.914	0.925	0.943	0.973	0.998	1.039	1.063	1.086	1.098											
9.0	0.918	0.930	0.950	0.985	1.013	1.061	1.084	1.095												
10.0	0.922	0.936	0.958	0.997	1.030	1.081	1.093													
12.0	0.931	0.949	0.976	1.024	1.067															
14.0	0.942	0.963	0.995	1.056	1.085															
16.0	0.953	0.978	1.016	1.078																
18.0	0.966	0.994	1.041																	
20.0	0.979	1.011	1.061																	
22.0	0.994	1.030																		
24.0	1.008	1.047																		
26.0	1.023	1.057																		
28.0	1.036																			
30.0	1.045																			

Based on data by Berger M. Published in Task Group 21, Radiation Therapy Committee, American Association of Physicists in Medicine. A protocol for the determination of absorbed dose from high energy photon and electron beams. Med Phys 1983;10:741.

TABLE A.5. STOPPING POWER RATIOS, $\left(\dfrac{\overline{L}}{\rho}\right)_{air}^{acrylic}$ **, FOR ELECTRON BEAMS** ($\Delta = 10$ keV)

Depth (g/cm²)	Electron Beam Energy (MeV)																			
	60.0	50.0	40.0	30.0	25.0	20.0	18.0	16.0	14.0	12.0	10.0	9.0	8.0	7.0	6.0	5.0	4.0	3.0	2.0	1.0
0.0	0.870	0.874	0.882	0.898	0.909	0.923	0.929	0.936	0.944	0.953	0.963	0.969	0.975	0.983	0.992	1.003	1.023	1.043	1.063	1.083
0.1	0.871	0.875	0.883	0.899	0.910	0.924	0.930	0.937	0.945	0.953	0.964	0.970	0.976	0.984	0.993	1.005	1.025	1.046	1.068	1.093
0.2	0.872	0.876	0.884	0.900	0.911	0.925	0.931	0.938	0.945	0.954	0.965	0.971	0.978	0.986	0.995	1.007	1.028	1.050	1.073	1.101
0.3	0.872	0.877	0.886	0.902	0.912	0.925	0.932	0.939	0.946	0.955	0.966	0.972	0.979	0.988	0.997	1.010	1.031	1.054	1.079	1.106
0.4	0.873	0.878	0.887	0.902	0.913	0.926	0.933	0.939	0.947	0.956	0.967	0.974	0.981	0.990	1.000	1.013	1.035	1.059	1.085	1.107
0.5	0.874	0.879	0.888	0.903	0.914	0.927	0.933	0.940	0.948	0.958	0.969	0.975	0.983	0.992	1.003	1.016	1.040	1.064	1.091	
0.6	0.875	0.880	0.889	0.905	0.915	0.928	0.934	0.941	0.949	0.959	0.970	0.977	0.985	0.994	1.006	1.020	1.044	1.069	1.095	
0.8	0.876	0.882	0.891	0.907	0.916	0.930	0.936	0.944	0.952	0.962	0.974	0.981	0.989	1.000	1.012	1.029	1.054	1.080	1.103	
1.0	0.877	0.883	0.893	0.909	0.918	0.932	0.938	0.946	0.954	0.964	0.977	0.985	0.994	1.006	1.020	1.038	1.064	1.089		
1.2	0.878	0.885	0.894	0.910	0.920	0.934	0.940	0.948	0.957	0.968	0.981	0.990	1.000	1.012	1.028	1.048	1.073	1.097		
1.4	0.880	0.886	0.896	0.912	0.922	0.936	0.943	0.951	0.960	0.971	0.986	0.995	1.006	1.020	1.037	1.057	1.083	1.103		
1.6	0.881	0.887	0.897	0.914	0.924	0.938	0.945	0.953	0.963	0.975	0.990	1.000	1.012	1.027	1.045	1.067	1.091			
1.8	0.882	0.889	0.899	0.915	0.926	0.940	0.947	0.956	0.966	0.978	0.995	1.006	1.019	1.035	1.054	1.076	1.098			
2.0	0.883	0.892	0.902	0.919	0.927	0.942	0.950	0.958	0.969	0.982	1.000	1.012	1.026	1.043	1.063	1.085	1.103			
2.5	0.886	0.895	0.906	0.923	0.932	0.948	0.956	0.965	0.977	0.992	1.014	1.028	1.044	1.063	1.085	1.101				
3.0	0.888	0.898	0.909	0.927	0.937	0.953	0.962	0.973	0.986	1.004	1.029	1.045	1.063	1.083	1.098					
3.5	0.891	0.900	0.912	0.931	0.941	0.959	0.968	0.980	0.996	1.016	1.045	1.063	1.082	1.096						
4.0	0.893	0.903	0.915	0.935	0.946	0.965	0.975	0.989	1.006	1.030	1.062	1.080	1.094							
4.5	0.895	0.905	0.918	0.939	0.951	0.971	0.983	0.998	1.018	1.045	1.079	1.092	1.097							
5.0	0.897	0.908	0.921	0.943	0.956	0.978	0.991	1.008	1.031	1.061	1.090	1.096								
5.5	0.900	0.910	0.924	0.947	0.962	0.986	1.000	1.020	1.045	1.075	1.095									
6.0	0.902	0.915	0.930	0.951	0.968	0.994	1.010	1.032	1.059	1.086										
7.0	0.905	0.920	0.937	0.957	0.981	1.012	1.033	1.058	1.083	1.092										
8.0	0.909	0.925	0.945	0.967	0.995	1.033	1.056	1.080	1.090											
9.0	0.913	0.931	0.953	0.979	1.011	1.055	1.077	1.088												
10.0	0.917	0.943	0.970	0.991	1.029	1.075	1.086													
12.0	0.926	0.957	0.989	1.018	1.067															
14.0	0.937	0.973	1.011	1.051	1.076															
16.0	0.948	0.989	1.036	1.071																
18.0	0.961	1.006	1.055																	
20.0	0.974	1.025																		
22.0	0.989	1.042																		
24.0	1.004	1.050																		
26.0	1.019																			
28.0	1.031																			
30.0	1.039																			

Based on data by Berger M. Published in Task Group 21, Radiation Therapy Committee, American Association of Physicists in Medicine. A protocol for the determination of absorbed dose from high energy photon and electron beams. Med Phys 1983;10:741.

TABLE A.6. RATIOS OF MEAN MASS-ENERGY ABSORPTION COEFFICIENTS, $\left(\dfrac{\overline{\mu}_{en}}{\rho}\right)_{air}^{med}$ FOR VARIOUS MATERIALS

Nominal Accelerating Potential (MV)	$(\overline{\mu}_{en}/\rho)_{air}^{med}$							
	Water	Polystyrene	Acrylic	Graphite	A-150	C-552	Bakelite	Nylon
2	1.111	1.072	1.078	0.992	1.100	1.000	1.051	1.090
^{60}Co-6	1.111	1.072	1.078	0.997	1.099	1.000	1.055	1.092
8	1.109	1.068	1.075	0.997	1.092	0.998	1.052	1.090
10	1.108	1.066	1.072	0.995	1.089	0.997	1.049	1.087
15	1.105	1.053	1.063	0.986	1.078	0.995	1.039	1.075
20	1.094	1.038	1.051	0.975	1.065	0.992	1.027	1.061
25	1.092	1.032	1.047	0.971	1.060	0.991	1.022	1.055
35	1.085	1.016	1.034	0.960	1.044	0.989	1.009	1.039
45	1.074	0.980	1.009	0.937	1.010	0.983	0982	1.000

The data are applicable to ionization measurements made in phantom.
From Johns HE, Cunning JR. *The physics of radiology,* 4th ed. Springfield, IL: Charles C Thomas, 1983; table published in Task Group 21, Radiation Therapy Committee, American Association of Physicists in Medicine. A protocol for the determination of absorbed dose from high energy photon and electron beams. *Med Phys* 1983;10:741, with permission.

TABLE A.7. PHOTON MASS ATTENUATION COEFFICIENTS, μ/ρ, AND MASS ENERGY-ABSORPTION COEFFICIENTS μ_{en}/ρ, IN m²/kg FOR ENERGIES 1 keV TO 20 MeV (MULTIPLY m²/kg BY 10 TO CONVERT TO cm²/g).

Photon Energy (eV)	Air, Dry $\overline{Z} = 7.78$ $\rho = 1.205$ kg/m³ (20°C) 3.006×10^{26} e/kg		Water $\overline{Z} = 7.51$ $\rho = 1000$ kg/m³ 3.343×10^{26} e/kg		Muscle $\overline{Z} = 7.64$ $\rho = 1040$ kg/m³ 3.312×10^{26} e/kg	
	μ/ρ	μ_{en}/ρ	μ/ρ	μ_{en}/ρ	μ/ρ	μ_{en}/ρ
1.0 + 03	3.617 + 02	3.616 + 02	4.091 + 02	4.089 + 02	3.774 + 02	3.772 + 02
1.5 + 03	1.202 + 02	1.201 + 02	1.390 + 02	1.388 + 02	1.275 + 02	1.273 + 02
2.0 + 03	5.303 + 01	5.291 + 01	6.187 + 01	6.175 + 01	5.663 + 01	5.651 + 01
3.0 + 03	1.617 + 01	1.608 + 01	1.913 + 01	1.903 + 01	1.828 + 01	1.813 + 01
4.0 + 03	7.751 + 00	7.597 + 00	8.174 + 00	8.094 + 00	8.085 + 00	7.963 + 00
5.0 + 03	3.994 + 00	3.896 + 00	4.196 + 00	4.129 + 00	4.174 + 00	4.090 + 00
6.0 + 03	2.312 + 00	2.242 + 00	2.421 + 00	2.363 + 00	2.421 + 00	2.354 + 00
8.0 + 03	9.721 − 01	9.246 − 01	1.018 + 00	9.726 − 01	1.024 + 00	9.770 − 01
1.0 + 04	5.016 − 01	4.640 − 01	5.223 − 01	4.840 − 01	5.284 − 01	4.895 − 01
1.5 + 04	1.581 − 01	1.300 − 01	1.639 − 01	1.340 − 01	1.668 − 01	1.371 − 01
2.0 + 04	7.643 − 02	5.255 − 02	7.958 − 02	5.367 − 02	8.099 − 02	5.531 − 02
3.0 + 04	3.501 − 02	1.501 − 02	3.718 − 02	1.520 − 02	3.754 − 02	1.579 − 02
4.0 + 04	2.471 − 02	6.694 − 02	2.668 − 02	6.803 − 03	2.674 − 02	7.067 − 03
5.0 + 04	2.073 − 02	4.031 − 03	2.262 − 02	4.155 − 03	2.257 − 02	4.288 − 03
6.0 + 04	1.871 − 02	3.004 − 03	2.055 − 02	3.152 − 03	2.045 − 02	3.224 − 03
8.0 + 04	1.661 − 02	2.393 − 03	1.835 − 02	2.583 − 03	1.822 − 02	2.601 − 03
1.0 + 05	1.541 − 02	2.318 − 03	1.707 − 02	2.539 − 03	1.693 − 02	2.538 − 03
1.5 + 05	1.356 − 02	2.494 − 03	1.504 − 02	2.762 − 03	1.491 − 02	2.743 − 03
2.0 + 05	1.234 − 02	2.672 − 03	1.370 − 02	2.966 − 03	1.358 − 02	2.942 − 03
3.0 + 05	1.068 − 02	2.872 − 03	1.187 − 02	3.192 − 03	1.176 − 02	3.164 − 03
4.0 + 05	9.548 − 03	2.949 − 03	1.061 − 02	3.279 − 03	1.052 − 02	3.250 − 03
5.0 + 05	8.712 − 03	2.966 − 03	9.687 − 03	3.299 − 03	9.599 − 03	3.269 − 03
6.0 + 05	8.056 − 03	2.953 − 03	8.957 − 03	3.284 − 03	8.876 − 03	3.254 − 03
8.0 + 05	7.075 − 03	2.882 − 03	7.866 − 03	3.205 − 03	7.795 − 03	3.176 − 03
1.0 + 06	6.359 − 03	2.787 − 03	7.070 − 03	3.100 − 03	7.006 − 03	3.072 − 03
1.5 + 06	5.176 − 03	2.545 − 03	5.755 − 03	2.831 − 03	5.702 − 03	2.805 − 03
2.0 + 06	4.447 − 03	2.342 − 03	4.940 − 03	2.604 − 03	4.895 − 03	2.580 − 03
3.0 + 06	3.581 − 03	2.054 − 03	3.969 − 03	2.278 − 03	3.932 − 03	2.257 − 03
4.0 + 06	3.079 − 03	1.866 − 03	3.403 − 03	2.063 − 03	3.370 − 03	2.043 − 03
5.0 + 06	2.751 − 03	1.737 − 03	3.031 − 03	1.913 − 03	3.001 − 03	1.894 − 03
6.0 + 06	2.523 − 03	1.644 − 03	2.771 − 03	1.804 − 03	2.743 − 03	1.785 − 03
8.0 + 06	2.225 − 03	1.521 − 03	2.429 − 03	1.657 − 03	2.403 − 03	1.639 − 03
1.0 + 07	2.045 − 03	1.446 − 03	2.219 − 03	1.566 − 03	2.195 − 03	1.548 − 03
1.5 + 07	1.810 − 03	1.349 − 03	1.941 − 03	1.442 − 03	1.918 − 03	1.424 − 03
2.0 + 07	1.705 − 03	1.308 − 03	1.813 − 03	1.386 − 03	1.790 − 03	1.367 − 03

TABLE A.7. (*continued*)

Photon Energy (eV)	Fat $\overline{Z} = 6.46$ $\rho = 920$ kg/m^3 3.34×10^{26} e/kg		Bone $\overline{Z} = 12.31$ $\rho = 1850$ kg/m^3 3.192×10^{26} e/kg		Polystyrene (C$_8$H$_8$) $\overline{Z} = 5.74$ $\rho = 1046$ kg/m^3 3.238×10^{26} e/kg	
	μ/ρ	μ_{en}/ρ	μ/ρ	μ_{en}/ρ	μ/ρ	μ_{en}/ρ
1.0 + 03	2.517 + 02	2.516 + 02	3.394 + 02	3.392 + 02	2.047 + 02	2.046 + 02
1.5 + 03	8.066 + 01	8.055 + 01	1.148 + 02	1.146 + 02	6.227 + 01	6.219 + 01
2.0 + 03	3.535 + 01	3.526 + 01	5.148 + 01	5.133 + 01	2.692 + 01	2.683 + 01
3.0 + 03	1.100 + 01	1.090 + 01	2.347 + 01	2.303 + 01	8.041 + 00	7.976 + 00
4.0 + 03	4.691 + 00	4.621 + 00	1.045 + 01	1.025 + 01	3.364 + 00	3.312 + 00
5.0 + 03	2.401 + 00	2.345 + 00	1.335 + 01	1.227 + 01	1.704 + 00	1.659 + 00
6.0 + 03	1.386 + 00	1.338 + 00	8.129 + 00	7.531 + 00	9.783 − 01	9.375 − 01
8.0 + 03	5.853 − 01	5.474 − 01	3.676 + 00	3.435 + 00	4.110 − 01	3.773 − 01
1.0 + 04	3.048 − 01	2.716 − 01	1.966 + 00	1.841 + 00	2.150 − 01	1.849 − 01
1.5 + 04	1.022 − 01	7.499 − 02	6.243 − 01	5.726 − 01	7.551 − 02	5.014 − 02
2.0 + 04	5.437 − 02	3.014 − 02	2.797 − 01	2.450 − 01	4.290 − 02	2.002 − 02
3.0 + 04	3.004 − 02	8.881 − 03	9.724 − 02	7.290 − 02	2.621 − 02	6.059 − 03
4.0 + 04	2.377 − 02	4.344 − 03	5.168 − 02	3.088 − 02	2.177 − 02	3.191 − 03
5.0 + 04	2.118 − 02	2.980 − 03	3.504 − 02	1.625 − 02	1.982 − 02	2.387 − 03
6.0 + 04	1.974 − 02	2.514 − 03	2.741 − 02	9.988 − 03	1.868 − 02	2.153 − 03
8.0 + 04	1.805 − 02	2.344 − 03	2.083 − 02	5.309 − 03	1.724 − 02	2.152 − 03
1.0 + 05	1.694 − 02	2.434 − 03	1.800 − 02	3.838 − 03	1.624 − 02	2.293 − 03
1.5 + 05	1.506 − 02	2.747 − 03	1.490 − 02	3.032 − 03	1.448 − 02	2.631 − 03
2.0 + 05	1.374 − 02	2.972 − 03	1.332 − 02	2.994 − 03	1.322 − 02	2.856 − 03
3.0 + 05	1.192 − 02	3.209 − 03	1.141 − 02	3.095 − 03	1.147 − 02	3.088 − 03
4.0 + 05	1.067 − 02	3.298 − 03	1.018 − 02	3.151 − 03	1.027 − 02	3.174 − 03
5.0 + 05	9.740 − 03	3.318 − 03	9.274 − 03	3.159 − 03	9.376 − 03	3.194 − 03
6.0 + 05	9.008 − 03	3.304 − 03	8.570 − 03	3.140 − 03	8.672 − 03	3.181 − 03
8.0 + 05	7.912 − 03	3.226 − 03	7.520 − 03	3.061 − 03	7.617 − 03	3.106 − 03
1.0 + 06	7.112 − 03	3.121 − 03	6.758 − 03	2.959 − 03	6.847 − 03	3.005 − 03
1.5 + 06	5.787 − 03	2.850 − 03	5.501 − 03	2.700 − 03	5.571 − 03	2.744 − 03
2.0 + 06	4.963 − 03	2.619 − 03	4.732 − 03	2.487 − 03	4.778 − 03	2.522 − 03
3.0 + 06	3.972 − 03	2.282 − 03	3.826 − 03	2.191 − 03	3.822 − 03	2.196 − 03
4.0 + 06	3.390 − 03	2.055 − 03	3.307 − 03	2.002 − 03	3.261 − 03	1.977 − 03
5.0 + 06	3.005 − 03	1.894 − 03	2.970 − 03	1.874 − 03	2.889 − 03	1.820 − 03
6.0 + 06	2.732 − 03	1.775 − 03	2.738 − 03	1.784 − 03	2.626 − 03	1.706 − 03
8.0 + 06	2.371 − 03	1.613 − 03	2.440 − 03	1.667 − 03	2.227 − 03	1.548 − 03
1.0 + 07	2.147 − 03	1.508 − 03	2.263 − 03	1.598 − 03	2.060 − 03	1.446 − 03
1.5 + 07	1.840 − 03	1.361 − 03	2.040 − 03	1.508 − 03	1.763 − 03	1.304 − 03
2.0 + 07	1.693 − 03	1.290 − 03	1.948 − 03	1.474 − 03	1.620 − 03	1.234 − 03

TABLE A.7. (*continued*)

Photon Energy (eV)	Lucite (C$_6$H$_8$O$_2$) $\overline{Z} = 6.56$ $\rho = 1180$ kg/m^3 3.248×10^{26} e/kg		Lithium Fluoride (LiF) $\overline{Z} = 8.31$ $\rho = 2635$ kg/m^3 2.786×10^{26} e/kg		Carbon $\overline{Z} = 6$ $\rho = 2265$ kg/m^3 3.008×10^{26} e/kg	
	μ/ρ	μ_{en}/ρ	μ/ρ	μ_{en}/ρ	μ/ρ	μ_{en}/ρ
1.0 + 03	2.803 + 02	2.802 + 02	4.096 + 02	4.095 + 02	2.218 + 02	2.217 + 02
1.5 + 03	9.051 + 01	9.039 + 01	1.432 + 02	1.431 + 02	6.748 + 01	6.739 + 01
2.0 + 03	3.977 + 01	3.967 + 01	6.540 + 01	6.529 + 01	2.917 + 01	2.908 + 01
3.0 + 03	1.211 + 01	1.203 + 01	2.086 + 01	2.076 + 01	8.711 + 00	8.644 + 00
4.0 + 03	5.129 + 00	5.066 + 00	9.072 + 01	8.991 + 00	3.643 + 00	3.589 + 00
5.0 + 03	2.618 + 00	2.565 + 00	4.705 + 00	4.639 + 00	1.844 + 00	1.798 + 00
6.0 + 03	1.507 + 00	1.460 + 00	2.739 + 00	2.682 + 00	1.057 − 00	1.016 + 00
8.0 + 03	6.331 − 01	5.953 + 01	1.161 + 00	1.117 + 00	4.422 − 01	4.089 − 01
1.0 + 04	3.273 − 01	2.944 − 01	5.970 − 01	5.607 − 01	2.298 − 01	2.003 − 01
1.5 + 04	1.077 − 01	8.083 − 02	1.847 − 01	1.576 − 01	7.869 − 02	5.425 − 02
2.0 + 04	5.616 − 02	3.232 − 02	8.646 − 02	6.352 − 02	4.340 − 02	2.159 − 02
3.0 + 04	3.006 − 02	9.391 − 03	3.687 − 02	1.788 − 02	2.541 − 02	6.411 − 03
4.0 + 04	2.340 − 02	4.500 − 03	2.471 − 02	7.742 − 03	2.069 − 02	3.265 − 03
5.0 + 04	2.069 − 02	3.020 − 03	2.012 − 02	4.470 − 03	1.867 − 02	2.360 − 03
6.0 + 04	1.921 − 02	2.504 − 03	1.787 − 02	3.184 − 03	1.751 − 02	2.078 − 03
8.0 + 04	1.750 − 02	2.292 − 03	1.562 − 02	2.370 − 03	1.609 − 02	2.029 − 03
1.0 + 05	1.640 − 02	2.363 − 03	1.440 − 02	2.222 − 03	1.513 − 02	2.144 − 03
1.5 + 05	1.456 − 02	2.656 − 03	1.260 − 02	2.330 − 03	1.347 − 02	2.448 − 03
2.0 + 05	1.328 − 02	2.872 − 03	1.145 − 02	2.483 − 03	1.229 − 02	2.655 − 03
3.0 + 05	1.152 − 02	3.099 − 03	9.898 − 03	2.663 − 03	1.066 − 02	2.869 − 03
4.0 + 05	1.031 − 02	3.185 − 03	8.852 − 03	2.734 − 03	9.545 − 03	2.949 − 03
5.0 + 05	9.408 − 03	3.204 − 03	8.076 − 03	2.749 − 03	8.712 − 03	2.967 − 03
6.0 + 05	8.701 − 03	3.191 − 03	7.468 − 03	2.736 − 03	8.058 − 03	2.955 − 03
8.0 + 05	7.642 − 03	3.115 − 03	6.557 − 03	2.670 − 03	7.077 − 03	2.885 − 03
1.0 + 06	6.869 − 03	3.014 − 03	5.893 − 03	2.583 − 03	6.362 − 03	2.791 − 03
1.5 + 06	5.590 − 03	2.751 − 03	4.797 − 03	2.358 − 03	5.177 − 03	2.548 − 03
2.0 + 06	4.796 − 03	2.530 − 03	4.122 − 03	2.170 − 03	4.443 − 03	2.343 − 03
3.0 + 06	3.844 − 03	2.207 − 03	3.320 − 03	1.940 − 03	3.562 − 03	2.045 − 03
4.0 + 06	3.286 − 03	1.992 − 03	2.856 − 03	1.731 − 03	3.047 − 03	1.847 − 03
5.0 + 06	2.919 − 03	1.840 − 03	2.554 − 03	1.612 − 03	2.708 − 03	1.707 − 03
6.0 + 06	2.659 − 03	1.729 − 03	2.343 − 03	1.527 − 03	2.469 − 03	1.605 − 03
8.0 + 06	2.317 − 03	1.578 − 03	2.069 − 03	1.414 − 03	2.154 − 03	1.467 − 03
1.0 + 07	2.105 − 03	1.481 − 03	1.903 − 03	1.345 − 03	1.960 − 03	1.379 − 03
1.5 + 07	1.819 − 03	1.348 − 03	1.687 − 03	1.254 − 03	1.698 − 03	1.259 − 03
2.0 + 07	1.684 − 03	1.285 − 03	1.592 − 03	1.217 − 03	1.575 − 03	1.203 − 03

TABLE A.7. (*continued*)

Photon Energy (eV)	Aluminum $\overline{Z} = 13$ $\rho = 2699$ kg/m^3 2.902×10^{26} e/kg		Copper $\overline{Z} = 29$ $\rho = 8960$ kg/m^3 2.749×10^{26} e/kg		Lead $\overline{Z} = 82$ $\rho = 1135$ kg/m^3 2.383×10^{26} e/kg	
	μ/ρ	μ_{en}/ρ	μ/ρ	μ_{en}/ρ	μ/ρ	μ_{en}/ρ
1.0 + 03	1.076 + 02	1.074 + 02	1.003 + 03	1.002 + 03	5.210 + 02	5.198 + 02
1.5 + 03	3.683 + 01	3.663 + 01	4.223 + 02	4.219 + 02	2.356 + 02	2.344 + 02
2.0 + 03	2.222 + 02	2.164 + 02	2.063 + 02	2.059 + 02	1.285 + 02	1.274 + 02
3.0 + 03	7.746 + 01	7.599 + 01	7.198 + 01	7.158 + 01	1.965 + 02	1.954 + 02
4.0 + 03	3.545 + 01	3.487 + 01	3.347 + 01	3.313 + 01	1.251 + 00	1.242 + 02
5.0 + 03	1.902 + 01	1.870 + 01	1.834 + 01	1.804 + 01	7.304 + 01	7.222 + 01
6.0 + 03	1.134 + 01	1.115 + 01	1.118 + 01	1.092 + 01	4.672 + 01	4.598 + 01
8.0 + 03	4.953 + 00	4.849 + 00	5.099 + 00	4.905 + 00	2.287 + 01	2.226 + 01
1.0 + 04	2.582 + 00	2.495 + 00	2.140 + 01	1.514 − 00	1.306 + 01	1.256 + 01
1.5 + 04	7.836 − 01	7.377 − 01	7.343 + 00	5.853 − 00	1.116 + 01	8.939 + 00
2.0 + 04	3.392 − 01	3.056 − 01	3.352 + 00	2.810 + 00	8.636 + 00	6.923 + 00
3.0 + 04	1.115 − 01	8.646 − 02	1.083 + 00	9.382 − 01	3.032 − 00	2.550 + 00
4.0 + 04	5.630 − 02	3.556 − 02	4.828 − 01	4.173 − 01	1.436 + 00	1.221 + 00
5.0 + 04	3.655 − 02	1.816 − 02	2.595 − 01	2.196 − 01	8.041 − 01	6.796 − 01
6.0 + 04	2.763 − 02	1.087 − 02	1.583 − 01	1.290 − 01	5.020 − 01	4.177 − 01
8.0 + 04	2.012 − 02	5.464 − 03	7.587 − 02	5.593 − 02	2.419 − 01	1.936 − 01
1.0 + 05	1.701 − 02	3.773 − 03	4.563 − 02	2.952 − 02	5.550 − 01	2.229 − 01
1.5 + 05	1.378 − 02	2.823 − 03	2.210 − 02	1.030 − 02	2.014 − 01	1.135 − 01
2.0 + 05	1.223 − 02	2.745 − 03	1.557 − 02	5.811 − 03	9.985 − 02	6.229 − 02
3.0 + 05	1.042 − 02	2.817 − 03	1.118 − 02	3.636 − 03	4.026 − 02	2.581 − 02
4.0 + 05	9.276 − 03	2.863 − 03	9.409 − 03	3.135 − 03	2.323 − 02	1.439 − 02
5.0 + 05	8.446 − 03	2.870 − 03	8.360 − 03	2.943 − 03	1.613 − 02	9.564 − 03
6.0 + 05	7.801 − 03	2.851 − 03	7.624 − 03	2.835 − 03	1.248 − 02	7.132 − 03
8.0 + 05	6.842 − 03	2.778 − 03	6.605 − 03	2.686 − 03	8.869 − 03	4.838 − 03
1.0 + 06	6.146 − 03	2.684 − 03	5.900 − 03	2.563 − 03	7.103 − 03	3.787 − 03
1.5 + 06	5.007 − 03	2.447 − 03	4.803 − 03	2.313 − 03	5.222 − 03	2.714 − 03
2.0 + 06	4.324 − 03	2.261 − 03	4.204 − 03	2.156 − 03	4.607 − 03	2.407 − 03
3.0 + 06	3.541 − 03	2.018 − 03	3.599 − 03	2.016 − 03	4.234 − 03	2.351 − 03
4.0 + 06	3.107 − 03	1.877 − 03	3.318 − 03	1.981 − 03	4.197 − 03	2.463 − 03
5.0 + 06	2.836 − 03	1.790 − 03	3.176 − 03	1.991 − 03	4.272 − 03	2.600 − 03
6.0 + 06	2.655 − 03	1.735 − 03	3.108 − 03	2.019 − 03	4.391 − 03	2.730 − 03
8.0 + 06	2.437 − 03	1.674 − 03	3.074 − 03	2.092 − 03	4.675 − 03	2.948 − 03
1.0 + 07	2.318 − 03	1.645 − 03	3.103 − 03	2.165 − 03	4.972 − 03	3.114 − 03
1.5 + 07	2.195 − 03	1.626 − 03	3.247 − 03	2.286 − 03	5.658 − 03	3.353 − 03
2.0 + 07	2.168 − 03	1.637 − 03	3.408 − 03	2.384 − 03	6.205 − 03	3.440 − 03

The numbers following + or − refer to the power of 10, e.g., *3.617 + 02* should be read as 3.617 × 10^2.
Data from Hubbell JH. Photon mass attenuation and energy-absorption coefficients from 1 keV to 20 MeV. *Int J Appl Radiat Isotopes* 1982;33:1269, with permission.

TABLE A.8. COLLISION MASS STOPPING POWERS, S/ρ, IN MeV cm²/g, FOR ELECTRONS IN VARIOUS MATERIALS

Electron Energy (MeV)	Carbon	Air	Water	Muscle	Fat
0.0100	2.014E + 01	1.975E + 01	2.256E + 01	2.237E + 01	2.347E + 01
0.0125	1.694E + 01	1.663E + 01	1.897E + 01	1.881E + 01	1.971E + 01
0.0150	1.471E + 01	1.445E + 01	1.647E + 01	1.633E + 01	1.709E + 01
0.0175	1.305E + 01	1.283E + 01	1.461E + 01	1.449E + 01	1.515E + 01
0.0200	1.177E + 01	1.157E + 01	1.317E + 01	1.306E + 01	1.365E + 01
0.0250	9.911E + 00	9.753E + 00	1.109E + 01	1.100E + 01	1.148E + 01
0.0300	8.624E + 00	8.492E + 00	9.653E + 00	9.571E + 01	9.984E + 00
0.0350	7.677E + 00	7.563E + 00	8.592E + 00	8.519E + 00	8.881E + 00
0.0400	6.948E + 00	6.848E + 00	7.777E + 00	7.711E + 00	8.034E + 00
0.0450	6.370E + 00	6.281E + 00	7.130E + 00	7.069E + 00	7.362E + 00
0.0500	5.899E + 00	5.819E + 00	6.603E + 00	6.547E + 00	6.816E + 00
0.0550	5.508E + 00	5.435E + 00	6.166E + 00	6.113E + 00	6.362E + 00
0.0600	5.177E + 00	5.111E + 00	5.797E + 00	5.747E + 00	5.979E + 00
0.0700	4.650E + 00	4.593E + 00	5.207E + 00	5.163E + 00	5.369E + 00
0.0800	4.247E + 00	4.198E + 00	4.757E + 00	4.717E + 00	4.903E + 00
0.0900	3.929E + 00	3.886E + 00	4.402E + 00	4.365E + 00	4.535E + 00
0.1000	3.671E + 00	3.633E + 00	4.115E + 00	4.080E + 00	4.238E + 00
0.1250	3.201E + 00	3.172E + 00	3.591E + 00	3.561E + 00	3.696E + 00
0.1500	2.883E + 00	2.861E + 00	3.238E + 00	3.210E + 00	3.330E + 00
0.1750	2.654E + 00	2.637E + 00	2.984E + 00	2.958E + 00	3.068E + 00
0.2000	2.482E + 00	2.470E + 00	2.793E + 00	2.769E + 00	2.871E + 00
0.2500	2.241E + 00	2.236E + 00	2.528E + 00	2.506E + 00	2.597E + 00
0.3000	2.083E + 00	2.084E + 00	2.355E + 00	2.335E + 00	2.418E + 00
0.3500	1.972E + 00	1.978E + 00	2.233E + 00	2.215E + 00	2.294E + 00
0.4000	1.891E + 00	1.902E + 00	2.145E + 00	2.129E + 00	2.204E + 00
0.4500	1.830E + 00	1.845E + 00	2.079E + 00	2.065E + 00	2.135E + 00
0.5000	1.782E + 00	1.802E + 00	2.028E + 00	2.016E + 00	2.081E + 00
0.5500	1.745E + 00	1.769E + 00	1.988E + 00	1.976E + 00	2.039E + 00
0.6000	1.716E + 00	1.743E + 00	1.956E + 00	1.945E + 00	2.005E + 00
0.7000	1.672E + 00	1.706E + 00	1.910E + 00	1.898E + 00	1.954E + 00
0.8000	1.643E + 00	1.683E + 00	1.879E + 00	1.866E + 00	1.921E + 00
0.9000	1.623E + 00	1.669E + 00	1.858E + 00	1.845E + 00	1.897E + 00
1.0000	1.609E + 00	1.661E + 00	1.844E + 00	1.830E + 00	1.880E + 00
1.2500	1.590E + 00	1.655E + 00	1.825E + 00	1.809E + 00	1.858E + 00
1.5000	1.584E + 00	1.661E + 00	1.820E + 00	1.802E + 00	1.849E + 00
1.7500	1.584E + 00	1.672E + 00	1.821E + 00	1.801E + 00	1.848E + 00
2.0000	1.587E + 00	1.684E + 00	1.825E + 00	1.804E + 00	1.850E + 00
2.5000	1.598E + 00	1.712E + 00	1.837E + 00	1.814E + 00	1.860E + 00
3.0000	1.611E + 00	1.740E + 00	1.850E + 00	1.826E + 00	1.872E + 00
3.5000	1.623E + 00	1.766E + 00	1.864E + 00	1.839E + 00	1.885E + 00
4.0000	1.636E + 00	1.790E + 00	1.877E + 00	1.851E + 00	1.897E + 00
4.5000	1.647E + 00	1.812E + 00	1.889E + 00	1.862E + 00	1.909E + 00
5.0000	1.658E + 00	1.833E + 00	1.900E + 00	1.873E + 00	1.920E + 00
5.5000	1.667E + 00	1.852E + 00	1.910E + 00	1.883E + 00	1.930E + 00
6.0000	1.676E + 00	1.870E + 00	1.919E + 00	1.892E + 00	1.939E + 00
7.0000	1.693E + 00	1.902E + 00	1.936E + 00	1.909E + 00	1.956E + 00
8.0000	1.707E + 00	1.931E + 00	1.951E + 00	1.924E + 00	1.972E + 00
9.0000	1.719E + 00	1.956E + 00	1.964E + 00	1.937E + 00	1.985E + 00
10.0000	1.730E + 00	1.979E + 00	1.976E + 00	1.949E + 00	1.997E + 00
12.5000	1.753E + 00	2.029E + 00	2.000E + 00	1.974E + 00	2.022E + 00
15.0000	1.770E + 00	2.069E + 00	2.020E + 00	1.995E + 00	2.042E + 00
17.5000	1.785E + 00	2.104E + 00	2.037E + 00	2.012E + 00	2.059E + 00
20.0000	1.797E + 00	2.134E + 00	2.051E + 00	2.026E + 00	2.073E + 00
25.0000	1.816E + 00	2.185E + 00	2.074E + 00	2.050E + 00	2.095E + 00
30.0000	1.832E + 00	2.226E + 00	2.092E + 00	2.068E + 00	2.113E + 00
35.0000	1.845E + 00	2.257E + 00	2.107E + 00	2.084E + 00	2.128E + 00
40.0000	1.856E + 00	2.282E + 00	2.120E + 00	2.097E + 00	2.141E + 00
45.0000	1.865E + 00	2.302E + 00	2.131E + 00	2.108E + 00	2.152E + 00
50.0000	1.874E + 00	2.319E + 00	2.141E + 00	2.118E + 00	2.161E + 00
55.0000	1.881E + 00	2.334E + 00	2.149E + 00	2.126E + 00	2.170E + 00
60.0000	1.888E + 00	2.347E + 00	2.157E + 00	2.134E + 00	2.178E + 00
70.0000	1.900E + 00	2.369E + 00	2.171E + 00	2.148E + 00	2.192E + 00

Electron Energy (MeV)	Bone	Polystyrene	Lucite	Aluminum	Lead
80.0000	1.911E + 00	2.387E + 00	2.183E + 00	2.160E + 00	2.203E + 00
90.0000	1.920E + 00	2.403E + 00	2.194E + 00	2.171E + 00	2.214E + 00
0.0100	2.068E + 01	2.223E + 01	2.198E + 01	1.649E + 01	8.428E + 00
0.0125	1.742E + 01	1.868E + 01	1.848E + 01	1.398E + 01	7.357E + 00
0.0150	1.514E + 01	1.621E + 01	1.604E + 01	1.220E + 01	6.561E + 00
0.0175	1.344E + 01	1.437E + 01	1.423E + 01	1.088E + 01	5.946E + 00
0.0200	1.213E + 01	1.296E + 01	1.283E + 01	9.845E + 00	5.453E + 00
0.0250	1.023E + 01	1.091E + 01	1.080E + 01	8.339E + 00	4.714E + 01
0.0300	8.912E + 00	9.485E + 00	9.400E + 00	7.288E + 00	4.182E + 00
0.0350	7.939E + 00	8.440E + 00	8.367E + 00	6.510E + 00	3.779E + 00
0.0400	7.190E + 00	7.637E + 00	7.573E + 00	5.909E + 00	3.463E + 00
0.0450	6.596E + 00	7.000E + 00	6.942E + 00	5.431E + 00	3.208E + 00
0.0500	6.112E + 00	6.481E + 00	6.429E + 00	5.040E + 00	2.997E + 00
0.0550	5.709E + 00	6.051E + 00	6.003E + 00	4.715E + 00	2.821E + 00
0.0600	5.370E + 00	5.688E + 00	5.644E + 00	4.439E + 00	2.670E + 00
0.0700	4.827E + 00	5.108E + 00	5.070E + 00	3.999E + 00	2.426E + 00
0.0800	4.412E + 00	4.666E + 00	4.631E + 00	3.661E + 00	2.237E + 00
0.0900	4.085E + 00	4.317E + 00	4.286E + 00	3.394E + 00	2.087E + 00
0.1000	3.820E + 00	4.034E + 00	4.006E + 00	3.178E + 00	1.964E + 00
0.1250	3.336E + 00	3.520E + 00	3.496E + 00	2.782E + 00	1.738E + 00
0.1500	3.010E + 00	3.172E + 00	3.152E + 00	2.514E + 00	1.583E + 00
0.1750	2.775E + 00	2.923E + 00	2.904E + 00	2.320E + 00	1.471E + 00
0.2000	2.599E + 00	2.735E + 00	2.719E + 00	2.175E + 00	1.387E + 00
0.2500	2.354E + 00	2.475E + 00	2.461E + 00	1.973E + 00	1.269E + 00
0.3000	2.194E + 00	2.305E + 00	2.292E + 00	1.840E + 00	1.193E + 00
0.3500	2.079E + 00	2.187E + 00	2.175E + 00	1.748E + 00	1.140E + 00
0.4000	1.996E + 00	2.101E + 00	2.090E + 00	1.681E + 00	1.102E + 00
0.4500	1.932E + 00	2.035E + 00	2.026E + 00	1.631E + 00	1.074E + 00
0.5000	1.883E + 00	1.984E + 00	1.975E + 00	1.594E + 00	1.053E + 00
0.5500	1.845E + 00	1.943E + 00	1.935E + 00	1.564E + 00	1.037E + 00
0.6000	1.815E + 00	1.911E + 00	1.903E + 00	1.541E + 00	1.026E + 00
0.7000	1.770E + 00	1.864E + 00	1.856E + 00	1.508E + 00	1.009E + 00
0.8000	1.740E + 00	1.832E + 00	1.825E + 00	1.487E + 00	1.000E + 00
0.9000	1.719E + 00	1.810E + 00	1.803E + 00	1.474E + 00	9.957E − 01
1.0000	1.705E + 00	1.794E + 00	1.788E + 00	1.466E + 00	9.939E − 01
1.2500	1.686E + 00	1.773E + 00	1.767E + 00	1.458E + 00	9.966E − 01
1.5000	1.680E + 00	1.766E + 00	1.760E + 00	1.460E + 00	1.004E + 00
1.7500	1.681E + 00	1.765E + 00	1.759E + 00	1.467E + 00	1.014E + 00
2.0000	1.684E + 00	1.768E + 00	1.762E + 00	1.475E + 00	1.024E + 00
2.5000	1.696E + 00	1.778E + 00	1.772E + 00	1.492E + 00	1.044E + 00
3.0000	1.709E + 00	1.791E + 00	1.784E + 00	1.509E + 00	1.063E + 00
3.5000	1.722E + 00	1.804E + 00	1.797E + 00	1.525E + 00	1.080E + 00
4.0000	1.735E + 00	1.816E + 00	1.809E + 00	1.539E + 00	1.095E + 00
4.5000	1.747E + 00	1.828E + 00	1.821E + 00	1.552E + 00	1.108E + 00
5.0000	1.758E + 00	1.839E + 00	1.832E + 00	1.563E + 00	1.120E + 00
5.5000	1.768E + 00	1.849E + 00	1.842E + 00	1.574E + 00	1.132E + 00
6.0000	1.778E + 00	1.859E + 00	1.851E + 00	1.583E + 00	1.142E + 00
7.0000	1.795E + 00	1.876E + 00	1.868E + 00	1.600E + 00	1.160E + 00
8.0000	1.810E + 00	1.891E + 00	1.883E + 00	1.614E + 00	1.175E + 00
9.0000	1.823E + 00	1.904E + 00	1.896E + 00	1.627E + 00	1.189E + 00
10.0000	1.835E + 00	1.916E + 00	1.908E + 00	1.638E + 00	1.201E + 00
12.5000	1.860E + 00	1.940E + 00	1.932E + 00	1.661E + 00	1.226E + 00
15.0000	1.879E + 00	1.960E + 00	1.952E + 00	1.679E + 00	1.246E + 00
17.5000	1.896E + 00	1.975E + 00	1.968E + 00	1.694E + 00	1.262E + 00
20.0000	1.909E + 00	1.989E + 00	1.982E + 00	1.707E + 00	1.277E + 00
25.0000	1.931E + 00	2.010E + 00	2.004E + 00	1.728E + 00	1.299E + 00
30.0000	1.949E + 00	2.027E + 00	2.022E + 00	1.744E + 00	1.318E + 00
35.0000	1.963E + 00	2.041E + 00	2.036E + 00	1.758E + 00	1.332E + 00
40.0000	1.976E + 00	2.053E + 00	2.049E + 00	1.770E + 00	1.345E + 00
45.0000	1.986E + 00	2.064E + 00	2.059E + 00	1.780E + 00	1.356E + 00
50.0000	1.996E + 00	2.073E + 00	2.069E + 00	1.789E + 00	1.365E + 00
55.0000	2.004E + 00	2.081E + 00	2.077E + 00	1.797E + 00	1.374E + 00
60.0000	2.012E + 00	2.089E + 00	2.085E + 00	1.804E + 00	1.381E + 00
70.0000	2.025E + 00	2.102E + 00	2.098E + 00	1.816E + 00	1.395E + 00
80.0000	2.037E + 00	2.113E + 00	2.109E + 00	1.827E + 00	1.406E + 00
90.0000	2.047E + 00	2.123E + 00	2.120E + 00	1.837E + 00	1.415E + 00

The numbers following E + or E − refer to the power of 10, e.g., *2.014E + 01* should be read as 2.014 × 10^1.
From Berger MJ, Seltzer SM. *Stopping powers and ranges of electrons and positrons,* 2nd ed. Washington, DC: U.S. Department of Commerce, National Bureau of Standards, 1983, with permission.

TABLE A.9.1. COBALT-60 PERCENT DEPTH DOSES: 80 cm SSD

	Field Size (cm) and Backscatter Factor[a]									
Depth (cm)	0 1.00	4 × 4 1.01$_4$	5 × 5 1.01$_7$	6 × 6 1.02$_1$	7 × 7 1.02$_5$	8 × 8 1.02$_9$	10 × 10 1.03$_6$	12 × 12 1.04$_3$	15 × 15 1.05$_2$	20 × 20 1.06$_1$
0.5	100.0	100.0	100.0	100.0	100.0	100.0	100.0	100.0	100.0	100.0
1	95.4	96.8	97.0	97.4	97.6	97.8	98.2	98.3	98.4	98.4
2	87.1	90.6	91.3	91.9	92.3	92.7	93.3	93.6	93.9	94.0
3	79.5	84.7	85.6	86.5	87.1	87.6	88.3	88.8	89.3	89.6
4	72.7	79.0	80.2	81.1	81.9	82.5	83.4	84.0	84.7	85.2
5	66.5	73.5	74.8	75.9	76.7	77.4	78.5	79.3	80.1	80.8
6	60.8	68.1	69.6	70.7	71.6	72.4	73.6	74.4	75.4	76.4
7	55.6	62.9	64.4	65.7	66.7	67.5	68.8	69.8	70.8	72.1
8	50.9	58.0	59.4	60.8	61.9	62.7	64.1	65.3	66.5	68.0
9	46.6	53.5	55.0	56.2	57.3	58.2	59.7	60.8	62.3	64.0
10	42.7	49.3	50.7	52.0	53.0	54.0	55.6	56.9	58.4	60.2
11	39.2	45.5	46.9	48.1	49.2	50.1	51.7	53.0	54.7	56.6
12	35.9	41.9	43.2	44.5	45.5	46.5	48.1	49.5	51.2	53.2
13	32.9	38.6	39.9	41.1	42.1	43.2	44.8	46.1	47.9	50.0
14	30.2	35.6	36.8	38.0	39.2	40.1	41.8	43.2	44.9	47.0
15	27.7	32.9	34.2	35.2	36.2	37.2	38.9	40.3	42.0	44.2
16	25.4	30.4	31.5	32.6	33.6	34.5	36.2	37.6	39.3	41.5
17	23.3	28.1	29.2	30.2	31.2	32.1	33.7	35.1	36.8	39.0
18	21.4	26.0	27.1	28.0	29.0	29.8	31.4	32.8	34.5	36.7
19	19.6	24.0	25.0	26.0	26.8	27.7	29.2	30.6	32.3	34.6
20	18.0	22.1	23.1	24.0	24.9	25.7	27.2	28.5	30.3	32.6
22	(15.3)	(18.9)	(19.8)	(20.6)	(21.4)	(22.1)	(23.7)	(24.9)	(26.5)	(28.8)
24	(12.9)	(16.1)	(16.9)	(17.7)	(18.4)	(19.1)	(20.5)	(21.8)	(23.2)	(25.4)
26	(10.8)	(13.7)	(14.4)	(15.1)	(15.8)	(16.5)	(17.8)	(18.9)	(20.4)	(22.5)
28	(9.1)	(11.7)	(12.3)	(12.9)	(13.6)	(14.2)	(15.5)	(16.5)	(17.9)	(19.9)
30	(7.7)	(10.0)	(10.6)	(11.1)	(11.7)	(12.3)	(13.5)	(14.4)	(15.7)	(17.5)

[a] Values in parentheses represent extrapolated data.
Data from Hospital Physicists' Association. Central axis depth dose data for use in radiotherapy. *Br J Radiol* 1978; [Suppl. 11], with permission.

TABLE A.9.2. COBALT-60 TISSUE-MAXIMUM RATIOS

	Field (cm) and S_p									
	0 × 0	**4 × 4**	**5 × 5**	**6 × 6**	**7 × 7**	**8 × 8**	**10 × 10**	**12 × 12**	**15 × 15**	**20 × 20**
Depth (cm)	**0.965**	**0.979**	**0.982**	**0.986**	**0.989**	**0.993**	**1.000**	**1.007**	**1.015**	**1.024**
0.5	1.000	1.000	1.000	1.000	1.000	1.000	1.000	1.000	1.000	1.000
1.0	0.966	0.980	0.982	0.986	0.988	0.990	0.994	0.995	0.996	0.996
2.0	0.904	0.939	0.946	0.952	0.957	0.961	0.967	0.970	0.973	0.975
3.0	0.845	0.898	0.908	0.917	0.924	0.929	0.937	0.942	0.947	0.951
4.0	0.792	0.857	0.870	0.880	0.808	0.895	0.905	0.911	0.919	0.925
5.0	0.741	0.815	0.829	0.841	0.851	0.858	0.870	0.879	0.889	0.898
6.0	0.694	0.771	0.788	0.801	0.811	0.820	0.834	0.843	0.855	0.867
7.0	0.649	0.728	0.745	0.759	0.771	0.781	0.796	0.808	0.820	0.835
8.0	0.608	0.685	0.702	0.717	0.730	0.741	0.757	0.770	0.786	0.804
9.0	0.570	0.645	0.663	0.677	0.690	0.701	0.719	0.733	0.750	0.772
10.0	0.534	0.607	0.624	0.638	0.651	0.662	0.682	0.690	0.717	0.740
11.0	0.501	0.571	0.588	0.602	0.615	0.627	0.646	0.663	0.683	0.709
12.0	0.469	0.537	0.553	0.567	0.581	0.592	0.613	0.630	0.651	0.679
13.0	0.439	0.504	0.520	0.534	0.547	0.559	0.581	0.598	0.620	0.649
14.0	0.412	0.474	0.489	0.502	0.516	0.530	0.551	0.569	0.592	0.621
15.0	0.386	0.446	0.461	0.476	0.487	0.499	0.521	0.540	0.563	0.594
16.0	0.361	0.420	0.434	0.447	0.460	0.471	0.493	0.512	0.536	0.567
17.0	0.338	0.395	0.409	0.422	0.434	0.445	0.467	0.485	0.510	0.541
18.0	0.317	0.372	0.386	0.399	0.410	0.421	0.442	0.460	0.485	0.517
19.0	0.296	0.350	0.363	0.375	0.387	0.397	0.418	0.436	0.461	0.494
20.0	0.278	0.328	0.340	0.352	0.363	0.374	0.395	0.413	0.437	0.472
22.0	0.246	0.290	0.302	0.313	0.323	0.333	0.351	0.371	0.395	0.428
24.0	0.215	0.256	0.266	0.276	0.286	0.296	0.313	0.331	0.356	0.388
26.0	0.187	0.225	0.234	0.243	0.252	0.261	0.279	0.296	0.310	0.352
28.0	0.164	0.198	0.207	0.215	0.222	0.230	0.247	0.264	0.286	0.319
30.0	0.144	0.175	0.182	0.190	0.198	0.204	0.220	0.236	0.257	0.287

Calculated from the percent depth dose data from Hospital Physicists' Association. Central axis depth dose data for use in radiotherapy. *Br J Radiol* 1978; [Suppl. 11], using Equation 10.5. S_p is the phantom scatter factor, calculated from Equation 10.1.

TABLE A.9.3. COBALT-60 SCATTER-MAXIMUM RATIOS FOR CIRCULAR FIELDS[a]

Depth *d* (cm)	Field Radius (cm)											
	1	2	3	4	5	6	7	8	9	10	11	12
0.5	0.007	0.014	0.019	0.026	0.032	0.037	0.043	0.048	0.054	0.058	0.063	0.067
1	0.013	0.025	0.037	0.048	0.058	0.066	0.073	0.078	0.084	0.089	0.094	0.098
2	0.023	0.045	0.064	0.080	0.091	0.102	0.110	0.116	0.122	0.127	0.133	0.139
3	0.032	0.061	0.084	0.103	0.118	0.130	0.139	0.147	0.154	0.161	0.166	0.172
4	0.038	0.071	0.099	0.121	0.137	0.151	0.162	0.170	0.179	0.186	0.191	0.197
5	0.041	0.076	0.107	0.134	0.152	0.166	0.178	0.189	0.198	0.206	0.212	0.218
6	0.042	0.080	0.114	0.141	0.160	0.176	0.190	0.201	0.211	0.219	0.226	0.234
7	0.042	0.081	0.115	0.143	0.164	0.181	0.196	0.209	0.220	0.229	0.239	0.246
8	0.041	0.080	0.114	0.142	0.165	0.185	0.199	0.214	0.225	0.236	0.246	0.254
9	0.040	0.078	0.112	0.140	0.164	0.183	0.200	0.216	0.228	0.240	0.251	0.260
10	0.038	0.075	0.109	0.136	0.161	0.181	0.199	0.215	0.229	0.242	0.252	0.262
11	0.036	0.071	0.104	0.132	0.157	0.178	0.197	0.213	0.227	0.241	0.252	0.262
12	0.035	0.069	0.099	0.128	0.153	0.174	0.194	0.210	0.225	0.239	0.251	0.261
13	0.034	0.066	0.095	0.124	0.149	0.170	0.190	0.207	0.223	0.237	0.249	0.260
14	0.032	0.063	0.092	0.120	0.145	0.168	0.186	0.204	0.220	0.235	0.247	0.258
15	0.031	0.060	0.089	0.116	0.140	0.162	0.182	0.200	0.216	0.231	0.244	0.255
16	0.030	0.058	0.086	0.112	0.136	0.157	0.177	0.196	0.212	0.227	0.240	0.252
17	0.029	0.056	0.083	0.108	0.132	0.153	0.172	0.191	0.207	0.223	0.236	0.248
18	0.027	0.054	0.080	0.104	0.128	0.148	0.167	0.186	0.202	0.218	0.232	0.244
19	0.026	0.052	0.077	0.101	0.124	0.144	0.162	0.181	0.197	0.213	0.226	0.239
20	0.024	0.049	0.074	0.097	0.119	0.139	0.157	0.176	0.192	0.207	0.221	0.234
22	0.022	0.044	0.067	0.088	0.109	0.128	0.146	0.163	0.180	0.194	0.208	0.222
24	0.020	0.040	0.060	0.080	0.099	0.118	0.136	0.152	0.168	0.182	0.196	0.208
26	0.018	0.036	0.054	0.073	0.091	0.108	0.125	0.142	0.156	0.170	0.184	0.196
28	0.016	0.032	0.049	0.067	0.083	0.098	0.115	0.132	0.156	0.159	0.172	0.184
30	0.015	0.030	0.045	0.061	0.076	0.089	0.105	0.121	0.134	0.146	0.159	0.170

	13	14	15	16	17	18	19	20	21	22	23	24	25
0.5	0.070	0.073	0.076	0.078	0.080	0.082	0.084	0.085	0.086	0.087	0.088	0.088	0.089
1	0.101	0.104	0.107	0.109	0.112	0.114	0.116	0.118	0.119	0.120	0.121	0.122	0.123
2	0.142	0.146	0.149	0.152	0.154	0.156	0.158	0.160	0.161	0.162	0.164	0.166	0.167
3	0.176	0.180	0.184	0.187	0.190	0.193	0.195	0.198	0.200	0.202	0.203	0.204	0.205
4	0.201	0.205	0.210	0.215	0.218	0.222	0.225	0.228	0.231	0.233	0.235	0.237	0.239
5	0.224	0.229	0.235	0.240	0.245	0.248	0.252	0.255	0.258	0.261	0.263	0.264	0.266
6	0.241	0.246	0.252	0.257	0.262	0.265	0.269	0.272	0.275	0.278	0.280	0.282	0.284
7	0.254	0.260	0.267	0.273	0.278	0.282	0.287	0.290	0.294	0.296	0.299	0.302	0.304
8	0.263	0.271	0.278	0.285	0.289	0.294	0.298	0.301	0.305	0.309	0.311	0.313	0.315
9	0.269	0.277	0.284	0.292	0.298	0.303	0.308	0.312	0.316	0.319	0.322	0.324	0.327
10	0.271	0.279	0.288	0.295	0.302	0.308	0.314	0.318	0.324	0.327	0.331	0.333	0.336
11	0.272	0.280	0.289	0.296	0.304	0.311	0.316	0.322	0.328	0.331	0.334	0.337	0.339
12	0.272	0.281	0.290	0.297	0.305	0.312	0.318	0.324	0.330	0.333	0.337	0.340	0.342
13	0.270	0.280	0.290	0.298	0.306	0.313	0.319	0.325	0.332	0.335	0.340	0.342	0.345
14	0.268	0.279	0.288	0.297	0.305	0.313	0.320	0.326	0.333	0.337	0.341	0.344	0.347
15	0.266	0.277	0.286	0.295	0.303	0.311	0.318	0.325	0.331	0.336	0.340	0.344	0.347
16	0.263	0.274	0.283	0.292	0.300	0.308	0.315	0.322	0.328	0.333	0.337	0.342	0.346
17	0.259	0.271	0.279	0.288	0.296	0.304	0.311	0.318	0.324	0.329	0.334	0.339	0.343
18	0.255	0.266	0.275	0.284	0.292	0.300	0.307	0.313	0.320	0.325	0.330	0.335	0.339
19	0.251	0.261	0.270	0.280	0.288	0.295	0.303	0.309	0.315	0.321	0.326	0.331	0.335
20	0.246	0.257	0.265	0.275	0.284	0.291	0.299	0.305	0.311	0.316	0.321	0.326	0.329
22	0.233	0.246	0.255	0.264	0.273	0.280	0.288	0.295	0.301	0.306	0.311	0.316	0.319
24	0.220	0.235	0.243	0.252	0.259	0.267	0.275	0.281	0.288	0.294	0.299	0.304	0.309
26	0.207	0.219	0.229	0.236	0.245	0.253	0.260	0.266	0.272	0.279	0.284	0.289	0.295
28	0.194	0.205	0.214	0.222	0.230	0.238	0.245	0.251	0.258	0.264	0.269	0.274	0.279
30	0.181	0.191	0.200	0.208	0.215	0.223	0.230	0.236	0.242	0.249	0.255	0.260	0.265

[a] As discussed in section 10.1D, SMRs are equal to SARs for cobalt-60. For higher energies, SARs cannot be as accurately measured.
SAR data from Johns HE, Cunningham JR. *The physics of radiology,* 4th ed. Springfield, IL: Charles C Thomas, 1983, with permission.

TABLE A.10.1. 4-MV X-RAY PERCENT DEPTH DOSES: 100 cm SSD

Depth (cm)	Field Size (cm) and S_p									
	0.0×0.0 0.97	4.0×4.0 0.98	6.0×6.0 0.99	8.0×8.0 0.99	10.0×10.0 1.00	12.0×12.0 1.00	15.0×15.0 1.01	20.0×20.0 1.01	25.0×25.0 1.02	30.0×30.0 1.02
1.0	100.0	100.0	100.0	100.0	100.0	100.0	100.0	100.0	100.0	100.0
2.0	93.2	96.5	97.0	97.2	97.4	97.4	97.4	97.7	97.9	97.9
3.0	86.9	91.3	92.3	92.7	92.9	93.2	93.6	94.0	94.4	94.3
4.0	81.1	85.4	87.3	88.0	88.5	89.1	89.4	90.2	90.5	90.3
5.0	75.6	81.1	83.1	84.3	84.8	85.2	85.4	86.4	87.0	86.9
6.0	70.5	76.0	78.4	79.6	80.3	80.9	81.6	82.6	82.9	83.1
7.0	65.9	71.1	73.8	75.4	76.4	77.0	77.8	78.8	79.3	79.7
8.0	61.4	66.4	69.4	71.3	72.5	73.3	74.1	75.2	75.9	76.5
9.0	57.4	62.1	65.1	67.1	68.6	69.5	70.3	71.6	72.4	73.2
10.0	53.5	58.0	61.0	63.1	64.8	65.8	66.7	68.2	69.1	70.0
11.0	50.1	54.6	57.4	59.6	61.3	62.3	63.3	64.8	65.9	66.8
12.0	46.9	51.3	54.0	56.2	57.9	58.9	59.9	61.5	62.7	63.8
13.0	43.7	48.1	50.8	53.0	54.6	55.7	56.7	58.3	59.7	60.9
14.0	40.7	45.0	47.6	49.8	51.5	52.5	53.6	55.2	56.7	58.1
15.0	38.2	42.1	44.7	46.8	48.5	49.6	50.7	52.5	54.0	55.4
16.0	35.7	39.2	41.8	43.9	45.6	46.7	48.0	49.9	51.4	52.7
17.0	33.3	36.4	39.1	41.1	42.7	43.9	45.3	47.3	48.8	50.1
18.0	31.0	33.8	36.5	38.4	40.0	41.3	42.8	44.9	46.3	47.5
19.0	29.1	31.8	34.3	36.2	37.8	39.0	40.5	42.6	44.1	45.5
20.0	27.2	29.9	32.2	34.0	35.6	36.8	38.2	40.4	42.0	43.5
21.0	25.4	28.0	30.2	31.9	33.5	34.6	36.0	38.2	40.0	41.6
22.0	23.7	26.2	28.2	29.9	31.4	32.5	33.9	36.2	38.0	39.7
23.0	22.3	24.6	26.6	28.2	29.6	30.7	32.1	34.3	36.1	37.7
24.0	20.9	23.1	25.1	26.6	27.9	28.9	30.2	32.4	34.1	35.7
25.0	19.5	21.7	23.6	25.0	26.2	27.1	28.5	30.7	32.3	33.7
26.0	18.2	20.3	22.1	23.4	24.6	25.4	26.8	28.9	30.4	31.8
27.0	17.1	19.1	20.8	22.1	23.2	24.1	25.3	27.4	28.9	30.4
28.0	16.0	17.9	19.6	20.8	21.9	22.7	23.9	25.9	27.5	29.0
29.0	15.0	16.7	18.3	19.5	20.6	21.4	22.5	24.4	26.1	27.7
30.0	14.0	15.6	17.2	18.3	19.3	20.1	21.2	23.0	24.8	26.4

SSD, source-surface distance; S_p, the phantom scatter correction factor (Eq. 10.2).
Data are from the University of Minnesota.

TABLE A.10.2. 4-MV X-RAY TISSUE-MAXIMUM RATIOS

Depth (cm)	Field Size (cm)									
	0.0 × 0.0	4.0 × 4.0	6.0 × 6.0	8.0 × 8.0	10.0 × 10.0	12.0 × 12.0	15.0 × 15.0	20.0 × 20.0	25.0 × 25.0	30.0 × 30.0
1.0	1.000	1.000	1.000	1.000	1.000	1.000	1.000	1.000	1.000	1.000
2.0	0.951	0.984	0.989	0.991	0.993	0.993	0.994	0.996	0.999	0.998
3.0	0.904	0.948	0.959	0.963	0.966	0.968	0.973	0.977	0.981	0.981
4.0	0.860	0.903	0.924	0.931	0.937	0.943	0.947	0.955	0.958	0.957
5.0	0.817	0.874	0.894	0.909	0.914	0.919	0.922	0.931	0.938	0.939
6.0	0.777	0.833	0.858	0.875	0.882	0.889	0.896	0.907	0.912	0.913
7.0	0.739	0.793	0.822	0.842	0.853	0.861	0.870	0.881	0.887	0.892
8.0	0.702	0.753	0.785	0.809	0.823	0.834	0.843	0.856	0.863	0.870
9.0	0.668	0.716	0.749	0.774	0.791	0.803	0.814	0.829	0.838	0.846
10.0	0.635	0.679	0.713	0.739	0.759	0.773	0.785	0.802	0.813	0.823
11.0	0.606	0.651	0.683	0.709	0.730	0.745	0.757	0.774	0.787	0.798
12.0	0.577	0.622	0.653	0.679	0.701	0.716	0.729	0.747	0.761	0.774
13.0	0.548	0.594	0.623	0.649	0.671	0.687	0.701	0.720	0.735	0.749
14.0	0.519	0.565	0.593	0.620	0.642	0.659	0.673	0.692	0.709	0.725
15.0	0.495	0.535	0.565	0.591	0.614	0.631	0.647	0.668	0.686	0.701
16.0	0.471	0.505	0.537	0.563	0.585	0.603	0.620	0.643	0.662	0.678
17.0	0.447	0.475	0.509	0.535	0.557	0.575	0.594	0.619	0.639	0.654
18.0	0.423	0.445	0.481	0.507	0.528	0.547	0.567	0.594	0.615	0.631
19.0	0.404	0.426	0.459	0.485	0.505	0.524	0.544	0.571	0.594	0.611
20.0	0.384	0.407	0.438	0.462	0.482	0.501	0.521	0.549	0.572	0.590
21.0	0.365	0.388	0.416	0.439	0.460	0.478	0.498	0.526	0.550	0.570
22.0	0.346	0.369	0.395	0.417	0.437	0.455	0.475	0.503	0.528	0.550
23.0	0.330	0.352	0.378	0.399	0.418	0.436	0.455	0.482	0.508	0.529
24.0	0.315	0.335	0.360	0.381	0.400	0.416	0.435	0.462	0.488	0.508
25.0	0.299	0.318	0.343	0.364	0.381	0.397	0.414	0.442	0.467	0.487
26.0	0.283	0.301	0.326	0.346	0.362	0.377	0.394	0.421	0.447	0.466
27.0	0.270	0.286	0.311	0.330	0.346	0.361	0.378	0.404	0.429	0.449
28.0	0.258	0.272	0.296	0.315	0.330	0.345	0.362	0.386	0.411	0.431
29.0	0.245	0.257	0.281	0.300	0.314	0.329	0.346	0.369	0.393	0.414
30.0	0.232	0.242	0.266	0.284	0.298	0.312	0.330	0.352	0.375	0.397

Calculated from data in Table A.10.1, using Equation 10.4.

TABLE A.10.3. 4-MV X-RAY SCATTER-MAXIMUM RATIOS FOR CIRCULAR FIELDS

Depth (cm)	Radius (cm)												
	2.0	4.0	6.0	8.0	10.0	12.0	14.0	16.0	18.0	20.0	22.0	24.0	26.0
1.0	0.000	0.000	0.000	0.000	0.000	0.000	0.000	0.000	0.000	0.000	0.000	0.000	0.000
2.0	0.035	0.039	0.042	0.042	0.041	0.043	0.052	0.049	0.045	0.040	0.036	0.032	0.027
3.0	0.039	0.059	0.062	0.068	0.071	0.074	0.079	0.077	0.076	0.074	0.073	0.071	0.069
4.0	0.045	0.070	0.080	0.086	0.092	0.098	0.100	0.099	0.097	0.095	0.093	0.092	0.090
5.0	0.048	0.093	0.099	0.102	0.109	0.117	0.124	0.122	0.120	0.118	0.116	0.114	0.112
6.0	0.048	0.095	0.108	0.118	0.126	0.133	0.135	0.136	0.137	0.138	0.139	0.140	0.141
7.0	0.049	0.098	0.111	0.125	0.137	0.147	0.154	0.155	0.156	0.157	0.159	0.160	0.161
8.0	0.046	0.101	0.126	0.139	0.148	0.156	0.161	0.166	0.170	0.174	0.179	0.183	0.187
9.0	0.042	0.098	0.131	0.145	0.154	0.163	0.171	0.175	0.178	0.182	0.186	0.190	0.193
10.0	0.048	0.096	0.131	0.148	0.160	0.171	0.179	0.185	0.192	0.198	0.204	0.210	0.216
11.0	0.048	0.097	0.131	0.150	0.163	0.175	0.185	0.191	0.198	0.204	0.210	0.217	0.223
12.0	0.041	0.092	0.127	0.150	0.163	0.176	0.188	0.195	0.202	0.209	0.215	0.222	0.229
13.0	0.043	0.093	0.129	0.153	0.167	0.179	0.191	0.200	0.209	0.218	0.227	0.236	0.244
14.0	0.043	0.091	0.131	0.152	0.165	0.178	0.191	0.201	0.211	0.221	0.231	0.241	0.251
15.0	0.036	0.084	0.122	0.147	0.165	0.180	0.193	0.200	0.206	0.212	0.218	0.224	0.230
16.0	0.031	0.080	0.119	0.145	0.164	0.180	0.195	0.203	0.211	0.220	0.228	0.236	0.244
17.0	0.036	0.080	0.119	0.143	0.160	0.178	0.196	0.208	0.219	0.229	0.240	0.251	0.262
18.0	0.033	0.075	0.112	0.140	0.159	0.177	0.193	0.203	0.213	0.222	0.232	0.241	0.250
19.0	0.033	0.074	0.113	0.140	0.158	0.175	0.193	0.202	0.211	0.220	0.229	0.238	0.247
20.0	0.029	0.072	0.109	0.138	0.156	0.175	0.193	0.203	0.213	0.222	0.232	0.242	0.251
21.0	0.030	0.068	0.104	0.131	0.151	0.171	0.189	0.203	0.216	0.229	0.242	0.255	0.268
22.0	0.025	0.063	0.098	0.126	0.145	0.164	0.184	0.198	0.212	0.226	0.241	0.255	0.269
23.0	0.031	0.061	0.093	0.123	0.142	0.159	0.178	0.191	0.202	0.214	0.226	0.237	0.249
24.0	0.029	0.061	0.092	0.122	0.138	0.153	0.172	0.187	0.202	0.216	0.230	0.245	0.259
25.0	0.026	0.055	0.086	0.115	0.135	0.152	0.169	0.182	0.195	0.207	0.220	0.233	0.246
26.0	0.028	0.057	0.085	0.108	0.126	0.145	0.167	0.178	0.190	0.201	0.212	0.223	0.234
27.0	0.026	0.051	0.080	0.108	0.128	0.146	0.162	0.174	0.185	0.196	0.208	0.219	0.231
28.0	0.025	0.052	0.079	0.104	0.120	0.137	0.159	0.171	0.183	0.194	0.205	0.216	0.228
29.0	0.021	0.049	0.075	0.098	0.115	0.133	0.152	0.165	0.177	0.189	0.201	0.214	0.226
30.0	0.023	0.048	0.072	0.096	0.111	0.126	0.145	0.160	0.174	0.189	0.204	0.219	0.234

Calculated from Table A.10.1, using Equation 10.6.

TABLE A.11.1. 10-MV X-RAY PERCENT DEPTH DOSES

Depth (cm)					A/P and Field Size (cm)					
	0 × 0	1.00 4 × 4	1.50 6 × 6	2.00 8 × 8	2.50 10 × 10	3.00 12 × 12	3.75 15 × 15	5.00 20 × 20	6.25 25 × 25	7.50 30 × 30
0	5.0	6.5	8.5	10.7	12.5	14.5	17.0	21.0	24.5	28.0
0.2	37.0	40.0	43.0	45.0	46.5	48.0	50.0	52.5	54.0	56.0
0.5	65.0	67.0	69.0	70.5	72.0	73.0	74.0	76.0	77.0	79.0
1.0	86.0	88.0	89.0	90.0	91.0	91.5	92.0	93.0	94.0	95.0
1.5	94.5	95.5	96.0	96.5	97.0	97.0	97.5	98.0	98.0	98.5
2.0	96.5	97.5	98.0	98.0	98.0	98.5	99.0	99.0	99.5	99.5
2.5	100.0	100.0	100.0	100.0	100.0	100.0	100.0	100.0	100.0	100.0
3.0	97.4	99.0	99.0	99.0	99.0	99.0	99.0	99.0	99.0	99.0
4.0	92.3	96.4	96.4	96.4	96.4	96.5	96.5	96.5	96.5	96.5
5.0	87.5	91.6	91.8	91.9	92.1	92.2	92.3	92.5	92.6	92.7
6.0	83.0	87.0	87.4	87.7	87.9	88.1	88.3	88.6	88.8	89.0
7.0	78.7	82.6	83.2	83.6	83.9	84.2	84.5	84.9	85.2	85.5
8.0	74.7	78.5	79.2	79.7	80.1	80.4	80.8	81.4	81.8	82.1
9.0	70.8	74.6	75.4	76.0	76.5	76.9	77.3	78.0	78.4	78.8
10.0	67.2	70.8	71.8	72.5	73.0	73.5	74.0	74.7	75.3	75.7
11.0	63.8	67.3	68.4	69.1	69.7	70.2	70.8	71.6	72.2	72.7
12.0	60.6	63.9	65.1	65.9	66.6	67.1	67.7	68.6	69.3	69.8
13.0	57.5	60.7	62.0	62.8	63.5	64.1	64.8	65.7	66.5	67.1
14.0	54.6	57.7	59.0	59.9	60.7	61.3	62.0	63.0	63.8	64.4
15.0	51.9	54.8	56.2	57.1	57.9	58.5	59.3	60.4	61.2	61.8
16.0	49.3	52.1	53.5	54.5	55.3	55.9	56.8	57.8	58.7	59.4
17.0	46.8	49.5	50.9	52.0	52.8	53.5	54.3	55.4	56.3	57.0
18.0	44.5	47.0	48.5	49.5	50.4	51.1	52.0	53.1	54.0	54.8
19.0	42.3	44.7	46.1	47.2	48.1	48.8	49.7	50.9	51.8	52.6
20.0	40.2	42.4	43.9	45.0	45.9	46.7	47.6	48.8	49.7	50.5
22.0	36.3	38.3	39.8	41.0	41.9	42.6	43.5	44.8	45.8	46.6
24.0	32.8	34.6	36.1	37.2	38.2	38.9	39.9	41.1	42.1	43.0
26.0	29.7	31.2	32.7	33.9	34.8	35.5	36.5	37.8	38.8	39.6
28.0	26.9	28.1	29.7	30.8	31.7	32.5	33.4	34.7	35.7	36.5
30.0	24.3	25.4	26.9	28.0	28.9	29.6	30.6	31.8	32.9	33.7

Data from Khan FM, Moore VC, Sato S. Depth dose and scatter analysis of 10 MV x-rays. *Radiology* 1972;102:165, with permission.

TABLE A.11.2. 10-MV X-RAY TISSUE-MAXIMUM RATIOS

Depth d (cm)	A/P and Field Size (cm)[a]									
	0 × 0	1.00 4 × 4	1.50 6 × 6	2.00 8 × 8	2.50 10 × 10	3.00 12 × 12	3.75 15 × 15	5.00 20 × 20	6.25 25 × 25	7.50 30 × 30
0	0.048	0.062	0.081	0.102	0.119	0.138	0.162	0.200	0.233	0.267
0.2	0.354	0.382	0.411	0.430	0.444	0.459	0.478	0.502	0.516	0.535
0.5	0.625	0.644	0.663	0.678	0.692	0.702	0.711	0.731	0.740	0.759
1.0	0.835	0.854	0.864	0.874	0.884	0.888	0.893	0.903	0.913	0.922
1.5	0.927	0.936	0.941	0.946	0.951	0.951	0.956	0.961	0.961	0.966
2.0	0.956	0.966	0.970	0.970	0.970	0.975	0.980	0.980	0.985	0.985
2.5	1.000	1.000	1.000	1.000	1.000	1.000	1.000	1.000	1.000	1.000
3.0	0.983	1.000	1.000	1.000	1.000	1.000	1.000	1.000	1.000	1.000
4.0	0.950	0.992	0.992	0.993	0.993	0.993	0.993	0.993	0.993	0.994
5.0	0.918	0.960	0.963	0.965	0.966	0.967	0.968	0.970	0.971	0.972
6.0	0.887	0.930	0.934	0.937	0.939	0.941	0.944	0.947	0.949	0.951
7.0	0.858	0.899	0.906	0.910	0.913	0.916	0.920	0.924	0.928	0.931
8.0	0.829	0.870	0.878	0.884	0.888	0.892	0.896	0.902	0.906	0.910
9.0	0.801	0.841	0.851	0.858	0.863	0.867	0.873	0.880	0.885	0.889
10.0	0.774	0.813	0.824	0.832	0.838	0.843	0.850	0.858	0.864	0.869
11.0	0.748	0.786	0.798	0.807	0.814	0.820	0.827	0.836	0.843	0.849
12.0	0.723	0.760	0.773	0.783	0.791	0.797	0.805	0.815	0.823	0.830
13.0	0.699	0.734	0.749	0.759	0.768	0.774	0.783	0.794	0.803	0.810
14.0	0.676	0.709	0.725	0.736	0.745	0.752	0.762	0.774	0.783	0.791
15.0	0.653	0.684	0.701	0.713	0.723	0.731	0.741	0.753	0.764	0.772
16.0	0.631	0.661	0.678	0.691	0.701	0.710	0.720	0.734	0.744	0.753
17.0	0.610	0.638	0.656	0.669	0.680	0.689	0.700	0.714	0.726	0.735
18.0	0.589	0.615	0.634	0.648	0.659	0.669	0.680	0.695	0.707˙	0.717
19.0	0.570	0.593	0.613	0.628	0.639	0.649	0.661	0.676	0.689	0.699
20.0	0.551	0.572	0.593	0.608	0.620	0.629	0.642	0.658	0.671	0.681
22.0	0.514	0.532	0.553	0.569	0.582	0.592	0.605	0.622	0.636	0.647
24.0	0.480	0.494	0.516	0.533	0.546	0.556	0.570	0.588	0.602	0.614
26.0	0.449	0.458	0.481	0.498	0.511	0.522	0.536	0.555	0.570	0.583
28.0	0.419	0.425	0.448	0.465	0.479	0.490	0.505	0.524	0.539	0.552
30.0	0.392	0.394	0.417	0.434	0.448	0.459	0.474	0.494	0.509	0.523

[a] Projected at depth d.
Data calculated from Table A.11.1 and are from Khan FM. Depth dose and scatter analysis of 10 MV x-rays [Letter to the Editor]. *Radiology* 1973;106:662, with permission.

TABLE A.11.3. 10-MV X-RAY SCATTER-MAXIMUM RATIOS

Depth d (cm)	Field Radius (cm) at Depth d												
	2	4	6	8	10	12	14	16	18	20	22	24	26
2.5	0	0	0	0	0	0	0	0	0	0	0	0	0
3.0	0.017	0.017	0.017	0.017	0.017	0.017	0.017	0.017	0.017	0.017	0.017	0.017	0.017
4.0	0.042	0.042	0.043	0.043	0.043	0.043	0.043	0.043	0.044	0.044	0.044	0.044	0.044
6.0	0.043	0.048	0.053	0.056	0.058	0.060	0.062	0.063	0.065	0.066	0.067	0.068	0.069
8.0	0.041	0.052	0.060	0.066	0.070	0.074	0.077	0.080	0.082	0.084	0.086	0.088	0.090
10.0	0.039	0.055	0.066	0.074	0.080	0.085	0.089	0.093	0.097	0.100	0.102	0.105	0.107
12.0	0.037	0.056	0.070	0.080	0.087	0.094	0.099	0.104	0.109	0.112	0.116	0.119	0.122
14.0	0.033	0.056	0.072	0.084	0.093	0.101	0.107	0.113	0.118	0.123	0.127	0.130	0.134
16.0	0.030	0.055	0.073	0.086	0.097	0.106	0.113	0.119	0.125	0.130	0.135	0.140	0.144
18.0	0.026	0.053	0.073	0.088	0.099	0.109	0.117	0.124	0.131	0.137	0.142	0.147	0.151
20.0	0.021	0.051	0.072	0.088	0.101	0.111	0.120	0.128	0.135	0.141	0.147	0.152	0.157
22.0	0.018	0.048	0.071	0.087	0.101	0.112	0.121	0.129	0.137	0.144	0.150	0.155	0.161
24.0	0.014	0.045	0.069	0.086	0.100	0.112	0.121	0.130	0.138	0.145	0.152	0.158	0.163
26.0	0.009	0.042	0.066	0.084	0.098	0.110	0.121	0.130	0.138	0.145	0.152	0.158	0.164
28.0	0.006	0.039	0.063	0.082	0.096	0.109	0.119	0.129	0.137	0.145	0.152	0.158	0.164
30.0	0.002	0.035	0.060	0.079	0.094	0.106	0.117	0.127	0.136	0.143	0.151	0.157	0.163

Data calculated from Table A.11.1 and are from Khan FM. Depth dose and scatter analysis of 10 MV x-rays [Letter to the Editor]. *Radiology* 1973;106:662, with permission.

TABLE A.12.1. PATTERSON-PARKER PLANAR IMPLANT TABLES

TABLE A.12.1A. MILLIGRAM-HOURS PER 1,000 R FOR DIFFERENT AREAS AND VARIOUS TREATING DISTANCES[a]

Area[b]	0.5[c]	1.0	1.5	2.0	2.5	3.0	3.5	4.0	4.5	5.0
0	30	119	268	476	744	1,071	1,458	1,904	2,412	2,976
1	68	171								
2	97	213	375	598	865	1,197	1,595	2,043	2,545	3,117
3	120	247								
4	141	278	462	698	970	1,305	1,713	2,168	2,665	3,243
5	161	306								
6	177	333	536	782	1,066	1,405	1,822	2,286	2,778	3,360
7	192	359								
8	206	384	599	855	1,155	1,500	1,924	2,395	2,883	3,472
9	221	408								
10	235	433	655	923	1,235	1,590	2,020	2,500	2,987	3,580
11	248	456								
12	261	480	710	990	1,312	1,673	2,112	2,603	3,087	3,682
13	274	502								
14	288	524	764	1,053	1,386	1,753	2,200	2,698	3,185	3,785
15	302	546								
16	315	566	814	1,113	1,460	1,830	2,283	2,790	3,280	3,883
17	328	585								
18	342	605	863	1,170	1,525	1,905	2,363	2,879	3,370	3,985
19	355	623								
20	368	641	910	1,225	1,588	1,979	2,445	2,965	3,461	4,080
22	393	674	960	1,280	1,650	2,049	2,522	3,047	3,550	4,174
24	417	707	1,008	1,335	1,712	2,117	2,598	3,126	3,639	4,267
26	442	737	1,056	1,388	1,768	2,188	2,670	3,200	3,724	4,356
28	466	767	1,100	1,438	1,826	2,254	2,742	3,275	3,804	4,446
30	490	795	1,142	1,487	1,880	2,320	2,817	3,348	3,883	4,534
32	513	823	1,185	1,537	1,936	2,380	2,888	3,420	3,966	4,620
34	537	854	1,226	1,587	1,992	2,442	2,956	3,490	4,047	4,700
36	558	879	1,268	1,638	2,048	2,502	3,022	3,559	4,125	4,783
38	581	909	1,308	1,685	2,100	2,562	3,088	3,627	4,198	4,863
40	603	934	1,346	1,732	2,152	2,620	3,150	3,695	4,273	4,942
42	624	962	1,384	1,780	2,203	2,677	3,215	3,762	4,348	5,020
44	644	990	1,420	1,825	2,255	2,733	3,275	3,826	4,423	5,096
46	665	1,015	1,457	1,870	2,305	2,788	3,335	3,890	4,494	5,174
48	685	1,043	1,490	1,915	2,354	2,843	3,395	3,954	4,565	5,250
50	705	1,072	1,522	1,958	2,402	2,897	3,455	4,018	4,633	5,327
52	725	1,098	1,554	2,004	2,450	2,950	3,513	4,080	4,702	5,400
54	744	1,125	1,588	2,047	2,500	3,003	3,569	4,142	4,768	5,475
56	762	1,152	1,618	2,092	2,548	3,055	3,625	4,205	4,835	5,548
58	781	1,177	1,650	2,137	2,597	3,106	3,678	4,267	4,903	5,620
60	800	1,206	1,682	2,180	2,646	3,160	3,735	4,328	4,970	5,690
62	818	1,230	1,712	2,222	2,692	3,212	3,790	4,389	5,037	5,760
64	837	1,260	1,740	2,262	2,736	3,262	3,845	4,447	5,105	5,830
66	855	1,285	1,769	2,302	2,782	3,310	3,900	4,505	5,171	5,900
68	873	1,313	1,798	2,342	2,828	3,360	3,950	4,562	5,232	5,967
70	890	1,340	1,827	2,380	2,875	3,410	4,001	4,618	5,294	6,033
72	908	1,367	1,857	2,420	2,922	3,460	4,053	4,675	5,355	6,098
74	927	1,394	1,887	2,455	2,968	3,510	4,105	4,733	5,417	6,162
76	945	1,421	1,915	2,490	3,013	3,560	4,158	4,791	5,480	6,225
78	963	1,446	1,941	2,527	3,058	3,608	4,210	4,846	5,542	6,288
80	981	1,473	1,966	2,562	3,103	3,657	4,260	4,900	5,600	6,350
84	1,016	1,524	2,020	2,630	3,192	3,755	4,360	5,014	5,720	6,473
88	1,052	1,572	2,075	2,698	3,282	3,849	4,462	5,126	5,838	6,598
92	1,087	1,620	2,130	2,765	3,371	3,943	4,560	5,235	5,954	6,720
96	1,122	1,668	2,186	2,828	3,459	4,033	4,657	5,340	6,068	6,842
100	1,155	1,716	2,238	2,890	3,545	4,120	4,750	5,445	6,180	6,956

[a] Filtration = 0.5 mm platinum.
[b] Area is in centimeters squared.
[c] Treating distance is in centimeters.
From Merredith WJ, ed. *Radium dosage. The Manchester system.* Edinburgh: Livingston, 1967, with permission.

TABLE A.12.1B. LARGER AREAS

Area[a]	0.5[b]	1.0	1.5	2.0
120	1,307	1,960	2,510	3,180
140	1,463	2,194	2,788	3,470
160	1,608	2,412	3,055	3,736
180	1,746	2,617	3,312	4,010
200	1,880	2,820	3,560	4,288
220	2,008	3,008	3,805	4,554
240	2,132	3,200	4,045	4,824
260	2,256	3,383	4,288	5,095
280	2,372	3,560	4,530	5,360
300	2,495	3,747	4,760	5,630
320	2,622	3,924	4,984	5,892
340	2,737	4,105	5,200	6,145
360	2,853	4,280	5,427	6,388
380	2,968	4,455	5,630	6,623
400	3,080	4,620	5,840	6,864

[a] Area is in centimeters squared.
[b] Treating distance is in centimeters.

TABLE A.12.1C. SOME FILTRATION CORRECTORS

Filter Used	Correction to Radium Used
0.3 mm. Pt.	+4%
0.6 mm. Pt.	−2%
0.7 mm. Pt.	−4%
0.8 mm. Pt.	−6%
1.0 mm. Pt.	−10%
1.5 mm. Pt.	−20%

TABLE A.12.2. PATERSON-PARKER VOLUME IMPLANT TABLES

TABLE A.12.2A.

Volume in Cubic Centimeters	Milligram-Hours per 1,000 R
1	34.1
2	54.1
3	70.9
4	85.9
5	99.7
10	158.3
15	207
20	251
25	292
30	329
40	399
50	463
60	523
70	579
80	633
90	685
100	735
110	783
120	830
140	920
160	1,005
180	1,087
200	1,166
220	1,243
240	1,317
260	1,390
280	1,460
300	1,529
320	1,595
340	1,662
360	1,726
380	1,788
400	1,851

Filtration = 0.5 mm platinum.
From Merredith WJ, ed. *Radium dosage. The Manchester System.* Edinburgh: Livingston, 1967, with permission.

TABLE A.12.2B.

Elongation Factor	Elongation Correction
1.5	+3%
2.0	6%
2.5	10%
3.0	15%

TABLE A.12.2C. USEFUL FILTRATION CORRECTORS

Filter Used	Correction to Radium Used
0.3 mm. Pt.	+4%
0.6 mm. Pt.	−2%
0.7 mm. Pt.	−4%
0.8 mm. Pt.	−6%

SUBJECT INDEX

Page numbers followed by *f* indicate figures; those followed by *t* indicate tabular material.

Blocking. *See also* Field blocks
  in electron beam therapy
    dose rate and, 332–333*f*, 332–333
Body contours
  in patient data acquisition, 228–229, 229*f*
Bohr's atomic model, 5–6
Bolus
  defined, 259
  in electron beam therapy
    treatment planning in, 327
Bombardment
  deuteron, 24–25, 55
  neutron, 25–26, 55
  proton, 24, 56
Bone
  collision mass stopping powers for, A-12
  corrections for
    absorbed dose and, 252–254, 253*f*, 254*t*
    dose reductions and, 252, 252*t*
    in electron beam therapy, 324
  electrons in, 71*t*
  energy absorption coefficients for, A-9
  f factor of, 110*t*
  photon mass attenuation coefficients for, A-9
Bone-tissue interface
  absorbed dose and
    corrections in, 254–255, 256*f*, 258*t*
Brachytherapy, 357–397
  computer dosimetry in, 384–387
    dose computation in, 387
    source localization in, 385–387
  dose distribution in, 369–377
    absorbed dose in tissue in, 372–373, 373*t*, 374*f*
    exposure rate in, 369–372*f*, 369–372
    isodose curves in, 376–377, 377*f*
    modular dose calculation model in, 373, 375–377*t*, 375–376
  dose specification in
    in cervical cancer, 390–396
  high dose rate, 521–537. *See also* High dose rate brachytherapy
  implant dosimetry in, 378–384
    computer system as, 383–384, 385*f*
    Memorial system as, 382
    Paris system as, 382, 383*t*, 384*f*
    Paterson-Parker system as, 378–381, 379*f*, 381*f*
    Quimby system as, 381–382
  implantation techniques in, 387–390
    interstitial, 387–389, 388*f*
    intracavitary, 389*f*, 389–390
    surface molds in, 387
  intensity-modulated therapy *versus*, 504
  intravascular, 548–559. *See also* Intravascular brachytherapy
  quality assurance in, 429–430, 444–445
  radiation protection in, 413–414
  radioactive sources in, 357–364, 358*t*, 429–420
    calibration of, 364–369
    cesium-137 as, 360–361
    cobalt-60 as, 361

    exposure rate and, 367–369, 368–369*f*
    gold-198 as, 361
    in intravascular brachytherapy, 549–550, 550*f*, 550*t*
    iodine-125 as, 362–363*f*, 362–363
    iridium-192 as, 361
    leak testing of, 414
    palladium-103 as, 363–364, 364*f*
    preparation of, 414
    quality assurance and, 444–445
    radium as, 357–360, 358–359*f*, 360*t*
    source strength and, 364–367
    storage of, 413
    transportation of, 414
  remote afterloading units in, 396–397
Bragg peak
  absence in electrons of, 75
  defined, 56, 74
  in heavy particles, 56, 56*f*, 74
  pions as, 57–58
Bragg-Gray cavity theory
  absorbed dose and, 113–118
    chamber volume in, 114–116, 116*f*
    effective point of measurement in, 116–118, 117*f*
    Spencer-Attix formulation of, 114, 119–122, 122*t*
    stopping power in, 113–114
Brain
  stereotactic radiosurgery in, 507, 515, 518–519, 519*f*
Bremsstrahlung
  defined, 33
  in linear accelerators, 45
  in physics of x-ray production, 33–34, 34*f*
  principles of electron, 298
Brown-Robert-Wells frame
  in stereotactic radiosurgery, 508–509, 510*f*
Build-up bolus
  defined, 259
Build-up cap
  in ion chambers, 111–112*f*, 111–116, 179, 179*f*
Build-up effect
  dose, 90
Build-up region
  beam quality and, 162–163
  dose distribution measurement in, 280

C

C-552
  energy absorption coefficients for, A-3, A-7
  stopping powers for, A-3
Calibration
  beam
    electron, 137–138
    in electron arc therapy, 337–338, 338*f*
    photon, 136–137
    in TRS 398 protocol, 140
  of brachytherapy sources, 364–369
    exposure rate and, 367–369, 368–369*f*
    high dose rate, 527, 531–532
    quality assurance in, 444–447
    source strength and, 364–367

  dose. *See* Dose calibration
  of equipment
    in teletherapy, 422
  of ionization chambers, 302
    quality assurance and, 431, 431*t*
  of thimble chambers, 83, 83*f*
Calibration phantom
  dose, 126, 133
Calorimetry
  in absorbed dose measurement, 142, 143*f*
  technical difficulties with, 302
Cancer
  cervical. *See* Cervical cancer
  prostate. *See also* Prostate implants
    implants for, 539–547
  uterine
    brachytherapy in, 390
Capintec dose calibrator
  in brachytherapy, 368, 369*f*
Capture γ rays
  defined, 25
Carbon
  collision mass stopping powers for, A-12
  electrons in, 71*t*
  energy absorption coefficients for, A-10
  photon mass attenuation coefficients for, A-10
Catheter-based systems
  in intravascular brachytherapy, 555–558
Cathode ray tube
  in ultrasound imaging, 239
Cathodes
  defined, 28
  in x-ray tubes, 30
Cavity-gas calibration factor, 123, 124*t*
  TG-21 protocol, 118–119
Central axis depth-dose curves
  in electron beam therapy, 307–308, 308–310*f*
Cerrobend
  in field blocks, 274–275*f*, 274–275, 279*f*
  multileaf collimators and, 279
Cervical cancer
  brachytherapy in, 390–396
    high dose rate, 537
    ICRU system in, 392–395*f*, 392–394, 393*t*
    implantation techniques in, 389*f*, 389–390
    Manchester system in, 390–392, 391*f*
    milligram-hours in, 390
Cervix
  cancer of uterine. *See* Cervical cancer
Cesium-137
  in brachytherapy, 360–361
    isodose curves for, 359*f*
  characteristics of, 51, 52*t*, 358*t*
  cobalt-60 *versus*
    half-life and, 15
Chain reaction
  in fission, 26
Chamber calibration factor, 123, 136
Chamber polarity effects
  in dose calibration, 135